Biotechnological Tools for Genetic Resources

The Editor

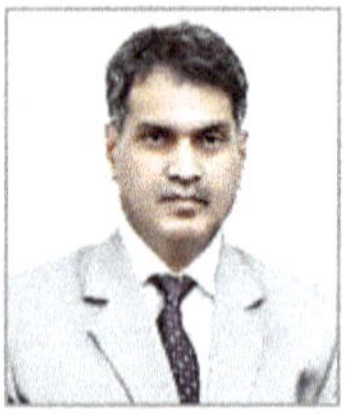

Prof. Pradip Chandra Deka obtained his Bachelor's degree from Assam Agricultural University, Jorhat and Master's and Doctorate degree in Genetics from Banaras Hindu University, Varanasi. He did his Post-Doctorate research in Molecular Genetics from University of Florida, Gainesville, USA and University of California, Berkeley, USA.

Prof. Deka started his career as Research Assistant at Bose Institute, Kolkata and then joined Assam Agricultural University, Jorhat as Assistant Professor. Thereafter he served as the Professor of Biotechnology and as the Dean, Faculty of Agriculture, Assam Agricultural University, Jorhat. He also served as the Visiting Professor at ETH, Zurich, Switzerland. In 2004, he joined as the Vice Chancellor, Tezpur Central University, Tezpur, Assam. Currently he is the Vice Chancellor, Sir Padampat Singhania University, Udaipur, Rajasthan. He has more than 36 years of teaching and research experience.

Prof. Deka served as Chairman/Members of Board of the Management and Academic Council of several State and Central Universities. He also served as one of the member of the Task Force on Education, Department of Biotechnology, Govt. of India.

His specialization is Plant Molecular Genetics and Plant Tissue Culture. He completed several research projects on various aspects of biotechnology and molecular genetics, sponsored by various agencies from India and abroad. He developed several biotechnology related protocols for the genetic improvement of agricultural, horticultural, floricultural and sericultural crops. He has published more than 190 research papers in reputed national and international journals, and authored five books on Biotechnology and Molecular Genetics. In September 2015 a Textbook entitled, "Molecular Biology: A Genetical Approach" authored by him and one of his colleagues has been published by Wiley.

Several eminent teachers/scientists obtained their Doctorate degrees under his supervision. Prof. Deka is life member of several National and International Professional Societies/Organizations.

Biotechnological Tools for Genetic Resources

— *Editor* —

Prof. Pradip Chandra Deka

Vice Chancellor
Sir Padampat Singhania University,
Udaipur – 313 601
Rajasthan (India)

2016

Daya Publishing House®

A Division of

Astral International Pvt. Ltd.

New Delhi – 110 002

Cataloging in Publication Data--DK
Courtesy: D.K. Agencies (P) Ltd. <docinfo@dkagencies.com>

Biotechnological tools for genetic resources / editor, Prof. Pradip Chandra Deka.
pages cm
Contributed articles.
Includes bibliographical references and index.

ISBN 978-93-5130-993-2 (International Edition)

1. Germplasm resources. 2. Biotechnology. I. Deka, Pradip Chandra, editor.

QH430.B56 2016 DDC 572.8 23

Published by : **Daya Publishing House®**
A Division of
Astral International Pvt. Ltd.
– ISO 9001:2008 Certified Company –
4760-61/23, Ansari Road, Darya Ganj
New Delhi-110 002
Ph. 011-43549197, 23278134
E-mail: info@astralint.com
Website: www.astralint.com

Laser Typesetting : **Classic Computer Services**, Delhi - 110 035

Preface

The idea of bringing out this book was conceived about two years ago, when I looked back into my academic career, and realized that several of my students have accomplished their academic excellence in the area of their specialization. Therefore, I thought that it would be worthwhile to bring out a book through their contributions. Accordingly I approached each one of them to contribute a review paper on the area of their expertise within biotechnology. The response was overwhelming and the present book is mostly the compilation of contributions of my students. They in turn associated their students for writing the review papers. Moreover, since few important areas remained uncovered, I approached my colleagues to contribute on these areas.

Biotechnology is a field which is advancing rapidly with constant flow of information. New areas of research have immersed leading to newer concepts. Therefore it is important to keep the students, researchers and the teaching community updated with the recent findings of this dynamic area of study. As the information grows in dimension, it becomes necessary to distil all such information and present in concise and understandable form for the students. To accomplish this goal, the authors have concentrated on most current information on some of the recently developed biotechnological tools and techniques applicable for identification and utilization of genetic resources. The authors have incorporated their knowledge with clear writing and with beautiful illustrations.

Proper identification of plant, animal and microbe has always been a challenge for the taxonomists. The conventional method is time consuming and not always reliable. With the development and refinement of DNA barcoding technique, it has now become possible to identify genetic resources at a much faster rate with authenticity. Similarly, development of Next Generation Sequencing Techniques has enhanced the process of nucleic acid sequencing at a much faster rate at low cost.

Development of plant derived vaccines has now become a reality. Similarly application of microRNAs for diagnosis of diseases in plants, animals and human has been recognised.

It has now been possible to associate specific genes to specific functions involved in secondary metabolite production. Application of high throughput molecular techniques in animal breeding has now been practiced regularly. Similarly application of microbial fuel cells for wastewater treatment and bioenergy production is becoming a possibility.

The topics included in the book shall cover the recent developments in the above topics, having potential for improvement and utilization of plants, animals microorganisms.

The book should be useful for the students and researchers pursuing post graduate degree programmes in biotechnology, molecular biology, genetics, microbiology, plant and animal breeding. I strongly believe that this book will contribute towards enriching the academic reservoir.

I would like to thank all the contributors for providing the manuscripts within the stipulated time. The facilities received from Sir Padampat Singhania University, Udaipur, Rajasthan during editing of the manuscript is thankfully acknowledged.

I feel immense pleasure in thanking Daya Publishing House, a division of Astral International Private Limited, New Delhi, India for bringing out the book in the present form.

Pradip C. Deka

Contents

List of Contributors

Ajit Kumar Shasany, Biotechnology Division, CSIR-Central Institute of Medicinal and Aromatic Plants, P.O. CIMAP, Lucknow – 226 015, U.P.

Akan Das, Department of Bioengineering and Technology, Institute of Science and Technology, Gauhati University, Guwahati – 781 014, Assam.

Albin M. Ahmed, School of Veterinary Medicine, University College Dublin, Belfield, Dublin 4, Ireland.

Ananya Borthakur, Department of Agricultural Biotechnology, Assam Agricultural University, Jorhat – 785 013, Assam.

Amita Misra, Biotechnology Division, CSIR-Central Institute of Medicinal and Aromatic Plants, P.O. CIMAP, Lucknow – 226 015, U.P.

Anindya Mukhopadhya, School of Agriculture and Food Science, University College Dublin, Belfield, Dublin 4, Ireland.

Archana Gajbhiye, Department of Biotechnology, Sir Padampat Singhania University, Udaipur – 313 601, Rajasthan.

Arghya Sett, Bioengineering Research Laboratory, Department of Biosciences and Bioengineering, Indian Institute of Technology, Guwahati – 781 039, Assam.

Bojlul Bahar, Institute of Food and Health, School of Agriculture and Food Science, University College Dublin, Belfield, Dublin 4, Ireland.

Deepika Singh, Bioengineering Research Laboratory, Department of Biosciences and Bioengineering, Indian Institute of Technology, Guwahati – 781 039, Assam.

Diganta Deka, Department of Agricultural Biotechnology, Assam Agricultural University, Jorhat – 785 013, Assam.

Jagajjit Sahu, Department of Agricultural Biotechnology, Assam Agricultural University, Jorhat – 785 013, Assam.

Jane P. Theophilus, Department of Zoology, Osmania University, Hyderabad – 500 007, Telengana.

Kamalakshi Devi, Department of Agricultural Biotechnology, Assam Agricultural University, Jorhat – 785 013, Assam.

M.A. Laskar, Biotechnology Department, St. Anthony's College, Shillong – 793 001, Meghalaya.

Manab Deka, Department of Applied Science, Institute of Science and Technology, Gauhati University, Guwahati – 781 014, Assam.

Mechuselie Kehie, School of Life Sciences, Jawaharlal Nehru University, New Delhi – 110 067.

Munmi Phukon, Department of Agricultural Biotechnology, Assam Agricultural University, Jorhat – 785 013, Assam.

Nirala Ramchiary, School of Life Sciences, Jawaharlal Nehru University, New Delhi – 110 067.

Pallavi Dwivedi, Biotechnology Department, Amity University, Mumbai-Pune Expressway, Somathne, Panvel, Mumbai – 410 206, Maharashtra

Paramananda Barman, Department of Botany, University of Delhi, Delhi – 110 007.

Pradip C. Deka, Vice Chancellor, Sir Padampat Singhania University, Udaipur – 313 601, Rajasthan.

Pragya Sharma, Department of Applied Science, Institute of Science and Technology, Gauhati University, Guwahati – 781 014, Assam.

Priyabrata Sen, Department of Agricultural Biotechnology, Assam Agricultural University, Jorhat – 785 013, Assam.

Ratna Kalita, Department of Agricultural Biotechnology, Assam Agricultural University, Jorhat – 785 013, Assam.

Sharmistha Barthakur, National Research Center on Plant Biotechnology, Pusa campus, New Delhi – 110 012.

Shubhra Rastogi, Biotechnology Division, CSIR-Central Institute of Medicinal and Aromatic Plants, P.O. CIMAP, Lucknow – 226 015, U.P.

Sushil Chhapekar, School of Life Sciences, Jawaharlal Nehru University, New Delhi – 110 067.

Tapan Kumar Mondal, Division of Genomic Resource, National Bureau of Plant Genetic Resource, Pusa, New Delhi – 110 012.

Utpal Bora, Bioengineering Research Laboratory, Department of Biosciences and Bioengineering, Indian Institute of Technology, Guwahati – 781 039, Assam.

Venkanna Bhanothu, Department of Zoology, Osmania University, Hyderabad – 500 007, Telengana.

:016, Biotechnological Tools for Genetic Resources Pages 1–18
:ditor: Pradip Chandra Deka
'ublished by: Daya Publishing House, NEW DELHI

Chapter 1

Next Generation Sequencing and Its Utilization for Managing the Plant Genetic Resources

Tapan Kumar Mondal* and Akan Das[2]

**Division of Genomic Resources,*
National Bureau of Plant Genetic Resources, Pusa, New Delhi – 110 012
[2]Department of Bioengineering and Technology,
Institute of Science and Technology, Gauhati University,
Guwahati – 781 014, Assam
**E-mail: mondaltk@yahoo.com*

ABSTRACT

Plant genetic resources (PGR) are the most important components of agro-biodiversity. Collection, management and utilisation of PGR gain paramount importance in agriculture to balance the genetic diversity of crop plant species. A total of ~1750 national and international gene banks worldwide preserve ~7 million accessions of advanced cultivars, landraces, and wild species relatives of plants that the world depends on for food, fiber, and fuel. However, duplicated samples of collected germplasm always create problem in marker studies to reach on a common panel of markers for a given species. The sample duplication problem can successfully be tackled using Next Generation Sequencing (NGS) technology without any shortcomings. Next Generation Sequencing technologies are suitable for fast and low-cost sequencing of core collection sets with low coverage to develop genome-wide markers which help in eliminating the duplication across genome populations. The integration of genomic data into genebank documentation systems and its correlation studies with taxonomic, phenotypic and ecological data will herald in a new era for the valorization of PGR. Hence, application of NGS will have a great impact not only on PGR conservation and management, but also on their utilization in genomics based application and breeding.

Keywords: *Next generation sequencing, High-throughput DNA sequencing, Plant genetic resources, Genomic data, Genebank, Germplasm.*

Introduction

Plant genetic resources (PGR) such as primitive forms of cultivated crop species and land-races, modern cultivars, obsolete cultivars, breeding lines *etc.* are the most important components of agro-biodiversity. Therefore, collection, management and utilisation of PGR gain paramount importance in agriculture which had already been made a huge impact in balancing the genetic diversity of the existing crop plant species and their application in genome based science. A total of ~1750 national and international gene banks worldwide preserve ~7 million accessions of advanced cultivars, landraces, and wild species relatives of plants that the world depends on for food, feed, fiber, and fuel. However, there is always a high degree of redundancy remain in the *ex situ* germplasm collections. These duplicated samples always create problem in marker studies to reach on a common panel of markers for a given species. The sample duplication problem can successfully be tackled using Next Generation Sequencing (NGS) technology without any shortcomings. However, sequencing of a large number of germplasm collections for eliminating the duplicated sample is practically not feasible. Hence, development of 'core germplasm' *i.e.* true representatives of the genetic resources of a crop for its genetic diversity is an alternative and better strategy. NGS technology will allow us for whole-genome re-sequencing of hundreds of individual plants. The integration of genomic data into genebank documentation systems and its correlation studies with taxonomic, phenotypic and ecological data will herald in a new era for the valorization of PGR. Hence, application of NGS will have great impacts not only on PGR conservation and management, but also on their utilization in genomics based application in breeding.

Brief Accout of different High Throughput Platform

The high–throughput DNA sequencing technologies are being used by researchers to address an increasingly diverse range of biological problems. In the study of plant genetic resources where genetic diversity is the central theme of research, needs robust high-throughput sequencing techniques to manage and harness the benefits of genetic diversity. During its short existence, the high-throughput sequencing science has witnessed the rise of many technologies capable of massive genomic analysis. In 1977, two first generation sequencing methods were developed, namely Sanger's and Maxam-Gilbert's method. The Sanger's method is a sequencing-by-synthesis (SBS) method that relies on a combination of deoxy- and dideoxy-labeled chain terminator nucleotides (Sanger *et al.*, 1977). The other method is based on chemical modification of DNA molecule followed by cleavage at specific sites (Maxam and Gilbert, 1977). However, due to technological simplicity, lower error rate, use of nonradioactive materials, and amenability to higher scale-up, Sanger's method moved forward so much so that it has become a highly automated technique. But, still there are so many shortfalls in first generation sequencing techniques such as low-throughput, involvement of bacterial cloning of the interested DNA sequence, lengthy procedure and labour intensiveness. In the last decade, new sequencing technologies have outperformed Sanger-based sequencing in throughput and overall cost, sequence length and error rate, of which some of them are described below (Kircher and Kelso, 2010).

The next generation high throughput sequencing platforms share three critical steps: DNA sample preparation, immobilization, and sequencing. In general, during sample preparation, genomic DNA is fragmented randomly to critical sizes and then defined sequences, known as "adapters", are added to the ends of these fragments. This preparation with common or universal nucleic acid ends is referred to as "sequencing library." The addition of adapters is required to anchor the DNA fragments of the sequencing library to a solid surface, thereby immobilizing the fragments at a fixed site to carry out the sequencing analysis. All high- throughput sequencing systems, except PacBio RS, require amplification of the sequencing library DNA to form spatially distinct and detectable sequencing features. Amplification is done *in situ* through PCR, in emulsion or in solution to generate clusters of clonal DNA copies. Sequencing is done either by using DNA polymerase synthesis for fluorescent nucleotides or by ligation of fluorescent oligonucleotides.

The NGS platforms integrate a variety of fluidic and optic technologies to perform and monitor the sequencing reactions. The platforms are also fitted with micro-liter scale fluidic devices to support DNA immobilization and sequencing using automated liquid dispensing systems. These equipments are also capable of maintaining automated flow of reagents onto the immobilized DNA fragments for cyclic interrogation of nucleotide sequence.

The second generation sequencing technologies include, Roche 454, Illumina/ Solexa, SOLiD system and Ion torrent. The sequencing chemistry of these technologies differs among them and eliminated the cloning step of the DNA sequence into the bacterial plasmid. Roche 454 is the first NGS technology to reach the market in the year 2005 (Ronaghi *et al.*, 1998). The 454 chemistry is known as "pyrosequencing," which is based on SBS method, where single fragments of DNA are hybridized to a capture bead array and the beads are emulsified with reagents necessary to PCR amplifying the individually bound template. This *in vitro* DNA amplification technique is known as 'Emulsion PCR'. Each bead in the emulsion acts as an independent PCR where millions of copies of template are produced and bound to the capture beads. The amplified copies serve as the templates for the subsequent sequencing reaction in which release of inorganic pyrophosphate is measured by chemiluminescence. The order of correct nucleotides that have been incorporated is detected on the basis of generated 'pyrogram'. However, this technology has difficulty quantifying homopolymers resulting in homopolymeric sequence stretches (*i.e.*, indels) and has an overall error rate of approximately 1 per cent (Glenn, 2011). The advantage of this technique is that it can perform the sequencing for longer read lengths but the disadvantage is being the higher cost per unit of sequence. Because of the advantage of sequencing longer read length, this technique is a choice for *de novo* sequencing.

Illumina technology, acquired by Illumina from Solexa uses solid-phase bridge amplification in which adapters are ligated to each end of a DNA template. The adapters hybridize to immobilize forward or reverse primers, creating a bridge that facilitates amplification, generating amplicons that remain attached to the substrate, thus forming clusters of identical templates, which enhance chemiluminescent detection (Straub *et al.*, 2012). The Illumina technique can generate sequence from opposite ends of a DNA fragment, so called paired-end (PE) reads. This technique has greater applications for studying epigenetic changes, ChIP-seq (identification of genomewide protein binding sequence of DNA), and the discovery of small noncoding RNA. Illumina sequencing is already a popular and the most suitable NGS platform for resequencing which can generate millions of reads. The flagship HiSeq2500 sequencing instrument from Illumina can generate up to 600 GB per run with a read length of 100 nucleotides and 0.1 per cent error rate (Kumar *et al.*, 2012).

The Applied Biosystems/Life Technologies, support oligonucleotide ligation detection (SOLiD) platform that utilizes emulsion PCR to immobilize the DNA library onto a solid support and cyclic sequencing-by-ligation chemistry (Shendure *et al.*, 2005). This process includes ligation, detection, and cleavage steps which are repeated several times during reaction for extending the complementary strand to a length determined by the number of cycles. This method is often used in re-sequencing studies, transcriptomics or in genomic sequencing alongside other technologies. This sequencing-by-ligation method in SOLiD-5500x1 platform generates up to 1,410 million PE reads of 75 + 35 nucleotides each with an error rate of 0.01 per cent (Kumar *et al.*, 2012).

The 'Ion Torrent' is another NGS technology where detection for sequencing is based on pH change as the result of the release of an H^+ ion upon nucleotide incorporation using semiconductor technology (Rothberg *et al.*, 2011). By sequentially adding nucleotides, the machine is able to detect which nucleotide has been incorporated into the growing strand. The advantage of this technology is that sample preparation cost is relatively low. This technique is also suitable for *de novo* sequencing of the genome with higher accuracy (Rothberg *et al.*, 2011, Ashley *et al.*, 2012).

Although second generation NGS technologies are widely accepted and used, these platforms suffer from certain shortfalls, such as amplification biases introduced by PCR and dephasing due to varying extension of templates (Kumar *et al.*, 2012). Therefore, third generation NGS technologies are being developed using single-molecule sequencing (SMS) method where prior amplification of DNA is not required. The advantages of this technology are: low cost, high-throughput, faster turnaround, and longer reads (Ashley *et al.*, 2012). These include Pacific Biosciences single molecule real time (SMART) and Heliscope true single molecule sequencing (tSMS) technologies. In PacBio system, DNA polymerase molecules are immobilized within a zero mode waveguide (ZMW) that spatially restricts the volume of nucleotides and light emission to a small area surrounding the DNA polymerase (Ashley *et al.*, 2012, Levene *et al.*, 2003). The PacBio sequencers can generate up to 140 MB of sequences per run (per smart cell) with reads of 2.5 Kbp at ~85 per cent accuracy. The heliscope sequencing is gaining popularity and has the advantage of using direct RNA sequencing where cDNA library construction step (the collection of all converted RNA molecules to its complementary DNA) is eliminated and ultimately reduced the cost of sample preparation. Heliscope sequencers can generate up to 28 GB of sequence data per run (50 channels) with maximum read length of 55 bp at ~99 per cent accuracy (Kumar *et al.*, 2012, Thompson and Steinmann 2012). However, NGS technologies are evolving at a very rapid pace to improve performance, accessibility, and accuracy of sequencing. Certain emerging "fourth-generation sequencing" technologies are being developed based on optical sequencing and nanotechnology, such as Visigene (Hardin, 2008) and Oxford Nanopore (Lieberman *et al.*, 2010) technology. These techniques are based on single-molecule real-time sequencing where read length will potentially be unlimited.

Different NGS Technique

NGS technologies are suitable for fast and low-cost sequencing of core collection sets with low coverage to develop genome wide markers which help in eliminating the duplication across genome populations (Ashley *et al.*, 2012, Davey *et al.*, 2012). Molecular markers are widely used in genetic research and breeding for the management and utilisation of plant genetic resources. There are numbers of methods developed in this regard, such as reduced-representation libraries (RRLs) (You *et al.*, 2011), complexity reduction of polymorphic sequences (CRoPS) (Van *et al.*, 2007), restriction site-associated DNA sequencing (RAD-seq) (Kakioka *et al.*, 2013), chromatin immunoprecipitation coupled with high throughput DNA Sequencing (ChIP-Seq) (Brandon *et al.*, 2011), genotyping-by-sequencing (GBS) (Huang *et al.*, 2009) and low-coverage sequencing for genotyping (Davey *et al.*, 2011, Bansal *et al.*, 2010). These methods are mostly applicable for the genetic analysis of non-model crop species, species with high levels of repetitive DNA and for breeding germplasms with low levels of polymorphism. These methods are currently applied for the comparison of Single Nucleotide Polymorphism (SNP) diversity within and between closely related plant species or within wild populations. Thus different techniques are discussed in the following section.

Reduced-Representation Libraries (RRLs)

The high throughput and ever decreasing cost of sequencing technologies makes reduced representation libraries (RRLs) an attractive choice for genome-wide SNP genotyping. The use of RRLs, that is, sequencing an enriched subset of a genome by eliminating a proportion of its repetitive fractions was first proposed in humans to efficiently find SNPs using sanger sequencing (You *et al.*, 2011). The reduction in genome complexity can be achieved through the construction of an RRL in two main steps: restriction digestion and size selection. The use of fragments from a size-selected digestion permits a similar subset of fragments to be obtained from different genotypes that can be deep-sequenced for accurate SNP discovery. The advantages of this technique is that the reduction of genome complexity can be altered by selecting different enzymes or size ranges, facilitates re-sampling and generates sufficient coverage for accurate SNP calling. In soybean (Hyten *et al.*, 2010) and sorghum (Nelson *et al.*, 2011), re-sequencing of RRLs using the SBS method has been performed for the purpose of SNP discovery.

Complexity Reduction of Polymorphic Sequences (CRoPS)

In CRoPS technology, tagged complexity-reduced libraries are prepared by amplified fragment length polymorphism (AFLP), preferably using a methylation-sensitive restriction enzyme (Davey *et al.*, 2011). The AFLP fragment libraries are then sequenced at 5 to 10-fold average redundancy in micro fabricated, high-density picoliter reactions using Genome Sequencer (GS). The generated sequences are clustered and aligned, and the aligned sequences are mined for SNPs using *in silico* analysis following stringent quality measures. The advantage of this technique is that irrespective of genome complexity and size, it can be applied to diverse organisms. Moreover, polymorphism discovery will become affordable in many organisms with high levels of repetitive DNA in the genome and/or low levels of polymorphism in the (breeding) germplasm without the need for prior sequence information by using CRoPS process. In maize, over 75 per cent of putative SNPs were discovered using CRoPS and successfully validated to be true SNPs derived from unique (single-copy) genome sequences (Van *et al.*, 2007).

Restriction-Site Associated DNA Sequencing (RAD-seq)

RAD-seqis, a recently developed powerful tool for targeted sequencing across the genomes of non-model species (Kakioka *et al.*, 2013). RAD-seq aims to explore SNPs adjacent to restriction endonuclease sites. The method relies on cutting DNA with a chosen restriction enzyme, ligating an adapter containing a molecular identifying sequence (MID) unique to each sample, and sequencing the DNA associated with each restriction site using the massively parallel sequencing technology (Stapley *et al.*, 2010). Thousands of RAD-tag markers are obtained, and the markers are genotyped simultaneously for multiple individuals. RAD-seq has broad potential for genetic analysis of non-model organisms including genotype-phenotype association mapping in crop plants (Ganal *et al.*, 2009), QTL analysis in barley (Chutimanitsakun *et al.*, 2011), linkage disequilibrium analysis rye (Li *et al.*, 2011), comparative genomics and genome assembly in several plant species (Ashley *et al.*, 2012).

Chromatin Immunoprecipitation Coupled with High-Throughput DNA Sequencing (ChIP-Seq)

Genome-wide identification of *in vivo* protein-bound genomic region is essential for a full understanding of transcriptional regulation. ChIP-Seq has emerged as one of the powerful tools for profiling protein-DNA binding sites and chromatin modifications on a genome-wide scale (Brandon *et al.*, 2011). The common approach to analyze the millions of short sequence reads obtained in a typical ChIP-seq experiment is to map them to a reference genome. There are several tools available for mapping, for example SOAPv2, Bowtie, or BWA (Ashley *et al.*, 2012). Reads that map to multiple locations in the genome *i.e.* 'multi-reads', are often discarded to avoid the ambiguity of their genomic origin. To account for varying sequencing depths among the different samples in an experiment, current methods typically standardize the number of mapped reads across all samples by scaling.

Till date, all works on ChIP-Seq technology are on model plants, *i.e. Arabidopsis thaliana* (Zhang *et al.*, 2007, Zhu *et al.*, 2012) and rice (Brandon *et al.*, 2011, Zhu *et al.*, 2012), but NGS will soon open this up to other organisms too. However, analyzing the large data sets generated by ChIP-Seq studies are highly challenging for most of the molecular biologists. A recent study was performed on H3K27me3 enrichment sites in rice young endosperm using the ChIP-Seq approach and analyzes the data using four peak calling algorithms, namely, FindPeaks, PeakSeq, USeq, and MACS (Brandon *et al.*, 2011). A detailed protocol of ChIP-ChIP or ChIP-seq technology, and a general guide for computational data analysis was developed and demonstrated successfully to identify direct target genes of the BZR1 Transcription Factor (TF) of the brassionosteroid signalling pathway in both *Arabidopsis* and rice (Zhu *et al.*, 2012).

Genotyping-by-Sequencing (GBS)

GBS is a recently developed highly cost effective approach for simultaneous SNP discovery and genotyping. It may be used for the discovery and identification of SNPs or as a screen for panels of thousands of known markers (Davey *et al.*, 2011). This technique is becoming increasingly important as a unique tool for association studies and genomics-assisted breeding in a range of plant species including those with complex genomes that lack a reference sequence. Although GBS is straightforward for small genomes, target enrichment or reduction of genome complexity must be employed for species with large genomes to ensure sufficient overlap in sequence coverage (Stapley *et al.*, 2010, Elshire *et al.*, 2011). Reducing genome complexity with restriction enzymes (REs) is an easy, quick, extremely specific and highly reproducible compared to the contemporary sequence capture approaches, such as various DNA hybridisation/sequence capture methods. The repetitive regions of genomes can be avoided and lower copy regions can be targeted by choosing appropriate restriction enzymes (RE's) with two to three fold higher efficiency. It simplifies the computationally challenging alignment problems in species with high levels of genetic diversity.

The GBS procedure was demonstrated with maize (IBM) and barley (Oregon Wolfe Barley) recombinant inbred populations where roughly 200,000 and 25,000 sequence tags were mapped, respectively (Elshire *et al.*, 2011). Sonah *et al.* (2013) have explored the use of GBS in soybean. A total of 10,120 high quality SNPs were obtained and the distribution of these SNPs mirrored closely the distribution of gene-rich regions in the soybean genome. A total of 39.5 per cent of the SNPs were present in genic regions and 52.5 per cent of these were located in the coding sequence. They demonstrated the use of selective primers to achieve a greater complexity reduction during GBS library preparation. The number of SNP calls could be increased by almost 40 per cent and their depth of coverage was more than doubled, thus opening the door to an increase in the throughput and a significant decrease in the per sample cost.

Low-Coverage Sequencing for Genotyping

Reductions in the cost of high throughput sequencing have enabled whole-genome sequencing to identify sequence variants segregating in a population. Low-coverage sequencing is a cost-effective and efficient approach to sequence many samples, then to combine data across samples to detect shared variants (Huang *et al.*, 2009, Elshire *et al.*, 2011, Andolfatto *et al.*, 2011). A recent study has presented a method to discover and genotype single-nucleotide polymorphism (SNP) sites from low-coverage sequencing data, making use of shared haplotype (linkage disequilibrium) information on various diploid samples (Le *et al.*, 2011). They collected SNP candidates based on independent sequence calls per site and then using a bioinformatics tool; called MARGARITA collected 20 ancestral recombination graphs (ARGs) from the genotype or phased haplotype data. By using a population genetic prior distribution on tree-branch length and Bayesian inference, they determined a posterior probability of the SNP being real and also the most probable phased genotype call for each individual.

Applications

The genomics technologies are paving the way to a new era of scientific discovery and make it easier than ever to explore the PGR for their proper management and utilisation. NGSs are making it more feasible to develop a large number of genetic markers, construct highly dense linkage maps, and exercises comparative genomics. Due to rapid climate change, deforestation, soil erosion and food security, importance of proper management and utilisation of PGR has increased, particularly in agriculture, plant diversity conservation and crop improvement (Ashley *et al.*, 2012, Huang *et al.*, 2009, Stapley *et al.*, 2010). In the backdrop of genetic erosion, conservation, utilization, and exploration of PGR should get the topmost priority. Utilization of the genomic resources can be enhanced at a much faster pace due to the advancement of high-throughput sequencing techniques.

Genome Wide SNP, SSR or Haplotype Discovery

Analysis of allelic differences or variations which can be detected by molecular markers such as SNPs or haplotypes (*i.e.*, groups of SNPs that are linked to a particular trait) is the main objective of studying genomics in PGR (Kumar *et al.*, 2010). SNPs are presently the marker of choice due to their abundance and stability compared to the other rapid markers, such as simple sequence repeats (SSR) (Ashley *et al.*, 2012). SNPs have been applied in areas including, marker assisted breeding, crop improvement, conservation, construction of genetic maps, assessment of genetic diversity, detection of genotype/phenotype associations and resource management. In functional genomics studies, SNP analysis is mainly focussed on those SNPs located within regulatory genes and transcripts. These studies have largely been improved by the automation of genome-wide SNP genotyping. Until recently, large scale SNP discovery and analysis in plants was mostly limited to maize, *Arabidopsis*, and rice. However, due to dramatic improvement of NGS technology, large scale SNPs has been discovered in several crops within few years. Genome-wide SNPs have been discovered in various model crop plants, such as wheat (Trebbi *et al.*, 2011), rice (McNally *et al.*, 2009, Yamamoto *et al.*, 2010), *Arabidopsis* (Jander *et al.*, 2002, Zhang and Borevitz 2009), barley (Close *et al.*, 2009), sorghum (Nelson *et al.*, 2011), soybean (Hyten *et al.*, 2010), potato (Hamilton *et al.*, 2011), maize (Jones *et al.*, 2009) etc. They have various applications such as construction of linkage map, genetic diversity analyses, association mapping, and marker assisted selection.

Allele Mining

Allele mining is a promising approach to dissect naturally occurring allelic variations at candidate genes level controlling important agronomic traits which has potential applications in utilisation and management of PGR. Allele mining can be effectively and efficiently used for the discovery of superior alleles, studying the rate of evolution of alleles, paving way for molecular discrimination among related species through development of allele-specific molecular markers, and facilitating introgression of novel alleles through Marker Assisted Selection (MAS) (Kumar *et al.*, 2010). Germplasms from wild or locally adapted landrace gene pools, conserved either *in situ* or *ex situ*, contain a rich repertoire of alleles that have been left behind by the selective processes of domestication, selection, and cross-breeding, which paved the way for today's elite cultivars. However, potential genetic resources of stored accessions in various gene banks remain underexplored due to lack of efficient strategies to screen, isolate, and transfer prospective alleles. Until recently, Sanger's sequencing was the only way to determine allelic richness at a given locus in a core collection set of species. NGS has now made allele determination via direct sequencing a cost-effective and realistic prospect (Huang *et al.*, 2009). Gene-specific allele mining was investigated recently in 336 oak (*Quercus robur*) and pedunculate oak (*Quercus petraea*) genotypes based on ten candidate genes. This study has reported 158 polymorphic sites among 8 genes (Homolka *et al.*, 2012).

Genome-Wide Association Studies (GWAS)

Traditionally, natural variation is the basis for selecting the parent for mapping populations. However, it always remains a challenge for the plant breeder to produce new mutants. Searching for mutants is always easier among the structured population in contrast to the identifying natural variants. Association mapping is an alternative and effective strategy over the traditional linkage mapping, which uses recombination events from many lineages. Association mapping is involved in unstructured populations that have been subjected to many recombination events (Abdurakhmonov and Abdukarimov 2008). Genome-wide dissection of complex traits was initially done by linkage mapping based on biparental progenies. Due to certain shortfalls of biparental based linkage mapping, association mapping comes into play for the identification of genes and quantitative trait loci QTL (Brachi *et al.*, 2011, Frary *et al.*, 2000). Later, it has been improved further combining the efforts of linkage mapping and association mapping.

This first genome-wide association studies (GWAS) was done in rice. By low genome coverage sequencing with NGS technology and imputation, 517 rice landraces were genotyped and high-density haplotype maps developed. GWA analyses identified 80 associations for 14 agronomic traits (Huang *et al.*, 2010). The potential of GWAS was demonstrated by the successful functional validation of the gene *ACCELERATED CELL DEATH6* (*ACD6*) in *A. thaliana*. Natural variation in *ACD6* was shown to underpin differences in vegetative growth and in resistance to pathogen and pest infestation (Brachi *et al.*, 2011). Wang *et al.* (2012) have reported GWAS of 32 morphologic and 10 agronomic traits in a collection of 615 barley cultivars which were genotyped by genome-wide polymorphisms from a recently developed barley oligonucleotide pool assay. Moreover, GWAS in diverse accessions promises new perspectives toward gene and allele discovery for agronomically important traits for understanding the genetic basis of complex QTL in plants. However, for GWAS effective genotyping techniques, high-density marker maps, phenotyping resources and even, if possible, high-quality reference genome sequence is required.

De novo Sequencing or Whole Genome Sequencing

Whole genome sequencing paved the way to the comparative genomics and speeds up the dissemination of genetic variations for a large number of germplasm collection in a short duration. After sequencing the genome of a plant, it can be used as a reference genome for the alignment of sequences of the same species or related species. High-throughput sequencing technology have made possible for the re-sequencing of numbers of plants or targeted re-sequencing of "core germplasm" (Ashley *et al.*, 2012). This has also made possible for the identification of rare alleles obtained through biparental mapping populations for the estimation of linkage disequilibrium and genetic relationships between accessions. The 1001 Genomes Project started in the year 2008 which aims re-sequencing of 1001 accessions of *Arabidopsis thaliana* for discovering various sequence variations (Cao *et al.*, 2011). Whole genome sequencing of *Arabidopsis* already have deciphered majority of common polymorphisms, numbers of insertions and deletions, gene functions and their patterns of local as well as global linkage among variants. Moreover, whole-genome resequencing of numbers of crops revealed various polymorphisms, such as SNPs in maize rice (McNally *et al.*, 2009) and soybean (Hyten *et al.*, 2010). These studies will help in selecting germplasm based on crop-specific markers for breeding programs.

Genome Wide Discovery of Small RNA and Degardome

Small RNAs constitute a major class of the small regulatory molecules that are involved in regulating the intrinsic normal growth and development of organisms as well as in maintaining the integrity of genomes. Although large numbers of small RNAs have been identified in various plants by direct cloning, the number of small RNAs discovered has increased significantly after the introduction of NGS due to the greater depth of sequencing. The use of NGS technology has also revealed that, on contrary to the fact, miRNAs were produced from a noncoding RNA that undergoes various steps to process mature miRNA (~22 bp long), miRNAs are also produced from the intronic region of some genes in *A. thaliana* and rice (Meng and Shao 2012). For understanding the biological roles of miRNAs, most of the miRNA targets were predicted using bioinformatics tools based on either the perfect or nearly perfect sequence complementarity between the miRNA and target genes or sequence conservation among different species in higher plants, however, due to the mismatches in miRNA-target pairing, it remains as a challenge. Out of the predicted targets, so far only a few targets have been validated experimentally. However, a new high-throughput technique called degradome sequencing has successfully been applied for screening miRNA targets (Yang *et al.*, 2013). Many novel miRNAs with low abundance and their targets have been identified and validated using NGS in conjunction with this technique (Addo-Quaye *et al.*, 2008, Li *et al.*, 2010b)

Due to the advancement of sequencing technology and bioinformatics, the last decade has witnessed remarkable progress in our knowledge of the biogenesis and activity of diverse classes of small RNAs. For example, Moxon *et al.* (2008) identified several conserved and non-conserved miRNAs and other short RNAs in tomato fruit and leaf using high-throughput pyrosequencing, such as SlymiR 156/157, SlymiR160. Expression of 25 miRNA families, such as miR156, miR390, miR529 in maize was verified by deep-sequencing of small RNA libraries (Zhang *et al.*, 2009). Conserved nature of miR444 in rice, maize, sorghum and sugarcane was also deciphered using NGS technology. In *Medicago truncatula*, 238 potential candidate miRNAs were identified, and among them 14 new miRNAs and 15 new members of known miRNA families whose complementary miRNAs were also detected (Wang *et al.*, 2011). Using small RNA sequencing followed by degradome sequencing, a total of seven miRNAs and eight *trans*-acting small interfering RNAs in wheat have also been discovered (Tang *et al.*, 2012). Numbers of stress associated miRNAs have also been discovered in several crop plant species, such as soybean (Kulcheski *et al.*, 2011), rice (Cao *et al.*, 2011), cowpea (Blanca *et al.*, 2011), and validated through real time PCR.

Methylome

DNA methylation is a major form of epigenetic modifications and is the most common covalent modification of DNA in eukaryotes. Genome-wide study of DNA methylation profile is critical for understanding the biological role of DNA methylation and their correlation with other epigenetic mechanisms (Zhang *et al.*, 2010). With the development of next-generation sequencing technologies, the ability to survey whole-genome methylation profiles has been enabled. NGS technologies have been applied in combination with bisulfite conversion of DNA for the characterisation of genome-wide methylation pattern in plants, using an application known as ultra-deep bisulphite DNA sequencing (BSSeq) (Cokus *et al.*, 2008). Bisulfite treatment is basically important for the conversion of unmethylated cytidine residues in DNA to uracil. Methylated fractions of genomes can also be sequenced using a combination of NGS and methyl-DNA immunoprecipitation (MeDIP) technique (Pomraning *et al.*, 2009). This approach is useful for generating detailed methylation maps of the genome, and one can address the ecologically and evolutionary important questions by comparing the genome wide methylation maps in different samples, such as genetic architecture of plants behind the differential gene expression during natural selection.

During the past decade, DNA methylation analysis has undergone a major technological revolution. A genome-wide DNA methylation profile was compared among 10 *A. thaliana* lines, derived from a common ancestor of 30 generations old. It was deciphered that around 30,000 cytosines in each strain were differentially methylated and larger regions of contiguous methylation were much more stable (Becker *et al.*, 2008). The same regions were often affected by differential methylation like an individual position in independent lines. Transposable elements and short interfering RNAs are rarely linked to DNA methylation. The biased distribution and frequent reversion of epimutations have important implications for the potential contribution of sequence-independent epialleles to plant evolution.

Differentially Expressed Transcriptome

There are numbers of methods for the identification of differentially expressed transcriptome, such as differential display of reverse transcriptase PCR (DDRT-PCR), microarrays, serial analysis of gene expression (SAGE), suppression subtractive hybridization (SSH), massive parallel sequence signatures, and cDNA-amplified fragment length polymorphisms (cDNA-AFLP), each of which present advantages and disadvantages. NGStechniques provide a better approach to gene expression profiling with several advantages. The power of NGS along with novel molecular techniques allows the investigator to perform gene expression studies to address various transcriptional complexities of an organism and answering several biological questions. The advancements of NGS technologies have highlighted the importance of sequencing-based approaches in transcriptome analysis. Although, SAGE was the first reported sequencing-based high-throughput method for gene expression profiling followed by massively parallel signature sequencing, microarray was employed widely by the researchers. The NGS technologies are used for whole-transcriptome sequencing (RNA-seq) or in combination with SAGE methods for transcriptome studies (Annadurai *et al.*, 2012, Robinson and Parkin 2008). RNA-seq gives unprecedented details about transcriptional features, such as novel transcribed regions, allele-specific expression, RNA editing, and a comprehensive capability to capture alternative splicing, for which it has become the popular choice to identify differentially expressed genes (Mizrachi *et al.*, 2010, Xia *et al.*, 2011). RNA-seq is quickly superceding the microarray based approaches for studying gene expression regarding greater quantitative and qualitative insight, and accuracy. RNA-seq combined with appropriate bioinformatics tools provides a better approach to study gene expression dynamics on a global scale in different cellular and biological contexts. However, appropriate bioinformatics and computational tools for analysing RNA-seq data remains as a challenge for the adoption of this technology.

Using RNA-seq technology, the transcriptional complexity and evolution of meiosis in *Arabidopsis* has been unravelled in two independent studies (Chen *et al.*, 2010, Yang *et al.*, 2011). The transcriptional analysis in maize identified 64.4 per cent of differentially expressed genes during leaf development (Li *et al.*, 2010a). Using Illumina sequencing, extensive analysis on gene expression and splice variants of grapevine during berry development was conducted (Zenoni *et al.*, 2010). Numbers of tissue specific genes were also identified in model legume crop, soybean (Libault *et al.*, 2010). Moreover, numbers of differentially expressed transcripts or transcriptional dynamics were identified and studied in several crop species, such as rice (Lu *et al.*, 2010), cucumber (Guo *et al.*, 2010), sweet orange (Xu *et al.*, 2010) and chickpea (Garg and Jain, 2011).

Conclusion

PGR and their diversity are the backbone of cultivar development. Huge in dimension, their sustainable management demands the high-throughput technologies. High-throughput phenotyping (Phenomics) as well as high-throughput genotyping cum sequencing are two landmarks discovery recently. NGS technology, although initial stage of application, it has already begun to reshape the ways in which plant science is portrayed. NGS technologies now allow millions of bases to be sequenced in one round, at a fraction of the cost relative to traditional Sanger sequencing. However, as costs and capabilities of these technologies continue to improve, we are only beginning to see the possibilities of NGS platforms for the management and utilisation of PGR. NGS technologies will give tremendous input in the identification of correct accessions, tracking of seed lots, varieties, and alleles, justification of adding new accessions in genbank, identification of core germplasm set, identification of diverse alleles located in diverse geographical areas, associate genotypes with phenotypes and choosing right plant material for breeding in an accurate and precise way at molecular level. It is expected that NGS technology will soon facilitate the development of need-based, region-specific cultivars to combat with climate change.

References

Abdurakhmonov I, Abdukarimov A. Application of association mapping to understanding the genetic diversity of plant germplasm resources. *Intl. J. Pl. Genomics*. 5: 1–18. 2008.

Addo-Quaye C, Eshoo TW, Bartel DP, Axtell MJ. Endogenous siRNA and miRNA targets identified by sequencing of the Arabidopsis degradome. *Curr. Biol*. 18: 758–762. 2008.

Andolfatto P, Davison D, Erezyilmaz D, Hu TT *et al.*, Multiplexed shotgun genotyping for rapid and efficient genetic mapping. *Genome Res*. 21: 610–617. 2011.

Annadurai RS, Jayakumar V, Mugasimangalam RC, Katta M *et al.*, Next generation sequencing and de novo transcriptome analysis of *Costus pictus* D. Don, a non-model plant with potent anti-diabetic properties. *BMC Genomics*. 13: 663, 2012.

Ashley NE, Jessica S, David MS. Applications of next-generation sequencing in plant biology. *Amer. J. Bot*. 99: 175-185. 2012.

Ball AD, Beckerman AP, Slate J. Adaptation genomics: the next generation. *Trends Ecol. Evol*. 25: 705-712. 2010.

Bansal V, Harismendy O, Tewhey R, Murray SS *et al.*, Accurate detection and genotyping of SNPs utilizing population sequencing data. *Genome Res*. 20: 537–545. 2010.

Becker C, Hagmann J, Müller J, Koenig D *et al.*, Spontaneous epigenetic variation in the *Arabidopsis thaliana* methylome. *Nature*. 480: 245-249. 2008.

Blanca EB-F, Gao L, Diop NN, Wu Z *et al.*, Identification and comparative analysis of drought-associated microRNAs in two cowpea genotypes. *BMC Pl. Biol.* 11: 127-138. 2011.

Brachi B, Morris GP, Borevitz JO. Genome-wide association studies in plants: the missing heritability is in the field. *Genome Biol.* 12: 232. 2011.

Brandon MM, Feng T, Susan MB, Zhaohua P. Comparison of four ChIP-Seq analytical algorithms using rice endosperm H3K27 trimethylation profiling data. *PLoS ONE*. 6: e25260, 2011.

Cao JK, Schneeberger S, Ossowski T, Günther SB *et al.*, Whole-genome sequencing of multiple Arabidopsis thaliana populations. *Nature Genet.* 43: 956–963. 2011.

Chen C, Farmer AD, Langley RJ, *et al.*, Meiosis-specific gene discovery in plants. RNA-Seq applied to isolated Arabidopsis male meiocytes. *BMC Pl. Biol.* 10. 280. 2010.

Chutimanitsakun Y, Nipper RW, Cuesta-Marcos A, Cistue L *et al.*, Construction and application for QTL analysis of a restriction site associated DNA (RAD) linkage map in barley. *BMC Genomics*. 12: 4. 2011.

Close TJ, Bhat PR, Lonardi S *et al.*, Development and implementation of high-throughput SNP genotyping in barley. *BMC Genomics*. 10: 582. 2009.

Cokus SJ, Feng S, Zhang X, Chen Z *et al.*, Shotgun bisulphite sequencing of the *Arabidopsis* genome reveals DNA methylation patterning. *Nature*. 452: 215-219. 2008.

Davey JW, Hohenlohe PA, Etter PD, Boone JQ *et al.*, Genome-wide genetic marker discovery and genotyping using next generation sequencing. *Nature Rev. Genet.* 12: 499-510. 2011.

Elshire RJ, Glaubitz JC, Sun Q, Poland JA *et al.*, A robust, simple genotyping-by-sequencing (GBS) approach for high diversity species. *PLoS ONE*. 6: e19379. 2011.

Frary A, Nesbitt TC, Frary A, Grandillo S *et al.*, fw2.2: A quantitative trait locus key to the evolution of tomato fruit size. *Science*. 289: 85–88. 2000.

Ganal MW, Altmann T, Röder MS. SNP identification in crop plants. *Curr. Opin. Pl. Biol.* 12: 211-217. 2009.

Garg R, Jain M. Pyrosequencing data reveals tissue-specific expression of lineage-specific transcripts in chickpea. *Pl. Sigl. Behavr.* 6: 2011. doi: 10.4161/psb/6.11.17879.

Glenn TC. Field guide to next-generation DNA sequencers. *Mol. Ecol. Resour.* 11: 759–769. 2011.

Guo S, Zheng Y, Joung JG, *et al.*, Transcriptome sequencing and comparative analysis of cucumber flowers with different sex types. *BMC Genomics*. 11: 384. 2010.

Hamilton JP, Hansey CN, Whitty BR *et al.*, Single nucleotide polymorphism discovery in elite north American potato germplasm. *BMC Genomics*, 12: 302. 2011.

Hardin SH. Real-time DNA sequencing. In: next generation genome sequencing: towards personalized medicine, (Janitz M, Weinheim Ed.). Germany. Wiley-VCH Verlag and Co. pp. 97–102. 2008.

Homolka A, Eder T, Kopecky D, Berenyi M *et al.*, Allele discovery of ten candidate drought-response genes in Austrian oak using a systematically informatics approach based on 454 amplicon sequencing. *BMC Res. Notes.* 5: 175-185. 2012.

Huang X, Wei X, Sang T, Zhao Q *et al.*, Genome-wide association studies of 14 agronomic traits in rice landraces. *Nature Genet.* 42: 961-967. 2010.

Huang XQ, Feng QQ, Zhao Q, Wang L *et al.*, High-throughput genotyping by whole-genome resequencing. *Genome Res.* 19: 1068–1076. 2009.

Hyten DL, Cannon SB, Song Q, Weeks N *et al.*, High-throughput SNP discovery through deep resequencing of a reduced representation library to anchor and orient scaffolds in the soybean whole genome sequence. *BMC Genomics.* **11:** 38. 2010.

Jander G, Norris SR, Rounsley D, Bush F *et al.*, Arabidopsis map-based cloning in the post genome era. *Pl. Physiol.* 129: 440–450. 2002.

Jones E, Chu WC, Ayele M *et al.*, Development of single nucleotide polymorphism (SNP) markers for use in commercial maize (*Zea mays* L.) germplasm. *Mol. Breed.* 24: 165-176. 2009.

Kakioka R, Kokita T, Kumada H, Watanabe K, Okuda N. A RAD-based linkage map and comparative genomics in the gudgeons (genus *Gnathopogon, Cyprinidae*). *BMC Genomics.* 14: 32. 2013.

Kircher M, Kelso J. High-throughput DNA sequencing-concepts and limitations. Bio. Essays. 32: 524–536. 2010.

Kulcheski FR, Oliveira LFV, Molina LG, Almerão MP *et al.*, Identification of novel soybean microRNAs involved in abiotic and biotic stresses. *BMC Genomics.* 12: 307-324. 2011.

Kumar GR, Sakthivel K, Sundaram RM, Neeraja CN *et al.*, Allele mining in crops: prospects and potentials. *Biotech. Adv.* 28: 451-461. 2010.

Kumar S, Banks TW, Cloutier S. SNP discovery through next-generation sequencing and its applications. *Intl. J. Pl. Genomics.* Article ID 831460, 2012. doi: 10.1155/2012/831460.

Le SQ, Durbin R. SNP detection and genotyping from low-coverage sequencing data on multiple diploid samples. *Genome Res.* 21: 952-960. 2011.

Levene MJ, Korlach J, Turner SW, Foquet M *et al.*, Zero-mode waveguides for single-molecule analysis at high concentration. *Science.* 299: 682-686. 2003.

Li P, Ponnala L, Gandotra N, *et al.*, The developmental dynamics of the maize leaf transcriptome. *Nature Genet.* 42: 1060–1067. 2010a.

Li Y, Haseneyer G, Schön CC, Ankerst D *et al.*, High levels of nucleotide diversity and fast decline of linkage disequilibrium in rye (*Secale cereale* L.) genes involved in frost response. *BMC Pl. Biol.* 11: 6–20. 2011.

Li YF, Zheng Y, Addo-Quaye C, Zhang L *et al.*, Transcriptome-wide identification of microRNA targets in rice. *Plant J.* 62: 742–759. 2010b.

Libault M, Farmer A, Joshi T, *et al.*, An integrated transcriptome atlas of the crop model *Glycine max*, and its use in comparative analyses in plants. *Plant J.* 63: 86–99. 2010.

Lieberman KR, Cherf GM, Doody MJ, Olasagasti F *et al.*, Possessive replication of single DNA molecules in a nanopore catalyzed by phi29 DNA polymerase. *J. Amer. Chem. Soc.* 132: 17961-17972. 2010.

Lu T, Lu G, Fan D, *et al.*, Function annotation of the rice transcriptome at single-nucleotide resolution by RNA-seq. *Genome Res.* 20: 1238–49. 2010.

Maxam AM, Gilbert W. A new method for sequencing DNA. *Proc. Natl. Acad. Sci. USA.* 74: 560–564. 1977.

McNally KL, Childs KL, Bohnert R *et al.*, Genomewide SNP variation reveals relationships among landraces and modern varieties of rice. *Proc. Natl. Acad. Sci. USA.* 106: 12273-12278. 2009.

Meng Y, Shao C. Large-scale identification of mirtrons in *Arabidopsis* and rice. *PLoS ONE*. 7: 31163–31170. 2012.

Mizrachi E, Ranik CA-HM, Joubert F, Myburg AA. De novo assembled expressed gene catalog of a fast-growing Eucalyptus tree produced by Illumina mRNA-Seq. *BMC Genomics.* 11: 681–687. 2010.

Moxon S, Jing R, Szittya G, Schwach F *et al.*, Deep sequencing of tomato short RNAs identifies microRNAs targeting genes involved in fruit ripening. *Genome Res.* 18: 1602–1609. 2008.

Nelson JC, Wang S, Wu Y, Li X *et al.*, Single-nucleotide polymorphism discovery by high-throughput sequencing in sorghum. *BMC Genomics.* **12:** 352. 2011.

Pomraning KR, Smith KM, Freitag M. Genome-wide high throughput analysis of DNA methylation in eukaryotes. *Methods.* 47: 142-150. 2009.

Robinson SJ, Parkin I AP. Differential SAGE analysis in *Arabidopsis* uncovers increased transcriptome complexity in response to low temperature. *BMC Genomics.* 9: 434. 2008.

Ronaghi M, Uhl´en M, Nyr´en P. A sequencing method based on real-time pyrophosphate. *Science.* 281: 363–365. 1998.

Rothberg JM, Hinz W, Rearick TM, Schultz J *et al.*, An integrated semiconductor device enabling non-optical genome sequencing. *Nature.* 475: 348-352. 2011.

Sanger F, Nicklen S, Coulson AR. DNA sequencing with chain-terminating inhibitors. *Proc. Natl. Acad. Sci. USA.* 74: 5463–5467. 1977.

Shendure J, Porreca GJ, Reppas NB *et al.*, Molecular biology: accurate multiplex polony sequencing of an evolved bacterial genome. *Science.* 309: 1728–1732. 2005.

Sonah H, Bastien M, Iquira E, Tardivel A *et al.*, An improved genotyping by sequencing (GBS) approach offering increased versatility and efficiency of SNP discovery and genotyping. *PLoS ONE.* 8: e54603. 2013.

Stapley J, Reger J, Feulner PG, Smadja C *et al.,* Navigating the tip of the genomic iceberg: next-generation sequencing for plant systematics. *Amer. J. Bot.* 99: 349-364. 2012.

Sunkar R, Zhou X, Zheng Y, Zhang W, Zhu JK. Identification of novel and candidate miRNAs in rice by high throughput sequencing. *BMC Pl. Biol.* 8: 25. 2008.

Tang Z, Zhang L, Xu C, Yuan S, *et al.,* Uncovering small RNA-mediated responses to cold stress in a wheat thermo-sensitive genic male sterile line by deep sequencing. *Pl. Physiol.* 159: 731-738. 2012.

Thompson JF, Steinmann KE. Single-molecule sequencing with a HeliScope genetic analysis system. *Curr. Proto. Mol. Biol.* 92: 1-14. 2010.

Trebbi D, Maccaferri M, Heer PD *et al.,* High-throughput SNP discovery and genotyping in durum wheat (*Triticum durum* Desf.). *Theo. Appl. Genet.* 123: 555–569. 2011.

Van O-NJ, Hogers RCJ, Janssen A, Yalcin F *et al.,* Complexity reduction of polymorphic sequences (CRoPS™): A novel approach for large-scale polymorphism discovery in complex genomes. *PLoS ONE.* 2: 1172–1182. 2007.

Wang M, Jiang N, Jia T, Leach L *et al.,* Genome-wide association mapping of agronomic and morphologic traits in highly structured populations of barley cultivars. *Theo. Appl. Genet.* 124: 233–246. 2012.

Wang T, Chen L, Zhao M, Tian Q, Zhang W-H. Identification of drought-responsive microRNAs in *Medicago truncatula* by genome-wide high throughput sequencing. *BMC Genomics.* 12: 367. 2011.

Xia Z, Xu H, Zhai J, Li D *et al.,* RNA-Seq analysis and *de novo* transcriptome assembly of *Hevea brasiliensis*. *Pl. Mol. Biol.* 77: 299-308. 2011.

Xu Q, Yu K, Zhu A, *et al.,* Comparative transcripts profiling reveals new insight into molecular processes regulating lycopene accumulation in a sweet orange (*Citrus sinensis*) red-flesh mutant. *BMC Genomics.* 10: 540. 2009.

Yamamoto T, Nagasaki H, Yonemaru JI *et al.,* Fine definition of the pedigree haplotypes of closely related rice cultivars by means of genome-wide discovery of singlenucleotide polymorphisms. *BMC Genomics.* 11: article 267. 2010.

Yang H, Lu P, Wang Y, *et al.,* The transcriptome landscape of *Arabidopsis* male meiocytes from high-throughput sequencing: the complexity and evolution of the meiotic process. *Plant J.* 65: 503-516. 2011.

Yang X, Wang L, YuanD, Lindsey K, Zhang X. Small RNA and degradome sequencing reveal complex miRNA regulation during cotton somatic embryogenesis. *J. Exptl. Bot.* 64: 1521–1536. 2013.

You FM, Huo N, Deal KR, Gu YQ *et al.,* Annotation-based genome-wide SNP discovery in the large and complex Aegilops tauschii genome using next-generation sequencing without a reference genome sequence. *BMC Genome.* 12: 59-78. 2011.

Zenoni S, Ferrarini A, Giacomelli E, *et al.*, Characterization of transcriptional complexity during berry development in *Vitis vinifera* using RNA-Seq. *Pl. Physiol.* 152: 1787–95. 2010.

Zhang L, Chia JM, Kumari S, Stein JC *et al.*, A genome-wide characterization of MicroRNA genes in maize. *PLoS Genet.* 5: 2009. doi: 10.1371/journal.pgen.1000716.

Zhang X, Borevitz JO. Global analysis of allele-specific expression in *Arabidopsis thaliana. Genetics.* 182: 943–954. 2009.

Zhang X, Clarenz O, Cokus S, Bernatavichute YV *et al.*, Whole-genome analysis of histone H3 lysine 27 trimethylation in Arabidopsis. *PLoS Biol.* 5: e129. 2007.

Zhang Y, Jeltsch A. The application of next generation sequencing in DNA methylation analysis. *Genes.* 1: 85-101. 2010.

Zhu JY, Sun Y, Wang ZY. Genome-wide identification of transcription factor-binding sites in plants using chromatin immunoprecipitation followed by microarray (ChIP-chip) or sequencing (ChIP-seq). *Methods. Mol. Biol.* 876: 173-88. 2012.

2016, Biotechnological Tools for Genetic Resources Pages 19–58
Editor: Pradip Chandra Deka
Published by: Daya Publishing House, NEW DELHI

Chapter 2

DNA Barcoding: Current Trends and Future Prospects

Deepika Singh[1], Arghya Sett[1], Pragya Sharma[2], Manab Deka[2] and Utpal Bora[1*]

[1]*Bioengineering Research Laboratory, Department of Biosciences and Bioengineering, Indian Institute of Technology, Guwahati – 781 039, Assam*

[2]*Department of Applied Science, Institute of Science and Technology, Gauhati University, Guwahati – 781 014, Assam*

**E-mail: ubora@iitg.ernet.in, ubora@rediffmail.com*

ABSTRACT

DNA barcoding has been evolved as an effective species-identification tool as compared to classical taxonomic system in diverse areas like phylogeny, ecology, population genetics, biodiversity etc. It has immense potential in identification of unexplored species which could provide insights into the taxonomic structure, function and composition. There is a remarkable increase in the barcode sequences of some taxa whereas some taxa are still under-described. DNA barcoding can not be a standalone discipline and has to be combined with morphological data for accurate taxonomic identification. Application of high throughput sequencing platforms in this approach has now been employed to unravel the diversity with rapid and error-free results. Here we present a comprehensive view of DNA barcoding approach in various taxa such as animals, plants, fungi, bacteria, virus and protists. The methodology, pros and cons, applications, current and future prospects of DNA barcoding have been discussed as well. Furthermore, we concluded that integrative approach combining morphological, molecular and the high throughput sequencing technologies which will rapidly unveil the diversity of various life forms.

Keywords: *Barcoding, Diversity, Taxonomy, Barcode, Integrative, Microbiome.*

Introduction

Identification and classification of species have traditionally been carried out by the researchers and professionals of taxonomic domain. Several aspects of classical taxonomy are far from complete understanding attributed to higher chances of species misidentification (Packer *et al.*, 2009). Traditional systematic based taxonomy suffers from complications in proper identification of organisms with phenotypic plasticity, genetic variability, immaturity and crypticity. Advanced alternative methods have emerged as essential tools for correct identification and to establish the field of taxonomy (Padial and De La Riva 2007, Padial *et al.*, 2009). DNA sequence-based analyses provide plethora of information that may be effective for distinguishing various hierarchial levels *i.e.* population to species and the deepest taxonomically hierarchial level. It has enabled the ecologists and evolutionary taxonomists to address the issues associated with morphological data analyses.

A molecular and bioinformatical tool termed as DNA barcoding was proposed in 2003 by Paul Hebert to aid in diagnosis of biodiversity. However it was not a novel concept. Earlier it had been used in the discrimination of microbial species and later been tested among various taxa (Eggert *et al.*, 2002, Floyd *et al.*, 2002).

This system circumvents the lapses associated with morphology based identification systems by providing a better taxonomic resolution. Moreover, it has gained considerable validation as a suitable tool to identify species, delimit species and define species boundaries (Hebert *et al.*, 2003). With the immense progress in DNA barcoding research area, the pros and cons have been emerged. DNA barcode based Next generation sequencing (NGS) is becoming new platform to enhance the level of identification and classification owing to its cost-effective and parallel sequencing at a single run.

DNA Barcoding and its Symbology

DNA barcoding is a rapid and accurate species identification tool that uses short, standardized, conserved gene regions as internal species tags called DNA barcodes. It performs species level identification by sequencing a specific barcode region derived from unknown specimens and comparing with the reference library of sequences of known specimens. Since every species most likely have a unique DNA signature code, this approach is based on the postulate that inter-species variation exceeds intra-species variation.

An ideal DNA barcoding system should serve following criteria:

1. Variation of barcode region between species but nearly identical within species.
2. Enough phylogenetic information for easy identification and classification of unknown species.
3. Robustness in highly conserved regions and highly consistent DNA amplifications and sequencing.
4. Short target gene that can amplify the degraded DNA.

The main goal of DNA barcoding is to identify unknown, cryptic, microscopic and other species with inaccessible or complex morphology as well as discovery of new species. It has proved to be effective amongst various groups of animals such as birds, fishes, spiders, lepidopteransetc. Apart from this, it has also been applied in plants, bacteria, fungi, mollusks, macroalgae and protists taxonomic classification (Hebert *et al.*, 2003, Taberlet *et al.*, 2007).

It is a broadly accepted species identification tool for budding researchers and specialists. It also complements taxonomy, molecular phylogenetics and population genetics. The integrated information on species distribution, structure and their genetic diversity will thus enhance the speed and efficacy of local population studies (Hajibabaei *et al.*, 2007).

Presently used DNA sequences are not amenable for documentation or data storage. Despite the development of variant barcode technology in manufacturing and retailing industries, no such type of barcode has been assessed for its suitability in representing the DNA barcode sequences. In contrast to one dimensional barcodes (1D), two dimensional barcodes (2D) have better potential in DNA barcoding applications. A study reveals that the use of PDF417 digital barcodes has high longevity for digital imaging of DNA sequences (Kumar *et al.*, 2008). Moreover, various 2D barcodes (*e.g.* Data Matrix, CodaBlock-F, the Aztec Code, PDF417, PDF417 Truncated, QR2005 code, and QR code) have been evaluated as symbology for barcoding by using five broadly accepted plant and animal barcodes sequences (COI, *rbcL*, *matK*, ITS2 and *psbA-trnH*). Among all, Quick Response (QR) code was reported as the most accurate symbology for DNA barcodes due to its good compression efficiency and ease of scanning and decoding (Liu *et al.*, 2012).

DNA Barcoding in Various Taxa

Selection of a suitable barcode region is an important prerequisite for DNA barcoding that varies amongst various taxa. Several mitochondrial, chloroplast and nuclear regions have been studied for their efficiency to fulfill the requirements of barcoding. Each region has its own advantages and disadvantages. The barcode markers for plants, fungi, bacteria, animals and other eukaryotes are enlisted in Table 2.1.

The schematic diagram representing DNA barcoding in animals, plants, fungi, virus, and bacteria is illustrated in Figure 2.1.

DNA Barcoding in Animals

The mitochondrial genome of animals is devoid of introns, has a limited exposure to recombination and haploid type of inheritance. Therefore, it is a better candidate for analysis than the nuclear genome (Saccone *et al.*, 1999). The universal primers enable the routine amplification of specific regions of the mitochondrial genome (Simmons and Weller 2001). The use of ribosomal sequence (12S and 16S) as universal barcode in the past phylogenetic studies is now constrained by the prevalence of insertions and deletions (indels). These indels complicate sequence alignment with the existing template sequences (Doyle and Gaut, 2000). A 650-base fragment of the 5′ end of the mitochondrial gene cytochrome c oxidase I (COI, *cox1*)

Table 2.1: Choice of DNA Barcode Markers in Various Taxa

Taxa	*Gene/Genomic Sequence*	*References*
Animals and many other eukaryotes	Mitochondrial gene cytochrome c oxidase subunit 1 (*COI*) gene	Hebert *et al.*, 2003
Plants	Chloroplast gene-*matK*	Lahaye *et al.*, 2008, Yu *et al.*, 2011,
	Chloroplast gene-*rbcL*	Newmaster *et al.*, 2006
	Chloroplast gene-*trnH-psbA*	Kress *et al.*, 2005
	rbcL+matK	Hollingsworth *et al.*, 2011
	Internal transcribed spacers of nuclear ribosomal DNA (nrDNA ITS)	Chen *et al.*, 2010
Fungi	Internal transcribed spacer (*ITS*) of nuclear DNA alone or in combination with *SSU* and *LSU*	Kress *et al.*, 2005, Chen *et al.*, 2010, Dumbrell *et al.*, 2011, Arfi *et al.*, 2012, Schoch *et al.*, 2012
Bacteria	Large subunit of ribosomal polymerase II (*RPB1* and *RPB2*)	Seifert 2009
	rpoB	Case *et al.*, 2007, Walsh *et al.*, 2012
	16S rRNA	Woo *et al.*, 2008
	COI	Michel *et al.* (1998)
	Cpn60	Links *et al.*, 2012
	SSU rRNA in some Archaea	Benlloch *et al.*, 2002
Viruses	No specific marker (S3-peptidase gene for some virus)	Cheng *et al.*, 1995, Kumar *et al.*, 2011
Protozoans	*COI* for amoebae	Kosakyan *et al.*, 2012
	ITS and *28S rRNA* (for *Piroplasma*)	Gou *et al.*, 2012
	18S rRNA (SSU)	Karnati *et al.*, 2003

Abbreviations: *16S rRNA*: 16S ribosomal RNA, *28S rRNA*: 28S ribosomal RNA, *COI:* cytochrome c oxidase I, *cpn60*: chaperonin-60, *rpoB*: RNA polymerase beta subunit, *matK*: maturase K, *rbcL*: ribulose-bisphosphate carboxylase, *LSU*: large subunit, *SSU*: small subunit, *ITS*: internal transcribed spacer, RPB1/RPB2: ribosomal polymerase B1/B2.

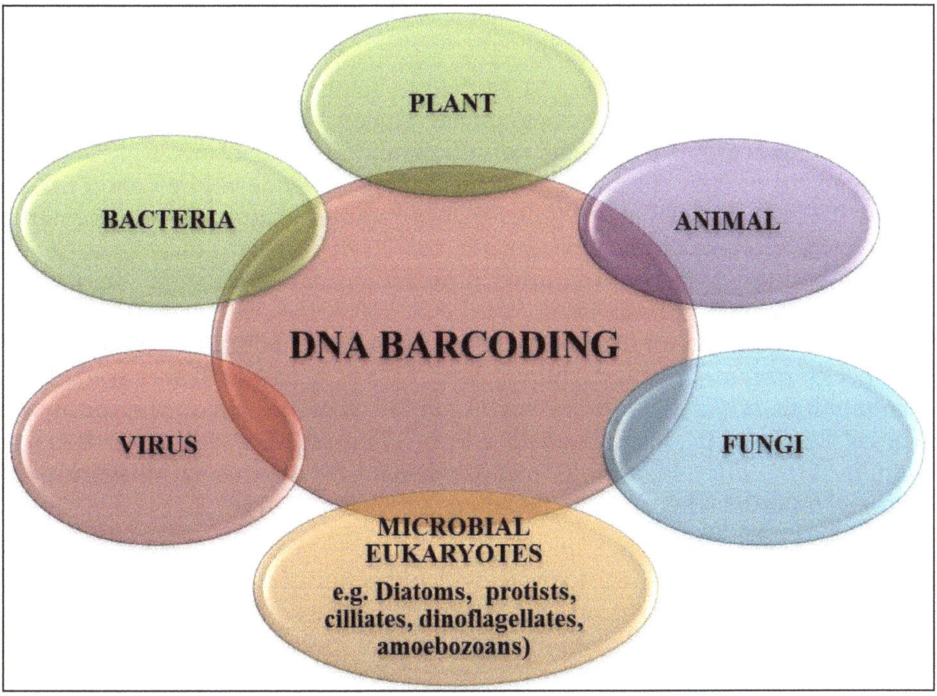

Figure 2.1: DNA Barcoding in Various Taxa.

has been considered as gold standard barcode region for animals (Hebert *et al.*, 2003, Folmer *et al.*, 1994) due to following advantages:

1. Robust universal primers for this gene.
2. Lack of insertions or deletion mutations, more conserved region of sequence.
3. A longer range of phylogenetic signal relative to ribosomal sequences (12S and 16S).

DNA barcoding resolves most of the animal species but some taxa have proved intractable. COI has been proved to be an ideal DNA barcode for most of the animal species, such as spiders, crustaceans, reptiles, fishes, birds, bryozoans, mammals *etc.* (Robinson *et al.*, 2009, Costa *et al.*, 2007, Huang *et al.*, 2015, Ivanova *et al.*, 2007, Hebert *et al.*, 2004, Kerr *et al.*, 2007, Gómez *et al.*, 2007, Bennett *et al.*, 2011). Taxonomically well-studied mammals have not been much focussed in DNA barcoding system (Wilson and Reeder, 2005). Barcoding on mammals has been epicentered on some groups such as rodents, bats and opossums (Borisenko *et al.*, 2008, Clare *et al.*, 2007).

Barcoding has also been applied for insect species, particularly Lepidopteran insects (Silva-Brandão *et al.*, 2009, Anslan and Tedersoo 2015). This is quite effective in the identification of moths, butterflies, mayflies *etc.* (Hebert *et al.*, 2003, Hebert *et al.*, 2004, Ball *et al.*, 2005). They have also been successfully employed for barcoding of psocids of family Liposcelididae and in closely related species of silkworm pests (Jinbo *et al.*, 2011, Yang *et al.*, 2013).

DNA barcoding has emerged in field of ichthyology where fishes show morphological diversity during development (Hubert *et al.*, 2008, Steinke *et al.*, 2009). Fish is the largest group of invertebrate with significant diversity in morphology and ecology (Nelson 2006). A campaign of International Barcode of Life Project (iBOL) *i.e.* Fish Barcode of Life Initiative (FISH-BOL) provides a platform for ichthyologists to accelerate species identification (Swartz *et al.*, 2008). The high efficiency of COI in species identification has been reported in Australian marine, Canadian marine and ornamental North American fishes (Ward *et al.*, 2005). The efficiency of this marker has also been checked for Cuban freshwater fish species, billfishes and freshwater fish species from rich Balkan ichthyofauna (Lara *et al.*, 2010, Hanner *et al.*, 2011, Triantafyllidis *et al.*, 2011). A successful amplification has been acheived in the fishes of Taal Lake, the third largest lake in the Philippines, using COI as a barcode (Aquilino *et al.*, 2011). Identification of problematic fish species *e.g.* Sillaginids has also been reported where COI alone failed (Kruck *et al.*, 2013).

Furthermore, DNA barcoding has been found to be effective using COI than 16S ribosomal RNA gene (*16S*) for species identification of endangered amphibians (Smith *et al.*, 2008). The shortcomings of existing primers direct to inception of new primer sets. They universally amplify COI region in species like salamanders, frogs, caecilians *etc.* (Che *et al.*, 2012).

The species identification in earthworms is difficult due to rapid diversity in the evolution and lack of expertise in this field (Martin *et al.*, 2000). Use of molecular markers paves a new way for identification of new taxa, juveniles, cryptic species and earthworm biodiversity (Decaens *et al.*, 2013). Several studies revealed the efficiency of 12S rRNA (~400 bp) and 16S rRNA in species identification, due to their markedly lower genetic distances. In contrary, the efficiency of COI gene has been studied in genetic lineages and discovering cryptic species (Klarica *et al.*, 2012).

Moreover, the use of *cox1*, *16S* and cytochrome b (COB) has also been explored in barcoding of primates with *cox1* showing largest amount of genetic variation (Lorenz *et al.*, 2005). Thus, COI has been proved as an ideal marker for accurate identification of primates and plays a key role in comparative primatology (Nijman *et al.*, 2010).

DNA Barcoding in Plants

The nuclear and plastid/chloroplast genomes could provide suitable barcode regions as they are variable enough to discriminate amongst species and have less intraspecific variation than interspecific variation (Chase *et al.*, 2005, Kress *et al.*, 2005). COI is not primarily used for species identification and new species discovery in plants. It is due to low substitution rate of mitochondrial genes than plastid or nuclear gene in plants (Palmer and Herbon 1988, Yang *et al.*, 1999).

Amongst all the nuclear regions, internal transcribed spacer (ITS) and regions of ITS could be used as potential barcode candidates in plant phylogenetic analysis. Although the presence of paralagous copies of ITS has been observed as a problem in some genera (Campbell *et al.*, 2005). ITS2 region has been proved to be the most promising universal barcode candidate for identification of medicinal plants (Chen *et al.*, 2010). ITS1/ITS2 has been found to be the most potential markers for assessment of diversity and species identification of Euphorbiaceae family (Pang *et al.*, 2010).

Apart from the nuclear genes, chloroplast genes could also be good candidates in plant barcoding. It has been observed that non-coding regions are appropriate than coding regions as they exhibit more variation and reduced functional constraints (Shaw *et al.*, 2005). The plastid *trnH-psbA* spacer (119 to >1000 bp) has been proposed as a promising candidate locus for high species level identification due to following criteria:

1. Short sequence length, easy DNA extraction and amplification.
2. Highly conserved priming sites.

However, alignment and analysis of *trnH-psbA* is one of major challenge which is not a strict criterion for DNA identification but a critical prerequisite for developing bioinformatics tools (Blaxter, 2004). It shows improved discriminatory power in the identification of closely related plant taxa (Bruni *et al.*, 2012). Studies showed the successful amplification of *trnH-psbA* spacer in gymnosperms, mosses, ferns, liverwort etc. but not in all angiosperms. The length variation due to multiple indels makes the alignment difficult or impossible (Yamashiro *et al.*, 2004). In addition, *atpF-atpH*, a noncoding spacer, has been proposed as a universal DNA barcoding marker for species-level discrimination of duckweeds, an aquatic monocot belonging to the family Lemnaceae (Wang *et al.*, 2010). It has also been reported that the ITS and *trnH-psbA* could be used as a pair of potential barcode for identifying most divergent angiosperm taxa but failed in the order *Cycadales* (Sass *et al.*, 2007).

The most characterized plastid coding region in GenBank *i.e. rbcL* has also been evaluated for molecular identification of plants due to its universality, ease of amplification and alignment (Newmaster *et al.*, 2006). Studies reveal that it had been previously rejected as a candidate gene for species identification by Gielly and Taberlet (1994), Renner (1999), and Salazar *et al.* (2003). But it is a broad spectrum candidate for all major groups and provides a good baseline for barcoding of land plants as compared to other plastid genes. The promising results have been obtained using *rbcL* as a barcode with less variation between the species and large interspecific variation. It can be used to resolve congeneric species and different populations of mosses. Moreover, its discriminatory power has been evaluated for many arid wild plants (Bafeel *et al.*, 2012). Apart from this gene as a potential barcode, other plastid regions may also provide greater utility in barcoding of plants.

The plastid gene, *matK* has higher substitution rates than *rbcL* in angiosperms/flowering plants but not in all bryophytes and ferns (Lahaye *et al.*, 2008, Yu *et al.*, 2011). It has high resolving power in river weeds of angiosperm family Podostemaceae (Kelly *et al.*, 2010). It has also been proposed as a barcode marker for land plants. The problem in amplification of *matK* region across the plant kingdom implied the need of multiple primer set rather than a single pair (Dunning *et al.*, 2010). The potential of *matK, trnH-psbA* and *rbcL* regions in designing enivronmental

DNA (eDNA) markers has been proposed as a surviellance tool in monitoring of invasive water plants (Scriver *et al.*, 2015).

No single plant marker can substitute COI and thus combination of different markers (*trnH-psbA, matK, rpoC, rpoB, rbcL*) is now being employed in the barcoding of plants (Kress *et al.*, 2007). Consortium for the Barcode of Life-Plant Working Group (CBOL) recommended a two-locus standard barcode (rbcL + matK), with 70 per cent discriminatory power, for barcoding of plant species based on two criteria: efficient recovery of good-quality sequences and high species discriminatory potential (Vijayan *et al.*, 2010). In a study, ITS and *trnH-psbA* are used as suitable barcode loci for DNA barcoding of tropical tree species of India. *rbcL* considered as best barcode marker failed to identify tropical tree species whereas *matK* too showed low amplification rate. The combination of *rbcL* and *matK* failed to discriminate tropical tree species (Tripathi *et al.*, 2013). But recently, the combination of markers (matK and rbcL) allowed the significant discrimination among the *Annona* species (Larranaga and Hormaza, 2015). In addition to two-locus barcodes, three-locus barcodes (rpoC1+rpoB+matK or rpoC1+matK+trnH-psbA) are also being employed by various reserachers to develop plant DNA barcodes. However development of a single universal locus for discrimination of plant species is still challenging.

DNA Barcoding in Bacteria

Since 1980s, molecular characterization of bacterial species has been performed using ribosomal RNA and DNA sequences which served as the standard for species identification (Busse *et al.*, 1996). 16S rRNA was established as the "gold standard" for assessing phylogenetic analyses and microbial diversity. It has advantages like non-variable function, 1500 bp size sufficient for informatics work, presence in almost all bacterial species makes it a frequently used market. However, its utility in some bacterial species identification has been found to be problematic due to ubiquitous distribution, lack of informative characters, intragenomic heterogeneity, difficulty in sequence alignment (presence of indels) (Kjer 1995, Bennasar *et al.*, 1996).

In addition, 16S rRNA does not permit the accurate species identification among some taxa such as Enterobacteriaceae (Martinez- Murcia *et al.*, 1992, Roux and Raoult 1995). To confront the above limitations, use of alternate markers (conserved protein coding genes) including *rpoB* (the beta subunit of DNA polymerase) *gyrB*, the structural gene for the DNA gyrase β subunit has been proposed for accurate species identification (Ade ´kambi *et al.*, 2009, Holmes *et al.*, 2004). Amongst all markers, *rpoB* offers several advantages as described below:

1. *rpoB* is typically present in a single copy within a genome.
2. High level of genetic divergence and more informative characters provides an enhanced basis for phylogenetic reconstruction. Higher resolution of *rpoB* marker can reveal molecular evolution down to the population level.
3. Easy interpretation of the data generated using this marker in an evolutionary framework.
4. Easy identification and removal of the sequence errors which can disrupt the reading frame.

There are an incessent number of studies using single-copy protein-encoding genes for assessment of subspecies diversity. *rpoB* has widely been exploited as a potential barcode marker for bacterial species identification (Case *et al.*, 2007, Vos *et al.*, 2012). To date, many studies reveal the efficiency of using *rpoB* gene sequences for the identification and taxonomic classification of bacterial species including *Bacillus, Mycobacterium, Legionella, Staphylococcus, Pseudomonas* and *Streptomyces* (Ki *et al.*, 2009, Richert *et al.*, 2007). It has been demonstrated that the polymorphism exhibited by this gene can be used to identify marine *Vibrio* isolates in marine waters. The phylogenetic relationship between the gram-positive *Actinobacteria* and *Firmicutes* has also been studied using *rpoB* as a marker gene. It has been found to be an alternative marker for phylogenetic analyses and species identification in Archaea and bacteria. A remarkable level of divergence has been seen among enteric bacteria as compared to *16S rRNA* gene (Mollet *et al.*, 1998).

For past few decades, novel, as yet to be cultured haloarchaeal isolated were isolated and identified using *SSU rRNA* (Benlloch *et al.*, 2002). *SSU rRNA* is a multi-copy gene present in a single genome. There is less divergence (<1 per cent) between these copies in most of the archaea and bacteria but not in many haloarchaea (Acinas *et al.*, 2004). Intragenomic heterogeneity is one of the problems associated with the study of taxonomy and molecular evolution in haloarchaea especially the genera *Haloterrigena* and *Natrinema* (Boucher *et al.*, 2004). Thus, *rpoB* has thus been proposed as an ideal phylogenetic marker to study the taxonomic diversity in haloarchaea due to its universal and conserved nature (Walsh *et al.*, 2012). The utility of COI has also been observed to discriminate *Wolbachia* species which are the common endosymbiotic bacteria (Smith *et al.*, 2012). Apart from the above regions, chaperonin-60 (*cpn60*) has been found to be a bacterial barcode of 555 bp length (Links *et al.*, 2012).Hence *COI, 16S rRNA, cpn60* and *rpoB* genes can be suitable for bacterial DNA barcode development process. These barcodes can be effective in the identification, characterization and exploration of microbiota of the organisms (probiotic microbes) having economic significance (Woo *et al.*, 2008, Michel *et al.*, 1998, Reva *et al.*, 2015).

DNA Barcoding in Fungi

The use of COI as a standard barcode has also been excluded in fungi due to its difficulty in amplification and insufficient variation (Schoch *et al.*, 2012). ITS, a multi-copy and easily amplified region of the ribosomal DNA is considered as the most ideal barcode for identification of most of the fungal taxa at species or lower level (Hillis 1991, Alvarez 2003). It comprises of ITS1 and ITS2 regions, distinguished by the 5.8S gene and is covered by the 18S (SSU) and 28S (LSU) genes in the nuclear rDNA repeat units (Figure 2.2).

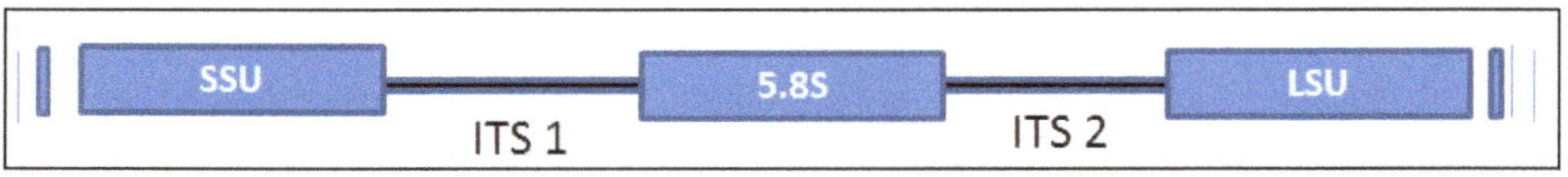

Figure 2.2: Map of Nuclear *rRNA* Genes and their ITS Regions in Fungi.

A major success has been achieved in the Basidiomycota division. However, multiple sequence alignments and subsequent phylogenetic analyses using this region are often hindered by its considerable variable length. Furthermore, ITS lacks species resolution, especially in the economically important microfungal groups in Ascomycota division, which constitute 60 per cent of the presently recognized fungal taxa (Seifert, 2009). So, there is an immense requirement of some other region which will allow the robust species identification in Ascomycota division.

To address all these issues, Assembling the Fungal Barcode of Life (AFTOL) project (2008) proposed the use of several protein coding genes *e.g.* ribosomal polymerase B2 (*rpb2*), β-tubulin for *Penicillium* and translation elongation factor 1-α for *Fusarium* for species identification and phylogenetic analyses in fungi particularly in Ascomycota division (Frisvad *et al.*, 2004, Schoch *et al.*, 2009, O'Donnell *et al.*, 2010). They provide better species level resolution in most of the fungi (Robert *et al.*, 2011). In Nectriaceous fungi, which are economically important and highly diverse fungi, beta-tubulin gene has been considered as a potential barcode marker (Zhao *et al.*, 2011). Among the protein coding genes, the largest subunit of RNA polymerase II (*RPB1*) has been proposed as a candidate barcode in Basidiomycota, Microsporidia and zygomycota and some protists due to the presence of single copy and comparatively low level of sequence variance (Garnica *et al.*, 2009). However, low PCR amplification rate than ITS might be a critical issue in its usage as a barcode candidate (McLaughlin *et al.*, 2009).

Presently, more than 130000 fungal ITS sequences have been submitted to the BOLD database and this number is growing exponentially (Table 2.2) (Hibbett *et al.*, 2011). ITS region is being employed as an ideal marker for identification of fungi in environmental samples (environmental DNA barcoding) (Nilsson *et al.*, 2009). The presence of multiple copies of ITS per cell (~250) makes it an ideal target for sequencing environmental templates having low quantity of DNA (Vilgalys *et al.*, 1990). In some environmental studies, the combination of ITS and LSU has been explored as candidate for barcoding (Geml *et al.*, 2009).

Table 2.2: List of Public Databases of DNA Barcoding

Databases	*Data Content*	*Website*
BOLD (Barcode of Life Data Systems)	Specimen Records: 5,800,485, Specimens with Barcodes: 4,353,038, Species with Barcodes: 245,957Animals 5201271, Plants 392238, Fungi 137666, Protists 23091	*http://www.boldsystems.org*
MMDBD (Medicinal Materials DNA Barcode Database)	1661 Medicinal species with 51375 sequences available.	*http://www.cuhk.edu.hk/icm/mmdbd.htm*
ITS2 Database Ribosomal RNA Database	ITS2 sequences and 25000 secondary structures for the known ITS sequences	*http://its2.bioapps.biozentrum.uni-wuerzburg.de*
The ITS2 Database III- sequences and structures for phylogeny	Identification of more than 160,000 correct full length and more than 50,000 partial structures	*http://its2.bioapps.biozentrum.uni-wuerzburg.de*

Besides ITS, the ribosomal subunits, small (SSU) and large (LSU) have also been reported for identification of novel fungal clade (Arfi *et al.*, 2012). The small subunit of rRNA (18S) is a conserved region with fewer hypervariable domains and is widely used in phylogenetic analyses in several Basidiomycota genera (Uhart *et al.*, 2007). The V6 and V9 domains of SSU displayed a high divergence level between *Tricholoma* species (Mouhamadou *et al.*, 2008). ITS1 and ITS2 gene regions have failed to infer for species identification in aquatic hyphomycetes where ITS1-5.8S-ITS2 rRNA gene has proved as a potential barcode (Seena *et al.*, 2010). Moreover, the combination of ITS along with SSU and LSU has been found to be a basis of DNA barcoding in arbuscular mycorrhizal fungi (Stockinger *et al.*, 2010). Thus for simultaneous species identification and phylogenetic studies, ITS supplemented with additional sequences such LSU or SSU should be used as barcoding markers (Toju *et al.*, 2012, Schoch *et al.*, 2012). DNA barcoding has thus proved to be useful in exploring the fungal diversity, studying pathogenicity, geographical and ecological roles.

DNA Barcoding in Viruses

The complexity of morphology-based system has led to the need of molecular methods for species identification in viruses (Ward 1993). DNA barcoding has been suggested as a new tool for species identification in viruses. Furthermore, it has been exploited as a tool for Avian influenza virus (AIV) isolation and identification of host bird species, thereby, helping to understand the AIV ecology, evolution and epidemiology in wild birds (Lee *et al.*, 2010). A 408 bps region encoding S3-peptidase located in structural gene of viral genome has been proposed as a hypothetical barcode which is yet to be confirmed (Cheng *et al.*, 1995, Kumar *et al.*, 2011). The viral DNA barcode records available on BOLD and the number of publications are negligible. No DNA or RNA marker has been developed to elucidate the complexity of the virus and studying viral diversity. Work has to be done in exploring a universal barcode region for accurate identification of viral taxa.

DNA Barcoding in Eukaryotic Microbes

DNA barcoding would be highly advantageous for the identification of eukaryotic microbes. This study is emerging as a new field for cataloguing species identification in microbial communities. COI was found to be efficient in species identification in different groups of eukaryotic microbes, such as ciliates, dinoflagellates, diatoms and amoebozoans (Lin *et al.*, 2009, Evans and Mann 2009, Heger *et al.*, 2011). Several DNA barcodes are being explored for identification of unknown and cyptic species of diatoms. Diatoms are the largest group of microalgae varying in shape, size and pattern during the life cycle with only <1 per cent species having full known cycle. *rbcL* and *LSU* rDNA have been proposed as universally acceptable barcode marker for diatoms (Mann *et al.*, 2010).

The identification of protistian lineages is quite promising due to lack of species-specific morphological traits. Single gene cannot be sufficient for proper identification of protists. DNA barcoding is a novel approach for species demilitation in protists using different genes such as COI, 18S rRNA, 28S rRNA and ITS as barcode regions (Karnati *et al.*, 2003). It has been reported that COI is as an ideal barcode for amoebae and ITS2 for *Piroplasma* (Kosakyan *et al.*, 2012, Gou *et al.*,

2012). An improved barcoding system has been proposed for rapid and accurate identification of cryptic species (Hoef-Emden 2012). It has also been exploited for identification of freshwater and marine red algae of order Rhodophyta using COI sequences (Rueness 2010).

Methodology for DNA Barcoding

DNA barcoding methodology is a sequential process comprising of following steps- collection, identification and preservation of specimens, extraction of DNA from tissues, amplification of target gene using universal primers, sequencing and data analysis followed by submission to the database. The schema of methodolgy is depicted in Figure 2.3.

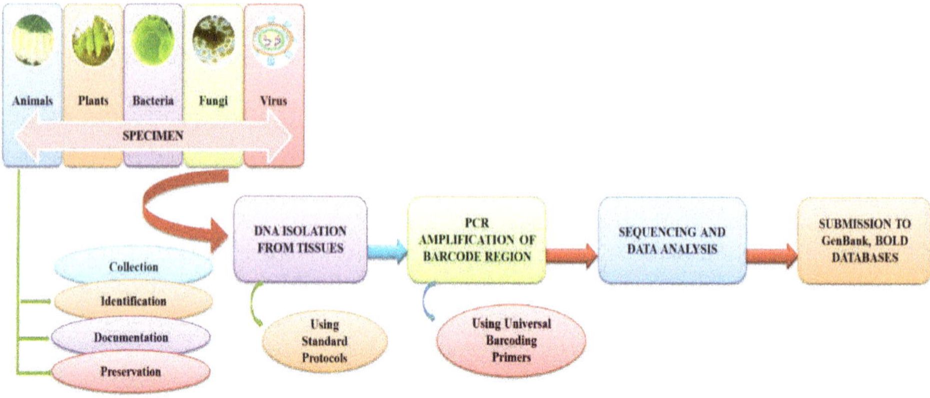

Figure 2.3: Schematic Representation of Methodology for DNA Barcoding.

Specimen Collection, Documentation and Preservation

Specimens (either fresh or preserved ones) can be collected from the repositories of biological materials such as natural history museums, herbaria, aquaria, seed banks etc and get identified through taxonomists. The identified specimens are then preserved with proper documentation (collection date, site, taxonomic description, photographic records etc.).

DNA Isolation

Total genomic/organellar DNA is isolated from the collected samples using standard DNA extraction protocols varying upon the type of specimen (Sharma *et al.*, 2010, Singh *et al.*, 2011). The quality of the extracted DNA is determined by gel electrophoresis and UV spectrophotometer in terms of A260/280 ratio. The ratio of 1.8, 2.0 and 0.6 indicates pure DNA, RNA and protein respectively. The extracted DNA can be stored at -20 °C for future use and in -80°C for longer storage.

PCR Amplification and Sequencing of Target Gene

Various universal barcoding primers have been reported for the amplification of the target gene. In case any of these primers fail to amplify, suitable primers can be designed from the conserved sequences registered in GenBank. The target genes/barcode regions are amplified by PCR using organelle-specific universal primers and then verified by gel electrophoresis. Concentration of the gel varies with the size of target barcode region. Generally, 1-2 per cent gel is preffered for quantitative and qualitative analysis of amplicons. The relevant PCR amplified products are then sequenced to obtain exact DNA barcode sequences from these specimens. The data are then analysed for subsequent submission in a public domain database (NCBI, BOLD *etc.*).

Submission to Database

Sequence analysis and phylogentic tree construction is done using various appropriate bioinformatics tools (BioEdit, ORFinder, CLUSTAL W, MEGA 5.2.2 etc.). After proper annotation, sequence is submitted to NCBI GenBank database (http://www.ncbi.nlm.nih.gov/WebSub/?tool=barcode) using sequence submission platform (Sequin/BanKit). The barcode sequences can also be submitted as projects in BOLD databases (http://www.boldsystems.org), which are characterized by an automatic submission tool for publishing sequences to GenBank. Conservation of entire morphological reference for species is one of the conditions for data submission to BOLD.

Analysis of DNA Barcode Data

The unknown specimens are identified by comparing the closest similar reference record in the database. A Data Analysis Working Group has been created by CBOL to develop the methods for analysing and maintainance of DNA barcode data.

Applications of DNA Barcoding

DNA barcodes can be useful in many fields such as ecology, biomedicine, epidemiology, evolutionary biology, biogeography, conservation biology, bio-industry and biomonitoring. Some of the applications of DNA barcoding are as follows:

1. It facilitates the discovery of many unknown species and identification of pathogenic species with ecological, medical and agronomical significance and thus serves as a promising tool in epidemiology studies (Ball and Armstrong 2006, Nzelu *et al.*, 2015, Gumiel *et al.*, 2015).
2. Further, barcoding system aids in recognition, detection and to trace dispersal of patented organisms in agro-biotechnology, either to certify the source organism *e.g.* truffles or to secure intellectual property rights for bio- resources (Rastogi *et al.*, 2007, Taberlet *et al.*, 2007).
3. DNA barcode is an important tool to associate adults with immature specimens (fish larvae, fungal sexual stage) and in cases, when morphological traits fail to discriminate species (*e.g.* red algal species and fungal species) (Pegg *et al.*, 2006, Shenoy *et al.*, 2007).

4. It is useful in identification of the cryptic species. The existence of many "cryptic" fungal species, which are morphologically alike, emphasizes that molecular information is essential (Sato *et al.*, 2008).
5. This approach helps in identification of species interactions. For example it has been used to study the host specificity of Australian beetles and their interaction with plants (Jurado-Rivera *et al.*, 2009).
6. It has been useful in identifying species-specific contaminants in fish consumed as food that may cause health problems (Lowenstein *et al.*, 2009).
7. Authentication of seafood species, which are commercially important having high market value, is one of the areas where DNA barcoding has been attempted. This approach aims to circumvent several issues related to food safety, species misbranding and accurate identification and conservation of wildlife and sustainable fishery fields (Pinto *et al.*, 2013).
8. It is widely used in food traceability to identify biological specimens for both raw and proceesed food (Galimberti *et al.*, 2013).
9. Authentication of natural health products (NHPs), derived from animals or plant origin has become possible by reliable DNA barcoding method. This reduces the chances of misrepresentstion and substitution of unprotected species in the commercial market (Wallace *et al.*, 2012).
10. 'Biomonitoring' or 'bioassessment' is the method of evaluation for overall ecological health of surrounding environment (*e.g.* streams, reservoirs, wetlands, estuaries) on the basis of change in the composition and structure of the benthic (bottom dwelling) community. DNA barcoding using COI has also recently gained much interest in the field of environmental biomonitoring by providing a level of data standardization that lacked in the previous environmental assessments using aquatic life forms such as in-stream alga (diatoms or soft-bodied algae) or benthic invertebrates (Sweeney *et al.*, 2011, Pilgrim *et al.*, 2011).
11. Authentication and quality control of aesthetically potent materials (plants or animals) can be executed during DNA barcoding tools. An integrated MMDBD (Medicinal Materials DNA Barcode Database) have been developed for the collection and storage of DNA barcodes of these materials and act as a resource for researchers of various fields such as conservation, forensic, systematic study and herbal industry (Lou *et al.*, 2010).
12. Identification of traditional medicinal plants can also be performed using barcodes which is essential for proper medicinal production, research and application (Huang *et al.*, 2015).

Current Status of DNA Barcoding

The concept of DNA barcoding gained immense support to revolutionize taxonomy and species discovery (Blaxter 2005). Till date, a total of 4353038 DNA barcode sequences have been recorded in BOLD that satisfied DNA barcoding criteria. A taxonomic bias has been observed in DNA barcoding due to limited research in search of universal barcode and classifying all live forms. The animal kingdom offered the maximum success rate (over 90 per cent) with Insecta representing around 46 per cent (Figure 2.4). Among insects, mostly, the progress has been made in the order Lepidoptera. Currently, more than 50000 barcode data have been collected which represent around 50 per cent of the total lepidopteran species (Lepidoptera-BOL). The proportion of barcode sequences is limited for plants, fungi and protists based on the BOLD results (BOLD search on 22-08-2015).

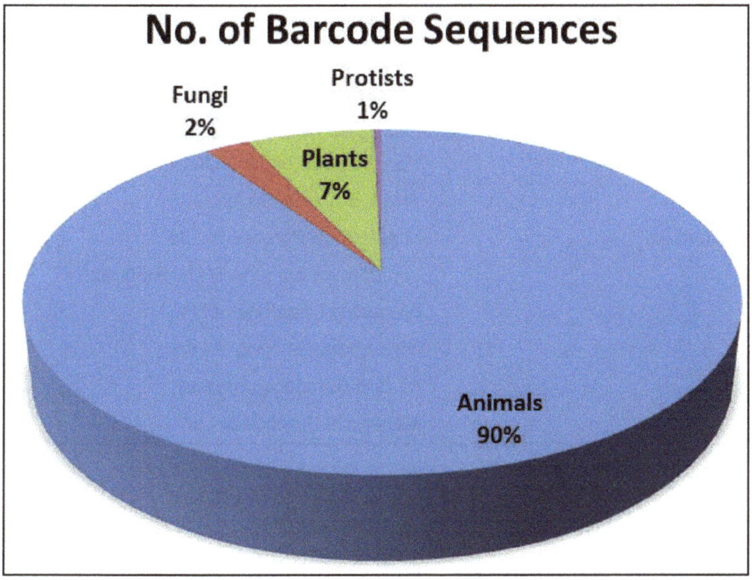

Figure 2.4: Taxonomic Bias in DNA Barcoding (Data obtained from BOLD database as on 22 August, 2015).

Presently, DNA barcoding is a global enterprise, operating three international databases (BOLD, CBOL and iBOL) for construction of DNA barcode libraries that will enable researchers for better understanding and biodiversity conservation. Several campaigns have been initiated for constructing DNA barcode libraries for various taxa (Table 2.3). Resolving technical, analytical and fundamental issues is a prerequisite for data submission in BOLD. Unlike other well-known sequence libraries (*e.g.* NCBI), the sequences deposited in BOLD can be revised and taxonomically classified.

There is a hefty progress in scientific assessment for efficient identification of earthworm using barcoding approach. "Barcoding Earthworm" campaign (Earthworm- BOL) assembles ~5000 barcode sequences representing 800 species from more than 50 different countries and this number is projected to rise by next few years (Decaëns *et al.*, 2013). To date, there are numerous publications on the topic with 2930 papers entitled 'DNA barcoding' (Figure 2.5).

Table 2.3: List of DNA Barcoding Consortium and Campaigns Initiated for Barcoding of Various Taxa

Main International DNA barcoding Consortium	
International Barcode of Life (iBOL)	Established in 2010 for rapid and automated identification of organisms based on DNA barcode library.
Consortium for the Barcode of Life (CBOL)	Established in 2004 that aims to enable development of DNA barcoding and to construct DNA barcoding libraries.
The Barcode of Life Data Systems (BOLD)	Established in 2005 that acts as an interface for submission of DNA sequences to GenBank.

Campaigns for DNA barcoding of various taxa launched by CBOL and iBOL

Organism	*Barcoding Campaigns*
Fishes	Fish Barcode of Life Initiative (Fish-BOL)
Sharks	Shark Barcode of Life
Moths and butterflies	Lepidoptera Barcode of Life
Saturniids	Lepidoptera barcode of life: Saturniidae
Ants	Formicidae Barcode of Life
Caddisflies	Trichoptera Barcode of Life
Birds	All Bird Barcoding Initiative
Mammals	Mammalia Barcode of Life

There are several studies which can demonstrate DNA barcoding as a tool to classify the biome distinctly. DNA barcoding separates 10 cryptic species from morphologically indistinguishable skipper butterflies (Hebert *et al.*, 2004). In another

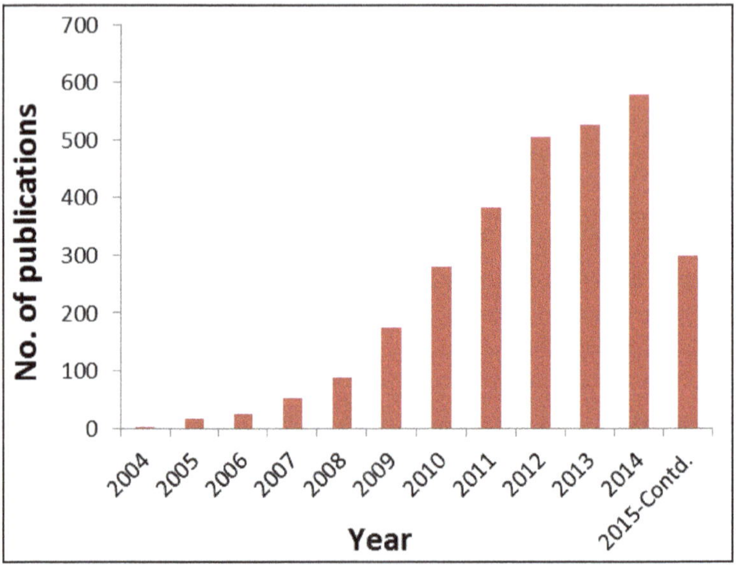

Figure 2.5: Trend of Publications Entitled 'DNA Barcoding' (Search from Scopus database as on 22 August, 2015).

study, it has identified cryptic species from morphologically identical parasitoid flies (Tachinidae) (Smith *et al.*, 2006). It can also be used to identify adult and larval stages within species (Rasmussen *et al.*, 2009).

So far, COI gene has been proved as a universal barcode for various taxa including gastropods, springtails, butterflies, mayflies, spiders, ants, birds, crustaceans, reptiles, fish and recently, diatoms and protists (Ward *et al.*, 2005, Smith *et al.*, 2005, Hajibabaei *et al.*, 2006, Costa *et al.*, 2007, Gou *et al.*, 2012, Huang *et al.*, 2015). It has also been used to effectively discriminate among species (>95 per cent) in three families of Lepidoptera- Hesperiidae (skipper butterflies), Sphingidae (sphinx moths), and Saturniidae (wild silk moths) (Hajibabaei *et al.*, 2006).

Use of a multi-locus approach, including COI- region and independent markers (*e.g.* nuclear subunit ribosomal RNA genes) is progressively emerging for species identification.

Advantanges of DNA Barcoding

The advantages of DNA barcoding are described in the following section.

Studying Species Biology and Ecology

DNA barcoding has emerged as an effective tool in ecology and species biology. This approach is now widely used for understanding species interactions and detecting the presence of elusive and endangered species (Pfenninger *et al.*, 2007). For example, long range wolf colonization of France and Switzerland has been found out using extracted DNA barcodes from faeces and hair samples (Valie're *et al.*, 2003).

Moreover, the tool is widely used to elucidate the transmission pathways to study the interactions among the beetles (Lecythidaceae) and their endosymbiotic yeasts (Berkov *et al.*, 2007). It allowed the detection of North American bullfrog (*Rana catesbeiana*), one of the world's worst invasive species in southwest France using water samples from ponds (Ficetola *et al.*, 2008). The ecology and biology of fungus, invasive plant species and microbes has also been studied using this powerful tool (Scriver *et al.*, 2015). Thus, DNA barcoding has immense potential to solve important ecological problems.

Barcoding : A Multidisciplinary and Technically Advanced Approach

The prerequisite of DNA barcoding approach is to assemble the reference DNA barcode data which in turn, depends on the conventional methods of DNA isolation, amplification followed by sequencing. The reference library is extremely useful in rapid identification of low taxonomic level taxa using specific short-DNA sequences *i.e.* mini-barcode 100 bp, 300 bp (Min and Hickey, 2007).

An increasing number of techniques (*e.g.* silicon-based microarrays, nylon-membrane-based macroarrays, bio-barcode amplification assay (BCA), fluorescent DNA barcode-based immunoassay and the Luminex system of DNA-tagged polystyrene beads (patented) sorted by flow cytometry) have recently been developed as a next step of DNA barcoding Silicon-platform microarray was first used to study fungal systems and BCA for virus systems (Summerbell *et al.*, 2005, Cao *et al.*, 2009, Yin *et al.*, 2011).

High-throughput sequencing enables the most efficient means of rapid barcode-based species identification (in case of mixed samples such as stomach contents, food, and blood or water columns). SASI-Seq (Sample assurance Spike-Ins) is one of the simple and inexpensive approaches to check the samples quality. Sample mix up or identification of cross-contaminants could be easily acheived through high throughput sequencing methods (Quail *et al.*, 2014). The full viral genome sequencing has also been carried out using multi-faceted approach that includes nucleic acid preparation, Illumina Seq and a novel iterative sequence classification algorithm (Cotten *et al.*, 2014).

Moreover, the use of cutting edge sequencing techniques in metagenomics could be promising in DNA barcoding as a new approach called metabarcoding (Hudson 2008, Reva *et al.*, 2015). It can be used for exploration of both culturable as well as non-culturable microbes. Conservation of entire morphological reference for species is one of the conditions for submission of data to BOLD database for which new techniques have been developed for extraction of non-destructive DNA from the specimens (Pook and McEwing 2005, Hunter *et al.*, 2008, Rowley *et al.*, 2007).

Limitations of DNA Barcoding

Inspite of the immense potential offered by DNA barcoding, it has some drawbacks which cannot be overlooked and are discussed in the following section.

Exploration of Microdiversity

Barcoding the microdiversity (*i.e.* archea, bacteria, unicellular fungi and protists) is one of the major challenges for the BOL objectives (Chantangsi *et al.*, 2007). The diversity of microscopic and sub-microscopic communities is masked by the dominant populations which lead to unexploration of microbes (Sogin *et al.*, 2006). It can be explored using COI-based identification system but for macroscopic life, multi-locus barcoding system may be needed (Blaxter *et al.*, 2005, Evans *et al.*, 2007).

The use of SSU has been reported in identification of human parasite *Blastocyctis hominis* (Scicluna *et al.*, 2006). Similarly other barcode regions (18S rRNA, 28S rRNA, ITS etc.) are being developed to study the diversity of protozoans, archea etc. Advanced methods such as metagenomics and community genomics have been emerging as new fields to study microdiversity, population studies and evolutionary relationships (DeLong 2004, Tringe *et al.*, 2005). But the expensive metagenomics approach makes DNA barcoding as a useful tool for studying microdiversity.

No Universal Barcode for Some Taxa

COI serves as a universal DNA barcode in animals but its utility in protists, fungi and plants is quite challenging. Amphibians have high variability in mtDNA and its COI priming sites and therefore large-scale effort is needed to barcode the amphibians using the same primary barcode region of COI (Smith *et al.*, 2008). COI fails to distinguish closely related animal species requiring nuclear regions *e.g. Cytb* and *Rhod* to identify all teleost fish species (Sevilla *et al.*, 2007).

In algae, there are shortcomings with the primers for COI and therefore, universal plastid amplicon (UPA) was reported as an alternative tool, although having a drawback of low interspecific divergence (Clarkston *et al.*, 2010). COI has failed in barcoding of some protists (some group of amoeba) and elicits the use of an alternative barcode (Gile *et al.*, 2010). It is also not suitable for DNA barcoding of plants and fungi due to low rate of molecular evolution (Chase and Fay, 2010).

To address all these issues, alternative stretches of DNA have been proposed as barcodes for the barcoding of these organisms. Combination of two plastid regions *matK* and *rbcL* is recommended as universal barcodes for terrestrial plants by CBOL Plant Working Group (2009). But it is not still widely accepted for all plant species (Hollingsworth *et al.*, 2011). Best results have been obtained using the internal transcribed spacer (ITS) region of the ribosomal DNA as a barcode for fungi. However, ITS offeres less remarkable result in the DNA barcoding of *Penicillium* moulds (Seifert *et al.*, 2007). Additional markers (single or in combination) are now being explored to resolve the fungal diversity. The development of universal barcode is need of the hour towards the exploration of biodiversity.

Barcoding of Formalin Preserved Specimens

Preserved tissues and specimens are vast repositories of genetic information which form the basis for construction and development of barcode libraries. Formalin-preserved specimens provide a great resource for this approach (Zhang *et al.*, 2010). However, extraction of DNA and amplification of the target gene from these specimens is quite challenging (Zimmermann *et al.*, 2008).

Tissue lysis is the primary obstacle for formalin preserved tissues which affect the integrity of the extracted DNA. Formalin preserves morphological structure more effectively by fixing proteins through peptide linkage conjugation but degrades DNA (Kolesárová *et al.*, 2012). It also affects the downstream applications such as PCR amplification and sequencing reactions due to the crosslink formations by formaldehyde.

Unfavourable preservation condition is a major constraint on DNA quality (Strutzenberger *et al.*, 2012). Use of alternative preservatives such as ethanol is preferred than formalin as it denatures proteins (at high concentration e"95 per cent) that may degrade DNA (Flournoy *et al.*, 1996). For DNA barcoding, ethanol at a concentration of 95 per cent is recommended for storage. Fresh sample and alcohol preservation is more preferable for DNA barcoding studies than formalin preservation to maintain maximum integrity (Nagy 2010, Baird *et al.*, 2011).

Presence of Barcoding Gaps

Constructing a database for DNA barcoding is essential where each taxon is optimally represented. Lack of reference data may lead to the mis-interpretation of barcode-based identification. Limited geographical sampling may lead to 'Barcoding gaps' which should be considered during the database construction phase. This may lead to failure of more recently diverged species (sister-species) identification (Meyer and Paulay 2005, Hebert *et al.*, 2003, Wiemers and Fiedler 2007). The unknown specimens may be problematic if belongs to under-described part of biodiversity (Rubinoff 2006, Rubinoff *et al.*, 2006). Collaboration with expert taxonomists for identification of undocumented voucher specimens is essential for proper construction of barcode database.

Delimitation of Species

Species delimitation refers to the process which determines the species boundaries and discovery of new species. The accuracy of species identification using DNA barcoding has been criticised by several taxonomists that depends on the overlap between intraspecific and interspecific variation (Moritz and Cicero 2004, Lee 2004, Ebach and Holdrege 2005, Rubinoff *et al.*, 2006). This approach is based on the hypothesis that intraspecific divergences will be less than interspecific divergences which is absent in several taxa (Meyer and Paulay 2005, Cognato 2006, Meier *et al.*, 2006, Whitworth *et al.*, 2007). This implies a query whether DNA barcoding can attain its goal to unravel the biodiversity. It is possible only if the target region is conserved among the members of a species and differs from others (Prendini 2005).

Utility of Mitochondrial Genome

The utility of a single mitochondrial gene in DNA barcoding to delineate species boundaries has also triggered several criticisms. Classifications solely based on the one character (*i.e.* mitochondrial gene) are inadequate for species identification (Rubinoff *et al.*, 2006). Nuclear loci is only required to resolve phylogenetic relationships in several cases where one host species can bear different symbionts which may lead to intraspecific (*i.e.* interpopulation) variation in mtDNA sequences (Hurst *et al.*, 1999).

Paraphyly, polyphyly, heteroplasmy (*e.g.* Mussels) or presence of nuclear pseudogenes in mitochondrial genome *i.e.* nuclear mitochonfrial DNA (NUMTs) are some of the artifacts associated with mitochondrial genes. This may cause the overestimation of sample divergence and thus obscure the real evolutionary history of organisms (Williams and Knowton 2001, Funk and Omland 2003, Meyer and Paulay 2005, Terranova *et al.*, 2007). It has been reported that heteroplasmy level differs among tissues and DNA extracted from large tissues displays less polymorphism (Magnacca and Brown, 2010).

Methodological Advances

There are two major drawbacks of DNA barcoding: (i) damage of specimen during DNA extraction method and (ii) nature of sample. A simple, rapid and reliable DNA extraction protocol is essential to obtain efficient yields of DNA for further process.

Various non-destructive DNA extraction protocols have been proposed which enable the determination of barcode with minimal damage of museum specimens or small insects (Acarina, Araneae, Coleoptera, Diptera, Hemiptera, Hymenoptera etc.) (Rowley *et al.*, 2007, Hunter *et al.*, 2008, Castalanelli *et al.*, 2010). However, these methods have been useful in some insects; DNA extraction is challenging in plants (*e.g.* Malvaceae, Asteraceae) having mucilaginous compounds, polysaccharides, phenolic compounds and other secondary metabolites. These compounds co-precipitate with DNA and thus hinder the extraction of high quality DNA. In addition, they complicate the downstream apllications such as polymerase chain reaction (PCR) or other enzymatic reactions.

To overcome these issues, several modified protocols have been reported that enable effective DNA extraction from problematic plant samples (Michiels 2003, Shepherd *et al.*, 2011, Kundu *et al.*, 2011, Souza *et al.*, 2012). Recent technical advancements such as highly efficient DNA polymerase and a DNA-repairing enzyme allow the extraction and amplification of DNA from historical museum specimens as well as fossilized samples (Hajibabaei *et al.*, 2005, Juen and Traugott, 2006, Ball and Armstrong, 2008).

Distance or Character Based Barcoding Analyses

Enumeration of molecular distance is proposed to be a standard method for barcode analysis (Hebert *et al.*, 2003). But it has lately been criticized and should not be considered as it is a phenetic measure non-indicative of common origin (Ward *et al.*, 2005, DeSalle *et al.*, 2005, Borisenko *et al.*, 2008, Kerr *et al.*, 2009).

On the contrary, character-based analysis has proven to be an effective tool for species identification and discrimination (Kelly *et al.*, 2007, Rach *et al.*, 2008, Bergmann *et al.*, 2009). It addresses all the objectives with no loss of information as multiple nucleotide differences are reduced to a single distance-based measure. This approach has been implemented through development of Characteristic Attributes Organization System (CAOS) software (Sarkar *et al.*, 2008). Some studies have been reported on character- based barcoding analysis but conflict still lies between distance and diagnostics (Locke *et al.*, 2010). However, the character- based barcoding is currently proposed to meet the requirement.

Conclusions and Future Prospects

DNA barcoding can be exploited to identify different species when it allows discriminating amongst closely related species, including sister taxa (Newmaster and Ragupathy 2009). Numerous studies focus on plethora of species with distant genetic relationships. It is still unclear whether this approach is restricted to species identification or species discovery and delimitation. Several studies are currently being performed for both intra- and inter species to clarify whether it can successfully delineate species rather than only higher taxonomic levels (*e.g.* genus or species groups).

In current era, data generation and analysis process is continuously evolving, especially from DNA and genomes which possibly transformed the biological sciences since past decades or so. But these advances have been incremental due to omnipresence of powerful computing system and market-driven activities to formulate cheaper and more advanced molecular biology procedures. Two paradigm shifts reported in the past decade have led to the advent of a new form of molecular systematics having a wide range of applications. These paradigms clarify how their convergence is influencing biodiversity studies and understanding of ecosystem (Hajibabaei, 2012).

The first paradigm shift occurred in 2003 employing 'DNA barcodes' for species identification. DNA barcoding has emerged as an initiative for the discovery of new species and retraining present era of taxonomy (DNA taxonomy). The paradigm shift lies in the transformation of the taxonomic method for unexplored microbiome, standardization of barcode although seen a significant advancement. This can be addressed by "Standard Signatures for DNA barcoding". Standards may continuously evolve over time, to address additional DNA information for resolving difficult taxonomic puzzles (Blaxter *et al.*, 2005, Ragupathy *et al.*, 2009, Pauls *et al.*, 2010).

Indeed, the use of only a single locus in barcoding research elicits contradictions and can result in the description of groups that are not monophyletic. It has been noted that DNA barcoding, in absence of other evidences can only suggest new species rather than outright discovering them (Goldstein and DeSalle 2011). Even a character-based methodology would struggle to identify the cryptic species. The advent of novel species using DNA barcoding is merely an iterative concept (Forister *et al.*, 2008). Thus, efforts should be made towards the improvements in this approach. Moreover, gold standard is yet to be developed with huge volume of data in order to create a genetic reference library (Lucking 2008, Packer *et al.*, 2009).

Barcoding- Towards Intergrative Taxonomy

The purpose of barcoding coincides with that of traditional taxonomy and therefore should supplement the morphological data rather than replacing it. Incorporation of DNA and morphological data as an integrated taxonomy would certainly be a solution to the current crisis generated by single data resources. One of the main aims of this initiative is the discovery and description of new taxa which is difficult to accomplish using only sequence based data (Ebach and Holdrege 2005). This initiative would be helpful in various fields like recognition of cryptic species, validation of taxonomy thus facilitating the better understanding of biodiversity (Smith *et al.*, 2008, Hamada *et al.*, 2010).

An integrative taxonomy has been proposed to delimit the diversity of live forms in terms of morphology, ecology, development, behaviour, phylogeography etc. Species that are under-described would be most benefitted from this proposal. Thus, identification and characterization of species in a manner which best reflects the biodiversity is one of the challenges for the future of taxonomy (Dayrat 2005).

Integrative taxonomy is not a new concept. Wilson's "encyclopedia of life", a database was created in 2003 that includes information on morphology, DNA (EOL, available at http://www.eol.org/) and natural history of every species. Later, the significance of integrative taxonomy was recognized by DNA barcoding community (Smith *et al.*, 2008, Fisher and Smith 2008). This approach facilitated comprehensive and detailed understanding of parasitoid diversity and host specificity on the combined basis of morphology, DNA barcoding and ecology. Also it enabled DNA barcoding for the collection and storage of voucher specimens andDor tissue samples for biodiversity research (Peterson *et al.*, 2007).

Thus the integration of information is an appropriate way to promote the scientific enterprise. The progress of an integrated approach is just one of the issues encountered by DNA barcoding that could be accelerated by the advent of NGS.

Application of NGS in DNA Barcoding

The second paradigm shift occurred by ground breaking advancements in DNA sequencing technologies. Traditional Sanger sequencing, invented in 1977, paves the way of breakthrough research in genomics, providing the provision of whole genome sequencing including the human genome. These technological advances minimized the labor-intensiveness and time for DNA sequencing, without altering the core Sanger-based method. But the emergence of NGS technologies revolutionized the DNA sequencing concept in the mid-2000s.

The advancement of novel technologies can perform parallel sequencing, producing thousands or millions of sequences at a single run. Several platforms like Roche 454 pyrosequencing, Illumina Hi Seq®, SOLiD sequencing, Helicos' HeliScope of modern era NGS are much relevant for DNA barcoding due to longer average read length. There is a huge difference in the amount of sequence information as compared to the classic Sanger method (Hall, 2007).

The technology has achieved some success in the investigation of single nucleotide polymorphisms, meiofaunal assemblages and microbial eukaryotes (Creer *et al.*, 2010, Stoeck *et al.*, 2010). The field of 'ecological genomics' has also been proposed to be an emerging discipline accessing the full genome data (Tautz *et al.*, 2010).

Furthermore, it has become the first and foremost choice for many areas of microbial research due to its ability to unveil the microbial communities (Schuster 2008). There is a rapid increment in the number of publications using high-throughput sequencing in fungal studies (Lim *et al.*, 2010, Dumbrell *et al.*, 2011). Now a steady flow of advancements allow DNA to be rapidly sequenced at ever-increasing volumes with simultaneous reduction in the cost per sequenced base.

DNA barcoding alone fails in the field of 'environmental barcoding' which aims at exploring large amount of environmental samples such as soil, water etc. With the increasing data generation (single or whole genome sequence) and lack of proper tools to organize, verify and analyse the data, the DNA barcoding cannot become a standalone discipline.

The utility of NGS for 'mini-barcodes' (even smaller fragments of DNA) in species identification have been suggested by DNA barcoding exponents, but this seems illogical particularly for species delimitation (Hajibabaei *et al.*, 2011). The Canadian Centre for DNA Barcoding *i.e.* the hub of the barcoding effort continues to support Sanger sequencing as one of the studies on techniques and logistics that focusses entirely on the 'high-throughput' 96-well microplates (Borisenko *et al.*, 2009).

Application of NGS in DNA barcoding will accelerate the process of exploration of diversity of various life forms. It has revolutionized the viral discovery using multiple barcodes for viral genome detection and discovery (Cotten *et al.*, 2014).

Also an emerging approach termed as "DNA metabarcoding" is being implied in the exploration of microbiome (both cultured and uncultured). It is a robust method which implies barcode based taxonomic structure, functional and composition exploration through high throughput sequencing technologies (Reva *et al.*, 2015).

Since the advent of NGS and ecological genomics technology might influence DNA barcoding with the risk of becoming irrelevant. It is thus essential to find a way to evolve their methods to encompass these emerging developmental tools. To that end, a combinatorial approach *i.e.* integration of taxonomic, molecular and application of NGS platforms can be a better solution to unravel the huge diversity among various taxa. This will facilitate easy and error-free analyses in areas like taxonomic profiling, phylogenetics, population genetics, computational biology etc.

Further Suggested DNA Barcoding Resources

Other DNA barcode resources are described in the following section.

DNA Barcode Databases

With the advancement of information technology, various databases and projects have been established for proper documentation of biodiversity, some of the public batabases are enlisted.

Barcode Related Websites

1. Barcodes of Life (http://www.barcodeoflife.org)
2. Canadian Centre for DNA Barcoding (http://www.dnabarcoding.ca/),
3. ECBOL - European Consortium for the Barcode of Life (http://www.ecbol.org/)
4. BOLNET.ca- Canadian Barcode of Life Network (http://www.bolnet.ca/)
5. iBOL-International Barcode of Life Project (http://www.dnabarcoding.org/)
6. All Birds Barcoding Initiative (http://www.barcodingbirds.org/)
7. FISH-BOL: Fish Barcode of Life Initiative (http://www.fishbol.org/)
8. All Leps - Barcode of Life (http://www.lepbarcoding.org/)
9. BOLD- Barcode of Life Database (http://www.barcodinglife.org/)
10. MarBOL - Marine Barcode of Life (http://www.marinebarcoding.org/)
11. Sponge Barcoding Project (http://www.spongebarcoding.org/)
12. Polar Barcode of Life (http://www.polarbarcoding.ca/)
13. Belgian Network for DNA Barcoding (http://www.bebol.myspecies.info)
14. CBOL- Consortium for the Barcode of Life (http://www.barcoding.si.edu)
15. NorBOL (http://dnabarcoding.no/en/)
16. MexBOL (http://www.mexbol.org/)
17. JBOLI (http://www.jboli.org/)

Books on DNA Barcoding

1. Miller FP, Vandome AF and McBrewster J. DNA barcoding: taxonomy, species, molecular phylogenetics, consortium for the barcode of life, identification (biology), eukaryote, mitochondrion. VDM Publishing. 2009.
2. Ortman BD. DNA Barcoding the Medusozoa and Ctenophora, Doctoral Dissertations. Paper AAI3345202. 2008.
3. Yu CR. Data Analysis for microarray experiment and DNA barcode of life. UMI Dissertation Publishing. 2008.
4. Ghosh SK. A textbook on DNA barcoding. Book Space, Kolkata. 2012.

References

Acinas SG, Marcelino LA, Klepac-Ceraj V, Polz MF. Divergence and redundancy of *16S rRNA* sequences in genomes with multiple *rrn* operons. *J. Bacteriol.* 186: 2629–2635. 2004.

Adekambi T, Drancourt M, Raoult D. The *rpoB* gene as a tool for clinical microbiologists. *Trends Microbiol.* 17: 37–45. 2009.

Alvarez I, Wendel JF. Ribosomal ITS sequences and plant phylogenetic inference. *Mol. Phylogenet Evol.* 29: 417–434. 2003.

Anslan S, Tedersoo L. Performance of cytochrome c oxidase subunit I (COI), ribosomal DNA Large Subunit (LSU) and Internal Transcribed Spacer 2 (ITS2) in DNA barcoding of Collembola. *Euro. J. Soil Biol.* 69: 1-7. 2015.

Aquilino SVL, Tango JM, Fontanilla IKC, Pagulayan RC *et al.*, DNA barcoding of the ichthyofauna of Taal Lake, Philippines. *Mol. Ecol. Resour.*, 11(4): 612–619. 2011.

Arfi Y, Bue´e M, Marchand C, Levasseur A *et al.*, Multiple markers pyrosequencing reveals highly diverse and host specific fungal communities on the mangrove trees *Avicennia marina* and *Rhizophora stylosa*. *FEMS Microbiol. Ecol.* 79: 433–444. 2012.

Bafeel SO, Arif IA, Bakir MA, Al Homaidan AA *et al.*, DNA barcoding of arid wild plants using *rbcL* gene sequences. *Genet. Mol. Res.* 11(3): 1934-1941. 2012.

Baird DJ, Pascoe TJ, Zhou X, Hajibabaei M. Building freshwater macroinvertebrate DNA-barcode libraries from reference collection material: formalin preservation vs specimen age. *J. North Amer. Benthol. Soc.* 30(1): 125-130. 2011.

Ball SL, Armstrong KF. DNA barcodes for insect pest identification: a test case with tussock moths (Lepidoptera: Lymantriidae). *Can. J. For. Res.* 36: 337– 350. 2006.

Ball SL, Armstrong KF. Rapid, one-step DNA extraction for insect pest identification by using DNA barcodes. *J. Econ. Entomol.* 101: 523–532. 2008.

Ball SL, Hebert PDN, Burian SK, Webb JM. Biological identifications of mayflies (Ephemeroptera) using DNA barcodes. *J. North Amer. Benthol. Soc.* 24: 508–524. 2005.

Benlloch S, Lopez-Lopez A, Casamayor EO, Øvreås L *et al.*, Prokaryotic geneti diversity throughout the salinity gradient of a coastal solar saltern. *Environ Microbiol.* 4: 349–360. 2002.

Bennasar A, Mora RR, Lalucat J, Moore ERB. *16S rRNA* gene sequence analysi relative to genomovars of *Pseudomonas stutzeri* and proposal of *Pseudomona balearica* sp nov. *Intl. J. Syst. Bacteriol.* 46: 200–205. 1996.

Bennett CE, Wilson BS, Desalle R. DNA barcoding of an invasive mammal species the small Indian mongoose (*Herpestes javanicus;* E. Geoffroy Saint-Hillaire 1818 in the Caribbean and Hawaiian Islands. *Mitochondrial DNA.* 22(1–2): 12–18. 2011

Bergmann T, Hadrys H, Breves G, Schierwater B. Character-based DNA barcoding a superior tool for species classification. Berliner Und Munchener Tierarztliche Wochenschrift. 122: 446–450. 2009.

Berkov A, Feinstein J, Small J, Nkamany M. Yeasts isolated from neotropical wood boring beetles in SE Peru. *Biotropica.* 39: 530–538. 2007.

Blaxter M, Mann J, Chapman T, Thomas F *et al.*, Defining operational taxonomic units using DNA barcode data. *Philos. Trans. R. Soc. Lond.* B. 360: 1935–1943. 2005.

Blaxter M. The Promise of DNA taxonomy. *Philos. Trans. R. Soc. Lond. B Biol. Sci.* 359: 669–679. 2004.

Borisenko AV, Lim BK, Ivanova NV, Hanner RH *et al.*, DNA barcoding in surveys of small mammal communities: a field study in Suriname. *Mol. Ecol. Resour.* 8: 471–479. 2008.

Borisenko AV, Sones JE and Hebert PDN. The front-end logistics of DNA barcoding challenges and prospects. *Mol. Ecol. Resour.* 9: 27–34. 2009.

Boucher Y, Douady CJ, Sharma AK, Kamekura M *et al.*, Intragenomic heterogeneity and intergenomic recombination among haloarchaeal ribosomal RNA genes. *J. Bacteriol.* 186(12): 3980-90. 2004.

Bruni I, De Mattia F, Martellos S, Galimberti A *et al.*, DNA Barcoding as an effective tool in improving a digital plant identification system: A Case Study for the Area of Mt. Valerio, Trieste (NE Italy). *Plos One.* 7(9): e43256. 2012.

Busse HJ, Denner EBM, Lubitz W. Classification and identification of bacteria: Current approaches to an old problem. Overview of methods used in bacterial systematics. *J. Biotech.* 47: 3–38. 1996.

Campbell CS, Wright WA, Cox M, Vining TF *et al.*, Nuclear ribosomal DNA internal transcribed spacer 1 (*ITS1*) in *Picea* (Pinaceae): sequence divergence and structure. *Mol. Phylogenet. Evol.* 35: 165–185. 2005.

Cao C, Dhumpa R, Bang DD, Ghavifekr Z *et al.*, Detection of avian influenza virus by fluorescent DNA barcode based immunoassay with sensitivity comparable to PCR. *Analyst.* 135: 337–342. 2009.

Case RJ, Boucher Y, Dahllof I, Holmstrom C *et al.*, Use of *16S rRNA* and *rpoB* genes as molecular markers for microbial ecology studies. *Appl. Envir. Microbiol.*, 173: 278–288. 2007.

Castalanelli MA, Severtson DL, Brumley CJ, Szito A *et al.*, A rapid non-destructive DNA extraction method for insects and other arthropods. *J. Asia Pacific Entomol.* 13: 243–248. 2010.

Chantangsi C, Lynn DH, Brandl MT, Cole JC *et al.*, Barcoding ciliates: a comprehensive study of 75 isolates of the genus *Tetrahymena*. *Intl. J. Syst. Evol. Microbiol.* 57: 2412–2425. 2007.

Chase MW, Fay MF. Barcoding of plants and fungi. *Science*. 325: 682-683. 2010.

Chase MW, Salamin N, Wilkinson M, Dunwell JM *et al.*, Land plants and DNA barcodes: short-term and long-term goals. *Philos. Trans. Royal Soc. Ser. B.* 360: 1889-1895. 2005.

Che J, Chen HM, Yang JX, Jin JQ *et al.*, Universal COI primers for DNA barcoding amphibians. *Mol. Ecol. Resour.* 12(2): 247-258. 2012.

Chen S, Yao H, Han J, Liu C *et al.*, Validation of the ITS2 Region as a Novel DNA Barcode for Identifying Medicinal Plant Species. *Plos One*. 5(1): e8613. 2010.

Cheng RH, Kuhn RJ, Olson NH, Rossman MG *et al.*, Nucleocapsid and glycoprotein organization in an enveloped virus. *Cell*. 80: 621-630. 1995.

Clare EL, Lim BK, Engstrom MD, Eger JL *et al.*, DNA bar-coding of Neotropical bats: species identification and discovery within Guyana. *Mol. Ecol. Notes*. 7: 184–190. 2007.

Clarkston BE, Saunders GW. A comparison of two DNA barcode markers for species discrimination in the red algal family Kallymeniaceae (Gigartinales, Florideophyceae), with a description of *Euthoratimburtonii* sp nov. *Botany-Botanique*. 88: 119–131. 2010.

Cognato AI. Standard percent DNA sequence difference for insects does not predict species boundaries. *J. Econ. Entomol.* 99: 1037-1045. 2006.

Costa FO, deWaard JR, Boutillier J, Ratnasingham S *et al.*, Biological identifications through DNA barcodes: the case of the Crustacea. *Can. J. Fish Aquat. Sci.* 64: 272-295. 2007.

Cotten M, Oude Munnink B, Canuti M, Deijs M *et al.*, Full genome virus detection in fecal samples using sensitive nucleic acid preparation, deep sequencing, and a novel iterative sequence classification algorithm. *PLoS ONE*. 9 (4): e93269. 2014.

Creer S, Fonseca VG, Porazinska DL, Giblin-Davis RM *et al.*, Ultrasequencing of the meiofaunal biosphere: practice, pitfalls and promises. *Mol. Ecol.* 19: 4–20. 2010.

Dayrat B. Towards integrative taxonomy. *Biol. J. Linn. Soc.* 85: 407–415. 2005.

Decaëns T, Porco D, Rougerie R, Brown GG *et al.*, Potential of DNA barcoding for earthworm research in taxonomy and ecology. *Appl. Soil Ecol.* 65: 35– 42. 2013.

DeLong EF. Microbial population genomics and ecology: the road ahead. *Environ. Microbiol.* 6 (9): 875–878. 2004.

DeSalle R, Egan MG, Siddall M. The unholy trinity: taxonomy, species delimitation and DNA barcoding. *Philosophil. Trans. Royal Soc. B-Biol. Sci.* 360: 1905–1916. 2005.

Doyle JJ, Gaut BS. Evolution of genes and taxa: a primer. *Plant Mol. Biol.* 42: 1–6. 2000.

Dumbrell AJ, Ashton PD, Aziz N, Feng G *et al.*, Distinct seasonal assemblages of arbuscular mycorrhizal fungi revealed by massively parallel pyrosequencing. *New Phytol.* 190: 794–804. 2011.

Dunning LT, Savolainen V. Broad-scale amplification of *matK* for DNA barcoding plants, a technical note. *Bot. J. Linnean Soc.* 164(1): 1-9. 2010.

Ebach, MC, Holdrege C. DNA barcoding is no substitute for taxonomy. *Nature.* 434: 697. 2005.

Eggert LS, Rasner CA, Woodruff DS. The evolution and phylogeography of the African elephant inferred from mitochondrial DNA sequence and nuclear microsatellite markers. *Proc. Royl. Soc. Lond. Ser. B-Biol. Sci.* 269: 1993–2006. 2002.

Evans KM, Mann DG. A proposed protocol for nomenclatural effective DNA barcoding of microalgae. *Phycologia,* 48: 70–74. 2009.

Evans KM, Wortley AH, Mann DG. An assessment of potential diatom "barcode" genes (*cox1, rbcL, 18S* and *ITS rDNA*) and their effectiveness in determining relationships in *Sellaphora* (Bacillariophyta). *Protist.* 158: 349–364. 2007.

Ficetola GF, Miaud C, Pompanon F, Taberlet P. Species detection using environmental DNA from water samples. *Biol. Lett.* 4: 423–425. 2008.

Fisher BL, Smith MA. A Revision of Malagasy Species of *Anochetus* Mayr and *Odontomachus* Latreille (Hymenoptera: Formicidae). *Plos One.* 3(5): e1787. 2008.

Flournoy LE, Adams RP, Pandy RN. Interim and archival preservation of plant specimens in alcohols for DNA studies. *Biotechniques.* 20: 657-660. 1996.

Floyd R, Abebe E, Papert A, Blaxter M. Molecular barcodes for soil nematode identification. *Mol. Ecol.* 11: 839–850. 2002.

Folmer O, Black M, Hoeh W, Lutz R *et al.*, DNA primers for amplification of mitochondrial cytochrome *c* oxidase subunit I from diverse metazoan invertebrates. *Mol. Mar. Biol. Biotechnol.* 3: 294–299. 1994.

Forister ML, Nice CC, Fordyce JA, Gompert Z *et al.*, Considering evolutionary processes in the use of single-locus genetic data for conservation, with examples from the Lepidoptera. *J. Insect Conserv.* 12: 37–51. 2008.

Frisvad JC, Samson RA. Polyphasic taxonomy of *Penicillium* subgenus *Penicillium*– a guide to identification of food and air-borne terverticillate penicillia and their mycotoxins. *Stud. Mycol.* 49: 1–173. 2004.

Funk DJ, Omland KE. Species-level paraphyly and polyphyly: frequency, causes, and consequences, with insights from animal mitochondrial DNA. *Ann. Rev. Ecol. Evol. S.* 34: 397-423. 2003.

Galimberti A, De Mattia F, Losa A, Bruni I *et al.*, DNA barcoding as a new tool for food traceability. *Food Res. Intl.* 50(1): 55-63. 2013.

Garnica S, Weiß M, Oertel B, Ammirati J *et al.*, Phylogenetic relationships in *Cortinarius*, section Calochroi, inferred from nuclear DNA sequences. *BMC Evol. Biol.* 9: 1. 2009.

Geml J, Laursen GA, Timling I, McFarland JM *et al.*, Molecular phylogenetic biodiversity assessment of arctic and boreal ectomycorrhizal *Lactarius Pers.* (Russulales; Basidiomycota) in Alaska, based on soil and sporocarp DNA. *Mol. Ecol.* 18: 2213–2227. 2009.

Gielly L, Taberlet P. The use of chloroplast DNA to resolve plant phylogeny: noncoding versus *rbcL* sequences. *Mol. Biol. Evol.* 11: 769–777. 1994.

Gile GH, Stern RF, James ER, Keeling PJ. DNA barcoding of chlorarachniophytes using nucleomorph ITS sequences. *J. Phycol.* 46: 743–750. 2010.

Goldstein PZ, DeSalle R. Integrating DNA barcode data and taxonomic practice: determination, discovery, and description. *Bioessays*, 33: 135–147. 2011.

Gómez A, Wright PJ, Lunt DH, Cancino JM *et al.*, Mating trials validate the use of DNA barcoding to reveal cryptic speciation of a marine bryozoan taxon. *Philos. Trans. Royl. Soc. B.* 274: 199–207. 2007.

Gou H, Guan G, Liu A, Ma M *et al.*, A DNA barcode for *Piroplasmea. Acta Trop.* 124: 92–97. 2012.

Gumiel M, Da Mota FF, Rizzo VDS, Sarquis O *et al.*, Characterization of the microbiota in the guts of *Triatoma brasiliensis* and *Triatoma pseudomaculata* infected by *Trypanosoma cruzi* in natural conditions using culture independent methods. *Parasites Vectors.* 8 (1): 245. 2015.

Hajibabaei M, deWaard J, Ivanova NV, Ratnasingham S *et al.*, Critical factors for assembling a high volume of DNA barcodes. *Philos. Trans. Royl. Soc. Lond. Series B.* 360: 1959–1967. 2005.

Hajibabaei M, Janzen DH, Burns JM, Hallwachs W *et al.*, DNA barcodes distinguish species of tropical Lepidoptera. *Proc. Natl. Acad. Sci. USA.* 103: 968–971. 2006.

Hajibabaei M, Singer GAC, Hebert PDN, Hickey DA. DNA barcoding: how it complements taxonomy, molecular phylogenetics and population genetics. *Trends Genet.* 23: 167–172. 2007.

Hajibabaei M. The golden age of DNA metasystematics. *Trends Genet.* 28(11): 535-537. 2012.

Hajibabaei MHM, Shokralla S, Zhou X, Singer GAC *et al.*, Environmental barcoding: a next-generation sequencing approach for biomonitoring applications using river benthos. *Plos One.* 6: e17497. 2011.

Hall N. Advanced sequencing technologies and their wider impact in microbiology. *J. Exp. Biol.* 210: 1518–1525. 2007.

Hamada N, Pepinelli M, Mattos-Glória A, Luz SLB. A new black fly species from Brazil, closely related to *Simulium guianense* Wise (Diptera, Simuliidae), revealed by morphology and DNA barcoding. *Zootaxa,* 2428: 22-36. 2010.

Hanner R, Floyd R, Bernard A, Collette BB *et al.*, DNA barcoding of billfishes. *Mitochondl. DNA.* 22(1): 27-36. 2011.

Hebert PDN, Cywinska A, Ball SL, deWaard JR. Biological identifications through DNA barcodes. *Proc. Royl. Soc. Lond. B. Bio.* 270: 313–322. 2003.

Hebert PDN, Penton EH, Burns JM, Janzen DH *et al.,* Ten species in one: DNA barcoding reveals cryptic species in the neotropical skipper butterfly *Astraptes fulgerator*. *Proc. Natl. Acad. Sci. USA*. 101: 14812–14817. 2004.

Heger TJ, Pawlowskid J, Larac E, Leandere BS *et al.,* Comparing potential *COI* and *SSU rDNA* barcodes for assessing the diversity and phylogenetic relationships of *Cyphoderiid testate* Amoebae (Rhizaria: Euglyphida). *Protist*. 162, 131–141. 2011.

Hibbett DS, Ohman A, Glotzer D, Nuhn M *et al.,* Progress in molecular and morphological taxon discovery in Fungi and options for formal classification of environmental sequences. *Fungal Biol. Rev.* 25: 38–47. 2011.

Hillis DM, Dixon MT. Ribosomal DNA: molecular evolution and phylogenetic inference. *Qtly. Rev. Biol.* 66: 411–453. 1991.

Hoef-Emden K. Pitfalls of establishing DNA barcoding systems in protists: the Cryptophyceae as a test case. *Plos One*. 7(8): e43652. 2012.

Hollingsworth PM, Graham SW, Little DP. Choosing and using a plant DNA barcode. *Plos One*. 6: e19254. 2011.

Holmes DE, Nevin KP, Lovley DR. Comparison of *16S rRNA*, *nifD*, *recA*, *gyrB*, *rpoB* and *fusA* genes within the family *Geobacteraceae* fam. nov. *Intl. J. Syst. Evolul. Microbiol.* 54: 1591–1599. 2004.

Huang Y, Zhang Y, Zhao C, Xu Y *et al.,* DNA barcoding and its utility in commonly-used medicinal snakes. *China J. Chinese materia medica*. 40(5): 868-874. 2015.

Hubert N, Hanner R, Holm E, Mandrak NE *et al.,* Identifying Canadian freshwater fishes through DNA barcodes. *Plos One*. 3(6): e2490. 2008.

Hudson ME. Sequencing breakthroughs for genomic ecology and evolutionary biology. *Mol. Ecol. Resour.* 8: 3–17. 2008.

Hunter SJ, Goodall TI, Walsh KA, Owen R *et al.,* Nondestructive DNA extraction from blackflies (Diptera: Simuliidae): retaining voucher specimens for DNA barcoding projects. *Mol. Ecol. Resour.* 8(1): 56-61. 2008.

Hurst GDD, Jiggins FM, von der Schulenburg JHG, Bertrand D *et al.,* Male-killing *Wolbachia* in two species of insect. *Proc. Roy. Soc. B.* 266: 735– 740. 1999.

Ivanova NV, Zemlak TS, Hanner RH, Hebert PDN. Universal primer cocktails for fish DNA barcoding. *Mol. Ecol. Notes*. 7: 544–548. 2007.

Jinbo U, Kato T, ITO M. Current progress in DNA barcoding and future implications for entomology. *Entomol. Sci.* 14(2): 107-124. 2011.

Juen A, Traugott M. Amplification facilitators and multiplex PCR: tools to overcome PCR-inhibition in DNA-gut-content analysis of soil-living invertebrates. *Soil Biol. Biochem.* 38: 1872–1879. 2006.

Jurado-Rivera JA, Vogler AP, Reid CA, Petitpierre E *et al.,* DNA barcoding insect-host plant associations. *Proc. Biol. Sci.* 276(1657): 639-648. 2009.

Karnati SK, Yu Z, Sylvester JT, Dehority BA *et al.*, Technical note: specific PCR amplification of protozoal 18S rDNA sequences from DNA extracted from ruminal samples of cows. *J. Animl. Sci.* 81: 812–815. 2003.

Kelly LJ, Ameka GK, Chase MW. DNA barcoding of African Podostemaceae (river-weeds): a test of proposed barcode regions. Taxon. 59(1): 251-260. 2010.

Kelly RP, Sarkar IN, Eernisse DJ, Desalle R. DNA barcoding using chitons (genus Mopalia). *Mol. Ecol. Notes.* 7: 177–183. 2007.

Kerr KCR, Lijtmaer DA, Barreira AS, Hebert PDN *et al.*, Probing evolutionary patterns in neotropical birds through DNA barcodes. *Plos One.* 4: e4379. 2009.

Kerr KCR, Stoeckle MY, Dove CJ, Weigt LA *et al.*, Comprehensive DNA barcode coverage of North American birds. *Mol. Ecol. Notes,* 7: 535–543. 2007.

Ki J-S, Zhang W, Qian P-Y. Discovery of marine *Bacillus* species by *16S rRNA* and *rpoB* comparisons and their usefulness for species identification. *J. Microbl. Methd.* 77: 48–57. 2009.

Kjer KM. Use of rRNA secondary structure in phylo-genetic studies to identify homologous positions: an example of alignment and data presentation from the frogs. *Mol. Phylogenet. Evol,* 4: 314–330. 1995.

Klarica J, Kloss-Brandstätter A, Traugott M, Juen A. Comparing four mitochondrial genes in earthworms – Implications for identification, phylogenetics, and discovery of cryptic species. *Soil Biol. Biochem.* 45: 23e30. 2012.

Koetschan C, Förster F, Keller A, Schleicher T *et al.*, The ITS2 Database III - sequences and structures for phylogeny. *Nucleic Acids Res.* 38: D275-9. 2010.

Kolesárová M, Herich R, Levkut M, Èurlík J *et al.*, Suitability of different tissue fixatives for subsequent PCR analysis of *Cysticercus ovis. Helminthologia.* 49: 67-70. 2012.

Kosakyan A, Heger TJ, Leander BS, Todorov M *et al.*, COI barcoding of Nebelid testate amoebae (Amoebozoa: Arcellinida): extensive cryptic diversity and redefinition of the Hyalospheniidae Schultze. *Protist.* 163: 415–434. 2012.

Kress WJ, Erickson DL. A two-locus global DNA barcode for land plants: the coding *rbcL* gene complements the non-coding *trnH-psbA* spacer region. *Plos One.* 2: e508. 2007.

Kress WJ, Wurdack KJ, Zimmer EA, Weigt LA *et al.*, Use of DNA barcodes to identify flowering plants. *Proc. Natl. Acad. Sci. USA.* 102: 8369–8374. 2005.

Kruck NC, Tibbetts IR, Ward RD, Johnson JW *et al.*, Multi-gene barcoding to discriminate sibling species within a morphologically difficult fish genus species (*Sillago*). *Fisheries Res.* 143: 39-46. 2013.

Kumar CP, John BA, Khan SA, Lyla PS *et al.*, Mutational patterns and DNA barcode for diagnosing chikungunya virus. *Intl. J. Virol.* 7: 42-52. 2011.

Kumar NP, Rajavel AR and Jambulingam P. Application of PDF417 symbology for DNA barcoding. *Comp. Methd. Prog. Biomed.* 90: 187–189. 2008.

Kundu A, Sarkar D, Bhattacharjee A, Topdar N *et al.*, A simple ethanol wash of the tissue homogenates recovers high-quality genomic DNA from *Corchorus* species characterized by highly acidic and proteinaceous mucilages. *Electro. J Biotech.* 14(1). 2011.

Lahaye R, van der Bank M, Bogarin D, Warner J *et al.*, DNA barcoding the floras of biodiversity hotspots. *Proc. Natl. Acad. Sci. USA.* 105: 2923–2928. 2008.

Lara A, de Leon JLP, Rodriguez R, Casane D *et al.*, DNA barcoding of Cuban freshwater fishes: evidence for cryptic species and taxonomic conflicts. *Mol. Ecol. Resourc.* 10(3): 421-430. 2010.

Larranaga N, Hormaza JI. DNA barcoding of perennial fruit tree species of agronomic interest in the genus *Annona* (Annonaceae). *Front. Plant Sci.* 6: 589. 2015.

Lee DH, Lee HJ, Lee YN, Lee YJ *et al.*, Application of DNA barcoding technique in avian influenza virus surveillance of wild bird habitats in Korea and Mongolia. *Avian Diseases.* 54(1): 677-681. 2010.

Lee MSY. The molecularisation of taxonomy. *Invertebr. Syst.*, 18: 1-6. 2004.

Lim YW, Kim BK, Kim C, Jung HS *et al.*, Assessment of soil fungal communities using pyrosequencing. *J. Microbiol.* 48: 284–289. 2010.

Lin S, Zhang H, Hou YB, Zhuang YY *et al.*, High-level diversity of dinoflagellates in the natural environment, revealed by assessment of mitochondrial *cox1* and *cob* genes for dinoflagellate DNA barcoding. *Appl. Environ. Microbiol.* 75: 1279–1290. 2009.

Links MG, Dumonceaux TJ, Hemmingsen SM, Hill JE. The chaperonin-60 universal target is a barcode for bacteria that enables de novo assembly of metagenomic sequence data. *PLoS One.* 7: e49755. 2012.

Liu C, Shi L, Xu X, Li H *et al.*, DNA Barcode goes two-dimensions: DNA QR Code web server. *Plos One.* 7(5): e35146. 2012.

Locke SA, McLaughlin JD, Marcogliese DJ. DNA barcodes show cryptic diversity and a potential physiological basis for host specificity among Diplostomoidea (Platyhelminthes: Digenea) parasitizing freshwater fishes in the St. Lawrence river, Canada. *Mol. Ecol.* 19: 2813–2827. 2010.

Lorenz JG, Jackson WE, Beck JC, Hanner R. The problems and promise of DNA barcodes for species diagnosis of primate biomaterials. *Philos. Trans. Royl. Soc. Lond. B Biol. Sci.* 360: 1869–1877. 2005.

Lou SK, Wong KL, Li M, But PP *et al.*, An integrated web medicinal materials DNA database: MMDBD (Medicinal materials DNA barcode database). *BMC Genomics.* 11: 402. 2010.

Lowenstein JH, Amato G, Kolokotronis SO. The real maccoyii: identifying tuna sushi with DNA barcodes – contrasting characteristic attributes and genetic distances. *Plos One.* 4: e7866. 2009.

Lucking R. Taxonomy: a discipline on the brink of extinction are DNA barcode scanners the future of biodiversity research? *Archives Des. Sci.* 61: 75–88. 2008.

Magnacca KN, Brown MJF. Mitochondrial heteroplasmy and DNA barcoding in *Hawaiian hylaeus* (Nesoprosopis) bees (Hymenoptera: Colletidae). *BMC Evol. Biol.* 10: 174. 2010.

Mann DG, Sato S, Trobajo R, Vanormelingen P *et al.*, DNA barcoding for species identification and discovery in diatoms. *Cryptogamie Algologie.* 31(4): 557-577. 2010.

Martin P, Kaygorodova I, Sherbakov DY, Verheyen E. Rapid evolving lineages impede the resolution of phylogenetic relationships among Clitellata (Annelida). *Mol. Phylogenet. Evol.* 15: 355–368. 2000.

Martinez-Murcia AJ, Benlloch S, Collins MD. Phylogenetic interrelationships of members of the genera *Aeromonas* and *Plesiomonas* as determined by 16S ribosomal DNA sequencing: lack of congruence with results of DNA-DNA hybridizations. *Intl. J. Syst. Bacteriol.* 42: 412-421. 1992.

McLaughlin DJ, Hibbett DS, Lutzoni F, Spatafora JW *et al.*, The search for the fungal tree of life. *Trends Microbiol.* 17: 488–497. 2009.

Meier R, Shiyang K, Vaidya G, NG PKL. DNA Barcoding and taxonomy in Diptera: a tale of high intraspecific variability and low identification success. *Syst. Biol.* 55(5): 715-728. 2006.

Meyer CP, Paulay G. DNA barcoding: error rates based on comprehensive sampling. *Plos Biol.* 3: 2229–2238. 2005.

Michel H, Behr J, Harrenga A, Kannt A. Cytochrome c oxidase: structure and spectroscopy. *Ann. Rev. Biophys. Biomol. Struct.* 27: 329–356. 1998.

Michiels A, Ende WV, Tucker M, Riet LV *et al.*, Extraction of high-quality genomic DNA from latex-containing plants. *Analytical Biochem.* 315: 85–89. 2003.

Min XJ, Hickey DA. Assessing the effect of varying sequence length on DNA barcoding of fungi. *Mol. Ecol. Notes.* 7: 365–373. 2007.

Mollet C, Drancourt M, Raoult D. Determination of *Coxiella burnetii rpoB* sequence and its use for phylogenetic analysis. *Gene.* 207: 97–103. 1998.

Moritz C, Cicero C. DNA barcoding: promise and pitfalls. *Plos Biol.* 2: 1529-1531. 2004.

Mouhamadou B, Carriconde F, Gryta H, Jargeat P *et al.*, Molecular evolution of mitochondrial ribosomal DNA in the fungal genus *Tricholoma*: Barcoding implications. *Fungal Genet. Biol.* 45: 1219–1226. 2008.

Nagy ZT. A hands-on overview of tissue preservation methods for molecular genetic analyses. *Organism Diversity Evol.* 10: 91-105. 2010.

Nelson JS. Fishes of the World, 4th ed., John Wiley and Sons, Hoboken, NJ. 2006.

Newmaster SG, Ragupathy S. Testing plant barcoding in a sister species complex of pantropical Acacia (Mimosoideae, Fabaceae). *Mol. Ecol. Resour.* 9 (1): 172–180. 2009.

Newmaster SG, Fazekas AJ, Ragupathy S. DNA barcoding in land plants: evaluation of *rbcL* in a multigene tiered approach. *Can. J. Bot.* 84: 335–341. 2006.

Nijman V, Aliabadian M. Performance of distance-based DNA barcoding in the molecular identification of Primates. *Comptes Rendus Biologies.* 333(1): 11-16. 2010.

Nilsson R, Ryberg M, Abarenkov K, Sjökvist E *et al.,* The ITS region as a target for characterization of fungal communities using emerging sequencing technologies. *FEMS Microbiol. Lett.* 296: 97-101. 2009.

Nzelu CO, Cáceres AG, Arrunátegui-Jiménez MJ, Lañas-Rosas MF *et al.,* DNA barcoding for identification of sand fly species (Diptera: Psychodidae) from leishmaniasis-endemic areas of Peru. *Acta Tropica,* 145: 45-51. 2015.

O'Donnell K, Sutton DA, Rinaldi MG, Sarver BA *et al.,* Internet-accessible DNA sequence database for identifying fusaria from human and animal infections. *J. Clinl. Microbiol.* 48: 3708–3718. 2010.

Packer L, Grixti JC, Roughley RE, Hanner R. The status of taxonomy in Canada and the impact of DNA barcoding. *Can. J. Zoology.* 87: 1097–1110. 2009.

Padial JM, De La Riva I. Integrative taxonomists should use and produce DNA barcodes. *Zootaxa,* 1586: 67-68. 2007.

Padial JM, Castroviejo-Fisher S, Köhler J, Vilà C *et al.,* Deciphering the products of evolution at the species level: the need for an integrative taxonomy. *Zool. Scripta,* 38: 431-447. 2009.

Palmer JD, Herbon LA. Plant mitochondrial DNA evolves rapidly in structure, but slowly in sequence. *J. Mol. Evol.* 28: 87–97. 1988.

Pang XH, Song JY, Zhu YJ, Xie CX *et al.,* Using DNA Barcoding to Identify Species within Euphorbiaceae. *Planta Medica.* 76(15): 1784-1786. 2010.

Pauls SU, Blahnik RJ, Zhou X, Wardwell CT *et al.,* DNA barcode data confirm new species and reveal cryptic diversity in *Chilean smicridea* (Smicridea) (Trichoptera: Hydropsychidae). *J. North Amer. Benthological Soc.* 29: 1058–1074. 2010.

Pegg GG, Sinclair B, Briskey L and Aspden WJ. MtDNA barcode identification of fish larvae in the southern great barrier reef. *Australian Sci.* 70: 7–12. 2006.

Peterson AT, Moyle RG, Nyari AS, Robbins MB *et al.,* The need for proper vouchering in phylogenetic studies of birds. *Mol. Phylogenet. Evol.* 45: 1042–1044. 2007.

Pfenninger M, Nowak C, Kley C, Steinke D *et al.,* Utility of DNA taxonomy and barcoding for the inference of larval community structure in morphologically cryptic *Chironomus* (Diptera) species. *Mol. Ecol.* 16: 1957–1968. 2007.

Pilgrim EM, Jackson S, Swenson S, Turcsanyi I *et al.,* Incorporation of DNA barcoding into a large-scale biomonitoring program: opportunities and pitfalls. *J. North Amer. Benthological Soc.* 30: 217–231. 2011.

Pinto AD, Pinto PD, Terio V, Bozzo G *et al.,* DNA barcoding for detecting market substitution in salted cod fillets and battered cod chunks. *Food Chem.* 141: 1757–1762. 2013.

Pook CE, McEwing R. Mitochondrial DNA sequences from dried snake venom: a DNA barcoding approach to the identification of venom samples. *Toxicon*. 46: 711–715. 2005.

Prendini L. Comment on "Identifying spiders through DNA barcodes". *Can. J. Zool.* 83: 481-491. 2005.

Quail MA, Smith M, Jackson D, Leonard S *et al.*, SASI-Seq: Sample assurance Spike-Ins, and highly differentiating 384 barcoding for Illumina sequencing. *BMC Genomics*. 15 (1): 110. 2014.

Rach J, DeSalle R, Sarkar IN, Schierwater B *et al.*, Character based DNA barcoding allows discrimination of genera, species and populations in Odonata. *Proc. Royl. Soc. Lond. Ser. B-Biol. Sci.* 275: 237–247. 2008.

Ragupathy S, Newmaster SG, Murugesan M, Balasubramaniam V. DNA barcoding discriminates a new cryptic grass species revealed in an ethnobotany study by the hill tribes of the western ghats in southern India. *Mol. Ecol. Resour.* 9 (1): 164–171. 2009.

Rasmussen RS, Morrissey MT, Hebert PDN. DNA barcoding of commercially important salmon and trout species (Oncorhynchus and Salmo) from north America. *J. Agril. Food Chem.* 57: 8379–8385. 2009.

Rastogi G, Dharne MS, Walujkar S, Kumar A *et al.*, Species identification and authentication of tissues of animal origin using mitochondrial and nuclear markers. *Meat Sci.*, 76: 666–674. 2007.

Ratnasingham S and Hebert PDN. Barcoding bold: The barcode of life data system (www.barcodinglife.org). *Mol. Ecol. Notes*. 1-10. 2007.

Renner SS. Circumscription and phylogeny of the Laurales: Evidence from molecular and morphological data. *Amer. J. Bot.* 86: 1301–1315. 1999.

Reva ON, Zaets IE, Ovcharenko LP, Kukharenko OE *et al.*, Metabarcoding of the kombucha microbial community grown in different microenvironments. *AMB Express*. 5 (1): 124. 2015.

Richert K, Brambilla E, Stackebrandt E. The phylogenetic significance of peptidoglycan types: Molecular analysis of the genera *Microbacterium* and *Aureobacterium* based upon sequence comparison of *gyrB, rpoB, recA* and *ppk* and *16S rRNA* genes. *Syst. Appl. Microbiol.*, 30: 102–108. 2007.

Robert V, Szöke S, Eberhardt U, Cardinali G *et al.*, The quest for a general and reliable fungal DNA barcode. *Open Appl. Inform. J.* 5: 55-71. 2011.

Robinson EA, Blagoev GA, Hebert PDN, Adamowicz SJ. Prospects for using DNA barcoding to identify spiders in species-rich genera. *Zookeys*. 16: 27-46. 2009.

Roux V, Raoult D. Phylogenetic analysis of the genus *Rickettsia* by *16S rDNA* sequencing. *Res. Microbiol*. 146: 85-396. 1995.

Rowley DL, Coddington JA, Gates MW, Norrbom AL *et al.*, Vouchering DNA-barcoded specimens: test of a non-destructive extraction protocol for terrestrial arthropods. *Mol. Ecol. Notes*. 7: 915–924. 2007.

Rubinoff D, Cameron S, Will K. Are plant DNA barcodes a search for the Holy Grail? *Trends Ecol. Evol.* 21: 1–2. 2006.

Rubinoff D. Utility of mitochondrial DNA barcodes in species conservation. *Conservn. Biol.* 20: 1026–1033. 2006.

Rueness J. DNA barcoding of select freshwater and marine red algae (Rhodophyta). *Cryptogamie Algologie.* 31(4): 377-386. 2010.

Saccone C, DeCarla G, Gissi C, Pesole G *et al.*, Evolutionary genomics in the Metazoa: the mitochondrial DNA as a model system. *Gene.* 238: 195–210. 1999.

Salazar GA, Chase MW, Arenas MAS, Ingrouille M. Phylogenetics of *Cranichideae* with emphasis on *Spiranthinae* (Orchidaceae, Orchidoideae): evidence from plastid and nuclear DNA sequences. *Amer. J. Bot.* 90: 777–795. 2003.

Sarkar IN, Planet PJ, Desalle R. CAOS software for use in character-based DNA barcoding. *Mol. Ecol. Resourc.* 8: 1256– 1259. 2008.

Sass C, Little DP, Stevenson DW, Specht CD. DNA barcoding in the Cycadales: testing the potential of proposed barcoding markers for species identification of Cycads. *Plos One.* 2: e1154. 2007.

Sato H, Murakami N. Reproductive isolation among cryptic species in the ectomycorrhizal genus *Strobilomyces*: Population-level caps marker-based genetic analysis. *Mol. Phyl. Evol.* 48: 326–334. 2008.

Schoch CL, Seifert KA, Huhndorf S, Robert V *et al.*, Nuclear ribosomal internal transcribed spacer (ITS) region as a universal DNA barcode marker for fungi. *Proc. Natl. Acad. Sci. USA.* 109: 6241–6246. 2012.

Schoch CL, Sung GH, López-Giráldez F, Townsend JP *et al.*, The Ascomycota tree of life: a phylum-wide phylogeny clarifies the origin and evolution of fundamental reproductive and ecological traits. *Syst. Biol.* 58: 224–239. 2009.

Schultz J, Müller T, Achtziger M, Seibel PN *et al.*, The internal transcribed spacer 2 database – a web server for (not only) low level phylogenetic analyses. *Nucleic Acids Res.* 34: W704-707. 2006.

Schuster SC. Next-generation sequencing transforms today's biology. *Nature.* 5: 16–18. 2008.

Scicluna SM, Tawari B, Clark CG. DNA barcoding of *Blastocystis*. *Protist.* 157: 77–85. 2006.

Scriver M, Marinich A, Wilson C, Freeland J. Development of species-specific environmental DNA (eDNA) markers for invasive aquatic plants. *Aquatic Bot.* 122: 27-31. 2015.

Seena S, Pascoal C, Marvanova L, Cassio F. DNA barcoding of fungi: a case study using *ITS* sequences for identifying aquatic hyphomycete species. *Fungal Diversity.* 44(1), 77-87. 2010.

Seifert KA, Samson RA, deWaard JR, Houbraken J *et al.*, Prospects for fungus identification using CO1 DNA barcodes, with *Penicillium* as a test case. *Proc. Natl. Acad. Sci. USA.* 104(10): 3901-6. 2007.

Seifert KA. Progress towards DNA barcoding of fungi. *Mol. Ecol. Resourc.* 9: 3-89. 2009.

Sevilla RG, Diez A, Noren M, Mouchel O *et al.*, Primers and polymerase chain reaction conditions for DNA barcoding teleost fish based on the mitochondrial cytochrome b and nuclear rhodopsin genes. *Mol. Ecol. Notes.* 7: 730–734. 2007.

Sharma P, Joshi N, Sharma A. Isolation of genomic DNA from medicinal plants without liquid nitrogen. *Ind. J. Exptl. Biol.* 48: 610-614. 2010.

Shaw J, Lickey EB, Beck JT, Farmer SS *et al.*, The tortoise and the hare: Relative utility of 21 noncoding chloroplast DNA sequences for phylogenetic analysis. *Amer. J. Bot.* 92: 142–166. 2005.

Shenoy BD, Jeewon R, Hyde KA. Impact of DNA sequence-data on the taxonomy of anamorphic fungi. *Fungal Diversity* 26: 1–54. 2007.

Shepherd LD, McLay TGB. Two micro-scale protocols for the isolation of DNA from polysaccharide-rich plant tissue. *J. Plant Res.*, 124: 311–314. 2011.

Silva-Brandão KL, Lyra ML, Freitas AVL. Barcoding Lepidoptera: current situation and perspectives on the usefulness of a contentious technique. *Neotropical Entomol.* 38: 441–451. 2009.

Simmons RB, Weller SJ. Utility and evolution of cytochrome *b* in insects. *Mol. Phylogenet. Evol.* 20: 196–210. 2001.

Singh HR, Unii BG, Neog K, Wann SB. Isolating silkworm genomic DNA without liquid nitrogen suitable for marker studies. *African J. Biotech.* 10(55): 11365-11372. 2011.

Smith MA, Bertrand C, Crosby K, Eveleigh ES *et al.*, *Wolbachia* and DNA barcoding insects: patterns, potential, and problems. *PLoS One.* 7: e36514. 2012.

Smith MA, Fisher BL, Hebert PDN. DNA barcoding for effective biodiversity assessment of a hyperdiverse arthropod group: the ants of Madagascar. *Philos. Trans Royl. Soc. Ser. B.* 360: 825–1834. 2005.

Smith MA, Poyarkov NA, Hebert PDN. CO1 DNA barcoding amphibians: take the chance, meet the challenge. *Mol. Ecol. Resourc.* 8(2): 235-246. 2008.

Smith MA, Woodley NE, Janzen DH, Hallwachs W *et al.*, DNA barcodes reveal cryptic host-specificity within the presumed polyphagous members of a genus of parasitoid flies (Diptera: Tachinidae). *Proc. Natl. Acad. Sci. USA.* 103: 3657-3662. 2006.

Sogin ML, Morrison HG, Huber JA, Welch DM *et al.*, Microbial diversity in the deep sea and the underexplored 'rare biosphere'. *Proc. Natl. Acad. Sci. USA.* 103: 12115–12120. 2006.

Souza HAV, Muller LAC, Brandão RL, Lovato MB. Isolation of high quality and polysaccharide-free DNA from leaves of *Dimorphandra mollis* (Leguminosae), a tree from the Brazilian Cerrado. *Genet. Mol. Res.* 11 (1): 756-764. 2012.

Steinke D, Zemlak TS, Hebert PDN. Barcoding Nemo: DNA-Based identifications for the ornamental fish Trade. *Plos One.* 4: e6300. 2009.

Stockinger H, Kruger M, Schussler A. DNA barcoding of arbuscular mycorrhiza fungi. *New Phytologist*. 187(2): 461-474. 2010.

Stoeck T, Bass D, Nebel M, Christen R *et al.*, Multiple marker parallel tag environmental DNA sequencing reveals a highly complex eukaryotic community in marine anoxic water. *Mol. Ecol.* 19: 21–31. 2010.

Strutzenberger P, Brehm G, Fiedler K. DNA barcode sequencing from old type specimens as a tool in taxonomy: a case study in the diverse genus *Eois* (Lepidoptera: Geometridae). *Plos One*. 7(11): e49710. 2012.

Summerbell RC, Lévesque CA, Seifert KA, Bovers M *et al.*, Microcoding: the second step in DNA barcoding. *Philos. Trans. Royl. Soc. Lond. B. Biol. Sci.* 360: 1897–1903 2005.

Swartz ER, Mwale M, Hanner R. A role for barcoding in the study of African fish diversity and conservation. *South African J. Sci.*, 104: 293–298. 2008.

Sweeney BW, Battle JM, Jackson JK, Dapkey T. Can DNA barcodes of stream macroinvertebrates improve descriptions of community structure and water quality? *J. North Amer. Benthological Soc.* 30: 195–216. 2011.

Taberlet P, Coissac E, Pompanon F, Gielly L *et al.*, Power and limitations of the chloroplast *trnL* (UAA) intron for plant DNA barcoding. *Nucleic Acids Res.* 35: e14. 2007.

Tautz D, Ellegren H, Weigel D. Next generation molecular ecology. *Mol. Ecol.* 19: 1–3. 2010.

Terranova MS, Brutto SL, Arculeo M, Mitton JB. A mitochondrial phylogeography of *Brachidontes variabilis* (Bivalvia: Mytilidae) reveals three cryptic species. *J. Zool. Syst. Evol. Res.* 45 (4): 289–298. 2007.

Toju H, Tanabe AS, Yamamoto S, Sato H. High-Coverage ITS Primers for the DNA-Based Identification of *Ascomycetes* and *Basidiomycetes* in Environmental Samples. *Plos One*. 7(7): e40863. 2012.

Triantafyllidis A, Bobori D, Koliamitra C, Gbandi E *et al.*, DNA barcoding analysis of fish species diversity in four north Greek lakes. *Mitochondl. DNA*. 22(1): 37-42. 2011.

Tringe SG, von Mering C, Kobayashi A, Salamov AA *et al.*, Comparative metagenomics of microbial communities. *Science*. 308: 554–557. 2005.

Tripathi AM, Tyagi A, Kumar A, Singh A *et al.*, The internal transcribed spacer (*ITS*) region and *trnhH-psbA* are suitable candidate loci for DNA barcoding of tropical tree species of India. *Plos One*. 8(2): e57934. 2013.

Uhart M, Sirand-Pugnet P, Labarere J. Evolution of mitochondrial *SSUrDNA* variable domain sequences and rRNA secondary structures, and phylogeny of the *Agrocybe aegerita* multispecies complex. *Res. Microbiol.* 158: 203–212. 2007.

Valière N, Fumagalli L, Gielly L, Miquel C *et al.*, Long-distance wolf recolonization of France and Switzerland inferred from non-invasive genetic sampling over a period of 10 years. *Animl. Conservn.* 6: 83-92. 2003.

Vijayan K, Tsou CH. DNA barcoding in plants: taxonomy in a new perspective. *Current Sci.* 99(1): 1530-1541. 2010.

Vilgalys R, Gonzalez D. Organisation of ribosomal DNA in the basidiomycete *Thanatephorus praticola. Current Genet.* 18: 277-280. 1990.

Vos M, Quince C, Pijl AS, de Hollander M *et al.*, A comparison of *rpoB* and *16S rRNA* as markers in pyrosequencing studies of bacterial diversity. *Plos One.* 7(2): e30600. 2012.

Wallace LJ, Boilard SMAL, Eagle SHC, Spall JL *et al.*, DNA barcodes for everyday life: Routine authentication of Natural Health Products. *Food Res. Intl* 49: 446–452. 2012.

Walsh DA, Bapteste E, Kamekura M, Doolittle WF. Evolution of the RNA polymerase B9 subunit Gene (*rpoB9*) in Halobacteriales: a complementary molecular marker to the *SSU rRNA* Gene. *Mol. Biol. Evol.* 21(12): 2340–2351. 2012.

Wang WQ, Wu YR, Yan YH, Ermakova M *et al.*, DNA barcoding of the Lemnaceae, a family of aquatic monocots. *BMC Plant Biol.* 10: 205. 2010.

Ward CW. Progress towards a higher taxonomy of viruses. *Res. Virol.* 144: 419-453. 1993.

Ward RD, Zemlak TS, Innes BH, Last PR *et al.*, DNA barcoding Australia's fish species. *Philos. Trans. R. Soc. Lond. B.* 360: 1847–1857. 2005.

Whitworth TL, Dawson RD, Magalon H, Baudry E. DNA barcoding cannot reliably identify species of the blowfly genus *Protocalliphora* (Diptera: Calliphoridae). *Proc. Royl. Soc. B.* 274: 1731-1739. 2007.

Wiemers M, Fiedler K. Does the DNA barcoding gap exist? – a case study in blue butterflies (Lepidoptera: Lycaenidae). *Frontiers Zool.* 4. 2007.

Williams ST, Knowlton N. Mitochondrial pseudogenes are pervasive and often insidious in the snapping shrimp genus *Alpheus. Mol. Biol. Evol.* 18: 1484-1493. 2001.

Wilson DE, Reeder DAM. Mammal species of the world: A taxonomic and geographic reference. 3rd ed. Johns Hopkins University Press, Baltimore, MA. 2005.

Woo PC, Lau SK, Teng JL, Tse H *et al.*, Then and now: use of 16S rDNA gene sequencing for bacterial identification and discovery of novel bacteria in clinical microbiology laboratories. *Clinl. Microbiol Infect.* 14: 908–934. 2008.

Yamashiro T, Fukuda T, Yokoyama J, Maki M. Molecular phylogeny of *Vincetoxicum* (Apocynaceae-Asclepiadoideae) based on the nucleotide sequences of cpDNA and nrDNA. *Mol. Phylogenet. Evol.* 31: 689-700. 2004.

Yang QQ, Zhao S, Kucerova Z, Stejskal V *et al.*, Validation of the 16S rDNA and COI DNA barcoding technique for rapid molecular identification of stored product psocids (Insecta: Psocodea: Liposcelididae). *J. Econ. Entomol.* 106(1): 419-425. 2013.

Yang YW, Lai KN, Li WH. Rates of nucleotide substitution in angiosperm mitochondrial DNA sequences and dates of divergence between *Brassica* and other angiosperm lineages. *J. Mol. Evol.* 48: 597–604. 1999.

Yin HQ, Jia MX, Shi LJ, Yang S *et al.*, Nanoparticle-based bio-barcode assay for the detection of bluetongue virus. *J. Virol. Methd.* 178: 225–228. 2011.

Yu J, Xue JH, Zhou SL. New universal *matK* primers for DNA barcoding angiosperms. *J. Syst. Evol.* 49(3): 176-181. 2011.

Zhang J. Exploiting formalin-preserved fish specimens for resources of DNA barcoding. *Mol. Ecol. Resourc.* 10(6): 935-41. 2010.

Zhao P, Luo J, Zhuang WY. Practice towards DNA barcoding of the nectriaceous fungi. *Fungal Diversity.* 46(1): 183-191. 2011.

Zimmermann J, Hajibabaei M, Blackburn DC, Hanken J *et al.*, DNA damage in preserved specimens and tissue samples: a molecular assessment. *Frontiers Zool.* 5: 18. 2008.

2016, Biotechnological Tools for Genetic Resources *Pages* 59–74
Editor: Pradip Chandra Deka
Published by: Daya Publishing House, NEW DELHI

Chapter 3

DNA Barcoding in Plants

Paramananda Barman[1] and M.A. Laskar[2]*

[1]Department of Botany, University of Delhi,
Delhi – 110 007
[2]Biotechnology Department, St. Anthony's College,
Shillong – 793 001, Meghalaya
**E-mail: laskar41@gmail.com*

ABSTRACT

DNA Barcoding is an approach where a short DNA sequence from a standardized locus is employed for species identification. DNA Barcoding is increasingly becoming popular as it is a simple, time and cost effective and an almost accurate technique. Selection of correct DNA marker is the main criterion for success in barcoding. DNA barcoding is difficult in plants than in animals as there are multiple consensuses about selection of barcoding markers for plant DNA barcoding. Some common plant barcoding markers are chloroplast genes matK, rbcL, rpoC1, rpoB and trnL; chloroplast intergenic spacers trnH-psbA, atpF-atpH and psbK-psbI; and the nuclear ribosomal internal transcribed spacer (ITS). These markers can be used alone or in combinations with other markers or spacers. Complete plastid genome and low or single copy nuclear genes are new potential candidates for plant DNA barcoding. In addition to species identification, DNA barcoding is also helpful in areas like biodiversity assessment, authentication and forensic science. International bodies like IBOL (the International Barcode of Life Project), CBOL (the Consortium for the Barcode of Life) and ECBOL (the European Consortium for the Barcode of Life); and databases like BOLD (the Barcode of Life Data Systems) and INSDC (International Nucleotide Sequence Database Collaboration) are dedicated for DNA barcoding services.

Keywords: *DNA barcoding, Chloroplast genes, Intergenic spacers, Internal transcribed spacer.*

Introduction

Exploring the tremendous biodiversity of our planet has been the major thrust area of Life Science researchers. The historical classification system was initiated by Carl Linnaeus 250 years before and in this long period, taxonomists were able to describe 1.7 million species and the number is increasing day by day (Casiraghi *et al.*, 2010). Although this number of species explored seems to be a huge one, it represents a tiny fraction of the actual biodiversity present (Vernooy *et al.*, 2010). Although traditional morphology based identification and classification is of sole importance, it becomes challenging many times when expert taxonomists are not available. Sometimes there might be only one expert worldwide to describe a particular group of organism, which increases the challenge. Identification becomes much difficult even in the presence of taxonomists, when the sample to be identified is not in intact shape or when a sample contains mixture of minute organism with very few identifiable traits (Chase and Fay, 2009). These shortcomings were addressed for the first time by Hebert *et al.* (2003). They reported that a small fragment of DNA can be successfully employed for identification of a species. Although the term barcoding was used in this sense for the first time in 1993 (Arnot *et al.*, 1993), the revolutionary finding of Hebert *et al.* (2003) of using the 648 base pair-long mitochondrial gene, *CO1* in animals as marker formed the basis of DNA Barcoding. DNA Barcoding can thus be defined as an approach where a short DNA sequence or sequences from a standardized locus (or loci) are employed as species identification tool.

The overwhelming popularity of Barcoding is not only because of its discrimination power itself, also because of joint use of three modern innovations of taxonomy: (a) molecularization: use of different molecular markers which are variable and thus useful as a discriminator; (b) computerization: The revolution in data storage, analysis, sharing and annotation and (c) standardization: application of the idea to vast groups of organisms which are not deeply related (Casiraghi *et al.*, 2010).

Barcoding Project has Multiple Components

The Barcode of Life Database (http://www.barcodeoflife.org/) recognises four basic components involved in a barcoding project:

1. **Specimens**: Specimen collection, storage still processing and proper description etc. are initial processes involved in a barcoding project. Stored identified specimens in museums, zoos, herbaria and seed bank *etc.* are the guidance source for description and identification of specimens.
2. **Analysis in laboratory**: Different barcoding protocols are necessary to obtain DNA barcode sequences from different specimens. The first task is to find an appropriate method of DNA isolation which is based on the type of the specimen to be processed. The second task is to select appropriate primers and PCR condition. This is followed by amplification of the region of interest and DNA sequencing. The process can be completed in few hours within a reasonable cost. One has to submit the sequence data obtained to a barcoding database for subsequent analysis.
3. **The Database**: The most crucial component of the Barcoding project is a common platform of a public reference library which is a repository of identified barcodes. This database can be used as a guide to identify unknown specimens based on known specimen information. Currently two major barcode databases serve this purpose.

The International Nucleotide Sequence Database (INSD): This is a collaborative approach maintained for a very long time by three leading sequence database groups of world which are GenBank in the U.S., the European Molecular Biology Lab (EMBL) in Europe and the DNA Data Bank of Japan (DDBJ). They have collaboration with Barcoding initiative CBOL (The Consortium for the Barcode of Life) and accepts the CBOL's data standards for barcode records.

Barcode of Life Database (BOLD): This is a huge barcoding database which guides barcoding researchers with information of existing projects, collection process, sample processing and primer information and to analyse barcoding data. This successful venture is maintained by University of Guelph in Ontario.

4. **Analysis of Barcoding DATA**: The new barcode isolated are identified by finding the closest matches in the reference record present in the barcoding databases. CBOL is working to improve the ways of barcoding data analysis, display and use and arranged a Data Analysis Working Group. A pipeline of a barcoding project is shown in Figure 3.1.

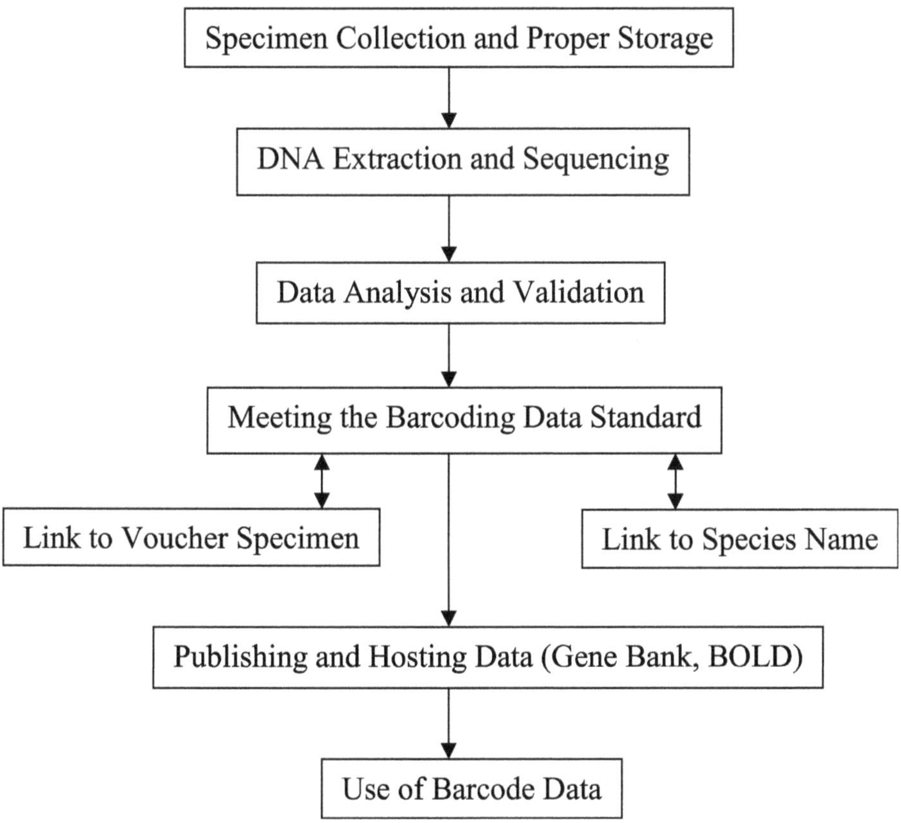

Figure 3.1: Step-wise Procedures to be Followed for DNA Barcoding.

Advantages of DNA Barcoding

Advantages of DNA barcoding are as follows:

- ☆ **Simple:** As evident from the components described above, DNA barcoding is a simple process where information and guidance about all the processes involved like DNA isolation, primers, PCR condition, data analysis etc. are in standardised form and available in public databases (Sandionigi *et al.*, 2012).
- ☆ **Accurate**: With some rare exceptions, DNA barcoding is generally accepted as an accurate tool for species identification. It is a regulatory tool used by the U.S. FDA.
- ☆ **Rapid:** Once the specimen to be worked with is available, getting a barcode sequence is a matter of few hours (Sandionigi *et al.*, 2012). Barcoding service providers like CCDB provides species identification in two-three days.
- ☆ **Cost Effective**: Getting a barcode within a reasonable cost is also a factor for wide acceptance of it. Sequencing services are rapid and reasonable and other factors involved can be managed in a reasonable amount of money.

Marker Selection for DNA Barcoding

Factors to be considered during selection of marker for DNA barcoding are described in the following section.

Universality of PCR Amplification

In a typical barcoding approach, universal primers are used for amplification of the DNA region of interest. Thus the ease of amplification with universal primer is a key factor guiding marker selection. Markers should have conserved flanking region for this purpose (Hollingsworth *et al.*, 2009). Universality also helps in sequencing.

Power of Species Differentiation

Although we want the flanking region to be conserved for universal primer binding, the internal region should be sufficiently variable for proper identification of a species. Low level of intraspecific variation is desirable to reduce confusion (KEW Web).

Length

A DNA marker should be short so that it can be amplified even in sub optimal conditions (Hollingsworth *et al.*, 2009). Short markers can be sequenced in one reaction as after a particular length poor quality chromatograms are obtained. Also short length marker can be isolated easily from degraded sample (Kew Web).

Variability

Marker should be less variable in length and structure. This reduces sequence quality and creates additional problems (Hollingsworth *et al.*, 2009).

Complementation among Markers

This is important for marker selection in plants and not in animals because for animals we have the universally accepted CO1 marker. Complementation is necessary in plants to increase the probability of correct identification (PCI) (Erickson *et al.*, 2008). Complementation in plant barcoding includes selection of unlinked marker to address the correlation problem in chloroplast markers. Complementation addresses the problems like low recovery or less sequence variation in one marker by using another marker that does not have these problems.

Bioinformatic Analysis

Markers should be easily alignable because sequence alignment is a key factor for comparisons and further analyses. They should have more substitutions than insertions and deletions (Erickson *et al.*, 2008).

Presence of a Reading Frame

This is only a desirable quality and does not matter much even if the criteria are not fulfilled. In this approach, the presence of nonsense substitutions can be used for evaluation of the quality of sequencing reactions and sequence editing (Chase *et al.*, 2007). This is also helpful for alignment purpose. A list of popular plant DNA Barcoding markers is presented in Table 3.1.

Different Markers Used for Plant DNA Barcoding

The mitochondrial *CO1* gene proved to be useful in DNA barcoding of various vertebrates and invertebrates, but this marker is not very useful for barcoding in plants, because in plants it evolves very slowly (Kress and Erickson 2007) and thus cannot provide necessary resolution. Plant barcoding is a complicated procedure with multiple consensuses about selection of barcoding markers. Various strategies have been proposed, such as use of a single chloroplast region (Kress *et al.*, 2005 and Lahaye *et al.*, 2008), nuclear ribosomal ITS region, which is fast evolving, and finally a combination of different regions (Kress *et al.*, 2007, Chase *et al.*, 2007).

Chloroplast Genes

Chloroplast genes comprise most of the plant DNA barcoding markers. They have various advantages such as:

1. They are present abundantly and thus isolation and amplification is easier.
2. Chloroplast primarily contains single copy genes and there are less chance of getting a mixed product.
3. The nucleotide substitution rate is conserved in chloroplast, and
4. With more and more chloroplast genome being sequenced, sufficient background information is available for chloroplast genome.

Some important chloroplast barcoding markers are described in the following section.

Table 3.1: Commonly Used DNA Barcoding Markers in Plants

Gene	*Primer*	*Direction*	*Sequence 5'-3'*	*Source*
matK	2.1	F	CCTATCCATCTGGAAATCTTAG	Kew Website
	2.1a	F	ATCCATCTGGAAATCTTAGTTC	Kew Website
	5	R	GTTCTAGCACAAGAAAGTCG	Kew Website
	3.2	R	CTTCCTCTGTAAAGAATTC	Kew Website
	matK 390 F	F	CGATCTATTCATTCAATATTTC	Cuenoud *et al.*, 2002
	1326R	R	TCTAGCACACGAAAGTCGAAGT	Cuenoud *et al.*, 2002
rpoC	1	F	GTGGATACACTTCTTGATAATGG	Kew Website
	2	F	GGCAAAGAGGGAAGATTTCG	Kew Website
	3	R	TGAGAAAACATAAGTAAACGGGC	Kew Website
	4	R	CCATAAGCATATCTTGAGTTGG	Kew Website
rpoB	1	F	AAGTGCATTGTTGGAACTGG	Kew Website
	2	F	ATGCAACGTCAAGCAGTTCC	Kew Website
	3	R	CCGTATGTGAAAAGAAGTATA	Kew Website
	4	R	GATCCCAGCATCACAATTCC	Kew Website
ITS	AB101	F	ACGAATTCATGGTCCGGTGAAGTGTTCG	Sun *et al.*, 1994
	AB102	R	TAGAATTCCCCGGTTCGCTCGCCGTTAC	Sun *et al.*, 1994
ITS2	ITS-S2F	F	ATGCGATACTTGGTGTGAAT	Chen *et al.*, 1010
	ITS4	R	TCCTCCGCTTATTGATATGC	White *et al.*, 1990
trn H– *psb*	psbAF	R	GTTATGCATGAACGTAATGCTC	Sang *et al.*, 1997
	trnH2	F	CGCGCATGGTGGATTCACAATCC	Tate and Simpson 2003
	psbA	R	CGAAGCTCCATCTACAAATGG	Hamilton 1999
	trnH (GUG)	F	ACTGCCTTGATCCACTTGGC	Hamilton, 1999
	psbA501f	R	TTTCTCAGACGGTATGCC	Cox *et al.*, 2004

Note: Additional information about different primers for barcoding can be retrieved from: http://www.boldsystems.org/index.php/Public_Primer_PrimerSearch.

matK

This gene is now extensively used for Barcoding and probably the best to be used. The *mat*K gene, which was known as *orf*K before (Hilu and Liang, 1997) is used very commonly as a reliable marker in plant molecular systematics and evolution (Johnson and Soltis 1994, 1995; Steele and Vilgalys, 1994, Liang and Hilu, 1996). This gene is located within two introns of the chloroplast gene *trn*K and approximately 1500 base pairs in length. One interesting fact about this gene is that it is present in parasitic *Epifagus*, a taxon that lost nearly 65 per cent of the chloroplast genes. The retaining of the matK gene proves its functional significance in plants (Hilu and Liang, 1997). Even the two exons of the *trn*K gene flanking the *mat*K region were lost, but matK is present with a large deletion in coding region (Wolfe *et al.*, 1992). Comparatively *matK* is one of the fast evolving plastid gene and successfully used for species discrimination among angiosperm species (Fazekas *et al.*, 2008, Lahaye *et al.*, 2008). About universality of *matK* primers, there are mixed reports ranging from successful amplification (Lahaye *et al.*, 2008) to intermediate kind of response (Kress *et al.*, 2007, Fazekas *et al.*, 2008). Thus a lack of consensus about universality leads to reservations about this locus by some researchers. The use of best currently available 'universal' primer pair for *matK* (3F/1R) on diverse samples sets results in PCR and sequencing success of 70 per cent in angiosperms (Hollingsworth *et al.*, 2011). Use of a secondary internal primer pair 390F/1326R (Cuenoud *et al.*, 2002) is reported to increase amplification and sequencing success by 10 per cent more than the existing one.

In gymnosperms the success rate (83 per cent) is reasonable but in cryptogams it is very limited (10 per cent) and not satisfactory even after use of multiple primer sets (Janzen *et al.*, CBOL, 2009). Amplification of matK has been reported to be problematic in many experiments (Hollingsworth, 2009).

rbcL

rbcL is the best characterized gene among all chloroplast genes. This gene is approximately 1430 base pairs in length. It is a single copy gene and generally free from length mutations except at the far 3′ end. The rate of evolution is conserved. The *rbc*L gene codes for the large subunit of ribulose 1, 5 bisphosphate carboxylase/ oxygenase (RUBISCO or RuBPCase). The sequence data of the *rbc*L gene are widely used in phylogenetic study throughout the seed plants. However, the resolution ability of *rbc*L below the family level is often very poor and thus not very suitable for species level phylogeny (Doebley *et al.*, 1990).

This coding gene has been proposed as a potential plant barcode by many research groups (Chase *et al.*, 2005, Newmaster *et al.*, 2006), usually in conjunction with one or more other markers (Fazekas *et al.*, 2008). Large amount of existing sequence in public databases is one of the additional advantage of this region. There are more than 10,000 *rbcL* sequences reported in GenBank (Chase *et al.*, 2005, Newmaster *et al.*, 2006). Universality of amplification is the most promising aspect of rbcL. Additional improvements in primer designing has made the recovery of high-quality bidirectional sequences possible across land plants (Fazekas *et al.*, 2008).

rpoC1

This is a slow evolving marker and thus bears less potential. However, it was able to discriminate among species in many groups of plants (Chase *et al.*, 2007). The universality of this marker with potential of amplification with limited range of PCR conditions and primer sets is a great advantage. Probably it is the only barcoding locus which can be routinely amplified and sequenced using a single primer pair and standard reaction conditions in all samples in all taxonomic groups (Hollingsworth *et al.*, 2009).

rpoB

This is regarded as a poor barcoding marker. It is amplifiable with a limited range of PCR conditions and primer sets. Although it is a slow evolving gene, it can discriminate among species in many groups of organisms particularly when used in combination (*e.g.*, *rpoC1*+*rpoB*+*mat*K) with other locus (Chase *et al.*, 2007).

trnL

(Have a P6 loop with great potential) The plastid intron in *trnL* region has also been suggested as an potential DNA barcoding (Taberlet *et al.*, 2007) sequence. However, slow rate of evolution, a genuine problem in chloroplast region leads to poor resolution (Shaw *et al.*, 2005). It is surprisingly highly conserved even after being a non-coding region. The presence of a small stem-loop structure called P6 loop within this intron (Taberlet *et al.*, 2007) bears great potential for species discrimination. P6 has a variable minibarcode of 10-143 base pairs which has conserved priming sites in both sides and thus bears great potential to be used for barcoding of degraded DNA samples (Hollingsworth *et al.*, 2011).

The collaborative approach of RBG, Kew has suggested six plastid coding regions (accD, matK, ndhJ, rpoB2, rpoC1, and ycf5) as potential plant barcodes (http://www. rbgkew. org.uk/barcoding/index. html), but comparisons of their effectiveness is not available (Kress and Erickson 2007). The three regions, *accD*, *ndhJ*, and *ycf5* were deleted from the list of proposed barcodes because of their absence from certain plant groups. The *ycf5* might have been deleted from the bryophyte plastid genomes and *accD* is missing in the grass family while *ndhJ* is found to be absent from *Pinus* and might be truncated or non-functional in some orchids. Many other regions are proposed but there is no single consensus about using one particular marker like CO1 in animals.

Chloroplast Intergenic Spacers

trnH-psbA

The non-coding trnH-psbA intergenic spacer is proposed to be the most viable candidate for a single-locus barcode for land plants (Kress *et al.*, 2005). This is one of the most variable non-coding regions in chloroplast genome of the angiosperms and contains the highest percentages of variable sites (Shaw *et al.*, 2007). Thus a high level of species discrimination is possible through this marker (Kress *et al.*, 2005, Shaw *et al.*, 2007). The potential problem is the presence of high rates of insertions/deletions which creates problem in sequence alignment. Great length variation is seen even within closely related taxa and no shared sequence remains in taxonomically distant taxa.

Very short (less than 300 bp) *psbA-trnH* spacer is reported in some taxa (Chase *et al.*, 2006), whereas in some genus like in orchids, the spacer is much longer because it contains copies of *rpl22* and *rps19* making it greater than 1,000 bp (Chang *et al.*, 2006). The pseudogene *rps19* is also found between *trnH* and *psbA* in maize, rice and wheat (Chang *et al.*, 2006). Various representatives of Commelinales, Dioscoreales, Liliales of Commelinales, Dioscoreales, Liliales and Zingiberales also have a copy of *rps19* in this position, but it is absent in representatives of Acorales or Alismatales (Chase *et al.*, 2007). Probably the *rps19-trnH* cluster was duplicated early in the evolution of monocots and in some monocots a copy of *rps19* is positioned between *trnH* and *psbA* (Chang *et al.*, 2006). The length of this spacer is more than 1000 base pairs and this might create a problem while isolating this marker from fragmented or degraded DNA (Chase *et al.*, 2007). Although this non-coding region is more rapidly evolving han genes, this is not true always. In some groups of mosses, *matK* and *rpoC1* was ound to contain more variable positions than this spacer (Chase *et al.*, 2007). Two ther spacers with potential application are *atpF-atpH* and *psbK-psbI*. The later one as good discriminatory power (Hollinsworth *et al.*, 2009).

;ombinations of Various Chloroplast Markers and Spacers

As no plant DNA barcoding marker is universally accepted because of various acunae, a combination of various markers was suggested by different working ;roups. Although the cost will increase, but this approach has the potential of roviding better results because markers will complement each other. The general rinciple of having a multi-locus barcode has been accepted by CBOL. Some popular ombinations used in this approach are as follows.

bcL + matK

The combination of chloroplast *rbcL* and *matK* marker was suggested as he standard barcode for land plants by the CBOL working group (Janzen *et l.*, 2009). This combination is preferred for its universality (rbcL), sequence uality, discrimination (matK), and comparatively lower cost involved. Species liscrimination was successful in 72 per cent of cases in this CBOL approach. Because f its great potential, this combination was provisionally adopted by the Consortium or the Barcode of Life.

bcL + trnH-psbA

The species discrimination success was increased to nearly 88 per cent using he combination of highly variable non-coding trnH-psbA spacer with coding loci ike rbcL. (Kress and Erickson, 2007). This is significant because no single marker as the ability to discriminate among species in a pair in more than 79 per cent of ;enera (Kress and Erickson, 2007).

poC1 + rpoB + matK

This three locus combination was suggested by Chase *et al.* (2005). Although low evolving, the markers *rpoC1* and *rpoB* are easily amplifiable and provide imited resolution. The *matK* region complements for it being more variable (Chase *t al.*, 2007).

poC1 + matK + trnH-psbA

Replacing rpoB with *trnH-psbA* might provide additional species level esolution. Size variation in *trnH-psbA* which creates problem in alignment and its ong length might be a hurdle for isolation from degraded samples (Chase *et al.*, .007).

Iuclear Markers

Theoretically barcoding should be based on nuclear DNA markers because hey are inherited from both parents. This might provide much more information han barcoding based on chloroplast DNA markers which are inherited from only ne parent (Chase and Fay, 2009). The nuclear ribosomal DNA (nrITS) is used outinely for DNA barcoding. nrITS is also popular phylogenetic marker and has a long record of its use for flowering plants (Baldwin, 1992). It is the desired choice when direct sequencing is possible (Thomas, 2009).

Issues with ITS

There are some issues which raise question about wide use of ITS marker. Presence of multiple, divergent paralogs makes nrITS unacceptable as a standard barcoding region across all land plants as it might be potentially misleading (Alveraez and Wendel 2003, Bailey *et al.*, 2003). The recovery rate (amplification and sequencing) might also not be satisfactory always. Another minor concern is that nrITS of fungal contaminants might get amplified (Alveraez and Wendel 2003).

Alternate Sources of Plant DNA Barcoding Markers

Several alternative source of plant DNA markers used for DNA barcoding are discussed in the following section.

Complete Plastid Genome

This alternative was suggested by various research groups (Parks *et al.*, 2009, Nock *et al.*, 2011). Getting a complete plastid genome sequence is not that difficult with next generation sequencing facility. The cost and assembly process might be the matter of concern but the potential of this approach cannot be ignored (Hollingsworth *et al.*, 2011).

Low or Single Copy Nuclear Genes

Nuclear markers for DNA barcoding might be a potential alternative solution (Hollingsworth *et al.*, 2011). Nuclear markers such as waxy, leafy, alcohol dehydrogenase and phytochrome genes etc. are being tried for phylogenetic studies in various groups with different degrees of success (Small *et al.*, 2004). The potential problems involved in this approach might be mutations in primer site, gene duplication, insertion of transposable elements, recombination and heterozygosity etc. (Hollingsworth *et al.*, 2011).

DNA Barcoding in Plant is more Challenging than in Animals

Finding a good marker in plants is a challenging task as there is no *CO1* like-alternative. Till now, there is no consensus has been made about a particular plant DNA barcoding marker. As mentioned above, various chloroplast genes, introns, spacers, nuclear markers and combination of various markers have been proposed. All of these have limitations. Thus search for a *CO1*-like marker is still desirable.

The low rate of nucleotide substitution in plant mitochondrial genomes restricts the use of *CO1* as a universal plant barcode (Fazekas *et al.*, 2008). In addition various factors in plant like polyploidy, hybridization, uniparental inheritance of chloroplast and mitochondria make it more complicated (Hollingsworth *et al.*, 2011).

Internaitonal Bodies working for DNA Barcoding

Consortia

The largest consortia for DNA Barcoding are as follows:

IBOL (The International Barcode of Life Project)

IBOL is the largest biodiversity genomics initiative ever undertaken. It includes hundreds of biodiversity experts in the fields of genomics; technologists and ethicists from 25 nations working together to construct a rich DNA barcode reference library. In their first phase of operations (2010-2015), IBOL has a plan to barcode five million specimens representing five lakh species. In the process of construction of the barcode library, other initiatives like biodiversity conservation, monitoring of ecosystem, forensics and agricultural pest control and invasive species *etc.* are also in focus.

CBOL (The Consortium for the Barcode of Life)

CBOL is an international initiative with a goal of developing DNA barcoding as a global standard for the identification of biological species. It was established in 2004 with support from the Alfred P. Sloan Foundation. CBOL promotes DNA barcoding through various working groups, networks, workshops, conferences, and training etc. CBOL is a huge initiative with 200 member organizations from 50 countries and operates from Washington, DC.

ECBOL (The European Consortium for the Barcode of Life)

ECBOL was established with the initiative of the European Distributed Institute of Taxonomy (EDIT).

Databases

There are two central DNA barcode databases:

BOLD (The Barcode of Life Data Systems)

At the University of Guelph is a public workbench for barcoding projects. In this platform, one can assemble, and analyze their data records in BOLD. BOLD is a very informative database where one can get information about existing barcode, suitable primers and published literature etc. (url: http://www.boldsystems.org/).

INSDC (International Nucleotide Sequence Database Collaboration)

It is a huge database which is a 18 year old collaboration of GenBank, EMBL and DDBJ. They are the permanent public repository for barcode data records in addition to many other resources. (url: http://insdc.org).

Other Organisation Working in the Field of DNA Barcoding

CCDB (Canadian Centre for DNA Barcoding)

It was established in 2006 within the Biodiversity Institute of Ontario (BIO) at the University of Guelph. CCDB is the world's first and largest high-throughput DNA barcoding facility. As per web site approximately 1,442,414 barcodes have been produced till now by CCDB (url: http://ccdb.ca/).

SwissBOL (Swiss Barcode of Life)

It is a national barcoding approach of Switzerland (url: http://www.swissbol.ch/).

RBG Kew

Kew is a member of CBOL. They have collaboration with ten other organizations and support from the Alfred P. Sloan and Gordon and Betty Moore Foundations, A huge collaborative work was initiated for investigating DNA regions for their potential as barcodes for all land plant species (url://www.kew.org/).

Application of Plant DNA Barcoding

DNA Barcoding is used for numerous different purposes. Some of them are as follows:

- ☆ Species identification: The main goal of Barcoding are identification of recognized species and discovery of novel genotypes that may form the basis of subsequent species discovery (Hebert *et al.*, 2004a, b).
- ☆ Biodiversity assessment: Barcoding is a useful tool for assessment of diversity for past and present organisms (Valentini *et al.*, 2008).
- ☆ Diet analysis: To understand the food chain and the functioning of the ecosystem as a whole (Valentini *et al.*, 2008).
- ☆ Complement other field of studies: The vast data generated in barcoding projects complements other area of studies like molecular phylogenetics and population genetics etc. (Hajibabaei *et al.*, 2007).
- ☆ Identification of poisonous plant: Barcoding is successfully employed for identification of poisonous plants, which very important for food safety (Bruni *et al.*, 2010).
- ☆ Authentication of natural health products: This application is important for legal, economic, health and conservation issue (Wallace *et al.*, 2012).
- ☆ Forensic science: Barcoding is successfully employed in Forensic science because only a small amount of DNA might help in solving cases.

Conclusion

The proposals for assignment of the keyword "barcode" to a DNA sequence region in the GenBank, must be accepted by CBOL, before GenBank accepts it. Till now, only *coxI* qualifies for that designation, which is not useful for plants and thus multiple loci and a different approach might be necessary for plants (Chase *et al.*, 2007).

Plant DNA barcoding is still in an infant stage (Chase and Fay 2009). All the reported markers and their combinations carry their own limitations. Plant Barcoding have various other issues which need to be addressed (Chase and Fay 2009). More rapidly evolving nuclear marker might be a potential solution to the problem. Information about DNA barcoding and current projects has been included in the review paper of Singh *et al.*, in this book.

References

Álvarez I, Wendel JF. Ribosomal ITS sequences and plant phylogenetic inference. *Mol. Phylogenet. Evol.* 29: 417–434.2003

Arnot D E., Roper C, Bayoumi RA. Digital codes from hypervariable tandemly repeated DNA sequences in the *Plasmodium falciparum* circumsporozoite gene can genetically barcode isolates. *Mol. Biochem. Parasitol.* 61, 15–24.1993.

Bailey CD, Carr TG, Harris SA, Hughes CE. Characterization of angiosperm nrDNA polymorphism, paralogy, and pseudogenes. *Mol. Phylogenet. Evolu.* 29: 435–455.2003.

Baldwin, B.G. Phylogenetic utility of the internal transcribed spacers of nuclear ribosomal DNA in plants: an example from the Compositae. *Mol. Phylogenet. Evol.* 1: 3–16. 1992.

Bruni I, Mattia FD, Galimberti A, Galasso G *et al.*, Identification of poisonous plants by DNA barcoding approach. *Intl. J. Legal Med.* 124: 595–603.2010.

Casiraghi M, Labra M, Ferri E,Galimbert A, Mattia FD. DNA barcoding: theoretical aspects and practical applications. Nimis P. L., Vignes Lebbe R. (eds.).*Tools for identifying biodiversity: progress and problems.* pp. 269-273. 2010.

Chase, MW, Salamin, N, Wilkinson, M, Dunwell, JM *et al.*, Land plants and DNA barcodes: short-term and long-term goals. *Philos. Trans. Ser. B.* 360: 1889–1895. 2005.

Chang CC, Lin HC, Lin IP *et al.*, Thechloroplast genome of *Phalaenopsis aphrodite* (Orchidaceae): comparative analysis of evolutionary rate with that of grasses and its phylogenetic implications. *Molec. Biol. Evol.* 23: 279–291. 2006.

Chase MW, Cowan RS, Hollingsworth PM, van den Berg C *et al.*, A proposal for a standardised protocol to barcode all land plants. *Taxon.* 56, 295–299.2007.

Chase M W, Fay M F. Barcoding of Plants and Fungi. *Science.* 325: 682-683. 2009.

Chen S, Yao H, Han J *et al.*, Validation of the ITS2 region as a novel DNA barcode for identifying medicinal plant species. *PLoS One.* 5: e8613.2010.

Cox CJ, Goffinet B, Shaw AJ, Boles SB. Phylogenetic relationships among mosses based on heterogeneous Bayesian analysis of multiple genes from multiple genomic compartments. *Syst. Bot.* 29: 234–250.2004.

Cuenoud P, Savolainen V, Chatrou LW, Powell M *et al.*, Molecular phylogenetics of Caryophyllales based on nuclear 18S rDNA and plastid rbcL, atpB, and matK DNA sequences. *Amer. J. Bot.* 89: 132–144.2002.

Doebley J, Durbin M, Golenberg EM, Clegg, MT, Ma DP.Evolutionary analysis of the large subunit of carboxylase (*rbc*L) nucleotide sequence among the grasses (Gramineae). *Evolution.* 44: 1097-1108. 1990.

Erickson D. L., Spouge J, Resch A, Weigt L A, Kress W J. DNA Barcoding in land plants: Developing standards to quantify and maximize. *Taxon.* 57(4): 1304–1316. 2008.

Fazekas AJ, Burgess KS, Kesanakurti PR, Graham SW *et al.*, Multiple multilocus DNA barcodes from the plastid genome discriminate plant species equally well. *PLoS ONE*. 3: e2802. 2008.

Fazekas AJ, Kesanakurti PR, Burgess KS *et al.*, Are plant species inherently harder to discriminate than animal species using DNA barcoding markers? *Mol. Ecol. Resour*. 9(1): 130–139.2009.

Fazekas AJ, Fuzmina ML, Newmaster SG, Hollingsworth PM. *DNA Barcoding methods for land plants*. Kress WJ and Erickson DL (eds.), Springer Sci. 223-252 LLC 2012.

Hajibabaei M, Gregory AC, Herbert PDN, Hickey DA. DNA barcoding: how it complements taxonomy, molecular phylogenetics and population genetics. *Trends Genet*. 23(4): 167-172.2007.

Hamilton MB.Four primer pairs for the amplification of chloroplast intergenic regions with intraspecific variation. *Mol. Ecol*. 8: 513–525.1999.

Hebert PDN, Cywinska A, Ball SL *et al.*, Biological identifications through DNA barcodes. *Proc. R. Soc. Lond. Biol. Sci. Ser. B*. 270: 313–321.2003.

Hebert PDN, Stoeckle MY, Zemlak TS, Francis CM. Identification of birds through DNA barcodes. *PLoS Biol*. 2: 312. 2004a.

Hebert PDN, Penton EH, Burns JM, Janzen DH, Hallwachs W. Ten species in one: DNA barcoding reveals cryptic species in the neotropical skipper butterfly Astraptes fulgerator. *Proc. Natl. Acad. Sci. USA*. 101: 14812—14817. 2004b.

Hilu KW, Liang H. The matK gene: sequence variation and applicationin plant systematics. *Amer. J. Bot*. 84: 830–839. 1997.

Hollingsworth ML, Clark A, Forrest LL, Richardson JR *et al.*, Selecting barcoding loci for plants: evaluation of seven candidate loci with species-level sampling in three divergent groups of land plants. *Mol. Eco. Resour*. 9: 439–457.2009.

Hollingsworth P M, Sean W. Graham, Damon P. L. Choosing and using a plant DNA barcode. *PLoS ONE*. 6 (5): 1-13.2011.

Janzen D. H., A DNA barcode for land plants. *Proc. Natl. Acad. Sci. USA*. 106: 12794-12797.2009.

Johnson LA, Soltis DE. *mat*K DNA sequences and phylogenetic reconstruction in *Saxifragaceae sensustricto*. *Syst. Bot*. 19: 143-156.1994.

Johnson LA, Soltis DE. Phylogenetic inference in *Saxifragaceae sensustricto* and *Gilia* (Polemoniaceae) using *mat*K sequences. *Annl. Mossouri Bot. Gard*. 82: 149-175.1995.

Kress WJ. Wurdack KJ, Zimmer EA, Weight LA, Janzen DH. Use of DNA barcodes to identify flowering plants. *Proc. Natl. Acad. Sci. USA*. 102: 8369–8374.2005.

Kress WJ, Erickson DL. A two-locus global DNA barcode for land plants: the coding rbcL gene complements the non-coding trnH-psbA spacer region. *PLoS ONE*. 2: e508.2007.

Lahaye R, van der Bank M, Bogarin D, Warner J *et al.*, DNA barcoding the floras of biodiversity hotspots. *Proc. Natl. Acad. Sci. USA*. 105, 2923–2928.2008.

Liang H, Hilu KW. Application of the *mat*K gene sequences to grass systematics. *Can. J. Bot*. 74: 125-134. 1996.

Newmaster SG, Fazekas, A.J, Ragupathy **S**. DNA barcoding in land plants: evaluation of *rbcL* in a multigene tiered approach. *Can. J. Bot*. 84: 335–34. 2006.

Nock CJ, Waters DLE, Edwards MA, Bowen SG *et al.*, Chloroplast genome sequences from total DNA for plant identification. *Plant Biotech. J*. 9: 328–333.2011.

Parks M, Cronn R, Liston A Increasing phylogenetic resolution at lowtaxonomic levels using massively parallel sequencing of chloroplast genomes. *BMC Biol*. 7: 84. 2009.

Sandionigi A, Galimberti A, Labra M, Ferri E *et al.*, Analytical approaches for DNA barcoding data – how to find a way for plants? *Plant Biosyst*. 146(4): 805–813.2012.

Sang T, Crawford DJ, Stuessy TF. Chloroplast DNA phylogeny, reticulate evolution and biogeography of *Paeonia* (Paeoniaceae). *Amer. J. Bot*. 84: 1120–1136.1997.

Small RL, Cronn RC, Wendel AS. Use of nuclear genes for phylogeny reconstruction in plants. *Australian Syst. Bot*. 17: 145–170. 2004.

Shaw J, Lickey EB, Beck JT, Farmer SB *et al.*, The tortoise and the hare II: relativeutility of 21 noncoding chloroplast DNA sequences for phylogenetic analysis. *Amer. J. Bot*. 92: 142–166.2005.

Shaw J, Lickey EB, Schilling EE, Small R.L. Comparison of whole chloroplast genome sequences to choose noncoding regions for phylogenetic studies in angiosperms. *Amer. J. Bot*. 94: 275–288.2007.

Steele KP, Vilgalys R. Phylogenetic analyses of Polemoniaceae using nucleotide sequences of the Plastid gene *mat*K. *Syst. Bot*. 19: 126-142.1994.

Sun Y, Skinner DZ, Liang GH, Hulbert SH. Phylogenetic analysis of Sorghum and related taxa using internal transcribed spacers of nuclear ribosomal DNA. *Theo. Appl. Gen*. 89: 26–32.1994.

Taberlet P, Coissac, E, Pompanon, F, Gielly L. Power and limitations of the chloroplast *trnL* (UAA) intron for plant DNA barcoding. *Nucleic Acid Res*. 35: e14.2007.

Tate JA, Simpson BB. Paraphyly of *Tarasa* (Malvaceae) and diverse origins of the polyploid species. *Syst. Bot*. 28: 723–737.2003.

Thomas C. Plant barcode soon to become reality. *Science*. 325: 526. 2009.

Valentini A, Franc¸ Pompanon1 O, Taberlet P. DNA barcoding for ecologists. *Trends Ecol. Evolu*. 30: 1-8.2008.

Vernooy R, Haribabu E, Muller MR, Vogel JH *et al.*, Barcoding life to conserve biological diversity: beyond the taxonomic imperative. *PLoS Biol*. 8(7): 1-5.2010.

Wallace LJ, Boilard SMAL, Eagle SHC, Spal JL *et al.*, DNA barcodes for everyday life: Routine authentication. *Natur. Health Prod. Food Res. Intl.* 49: 446–452.2012

White TJ, Bruns T, Lee S, Taylor J. Amplification and direct sequencing of fungal ribosomal RNA genes for phylogenetics. In: Innis MA, Gelfand DH, Sninsky JJ, White TJ (eds). *PCR protocols: a guide to methods and applications*. Acad. Press New York. pp.315–322. 1990.

Wolfe KH, Morden, CW Palmer JD. Function and evolution of a minimal plastid genome from a nonphotosynthetic parasitic plants. *Proc. Natl. Acad. Sci. USA* 89: 10648-10652. 1992.

2016, Biotechnological Tools for Genetic Resources Pages 75–125
Editor: Pradip Chandra Deka
Published by: Daya Publishing House, NEW DELHI

Chapter 4

MicroRNAs in Plants and Humans

Kamalakshi Devi, Ratna Kalita, Munmi Phukon, Jagajjit Sahu, Ananya Borthakur, Diganta Deka and Priyabrata Sen*

Department of Agricultural Biotechnology, Assam Agricultural University, Jorhat – 785 013, Assam
**E-mail: pbsen14@yahoo.co.in*

ABSTRACT

MicroRNAs (miRNAs) are the family of small, endogenous, non-coding RNAs having huge impact on gene expression and can be regarded as one of the key player in gene regulation. They play important roles in post-transcriptional gene regulation by targeting mRNAs either by cleavage or by translation repression both in plants and animals. However, plant miRNAs are substantially different from animal miRNAs in terms of their sequence, precursor structure, evolutionary origin and biogenesis mechanism. MicroRNAs are recently emerged as powerful regulators of diverse cellular processes viz. cell growth, proliferation, metastasis, apoptosis, and drug resistance with significantly important roles in many human diseases including human Prion brain diseases, Alzheimer, cancer and tissue remodelling. In case of plant, miRNAs are reported to be involved at different stages of development, tissue differentiation, signal transduction, protein degradation, response to different environmental stress and pathogen invasion, and also regulate their own biogenesis. But the aberrant expression of miRNAs, rise through different genomic abnormalities and epigenetic regulation, can cause many adverse effects in the cell or in the organism as a whole. A complete understanding of the mechanism of actions of miRNAs depends on its target genes or transcription factors. Identification of entire sets of miRNAs and their targets will lay the foundation to unravel the complex miRNA mediated regulatory networks that controls entire physiological processes of any organism. Till date, a large number of miRNAs are identified from a wide range of species using expressed sequence tag (EST) and genome survey sequence (GSS) approach. A total of 28,645 hairpin precursor miRNAs from 223 species have been identified and deposited in the publicly available miRNA database, miRBase. The comparative genomics study across a huge number of taxa has shown that many miRNAs are highly conserved through the evolutionary process both in the plant and animal kingdom. This review highlights the current knowledge of how the miRNAs are involved in plant and animal system, genomics, biogenesis, regulatory mechanisms, and their roles in gene regulatory pathways.

Keywords: *miRNA in plants, miRNA in human, Genetic abnormalities, Genomics, Gene regulation, Biogenesis, Regulatory mechanisms.*

Introduction

MicroRNA encompasses an important class of small regulatory molecule that can play fundamental role in regulation and expression of many other gene(s) either by direct cleavage of the mRNA or by translational repression. These small regulatory molecules are ~22-23 nucleotides in length and are known to be involved in myriad physiological processes and as such their deregulation may leads to onset of diseases. Originally identified as moderate biological modifiers, microRNAs have recently emerged as powerful regulators of diverse cellular processes with significantly important roles in disease and tissue remodelling (Rooij, 2011). They can also contribute to human disease as some mRNAs are elevated in certain tumors. Additionally, more than 60 per cent of human protein coding genes are predicted to contain miRNA binding sites within their 3′ untranslated regions (UTRs) (Selbach *et al.*, 2008, Friedman *et al.*, 2009). The diversity and number of miRNAs suggests that a vast number of normal and pathological outcomes may be controlled, at least in part, through miRNA-mediated repression (Davis and Hata, 2009). But to better understand how miRNAs influence various cell activities, it is important to know which miRNAs are acting upon which genes. Considering their sheer number and the fact that each single miRNA can regulate hundreds of target genes, it remains a big challenge. Thus studying the diverse regulatory task performed by these tiny pieces of nucleic acid molecules needs a huge effort and deep understanding of the cross talk between various genes at different levels of their expression.

The miRNA are the key player in post transcriptional gene silencing (PTGS) and the concealed reason of the phenomenon of co-suppression or RNA interference (RNAi). The phenomenon of plant co-suppression was accidentally discovered during attempts to alter the pigmentation of commercial petunia flowers using a genetic transformation approach (Napoli *et al.*, 1990). It was presumed that deeper flower colors might be the result of overexpression of a chalcone synthase gene driven by the constitutive 35S promoter. Instead, both endogenous and transgenic chalcone synthase genes were silenced in these plants, resulting in mosaic flowers with unpigmented white sectors (Napoli *et al.*, 1990). The first miRNA, lin-4, was discovered in 1993 as a small noncoding RNA that regulates *Caenorhabditis elegans* development by negative regulation of lin-14 protein expression (Lee *et al.*, 1993). Since the discovery of the first miRNA gene, *lin-4*, in the nematode *Caenorhabditis elegans*, many more of these short regulatory RNA genes have been identified in flowering plants, worms, flies, fish, frogs and mammals (Alvarez-Garcia and Miska 2005).

The term microRNA was coined in 2001 (Ruvkun 2001). Mature microRNAs (miRNAs) are a class of naturally occurring, endogenous, small non-coding single-stranded RNA molecules, about 21–25 nucleotides in length. MicroRNAs are partially complementary to one or more messenger RNA (mRNA) molecules, and their main function is to down-regulate gene expression in a variety of manners, including translational repression, mRNA cleavage, and deadenylation.

Recently, the miRNA research is proliferated in multidimensional fields. That includes studying its existence in various living systems starting from bacteria to human and plants to animals; its use in cellular process regulation, in cancer studies, virus protection in plant and other systems, drug discovery, on various medical use and therapeutic potential etc. In this chapter application of miRNA and recent advancements in plants and humans are discussed.

Processing of miRNA

The discovery of miRNA revealed that this is a natural phenomenon that is present in almost all organisms at various intensities. Then efforts were made to understand the biogenesis of miRNA in a living system. Various researchers reported that miRNAs are produced from either their own genes or from introns (Volk and Shomron 2011). The majority of the characterized miRNA genes are intergenic or oriented antisense to neighboring genes and are therefore suspected to be transcribed as independent units (Lee and Ambros 2001, Lagos *et al.*, 2001, Lau *et al.*, 2001, Lee *et al.*, 2004). The primary transcript produces a large primary (pri) and precursor (pre) transcripts that undergo various processing steps along their biogenesis pathway till they reach their mature and functional form. MicroRNA genes are transcribed in most cases by RNA polymerase II into primary miRNA transcripts (pri-miRNA) (Borchert *et al.*, 2006). The primary microRNA (pri-miRNA) is then cleaved into 70–110 nucleotide long precursor miRNA (pre-miRNA) by a complex called the microprocessor that contains DROSHA and DGCR8 (DiGeorge critical region 8) as well as additional proteins. DROSHA is an RNase III enzyme and DGCR8 is a protein that is essential for miRNA processing (also known as Pasha) (Lee *et al.*, 2003). After nuclear processing, Exportin-5 in a complex with Ran-GTP61 exported the pre-miRNA to the cytoplasm (Yi *et al.*, 2003). Once the pre-miRNA reached the cytoplasm the RNase III protein Dicer cleaves off the loop of the pre-miRNA and generates a roughly 22-nucleotide miRNA duplex. The functional strand of the mature miRNA is loaded together with Argonaute (Ago2) proteins into RISC complex (RNA induced silencing complex) (Chendrimada *et al.*, 2005). However, it is not clear, whether all miRNAs are processed similarly or not. Volk and Shomron (2011) reported that the ratio between pre-miRNA and mature miRNA forms varies between different miRNAs. Moreover, over-expression of several factors involved in miRNA biogenesis, including Exportin-5, DROSHA, NF90a, NF45 and KSRP, displayed bidirectional effects on pre/mature miRNA ratios, suggesting their intricate biogenesis sensitivity. Thus, they suspected the presence of some additional factors that differentially regulate the expression of various miRNAs. In an experiment to identify additional factors that might explain the versatility in miRNA biogenesis they have analyzed the contribution of two hnRNP family members, hnRNPH1 and hnRNPR. Knock-down or over-expression of these genes suggested that hnRNPR inhibits, whereas hnRNPH1 facilitates, miRNA processing. Overall, threir results emphasize that miRNA biogenesis is versatile.

Biogenesis of miRNA

The biogenesis of miRNA and its functioning is a highly regulated phenomenon. Widespread use of miRNA arrays to profile microRNA expression has indicated that the levels of many miRNAs are altered during development and disease. These findings have prompted a great deal of investigation into the mechanism and function of miRNA-mediated repression. However, the mechanisms which govern the regulation of microRNA biogenesis and activity are just beginning to be uncovered. The miRNA are generated through the concerted action of multi-subunit complexes which promote the sequential cleavage, export, and loading of miRNA into silencing complexes following transcription. It is increasingly clear that miRNA biogenesis does not proceed in a disambiguous manner. But, with increasing number of reports, it become more and more evident that each of these steps serves as a potential point of regulation, and therefore provides additional complexity to miRNA-dependent gene regulation, as well as, individual classes of miRNAs are differentially regulated through the association of regulatory factors with the core miRNA biogenesis machinery (Davis and Hata, 2009).

The activity of miRNA-mediated repression is highly regulated by diverse factors. The use of proteomics approaches have identified dozens of Ago associated proteins, and the differential association of these proteins allows for the modification of RISC activity (Hock *et al.*, 2007). For example, the members of the TRIM-NHL family of proteins, including TRIM32 in mouse (Schwamborn *et al.*, 2009), and NHL-2 in *C. elegans* (Hammell *et al.*, 2009), associate with RISC components and enhance the activity of miRNA. Interestingly, sequencing of TRIM32-associated miRNAs indicates that only a subset of miRNAs, including let-7a, interact with TRIM32. These findings emphasize that miR-mediated repression could be regulated by alterations in the biogenesis as well as the activity of RISCassociated miRNA. Further, the association of miRNA with specific RISC factors can result in increased translation of target genes (Vasudevan and Steitz 2007, Vasudevan *et al.*, 2007). The biological function of miRNA can also be altered indirectly by modification of the mRNA target site. For instance, the ability of a miRNA to repress a given mRNA is limited by the presence of miRNA binding sites within the 3′UTR. Analysis of alternative 3′UTR isoforms indicates a global reduction of 3′UTR length in proliferating cells (Sandberg *et al.*, 2008), while differentiating cells express mRNAs with longer 3′UTRs (Ji *et al.*, 2009). As shortened 3′UTRs contain fewer miRNA binding sites, mRNAs in proliferating cells are more resistant to miRNA-dependent repression (Sandberg *et al.*, 2008). It is speculated that the effects of both reduced expression of miRNAs, and increased expression of mRNAs with shorter 3′UTRs may synergistically contribute to pathogenesis of some human diseases, such as cancer.

Methods for Identification of miRNA

The discovery of miRNA have been done mainly using two major approaches: Genetic approach and Computational approach. Genetic approaches largely rely on two main strategies: (i) forward genetics (ii) direct cloning. The first ever miRNAs lin-4 and let-7 were identified in *Caenorhabditis elegans* using forward genetics method (Lee and Ambros 2001, Lau *et al.*, 2001). Forward genetics is the classical technique based on clear phenotypes where the phenotype is known but the DNA sequence coding for that phenotype is unknown (Kim and Nam, 2006).

Direct cloning methods deals with the cloning and sequencing of small RNA by construction of cDNA library for endogenous small RNAs (Chen *et al.*, 2005). The main pitfall of using this method is that while cDNA cloning, fragments of other non-coding RNAs besides miRNAs (such as rRNA, tRNA, SnRNA) and also mRNAs are cloned from size fractionated RNA samples. Hence this process is limited only fior highly expressed miRNAs as low expressed miRNAs are hard to clone (Ambros 2004). Repeats showed that most of the miRNAs are tissue and time specific with a low expression level and also in most cases their expression is specific to the environment stimuli. Sometimes they coexist with their cleaved and degraded target mRNAs.

The genetic approaches are limited as these are expensive, time consuming and dominated by chance and serendipity (Lai, 2003). To overcome these limitations, computational (bioinformatics) approaches were used to identify miRNAs. The basic principle that made computational approaches widely used is that miRNA are conserved across different species. Using computational tools and databases the homologus miRNAs can be identified in other species using preliminarily identified miRNA sequences (Weber, 2005). The exponentially growing sequence data in the public repositories also makes the computational approaches the best.

Bioinformatics Approach

The bioinformatics approaches uses computational tools and databases for discovering miRNA information. Broadly it is done in three steps: (i) Identification of miRNAs, (ii) Secondary structure analysis, (iii) Target prediction.

Several standalone and web-based software are available for identification of miRNAs in nucleotide sequences. The underlying principle in most of the tools is the conservation of miRNA sequences within and between species. The best way to identify miRNA is by comparing the nucleotide sequences with the known miRNA sequences and finding the homologs. Numerous public repositories have been reported which contains information regarding miRNAs identified with the help of genetic approaches. The most widely used public repository, miRBase is a searchable database of published miRNA sequences and annotation (Kozomara and Griffiths-Jones 2011). Users can easily search and download both hairpin and mature sequences available in the database. Each sequence entry in the miRBase represents a predicted hairpin portion of a miRNA transcript (termed mir), with information on the location and sequence of the mature miRNA sequence (termed miR). Another database, deepBase is a platform for annotating and discovering small and long ncRNAs (microRNAs, siRNAs, piRNAs) from next generation sequencing data (Yang *et al.*, 2009). This database allows the mapping, storage, retrieval, analysis, integration, annotation, mining and visualization of next generation sequencing data from different technological platforms, tissues and cell lines of different organisms. MicroRNA.org (http://www.microrna.org) is a comprehensive resource of microRNA experimentally observed microRNA expression patterns and predicted microRNA targets and target down regulation scores (Betel *et al.* 2008). Various other databases available for easy identification of miRNAs such as miRGen 2.0: a database of microRNA genomic information and regulation (Alexiou *et al.*, 2010), miRNAMap: genomic maps of microRNA genes and their target genes in mammalian genomes (Hsu *et al.*, 2008), PMRD: plant microRNA database (Zhang *et al.*, 2010) *etc.*

Generally BLAST is used for sequence similarity of given nucleotide sequences with the known miRNA sequence. A standalone BLAST program can be downloaded from the NCBI website and can be configured on a local server or personal computer for betterment of the comparison of sequences. There is other software like C-mii (Numnark *et al.*, 2012) which identifies the mature miRNA sequences in the nucleotide sequences with BLAST algorithm underlying.

Secondary Structure Analysis

MicroRNAs come from endogenous transcripts that can form single molecule fold-back (hairpin) structures. Generally after the homologous sequence are found, using computational tools the secondary structures are analysed for a hairpin structure. There are a number of RNA secondary structure prediction tools. The mfold package consists of a group of programs written in FORTRAN or C, and a group of Bourne shell or perl scripts (Zuker 2003). Both web and standalone versions are available for this tool. Upon input of a nucleotide sequence the output results with probable secondary structures with free energy.

All the structures should satisfy the criteria given below to make sure that they are different from all other small RNAs (Wang *et al.*, 2005).

1. The newly identified mature miRNA sequences should not have more than 4 mismatches with the respective previously known miRNA.
2. Precursor miRNA sequence should form a stem loop structure with mature miRNA at one arm.
3. No more than 6 mismatches between the potential mature miRNA sequence and the opposite miRNA*.
4. Minimal Free Energy (MFE) of secondary structures should have a higher negative value.

Target Prediction

Initially classical genetic techniques were being used to predict the miRNA targets (Lee *et al.*, 1993). To overcome the labour-intense and time consuming methods, researchers started to use computational approaches to predict miRNA targets. Most studies have found that miRNAs bind to the 3′-untranslated region (3′UTR) of their target mRNAs to suppress the translation. Thus, for miRNA target prediction, the computational tools depend heavily on complementarily between the mature miRNA sequence and the target sequence. In order to maximize the specificity, the prediction method combine 5′ seed matches, thermodynamic stability and evolutionary conservation analysis. However, the mechanism may be further modified in a specific manner depending upon the species (Bartel 2004, Lai 2004). Plant miRNAs have perfect or nearly perfect complementarities whereas in the case of animals the complementarities are limited. So the target prediction for animal miRNAs is relatively complicated and unspecific compared to plant miRNAs (Watanabe *et al.*, 2007).

Several methods have been subsequently developed for computational identification of miRNA targets. Lewis *et al.* (2003) developed TargetScan, an algorithm employing thermodynamics-based modelling of miRNA-mRNA interactions and comparative sequence analysis for the prediction of miRNA targets conserved across multiple genomes such as human, mouse, rat and pufferfish (Lewis *et al.*, 2003). Originally developed for the prediction of miRNA target genes in *D. melanogaster* (Enright *et al.*, 2003), miRanda algorithm was later improved by John *et al.* (2004). A strict model using dynamic programming to search for optimal sequence complementarities between a set of mature microRNAs and a given mRNA was employed for miRNA target prediction. Kiriakidou *et al.* (2004) used Diana-microT, one of the first target prediction tools and experimental approaches to identify human microRNA targets (Kiriakidou *et al.*, 2004). The tool was also able to work successfully in all validated *C. elegans* miRNA targets. Based on sequence complementarities, thermodynamic stability calculations, and evolutionary conservation among species, various other methods were also developed to determine the likelihood of a productive miRNA:mRNA duplex formation (Bartel 2004, Lai 2004). Another algorithm RNAhybrid (Rehmsmeier *et al.*, 2004, Kruger and Rehmsmeier 2006) is an extension to a RNA secondary structure prediction algorithm like the Mfold program (Zuker 2003) and RNAfold (Hofacker and Stadler 2003) which determines the most favourable hybridization site between two sequences. The basic principle in this method was to use an artificial linker between miRNA and binding site as the classical methods were designed for single sequence folding which sometimes lead to artefacts in prediction and intramolecular hybridizations or hybridization of the target and miRNA sequence with the linker. Grun *et al.* (2005) first used PicTar for predicting miRNA targets across seven Drosphila species. Unlike the methods like TargetScan which requires a seed match at exactly corresponding positions in a cross-species UTR alignment, PicTar filters binding sites based on thermodynamic stability, hidden Markov model (HMM) maximum likelihood scores and statistical methods to reduce false positives. Krek *et al.* (2005) predicted 13 targets using PicTar and validated 7 out of them experimentally. They also suggested that on the average, each vertebrate miRNA has approximately 200 targets. Also in another study a modified version of PicTar and sequence alignments of three nematodes were used for genome-wide search of miRNA targets in C. Elegans which showed that at least 10 per cent of the genes are predicted miRNA targets (Lall *et al.*, 2006).

Target Prediction Issues

However, there are a few issues associated with the miRNA target prediction which hampers the analysis. The short length of miRNA makes the ranking and scoring of the targets difficult as most of the conventional sequence alignment algorithm and statistical techniques require longer sequences (Karlin *et al.*, 1990). Identification of 3′ UTRs is a vital step for the prediction of targets which greatly depends on the knowledge of species specific 3′UTR information. Though in *Drosophila* and human, the transcripts are well defined, in other mammals, the location, extent or splice variation of 3′UTRs are still poorly understood (Hubbard *et al.*, 2002). In a large scale analysis such as prediction of targets in a whole genome, a higher degree of specificity (few false positives) is more important than sensitivity (few false negatives). But if the prediction is for a gene of interest or so, then the sensitivity is the most important criteria (Lai, 2004). So while performing the prediction the criteria of choice changes according to the cases.

To make the prediction of miRNA targets more vivid, researchers are developing web-based server which integrates prediction tools and various repositories such as miRBase, Ensembl, Swiss-prot, UCSC genome browser, KEGG pathway, etc. This combination predicts miRNA targets and several other associated information such as functions, pathways etc. TarBase 5.0 stores the experimentally validated miRNA targets and extensive information by linking to databases like Ensembl, Swiss-prot, Hugo and HGNC (Sethupathy *et al.*, 2006, Papadopoulos *et al.*, 2009). Another database miRGator contains information regarding functions, gene expression data and genome annotation and for the prediction of targets uses Boolean logic to combine the results of TargetScan, miRanda and PicTar (Nam *et al.*, 2008). For target prediction and ontology clustering in human miRNAs, GOmir was developed (Roubelakis *et al.*, 2009). It contains two java models *i.e.* JTarget consisting of 4 prediction tools (TargetScan, miRanda, RNAHybrid, PicTar) and TargBase, an experimental database and TAGGO performs GO clustering with the common genes resulted from JTarget. Hausser *et al.* (2009) developed MirZ, a web server which incorporates smiRNAdb miRNA expression atlas (Landgraf *et al.*, 2007) and the EIMMo miRNA target prediction algorithm (Gaidatzis *et al.*, 2007). Nam *et al.* (20009) developed a web server named MIMA (miRNA and mRNA integrated analysis) which selects up- and down-regulated miRNAs from input data and predicts the targets using TargetScan, PicTar or PITA (Probability of Interaction by Target Accessibility). Kertesz *et al.*, 2007) and the final output contains information regarding associated diseases, transcription factors, GO terms, KEGG pathways. Another successful online database system is miRDB (Wang, 2008). It uses a wiki interface with editable section for miRNA functional annotations and uneditable official sections containing miRNA names, Sanger accessions, sequences and genomic locations and target predictions which are predicted using MirTarget2 (Wang and Ei Naqa 2008).

MicroRNA in Plants

MicroRNAs in plants were identified about a decade ago. They are a large class of highly conserved small RNAs (21 nucleotides long) and are produced from nonprotein-coding genes. Initially RNA polymerase II-mediated transcription yields capped and polyadenylated primary miRNA precursors (pri-miRNA) which contain typical stem-loop regions. The pri-miRNA precursors are processed in two steps by the RNAse III enzyme Dicer-like 1 (DCL1) and its double-strand RNA binding (DRB) partner HYL1. A double-stranded miRNA intermediate (duplex miR:miR*) is yielded (Bartel 2004, Jones-Rhoades *et al.*, 2006, Mallory *et al.*, 2008, Vazquez 2006) which is then methylated by HEN1 (Yu *et al.*, 2005). Recently evolved MIR genes involve the use of DCL4 and other DCL proteins for production of miRNAs (Rajagopalan *et al.*, 2006, Vazquez *et al.*, 2008). The miRNA duplex consists of the mature miRNA and an almost complementary miRNA* strand (Jones-Rhoades *et al.*, 2006). The miRNAs are transferred from the nucleus to the cytoplasm via the transporter HASTY. The single stranded mature miRNAs are then incorporated into an RNA-induced silencing complex (RISC) which contains a protein of the ARGONAUTE (AGO) family. In this complex they serve as a guide for sequence-specific recognition of protein-coding mRNAs, mediate their cleavage and/or inhibit their translation (Brodersen *et al.*, 2008, Lanet *et al.*, 2009). Once the mature miRNA is recruited by the RISC (RNA-Induced Silencing Complex), the miRNA* strand gets degraded (Jones-Rhoades *et al.*, 2006). MicroRNA-targeted genes are very essential for transcription factors and F-box proteins in plants.They play crucial roles at major stages of development and regulate the expression of some key developmental as well as stress-related genes. The miRNA functions in plants include control of tissue (leaf, root, stem and flower) differentiation and development, phase switch from vegetative growth to reproductive growth, signal transduction and response to different biotic and abiotic stress (*e.g.* salinity, drought and pathogens) (Chen 2005, Zhang *et al.*, 2006c). The plant miRNAs occur in gene families (Jones-Rhoades *et al.*, 2006) and it appears that most plant miRNAs are produced from their own transcriptional units and are generally not located within protein-coding genes (Reinhart *et al.*, 2002). Isolation and cloning of small RNAs from biological samples have helped to identify small plant RNAs (Llave *et al.*, 2002, Mette *et al.*, 2002, Park *et al.*, 2002, Reinhart *et al.*, 2002, Sunkar *et al.*, 2005, Sunkar and Zhu 2004, Griffiths-Jones 2004). Several hundred miRNAs have been identified in plants through direct cloning and sequencing of small cellular RNAs or comparative genomics (Griffiths-Jones *et al.*, 2006, Zhang *et al.*, 2006b). Among them 184 were from *Arabidopsis thaliana*, 242 from rice, 215 from *Populus trichocarpa* (Griffiths-Jones *et al.*, 2006) and 118 from maize (Zhang *et al.*, 2006a). Very few reports are available on the identification of mutations at miRNA loci in genetic screens. Forward genetic screens helped to identify a plant miRNA responsible for loss-of-function allele, which resulted in flowers with extra petals in *Arabidopsis* (Baker *et al.*, 2005). Three plant miRNAs namely, miR319, miR172 and miR166 were identified and isolated in overexpression screens for dominant mutants (Aukerman and Sakai 2003, Kim *et al.*, 2005, Palaknik *et al.*, 2003, Williams *et al.*, 2005). Several groups also devised bioinformatic approaches specific to plant miRNA identification (Adai *et al.*, 2005, Bonnet 2004, Jones-Rhoades and Bartel 2004, Wang *et al.*, 2004) and were able to identify targets for nearly all miRNAs.

Zhang *et al.* (2008b) used the publicly available miRNAs identified in nine plant species to search the conserved tomato miRNA homologues in the EST, GSS, CoreNucleotide databases and BACs sequences. By this method they were able to predict a total of 13 potential miRNAs. Tomato RNAs from NCBI was further blasted using these potential miRNA sequence and 23 potential target genes were found which were mostly associated with the phase change from vegetative to generative growth, flower development and with responding to plant hormone and virus stress.

Cuperus *et al.* (2010) found that the miRNAs in this family are largely 22 nucleotides long and are known to be associated with the ability to generate secondary trans-acting siRNAs. The generation of secondary siRNAs and accumulation of cleaved target mRNAs in phase with R482 provided direct evidence of a cascade of miR482-mediated regulation of NBS-LRR gene expression.

Solanaceous Species

Kim *et al.* (2011) identified miRNAs and their target genes by analyzing expressed sequence tag (EST) data from five different Solanaceae species. Bioinformatic analysis of the EST data of these species revealed the presence of at least 11 miRNAs and 54 target genes in pepper (*Capsicum annuum* L.), 22 miRNAs and 221 target genes in potato (*Solanum tuberosum* L.), 12 miRNAs and 417 target genes in tomato (*Solanum lycopersicum* L.), 46 miRNAs and 60 target genes in tobacco (*Nicotiana tabacum* L.), and 7 miRNAs and 28 target genes in *Nicotiana benthamiana*.

Computational prediction of potential miRNAs from potato revealed 71 miRNAs belonging to 48 families (Yang *et al.*, 2010). Specific stem-loop RT primers were designed for verification of the predicted miRNAs and real-time PCR assays were used to profile the expression levels of seven miRNAs from different tissues of potato. The results showed that most of the selected miRNAs had their highest expression levels in leaves. Xie *et al.* (2011) used a newly modified comparative genome strategy and identified a total of 202 potential potato miRNAs which belong to 78 families. A total of 1094 miRNA targets were predicted which encode transcription factors as well as genes that function in stress response, signal transduction, and a variety of other metabolic processes. Gene ontology (GO) analysis implicated that these miRNA targets were involved in 545 biological processes. Twenty eight of these targets were involved in processes related to potato defence mechanisms against bacteria, viruses, and fungi, the metabolism of molecules such as carbon, sucrose, starch, and lipid, and the development of primary and lateral roots. Again pathway enrichment analysis, based on the Kyoto Encyclopedia of Genes and Genomes (KEGG), demonstrated that the identified miRNAs participated in 98 metabolism networks which include sucrose metabolism, fatty acid metabolism, amino acid metabolism, carbon fixation, and the biosynthesis of plant hormones.

Zhang *et al.* (2009) identified 48 potential miRNAs in potato, using previously known miRNAs from *Arabidopsis*, rice and other plant species against expressed sequence tags (ESTs), genomic survey sequence (GSS) and nucleotide databases. These miRNAs may regulate 186 potential targets involved in floral, leaf, root, and stem development, signal transduction, metabolism pathways, and stress responses. A RT-PCR analysis was performed to validate the prediction of the miRNAs it was found that potato miRNAs have diverse expression patterns during development.

Cotton

In cotton, thirty potential cotton miRNAs were found using a comparative genomic approach based on genomic survey sequence analysis and miRNA secondary structure which belong to 22 miRNA families. At least 3 miRNA families miR 396, 414, and 782) target transcriptional factors like callous synthase, fiber protein Fb23, and fiber quinoneoxidoreductase, suggesting that miRNAs play an important role in cotton fiber differentiation and development (Zhang *et al.*, 2007).

Soybean

Zhang *et al.* (2008a) identified 69 miRNAs belonging to 33 families in the domesticated soybean (*Glycine max*) and five miRNAs in the two wild species of soybean *viz. Glycine soja* and *Glycine clandestine* using comparative genomics. TaqMan(R) miRNA Assay analyses demonstrated that these miRNAs were differentially expressed in soybean tissues. A detailed sequence analyses also revealed that soybean pre-miRNAs vary in length from 44 to 259 nt, harbor mature miRNAs that differ in their physical location within the pre-miRNAs, and encode more than a single mature miRNA. A comparative sequence analyses of soybean miRNA sequences demonstrated that uracil is the dominant base in the first position at the 5′ end of the mature miRNAs while cytosine is dominant at the 19th position. This is indicative of the fact that these two bases may have important roles in miRNA biogenesis and/or miRNA-mediated gene regulation. Five antisense miRNAs were identified and their sense partners from soybean belonged to three miRNA families (miR-157, miR-162 and miR-396). A total of 152 miRNA-targeted mRNAs were predicted based on previously established *in silico* methods. This included mRNAs that encode transcription factors that regulate plant growth and development and mRNAs that encode environmental signal transduction proteins and central metabolic processes.

Wheat

In wheat (*Triticum aestivum*), computational identification of miRNAs from EST sequences was carried out by using the in-house program GenomicSVM, a prediction model for miRNAs. This study resulted in the discovery of 79 miRNA candidates. Twenty two miRNA representatives were randomly selected from the 79 miRNA candidates and 9 of them were experimentally validated with Northern blotting, which indicated that prediction accuracy is about 40 per cent. For these 9 validated miRNAs, 59 wheat ESTs were predicted as their putative targets (Jin *et al.*, 2008).

Apple

In apple (*Malus domestica*) cv Royal Gala about 120,000 expressed sequence tags (ESTs) were analysed which led to the identification of 10 distinct sequences that could be classified into 7 conserved plant miRNA families (miR156, miR159, miR162, miR167, miR172, miR393 and miR398). The secondary structure predictions indicated that these sequences have the characteristic fold-back structures of precursor miRNAs. Northern analysis validated the presence of these miRNA families within Royal Gala tissues. Some of the miRNAs were expressed constitutively in all the tissues tested (miR159, miR162 and miR172), while the others showed more restricted patterns of expression; some of them being expressed primarily in leaf (miR398), some expressed in leaf and floral bud tissue but down-regulated during fruit development (miR156 and miR167) or expressed in fungal pathogen-infected leaf tissue (miR393). The potential targets for six of the miRNA families were identified from the EST dataset and completely sequenced complementary deoxyribonucleic acids (Gleave *et al.*, 2008). Yu *et al.* (2011) discovered 31 potential miRNAs which belong to 16 miRNA families from more than 324 000 EST sequences of apple (*Malus domestica*). Precise sequences were validated by miR-RACE which is a newly developed method for the determination of the potential miRNAs predicted computationally. The expression of the 16 microRNAs were detected in apple young leaf, old leaf, young stem, flower bud, flower and developing fruits by quantitative RT-PCR (qRT-PCR). Some of them showed tissue-specific expression. Fifty-six potential targets were identified for the 16 apple miRNAs. Most of them were transcription factors that play important roles in apple development. Twelve target genes were experimentally verified by qRT-PCR.

Taxus Chinensis

High thoroughput Illumina sequencing was employed to identify miRNAs from *Taxus chinensis* and the effect of the taxoid elicitor methyl jasmonate (MJ) on miRNA expression was investigated by Qiu *et al.* (2009).

Switchgrass

In switchgrass, 121 potential miRNAs were identified which belong to 44 families, using a well-defined comparative genome-based computational approach. MicroRNA clusters and antisense miRNAs in switchgrass expressed sequences tags were also identified which potentially target 839 protein-coding genes, which can act as transcription factors, and take part in multiple biological and metabolic processes. The Gene ontology (GO) analysis of these targets, showed that 527 biological processes were involved and twenty-five of these processes were demonstrated to participate in the metabolism of carbon, glucose, starch, fatty acid, and lignin and in xylem formation (Xie *et al.*, 2010).

Citrus

Song *et al.* (2010) developed a comprehensive strategy for identifying new miRNA homologues by mining the repository of available citrus expressed sequence tags (ESTs). They were able to identify a total of 38 potential miRNAs. Nine of them were identified in *Citrus trifoliata* (ctr-miRNAs), 5 in *C. clementina* (ccl-miRNAs), 9 in *C. reticulata* (crt-miRNAs) and 15 in *C. sinensis* (csi-miRNAs) from more than 430,000 EST sequences in citrus. Using the potential miRNA sequences, and with the help of A further BLAST search of the mRNA database, six potential target genes in these citrus species were found. Eight of these miRNAs were selected to verify their existence in citrus using Northern blotting. These miRNAs may regulate expression of their target genes by cleavage, which is the most common situation in gene regulation mediated by plant miRNAs.

Brassica

In *Brassica rapa* L. 186 miRNAs belonging to 55 families were identified using comparative genomics. The mature and pre-miRNAs identified ranged in length from 18-22 and 66-305 nucleotides, respectively. A comparison of 4 nucleotides revealed that uracil is the predominant base in the first position of *B. rapa* miRNA.

This suggests that it plays an important role in miRNA-mediated gene regulation. Adenine and guanine were found to be predominant in mature miRNAs, whereas adenine and uracil were predominant in pre-miRNA sequences. One DNA sequence belonging to the BrMiR 399 family was identified which produce both sense and antisense mature miRNAs. This sequence differs by 1 nucleotide at the 20th position. *In silico analyses* predicted the presence of 66 miRNA target mRNAs for 33 miRNA families. Northern blot and qRT-PCR analyses of RNA samples prepared from different tissues for 17 miRNA families indicated that miRNAs are differentially expressed in different tissues of *B. rapa* (Dhandapant *et al.*, 2011). In Chinese cabbage 168 potential miRNAswere identified which were derived from 22 EST and 119 GSS sequences and classified into 38 miRNA families by well-defined computational analysis.Most of the miRNAs belonged to the miRNA1533, miRNA156, and miRNA2911 families. There were 129 identified miRNAs potentially targeting 1386 Chinese cabbage EST genes playing important roles in multiple biological and metabolic processes including metabolism, cell growth, signal transduction, stress response, and plant development. The gene ontology analysis which was carried out based on these target proteins, showed that 688 genes were involved in molecular functions, 532 in biological processes and 287 in cellular components. The Kyoto Encyclopedia of Genes and Genomes (KEGG) pathway analysis demonstrated that these miRNAs participated in 214 metabolism pathways which include plant-pathogen interaction, fatty acid metabolism, amino acid metabolism, nitrogen metabolism, plant hormone signal transduction (Wang *et al.*, 2011). Wang *et al.* (2012) identified 193 potential miRNA candidates from 17 expressed sequence tag (ESTs) and 152 genome survey sequences (GSSs) in *Brassica oleracea*. These miRNA candidates were classified into 70 families which were carried out using a well-defined comparative genome-based computational analysis. Most of the miRNAs belong to the miRNA169, miR5021, miR156 and miR158 families. Thirty Six of the miRNA families were found for the first time in *Brassica* species. About 1393 *B. oleracea* genes were predicted to be as candidate targets of 175 miRNAs. This mutual relationship between miRNAs and the candidate target genes was verified using quantitative real-time polymerase chain reaction (qRT-PCR) and 52 RLM-RACE analyses and the expression patterns in different tissues (*i.e.*, roots, young leaves, mature stems, and flowers) was analyzed. Gene Ontology (GO) analysis showed that the 818, 514, and 265 target 818 target genes are involved in molecular functions, 514 in biological processes, and 265 in cellular component respectively. The Kyoto Encyclopedia of Genes and Genomes (KEGG) Pathway enrichment analysis suggested that these miRNAs may regulate 186 metabolic pathways which including those of lipid, energy, starch and sucrose, fatty acid and nitrogen.

Lettuce

In the Asteraceae family, conserved miRNAs in lettuce (*Lactuca sativa*) were identified by using EST (expressed sequence tag) analysis (Han *et al.*, 2010). All previously known miRNAs in other plant species were blasted against lettuce EST sequences and novel miRNAs were selected in lettuce by following a series of filtering criteria. A total of 21 conserved miRNAs belonging to 12 miRNA families and 63 potential target genes were found in lettuce. The conservation and evolution of lettuce miRNAs and their counterparts in other plant species were analyzed. This revealed that inspite of miRNAs being highly conserved, some specific sites are likely to mutate. An RT-PCR approach was employed to confirm the expression of identified miRNAs in lettuce. Eight out of the 12 miRNA families could be detected which suggest that these 8 miRNA families do exist in lettuce. All the identified lettuce miRNAs were used to search their potential target genes by miRU web-server from TIGR database available at http://www.tigr.org. Some of the miRNA targets were transcription factors which were involved in lettuce growth and development, metabolism, and stress responses.

Safflower and Sunflower

High-throughput Illumina sequencing technology was used to the small RNA transcriptomes of safflower (*Carthamus tinctorius* L.) seed, flower, and leaf. It was found that at least 236 known miRNAs were expressed in safflower, out of which 100 miRNAs with relatively high expression abundance exhibited evolutionary conservation across multiple plants. A comparison of the expression of abundance of these miRNAs among different tissues showed that a total of 116, 133, and 128 miRNAs were differentially expressed with higher abundance or lower abundance between safflower seed/leaf, seed/petal, and leaf/petal. Moreover, 13 putative novel miRNAs had also been identified in safflower. The small RNA transcriptomes thus obtained in this investigation paved the way for further investigation of the physiological roles of identified miRNAs in safflower (Li *et al.*, 2011). Expressed sequence tag (EST) analysis was also used to identify potential conserved miRNAs and their putative target genes in the Asteraceae. Quantitative Real-Time PCR (qRT-PCR) was applied to confirm the expression of eight potential miRNAs in safflower (*C. tinctorius*) and sunflower (*Helianthus annuus*). Five out of eight miRNAs are differentially expressed during cotyledon development. These findings suggest that miRNAs may be involved in the regulation of gene expression during seed germination and the formation of the cotyledons in the Asteraceae. Using qRT-PCR analysis the differential expression pattern of five newly identified miRNAs during five different cotyledon growth stages in safflower was also investigated. These methods helped to identify and characterize 151 potentially conserved miRNAs, belonging to 26 miRNA families, in 11 genus of Asteraceae. The EST analysis predicted that the newly identified conserved Asteraceae miRNAs target 130 total protein-coding ESTs in sunflower and safflower, and 433 additional target genes in other plant species. The existence of seven predicted miRNAs, (miR156, miR159, miR160, miR162, miR166, miR396 and miR398) was confirmed experimentally in safflower and sunflower seedlings (Feshani *et al.*, 2012).

Aquilaris sinensis

Gao *et al.* (2012) employed the small RNA high-throughput sequencing and 454 transcriptome data to identify conserved as well as novel miRNAs in *Aquilaria sinensis*. A total of 27 novel miRNAs were discovered by in silico analysis of the small RNA deep sequencing data and transcriptome data. Again, 74 putative conserved miRNAs were identified based on the mature miRNA sequence conservation. Ten of them were confirmed with hairpin forming precursor. A novel miRNA sequence was determined to be the miRNA* of asi-miR408, but with accumulation much higher than asimiR408. This high accumulation of miRNA* of asi-miR408 implied thar miRNA*s would be functional in plants alongwith the miRNAs. The expression levels of ten stress-responsive miRNAs were also examined after wound treatment. Eight of them were found to be wound-responsive.

A total of 58 miRNAs were identified belonging to 25 miRNA families. Fifty six of them were conserved between angiosperms and gymnosperms. Two of them appeared to be gymnosperm-specific. MJ treatment showed significantly changed abundance in the expression of specific miRNAs. Fourteen miRNAs from 7 different families (miR156, miR168, miR169, miR172, miR396, miR480 and mir1310) were downregulated and 3 miRNAs from 2 families (miR164 and miR390) were upregulated. Legrand *et al.* (2010) predicted 18 conserved miRNAs in a clary sage (*Salvia sclarea* L) calyx EST library using 454pyrosequencing technology. Fifteen of them were present in most studied plant species and the others only shared limited or discrete plant lineages. Data mining was separately conducted for the same clary sage EST library and this suggested the presence of 19 potential target genes to the 18 predicted conserved miRNAs. These miRNAs coded for only 6 transcription factors or F-box proteins, 11 metabolism or abiotic stress response related proteins and 2 products were with no known predicted function.

Role of microRNA in Stress Regulation in Plants

Due to their sessile nature, plants face a myriad of adverse factors (both abiotic and biotic) in their natural environment, affecting cellular growth, development, and productivity. Abiotic conditions, such as drought, flooding, cold, heat, below and above normal illumination, low oxygen availability, heavy metals, radiation, nutrient deficiency, high salinity, and mechanical damage, are among the main factors that cause stress to plants, either alone or in combination (Boyer 1982). Among the biotic factors pathogen attack is the main problem which has a major impact on growth, development, and productivity of crop plants. To cope with all these stress conditions, plants have evolved highly complex and well-honed responses that include reprogramming gene expression, readjusting metabolism and water relations, and protecting cellular structures from the damages of stresses (Zhu 2002). The expression of a large set of genes is usually affected in response to stresses, indicating that stress responses involve a complex regulatory network. Within this network, gene expression is temporally and spatially coordinated at the transcriptional, post-transcriptional, and translational levels.

Recently, there has been strong evidence leading to the proposal that miRNAs are hypersensitive to abiotic or biotic stress as well as to diverse physiological processes (Lu *et al.*, 2005a, Sunkar and Zhu, 2004). MicroRNAs in plants are known to regulate the expression of a number of key developmental and stress-related genes and they play an important role in plant stress response by regulating gene expression in a sequence-specic manner. They are an integral component of the stress response network because they regulate the expression of their target protein coding genes, many of which encode transcription factors that regulate the expression of other genes. In addition, the expression of miRNA genes themselves is regulated by upstream transcription factors.

Sunkar and Zhu (2004) found that miRNA393, miR402, and miR319c were induced by cold, dehydration, salt, and plant stress hormone abscisic acid (ABA), whereas miR398 was downregulated. It was later revealed that miR398 was downregulated by oxidative stress (Sunkar *et al.*, 2006). miR398 regulates the expression of two homologous Cu/Zn superoxide dismutase genes that are involved in protecting cells from damage of toxic superoxide radicals.

Further studies showed that miR399 was upregulated by inorganic phosphate starvation (Chiou *et al.*, 2006), miR169 was downregulated by drought stress (Li *et al.*, 2008) and nitrogen starvation (Zhao *et al.*, 2011) in *Arabidopsis*, and several miRNAs were regulated by mechanical stresses in *Populus* (Lu *et al.*, 2005b). Lu *et al.* (2005a) identified 48 miRNA sequences from the Populus genome. Majority of these *Populus* miRNAs showed their target as developmental and stress/defence related genes.

A recent study has identified the involvement of miRNA in relation to submergence tolerance (Zhang *et al.*, 2008). At low-sulfur conditions, the ATP sulfurylase APS4 and the sulfate transporter AST68 are accumulated and both of these genes are regulated by miR395 (Allen *et al.*, 2005, Jones-Rhoades and Bartel 2004). miRNAs have emerged as important modulators in drought tolerance and avoidance via control of the expression of drought-responsive genes (Covarrubias and Reyes 2010, Martin *et al.*, 2010, Shuai *et al.*, 2013). In rice, miR169g was showed as the only member induced by drought stress among the miR169 family (Zhao *et al.*, 2007). Drought-induced miRNAs downregulate their target mRNAs, which may be negative functional proteins involved in drought response. Conversely, other miRNAs are downregulated, leading to the accumulation of their target mRNAs that contribute positively to stress adaption. It is important to note that most of these miRNAs target genes encoding transcription factors, which place miRNAs at the centre of gene regulatory networks. Zhou *et al.* (2007) predicted 21 miRNAs of *Arabidopsis* which were associated under UV-B stress condition. In another study using EST analyses, 25.8 per cent of ESTs containing miRNAs were found in stress-induced plant tissues (Zhang *et al.*, 2005).

In the case of adverse biotic conditions miRNA plays an interesting role in plants. *Arabidopsis* miR393 was the rst miRNA reported to play a role in plant antibacterial PTI (pattern triggered immunity) by regulating the auxin signaling pathway. miR393 was induced by a bacterial PAMP (pattern associated molecular pattern) peptide g22 post-treatment (Navarro *et al.*, 2006). Using small RNA-expression proling on *Arabidopsis* leaves collected at 1 and 3 h post-inoculation (hpi) with Pst DC3000 hrcC, Fahlgren *et al.* (2007) identied three miRNAs (miR160, miR167, and miR393) that were highly induced and one that was downregulated (miR825) after infection. The role of miRNAs in plant basal defence was further supported by the nding that *Arabidopsis* miRNA-decient mutants dcl1 and hen1 showed enhanced growth of the bacterium Pst DC3000 hrcC and several bacteria strains that are non-pathogenic to *Arabidopsis*, including *Pseudomonas syringae* pv. phaseolicola, *P. uorescens*, and *Escherichia coli* (Navarro *et al.*, 2008). Navarro *et al.*

2008) showed that the induction of g22-responsive pri-miR393 and pri-miR396 in Arabidopsis was suppressed by the virulent strainPst DC3000 but not by the TTSS mutant strainPst DC3000 hrcC. miR398 in *Arabidopsis* was downregulated by infection of with Pst (avrRpm1) and Pst (avrRpt2) but was unaffected by Pst DC3000 inltration (Jagadeeswaran *et al.*, 2009). In *Arabidopsis*, miR156 and miR164 were induced by infection with the virus TYMV p69 and were induced in transgenic *Arabidopsis* plants expressing the viral silencing suppressor P1/HC-Pro (Kasschau *et al.*, 2003). miR156, miR160, and miR164 were induced after virus infection in tobacco (Navarro *et al.*, 2008). Upon virus infection, new miRNAs (miR158 and miR1885) were identied in Brassica; miR158 and miR1885 were specically induced by turnip mosaic virus but not by cucumber mosaic virus or tobacco mosaic virus (He *et al.*, 2008). Various miRNA families were differentially expressed in response to infection by the rust fungus *Cronartium quercuumf.* sp. fusiforme, which causes fusiform rust disease in pines. Ten out of eleven miRNA families were downregulated, including seven that were pine specic (Kasschau *et al.*, 2003). For example, miR156 and miR160 were repressed in pine stems infected with the rust fungus (Lu *et al.*, 2007). It was also indicate that miRNAs may affect the response of wheat (*Triticum aestivum* L.) to powdery mildew infection; some of the conserved miRNAs showed differential expression patterns in response to powdery mildew infection: miR156, miR159, miR164, miR171, and miR396, were downregulated and miR393, miR444, and miR827, were upregulated (Xin *et al.*, 2010). In addition, a negative correlation between miRNA abundance and their targets was observed in roots infected by the plant-parasitic nematode *Heterodera schachtii*, which confirmed that miRNAs are involved in plant–nematode interactions (Bazzini *et al.*, 2007). In response to *H. schachtii* infection, miR161, miR164, miR167a, miR172c, miR396a,b, and miR398a were downregulated. Expression of miR156 and miR160 was substantially repressed in the galled stem.

Several miRNA families target genes encoding nucleotide binding site–leucine-rich repeat (NBS-LRR) plant innate immune receptors in legumes (Zhai *et al.*, 2011) and in the Solanaceae (Li *et al.*, 2012). Shivaprasad *et al.* (2012) demonstrated that the miR482/2118 family of miRNAs targets numerous NBS-LRR mRNAs encoding disease resistance proteins in tomato (*Solanum lycopersicum*) and other members of the Solanaceae family. This miRNA-mediated silencing of disease resistance mRNAs is shown to be lost in virus- and bacteria-infected plants, thereby resulting in a mechanism for pathogen-induced expression of NBS-LRR defense-related genes. This result suggests that the miR482/2118 superfamily may be a master regulator of diseases resistance in tomato. Shivaprasad *et al.* (2012) found the miR482/2118 superfamily to be highly variable both in sequence and in expression level across a wide range of plant families and especially abundant in the Rutaceae, Solanaceae, and Fabaceae. In all these cases there is a cascade of miR482-mediated regulation of NBS-LRR gene expression. They also propose that miRNA regulation of NBS-LRR gene expression might create a role for NBS-LRR proteins in non-race-specific immunity. In this case pathogen-encoded suppressors of RNA silencing mechanisms in the plant might trigger the loss of miR482/2118- mediated suppression of NBS-LRR genes in a non-race-specific manner, resulting in the induction of multiple

NBS-LRR defence proteins. Thus miRNA regulation of innate immunity is a new weapon to the arsenal of defence mechanisms in plants.

A complete understanding of the actions of miRNAs depends on the identification of the target genes. Identification of entire sets of miRNAs and their targets will lay the foundation that is needed to unravel the complex miRNA mediated regulatory networks controlling development and other physiologica processes. Given that miRNAs are crucial components of gene regulatory networks a complete understanding of the functions of miRNAs will greatly increase our understanding of plant tolerance to biotic and abiotic stresses.

MicroRNAs in Human

Currently, about 2 per cent of the known human genes encode miRNAs. Such miRNAs exhibit a developmental stage- and tissue-specific expression patterns. They are also present in complex regulatory circuits to regulate stem cells function tissue differentiation and maintenance of cell identity during embryogenesis and adult life. Recently, the deregulation of miRNAs expression and activity has been correlated with the pathogenesis of various human diseases and cancer (Fazi and Blandino 2013).

Human miRNA Targets

MicroRNAs interact with target mRNAs at specific sites to induce cleavage of the message or inhibit translation. The specific function of most mammalian miRNAs is unknown. John *et al.* (2011) reported that about 2,000 human genes with miRNA target sites have been conserved in mammals, and predicted target sites on the 39 untranslated regions (UTRs) of human gene transcripts for already known 218 mammalian miRNAs. Their analysis suggested that miRNA genes, which are about 2 per cent of all human genes, regulate protein production of 10 per cent or more of all human genes.

Role of miRNAs in Human Disease

Role of miRNA in regulating several human diseases has been documented convincingly. Many of the functional roles of miRNAs hint at the potential involvement of miRNAs in human disease. Important findings are presentd.

MicroRNA and Human Prion Brain Disease

Several processes are influenced and regulated by prion gene-associated miRNAs in human. These include: cell death, neuronal differentiation, development, synapse function, neurogenesis, as well as neurodegeneration and neuropathogenesis. Studies in mouse brains indicated that prion disease results in deregulation of miRNAs. For example, MiR-342-3p, miR-146a, miR-139-5p, miR-320, miR-128, miR-328, and let-7b miRNAs were up regulated; whereas miR-337-3p and miR-338-3p miRNAs were down regulated. Gene promoters that were cognate to several of these miRNAs included E2F-1 (cell cycle re-entry and neurodegeneration), PAX6 (neurogenesis), KROX (transcription factor), MAZ (inflammatory response transcription factor), and Early Growth Response 1 (EGR1), a Nerve Growth Factor-Induced Protein. Additional work indicated effects on Nmethyl- D-aspartic acid (NMDA), receptor glutamate receptor (ionotropic, N-methyl D-aspartate 2A, GRIN2A) as well (Saba *et al.*, 2012, Majer *et al.*, 2012). MicroRNAs also participate in neuronal development, dendrite, spine, and synapse, as well as neuron sub-type specificity and they are involved in CNS ischemia, recovery from ischemia, spinal cord injury, and traumatic brain injury (Bellingham *et al.*, 2012). In addition to prion diseases, miRNAs are involved in Parkinson's and Huntington's diseases (Leidinger *et al.*, 2013).

Human prion brain disease has been studied intensely since 1920. Examples of such diseases are Creutzfeldt-Jakob disease (CJD), fatal familial insomnia, Gerstmann-Straussler-Scheinker disease, and Kuru. Central in the epidemiology and pathogenesis of prion diseases is the prion protein itself and the gene for this protein resides on chromosome 12, at locus 20pterp12. The prion protein is termed as PRNP, has a monomer molecular weight of 22-36 Kd and is linked to glycosylphosphatidyl- inositol (GPI) on cell surfaces (Paul 2013).

MicroRNA and Alzheimer Disease

Alzheimer disease (AD) is the most common form of dementia but the identification of reliable, early and non-invasive biomarkers remains a major challenge. Leidinger *et al.* (2013) have introduced a novel miRNA-based signature for detecting AD from blood samples. They reported that the differentiation of AD from other neurological diseases is possible with accuracies between 74 per cent and 78 per cent. The differentiation of the other central nervous system (CNS) disorders from controls yields even higher accuracies. These data indicate that deregulated miRNAs in blood might be used as biomarkers in the diagnosis of AD or other neurological diseases.

Kloting *et al.* (2009) reported that miRNA expression differences may contribute to intrinsic differences between omental and subcutaneous adipose tissue. In addition, human adipose tissue miRNA expression correlates with adipocyte phenotype, parameters of obesity and glucose metabolism.

MicroRNA and Cancer

Many human miRNAs are located at genomic regions linked to cancer (Calin *et al.*, 2004b, McManus 2003). Of particular interest is the *mir-17* miRNA cluster, which is in a region on human chromosome 13 that is frequently amplified in B-cell lymphomas (He *et al.*, 2005). Overexpression of the *mir-17* cluster was found to co-operate with *Myc* to accelerate tumour development in a mouse B-cell lymphoma model. Further evidence for such a link between *Myc* and the *mir-17* cluster has come from microarray expression studies, which showed that *mir-17* cluster gene expression was induced by the overexpression of Myc (O'Donnell *et al.*, 2005). Predicted targets for the *mir-17* cluster miRNAs include members of the E2F and retinoblastoma families (Lewis *et al.*, 2003). Further, *mir-17* cluster miRNAs have been found to downregulate E2F1 expression (Alvarez-Garcia and Miska 2005, O'Donnell *et al.*, 2005).

Another potential link between miRNAs and human disease can be drawn from the identification of an essential co-factor for the miRNA biogenesis enzyme

DROSHA. This cofactor is encoded by DGCR8 gene (DGCR8 microprocessor complex subunit gene), which maps to chromosomal region 22q11.2, commonly deleted in DiGeorge syndrome (Denli *et al.*, 2004, Gregory *et al.*, 2004, Han *et al.*, 2004, Landthaler *et al.*, 2004, Lee *et al.*, 2003, Lindsay 2001, Shiohama *et al.*, 2003). Haploinsufficiency of this region accounts for over 90 per cent of individuals with DiGeorge syndrome, a disorder that affects 1 in 3,000 live births and results in heterogeneous defects including heart defects, immunodeficiency, schizophrenia and obsessive-compulsive disorder, among others.

The miRNAs might also be involved in immune defence system. A cellular miRNA, miR-32, can regulate primate foamy virus type 1 (PFV-1) proliferation in cell culture (Lecellier *et al.*, 2005). In addition, large DNA viruses of the herpesvirus family, including EBV (Pfeffer *et al.*, 2004, Pfeffer *et al.*, 2005) and SV40 (Sullivan *et al.*, 2005), encode viral miRNA genes. These viral miRNAs have no apparent homologues in host genomes and their function is currently not understood.

Nuclear protein "Wee1" that delays mitosis, by regulating the corresponding genes, was recognized as a tumor suppressor gene. Butz *et al.* (2010) reported that "Wee1" protein expression was decreased in nonfunctional pituitary adenomas (NFAs) and GH-producing tumors with or without prolactin production, but no change in mRNA expression was observed with qRT-PCR. A specific subset of five miRNAs revealed by *in silico* target prediction was significantly overexpressed in NFA samples; three miRs (miR-128a, miR-155, and miR-516a-3p) targeted the 3′-untranslated region of the *Wee1* transcript, and exogenous overexpression of these miRs inhibited Wee1 protein expression and HeLa cell proliferation.

MicroRNA regulates human vitamin D receptor (VDR). 1α,25-Dihydroxyvitamin D_3 [1,25$(OH)_2D_3$ or calcitriol], a biologically active metabolite of vitamin D3, known as a classical regulator of calcium and bone homeostasis (Mohri *et al.*, 2009, Dusso *et al.*, 2005, Nagpal *et al.*, 2005). Vitamin D deficiency is linked to rickets and osteoporosis. Additional roles have been found for vitamin D in the regulation of cell processes such as cell growth, differentiation and apoptosis. Since the vitamin D system has relevance for the prevention and treatment of cancer (Garland *et al.*, 2006), the development of a number of novel synthetic vitamin D analogues as a therapeutic agent in cancer has been attempted by Mohri *et al.* (2009).

Most of the biological effects of 1α, 25-dihydroxy vitamin D_3 (1,25$(OH)_2D_3$) are elicited by the binding to VDR, which regulates gene expression. Earlier studies reported no correlation between the VDR protein and mRNA levels, suggesting the involvement of posttranscriptional regulation. In the 30-untranslated region of human VDR mRNA, a potential miR-125b recognition element (MRE125b) was identified. It was reported that miR-125b posttranscriptionally regulated human VDR. Since the miR-125b level is known to be downregulated in cancer, such a decrease may result in the upregulation of VDR in cancer and augmentation of the antitumor effects of 1,25$(OH)_2D_3$.

MicroRNAs can function as regulatory molecules. Different miRNAs involved in such activities in the development of breast cancer is shown in Figure 4.1. It is interesting to note that some miRNAs may have dual functions as both tumor suppressor and oncogenes (Gebeshuber *et al.*, 2009). Amplification or over-expression of miRNAs can down-regulate tumor suppressors or other genes involved in cell differentiation, thereby contributing to tumor formation by stimulating proliferation, angiogenesis, and invasion, *i.e.*, they act as oncogenes (Shenouda and Alahari 2009, Garzon *et al.*, 2010, Hanahan and Weinberg 2011). Because of the small size of miRNAs, loss-of-function or gain-of-function point mutations represent rare event. The overall effects in the case of miRNA inactivation is the over-expression of target mRNAs, while miRNA activation will lead to down-regulation of target mRNAs involved in apoptosis, cell cycle, invasion, or angiogenesis (Alvarez-Garcia and Miska 2005, Di *et al.*, 2006).

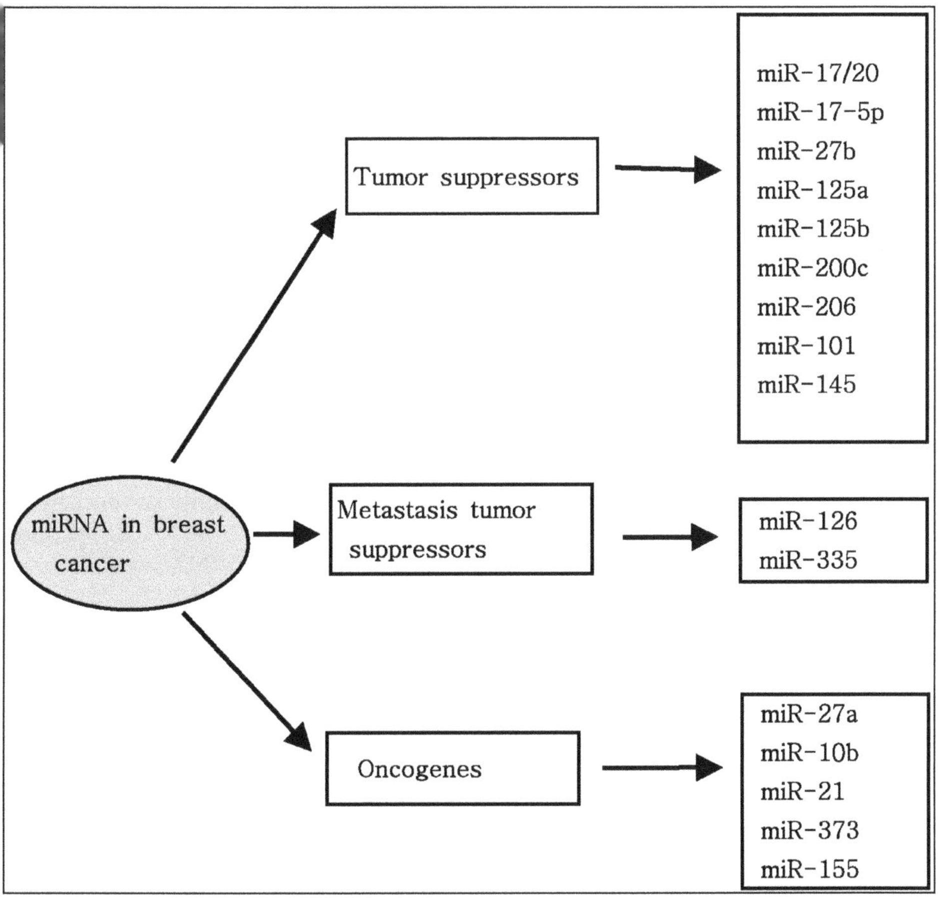

Figure 4.1: miRNAs Function as both Tumor Suppressor including metastasis suppressor miRNA, and Oncogene in Breast Cancer.

There has been an explosion of literature focusing on the role of regulatory T (Treg) cells in cancer immunity and miRNAs are highly expressed in Treg cells (Lu *et al.*, 2005, Ha 2011). Also, over the past many years, it has become clear that alteration in the expression of miRNA genes contribute to the pathogenesis of most-if not all-human malignancies (Schetter *et al.*, 2010, Calin and Croce, 2006). These alterations can be caused by various mechanisms, such as deletions, amplifications, mutations involving miRNA loci, epigenetic silencing or the dysregulation of transcription factors that targets specific miRNAs (Schetter *et al.*, 2010, Calin and Croce, 2006). Because malignant cells show dependence on the dysregulated expression of miRNA genes, which in turn control or are controlled by the dysregulation of multiple protein-coding oncogenes or tumor suppressor genes, these small RNAs provide important opportunities for the development of future miRNA-based therapies (Liston *et al.*, 2010, Croce 2009).

In cancer, the loss of tumour suppressive miRNAs enhances the expression of target oncogenes, whereas increased expression of oncogenic miRNAs can repress target tumour suppressor genes. This new wealth of knowledge points to miRNAs as being novel cancer genes and biomarkers relevant to the pathogenesis, diagnosis and prognosis of disease that may be useful for control strategy for human cancer. For example, miRNA expression profiles are now used to classify tumours based on the tissue type and stage of disease since they better reflect the developmental lineage and differentiation state of cancer (Fazi and Blandino, 2013).

In an attempt to study the miRNA expression profiles to classify human cancers, Lu *et al.* (2005) obtained unexpected findings with extraordinary level of diversity in miRNA expression across cancers, and the large amount of diagnostic information encoded in a relatively small number of miRNAs. For the experiment, they have used a bead-based flow cytometric miRNA expression profiling method to present a systematic expression analysis of 217 mammalian miRNAs from 334 samples, including multiple human cancers. Unlike with mRNA expression, a modest number of miRNAs (~200 in total) might be sufficient to classify human cancers. They did not observe substantial decreases in the mRNAs encoding components of the miRNA processing machinery (Dicer, Drosha, Argonaute 2 or DGCR8) (Cullen 2004, Tavazoie *et al.*, 2008), but clearly other mechanisms of miRNA regulation are possible (Lu *et al.*, 2005).

The miRNA profiles found to be surprisingly informative, reflecting the developmental lineage and differentiation state of the tumours. A general downregulation of miRNAs in tumours compared with normal tissues was observed. Furthermore, they were able to successfully classify poorly differentiated tumours using miRNA expression profiles, whereas messenger RNA profiles were highly inaccurate when applied to the same samples. These findings highlight the potential of miRNA profiling in cancer diagnosis.

To study A miRNA expression signature of human solid tumors that might defines cancer gene targets, Volinia *et al.* (2006) performed a large-scale miRnome analysis on 540 samples including lung, breast, stomach, prostate, colon, and pancreatic tumors, and identified a solid cancer miRNA signature composed by a large portion of overexpressed miRNAs. Among these miRNAs are some with well characterized cancer association, such as *miR-17-5p*, *miR-20a*, *miR-21*, *miR-92*, *miR-106a*, and *miR-155*. The predicted targets for the differentially expressed miRNAs are significantly enriched for protein-coding tumor suppressors and oncogenes ($P < 0.0001$). Volinia *et al.* (2006) first identified the six tissue-specific cancer signatures by performing independent prediction analysis of microarray tests and then selected the miRNAs shared among the different histotypes miRNA signatures (Table 4.1).

Table 4.1: The miRNAs Shared by the Signatures of the different Solid Cancers

miRNA	*Number of difreent Cancers Shared*	*Type of Cancer*
miR-21	6	Breast, colon, lung, prostrate, pancrease, stomach
miR-191	5	Breast, colon, lung, prostrate, pancrease
miR-17-5p	5	Colon, lung, prostrate, pancrease, stomach
miR-223	4	Breast, colon, prostrate, pancrease
miR-29b-2	4	Breast, colon, prostrate, pancrease
miR-221	3	Colon, pancrease, stomach
miR-214	3	Prostrate, pancrease, stomach
miR-199a-1	3	Lung, prostrate, pancrease
miR-181b-1	3	Breast, prostrate, pancrease
miR-155	3	Breast, colon, lung
miR-146	3	Breast, prostrate, pancrease
miR-107	3	Colon, pancrease, stomach
miR-106a	3	Colon, prostrate, pancrease
miR-92-2	3	Prostrate, pancrease, stomach
miR-32	3	Colon, prostrate, pancrease
miR-30c	3	Colon, prostrate, pancrease
miR-25	3	Prostrate, pancrease, stomach
miR-24-1	3	Colon, pancrease, stomach
miR-24-2	3	Colon, pancrease, stomach
miR-20a	3	Colon, prostrate, pancrease

A number of the predicted targets, including the tumor suppressors RB1 (Retinoblastoma 1) and TGFBR2 (transforming growth factor, beta receptor II) genes were confirmed experimentally. Their results indicated that miRNAs are extensively involved in cancer pathogenesis of solid tumors and support their function as either dominant or recessive cancer genes.

Epigenetic Control of miRNAs Expression in Cancer Cells

Dysregulation of miRNAs in cancer can occur through epigenetic changes and genetic alterations, which can affect the production of the primary RNAs, their processing to their mature miRNA form, and/or interactions with mRNA targets. There are three main epigenetic events that regulate tumor-associated genes:

1. The aberrant hypermethylation of tumor suppressor genes,
2. Global DNA hypomethylation and
3. Post-translational modifications of histones.

An extensive analysis of genomic sequences of microRNA genes suggests that approximately half of them are associated with CpG islands. Therefore these epigenetic events can also affect miRNA expression. In addition, some miRNAs are up-regulated, (i) upon the exposure of cells to the agent 5-aza- 20-deoxycytidine, (ii) upon mutation of methyltransferases (DNMTs), or (iii) upon histone deacetylase inhibitor treatment. Melo *et al.* (2010) reported that some miRNAs are repressed by CpG island hypermethylation in cancers relative to normal tissue. Some examples include miR-9-1 in breast cancer and miR-124a in colorectal tumors. The miR 203 locus also frequently undergoes DNA methylation in T-cell lymphoma but not in normal T lymphocytes. The epigenetic changes complemented by genetic inactivation due to mutation or deletion are also a possible mechanism that partially account for miRNA deregulation in cancer cells.The recent ndings of genetic defects in cancer-associated genes of the miRNA processing machinery, such as TARBP2 (Melo *et al.*, 2009), Dicer (Hill *et al.*, 2009), and XPO5 (Melo *et al.*, 2010) has strongly highlighted the relevance of these pathways in cellular transformation, where such defects contribute to a global dysregulation of miRNAs in cancer.

MicroRNA as Oncogenes and Tumor-Suppressor Genes

MicroRNAs can function both as oncogenes or tumor-suppressor genes (Ventura and Jacks, 2009). Chromosomal regions encompassing microRNAs involved in the negative regulation of a transcript encoding a known tumour suppressor gene can be amplied in cancer development. This amplication would result in the increased expression of the microRNA and consequent silencing of the tumour suppressor gene. These miRNAs could undergo loss of function in tumors due to chromosomal rearrangements, deletions or mutations. This has been shown for several miRNAs, including the let-7 family, whose expression can impair tumorigenesis through inhibition of oncogenes like the RAS family and HMGA2 (Esquela-Kerscher *et al.*, 2008). Conversely, microRNAs repressing oncogenes are often located in fragile loci, where deletions or mutations can occur and result in reduced microRNA levels and overexpression of the target oncogene. Oncogenic miRNAs can undergo a gain of function in tumors due to genomic amplifications example, miR-192 cluster, whose amplification in B-cell lymphomas promotes their development (He *et al.*, 2005). Different miRNAs that are functionally involved in cancer progression are shown in Table 4.2.

Consequences of Aberrant miRNA Expression in Cancer

MiRNAs regulate the expression of their targets, so over- or underexpression of miRNAs is expected to result in down- or up regulation, respectively, of the protein product of the target mRNAs. It is not difficult to associate a miRNA with cancer if a direct target of a miRNA is an oncogene or a tumor-suppressor genemiRNAs were linked to cancer was first reported in 2002 by Calin *et al.*, showing that miR-15 and miR-16 are located at chromosome 13q14, a region deleted in more than half of B cell chronic lymphocytic leukemias (B-CLL) (Calin *et al.*, 2002). Both of the miRNAs are deleted or down-regulated in approximately 68 per cent of CLL patients. Their further study mapping 186 miRNA locations in the genome indicated that 52.5 per cent of miRNA genes are located at cancer-associated genomic regions or in fragile

Table 4.2: MicroRNAs Functionally Involved in Cancer Progression. MicoRNAs with characterized functions in tumorigenesis, drug resistance, and metastasis during cancer progression are summarized as oncogenic or tumor suppressive miRNAs.

Tumorigenesis		*Drug Resistance*		*Invasion/ Metastasis*
		Oncogenic miRNAs		
miR-17-92 cluster	miR-21	miR-125b	miR-212	miR-9
miR-21	miR-27	miR-130a	miR-221/222	miR-10b
miR-107	miR-29b,c	miR-148a	miR-320	miR-107
miR-155	miR-34a	miR-181a	miR-328	miR-143
	miR-122	miR-199a-3p	miR-328	miR-151
		miR-200c	miR-451	miR-373
		miR-204	miR-512	miR-375
		miR-205		miR-520h
		Tumor suppressive miRNAs		
Let-7 family	miR-1		mi-200c	miR-29b
miR-15a/16-1	miR-15a/16-1		miR-214	miR-145
	miR-98		miR-215	miR-146a
	miR-140		miR-424	miR200c
	miR-143		miR-519c	miR-218
	miR-155			miR-335
	miR-192			miR-372
				miR-520c

sites. Iorio *et al.* (2005) identified 29 miRNAs with aberrant expression in human breast cancer by microarray and northern blot analyses on 76 breast tumor samples and 14 human breast cell lines and found that miR-125b, miR-145, miR-21 and miR-155 were significantly reduced in breast cancer tissues. Most importantly, they also observed that expression patterns of miRNAs were correlated with tumor stage, proliferation index, estrogen and progesterone receptor expression and vascular invasion. Jiang *et al.* (2005) detected 222 human miRNA precursors in expression profile of 32 human cell lines from lung, breast, colorectal, hematologic, prostate, pancreatic, and head and neck cancers. Several miRNAs had tissue specific aberrant expression including miR-205 which showed 36 times higher abundance in head and neck cancer cell lines than other cell lines. In 2006, Zhang and colleagues performed an analysis of 283 known human miRNA genes by array based comparative genomic hybridization in 227 human ovarian cancer, breast cancer, and melanoma specimens demonstrating the high-frequency gene copy number abnormality of miRNA-containing regions throughout the genome in human ovarian cancer (37.1 per cent), breast cancer (72.8 per cent), and melanoma (85.9 per cent). Colorectal neoplasia is also characterized by alterations in miRNAs expression. MiR-145 and miR-143 are frequently reduced at the adenomatous and cancer stages of colorectal neoplasia (Michael *et al.*, 2003). However, it was also described that the levels of pre-miR-143 and pre-miR-145 are not altered in precancerous and neoplastic colorectal tissue, suggesting that post-transcriptional control is the cause for the reduced mature miRNA levels. Table 4.3 shows the location of miRNAs in specific chromosome and their association with specific cancer.

Table 4.3: Location of miRNA in the Chromosome and their Association with Specific Human Cancer

miRNA	*Gene Loci*	*Cancer Involvement*
miR-15a, miR-16-1	Chromosome 13q14	Downregulated in B-cell chronic lymphocytic leukemia; negatively regulates the antiapoptotic gene BCL2
miR-143, miR-145	Chromosome 5q32–33	Decreased abundance in colorectal cancer; downregulated in,breast, prostate,cervical and lymphoid cancer cell lines; miR-145 is decreased in breast cancer
miR-21	Chromosome 17q23.2	Anti-apoptotic factor; upregulated in glioblastomas and breast cancer
let-7 family members	Multiple loci	Negatively regulate the Ras oncogenes; direct cell proliferation and differentiation; decreased abundance in lung cancer
miR-142	Chromosome 17q22	A t(8;17) translocation that places the MYC oncogene downstream of the mir-142 hairpin, resulting in an aggressive B-cell leukemia that is due to MYC overexpression
BIC/miR-155	Chromosome 21q21	Upregulated in paediatric Burkitt, Hodgkin, primarymediastinal and diffuse large-B-cell lymphomas;upregulated in human breast cancer
miR-17–19b cluster	Chromosome 13q31–32	Upregulated by MYC; negatively modulates the E2F1 oncogene; loss of heterozygosity of this cluster is found in hepatocellular carcinoma; overexpressed in B-cell lymphomas

Role of miRNA in Specific Human Cancer

Association of miRNA with specific human cancer has been well documented. Some of these associations are described in the following section.

MicroRNA in Hematopoiesis and Leukemia

MicroRNAs are involved in the management of hematopoiesis. These small regulatory RNAs are master regulators of developmental processes that modulate expression of several target genes post-transcriptionally. Various miRNAs are up-regulated at specific stages during hematopoietic development and the functional relevance of miRNAs has been proven at many different stages of line. Knockout of specific miRNAs can produce dramatic phenotypes leading to severe hematopoietic defects. Furthermore, several studies demonstrated that specific miRNAs are differentially expressed in hematopoietic stem cells (Figure 4.2). However, the emerging picture is extreamly complex due to differences between species, cell type dependent variation in miRNA expression and differential expression of diverse target genes that are involved in various regulatory networks. There is also evidence that miRNA play a role in cellular aging or in the inter-cellular crosstalk between hematopoietic cells and their microenvironment.

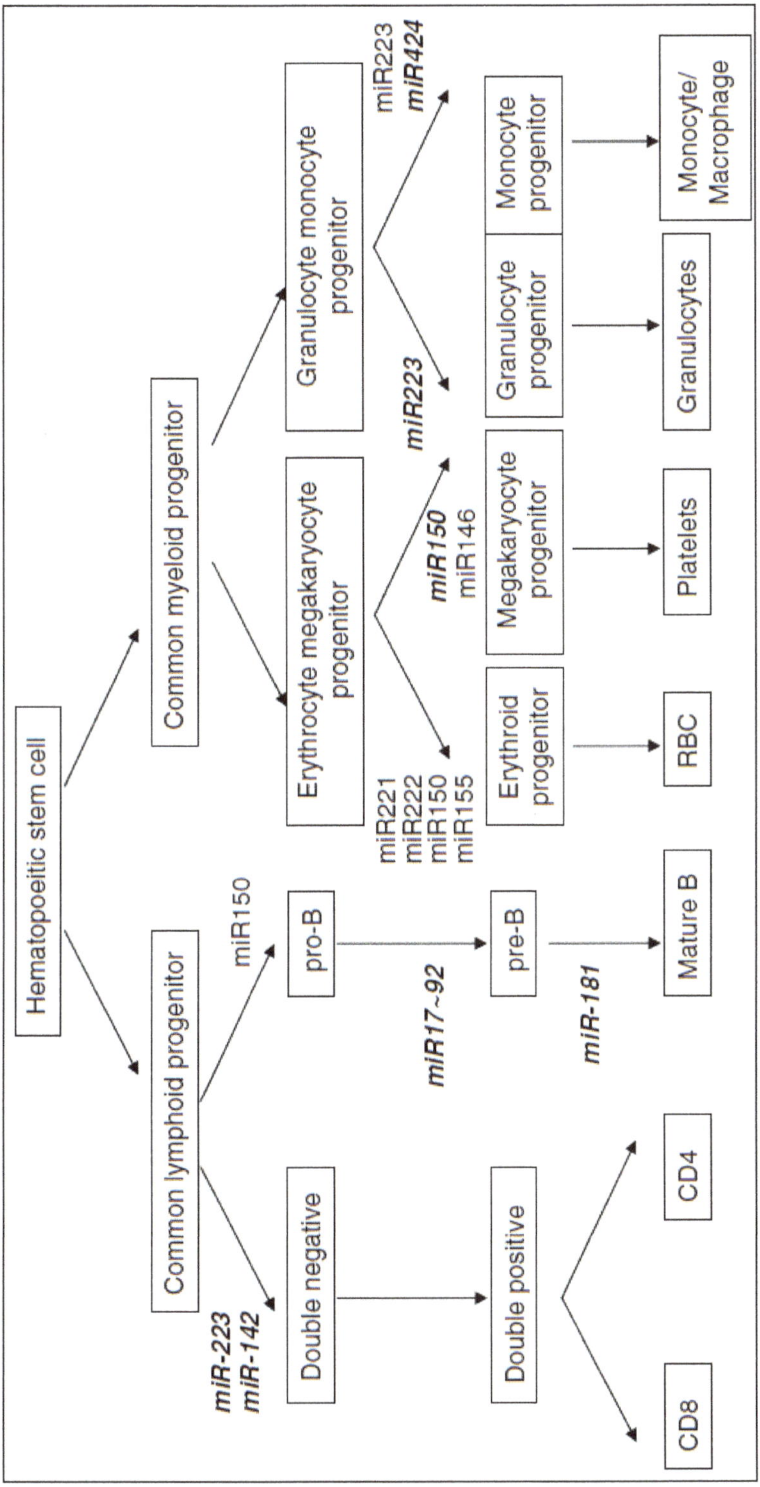

Figure 4.2: Some of the known miRNA that Regulate Hematopoeisis. The miRNA in bold italics are known to promote differentiation along the pathway. Whereas, the miRNA in regular font are known to inhibit differentiation along the pathway.

In the past few years there has been a significant expansion of the understanding of the role of miRNA in the pathogenesis of leukemia. It has been realized that miRNA dysregulation cause disruption of the hematopoietic system and may lead to leukemia development. Aberrant miRNA expression is a feature of leukemia. Morris *et al.* (2013) have identified miRNAs expressed differentially in AML (acute myeloid leukemia) and BC CML (blast crisis chronic myeloid leukemia) and also identified a new role for miR-150 in myeloid differentiation. Expression of miR-150 was low or absent in AML and BC CML patient samples and cell lines. Whereas in healthy individuals expression of miR-150 was normal. It was also suggested that miR-150 promotes myeloid differentiation, and that absence or low miR-150 expression contributes to blocking myeloid differentiation in acute leukemia cells.

MircoRNA and Breast Cancer

Interestingly, miRNA aberrant expression has been found in human breast cancer, where miRNA signature was associated with specific clinicobiological features (Tai-You 2011, Iorio *et al.*, 2005). Compared with normal breast tissue, miRNAs are aberrantly expressed in human breast cancer. Overall miRNA expression could clearly separate normal versus cancer tissues, with the most significantly deregulated miRNAs being miR-125b, miR-145, miR-21, and miR-155 (Tai-You 2011, Iorio *et al.*, 2005). Tavazoie *et al.*, showed that restoring the expression of some miRNAs in malignant cells suppresses lung and bone metastasis by human cancer cells in vivo (Tai-You 2011, Tavazoie *et al.*, 2008).

MicroRNA and Pancreatic Cancer

A miRNA expression signature has been found to be associated with pancreatic cancer and this has been accomplished with the application of real-time PCR profiling of 200 miRNA precursors on specimens of human pancreatic adenocarcinoma, paired benign issue, normal pancreas, pancreatitis and cell lines (Tai-You 2011, Lee *et al.*, 2007). Lee *et al.* (2007) showed that one hundred miRNA precursors were aberrantly expressed in pancreatic cancer or desmoplasia, including miRNAs previously reported as differentially expressed in other human cancers (miR-155, miR-21, miR-221, and miR-222) as well as those not previously reported in cancer (miR-376a and miR-301) (Tai-You 2011). They also demonstrated that most of the top aberrantly expressed miRNAs displayed increased expression in tumor and that three of the top differentially expressed miRNAs (miR-221, miR-221, miR-301) were localized to tumor cells and not to stroma or normal acini or ducts. They noted that aberrant miRNA expression may offer new clues to pancreatic tumorigenesis and may provide diagnostic biomarkers for pancreatic adenocarcinoma. It is well established that many tumor suppressor genes in human cancer are silenced by chromatin alterations, including promoter methylation and histone deacetylation (Tai-You 2011, Lee *et al.*, 2009).

MicroRNA and Colorectal Cancer (CRC)

A well-known tumor suppressor gene, p53 is mutated in about 50-75 per cent of all CRCs and many other human tumors. p53 responds to DNA damage or deregulation of mitogenic oncogenes through the induction of cell cycle checkpoints, apoptosis, or cellular senescence (Slaby *et al.*, 2009, Fearon and Vogelstein 1990). Although p53 is clearly a transcriptional activator, numerous reports have indicated that p53 also represses the expression of specific genes either directly or indirectly (He *et al.*, 2007). The manner in which this occurred was obscure, with both transcriptional and post-transcriptional suppression as possible mechanisms (Slaby *et al.*, 2009). In the latter case, the discovery of an extensive regulatory network of miRNAs offered the possibility that p53-mediated control of miRNA expression could allow it to act indirectly to repress target gene expression at the post-transcriptional level. Recently, several groups have unraveled important aspects of the connection between p53 and the miRNA network (Hermeking 2007). The conserved *miR-34a-c* family was found to be direct transcriptional targets of p53 (Slaby *et al.*, 2009). Significant changes of miRNA expression levels in CRC tissue in comparison to colorectal epithelium, and these have identified groups of miRNAs enabling prognostic stratification of CRC patients and prediction of their responses to selected chemotherapeutic regimens and radiotherapy.

In colon cancer, the VDR mRNA and protein expression levels are gradually increased in the early stages of cancerogenesis, but the VDR mRNA decreases subsequently to lower levels during advancement (Cross *et al.*, 2001). Mohri *et al.* (2009) concluded that the VDR expression is upregulated in cancers, although the expression levels seem to change during disease progression and in response to therapies. MicroRNAs recognize the 30-untranslated region (30-UTR) of the target mRNA and cause translational repression or mRNA degradation (Bartel, 2004).

MicroRNA and Lung Cancer

Lung cancer is the leading cause of death from cancer in the world. Although the molecular network of lung carcinogenesis has been partly known at the levels of genes and proteins, and personalized therapy based on the genetic changes has made considerable progress in the last decade, the high mortality rate is not markedly changed (Wang *et al.*, 2009).

Expression patterns of miRNAs, in lung, vary from fetal to adult, from normal to lung cancer. Specific miRNAs may have multi-functions in lung development and aberrant expression of miRNAs could induce lung tumorigenesis (Lu *et al.*, 2008, Johnson *et al.*, 2007). For mammals, miRNAs are specifically expressed or greatly enriched in a particular organ such as lung, implying an organ- or tissue-specific function. First, it is found that lung is one of the tissues with the most abundant expression of *let-7* (Fire *et al.*, 1998), which is reconfirmed by other researchers (Johnson *et al.*, 2007). Then, six lung-specific miRNAs are identified in the adult mice by using northern analysis (Sempere *et al.*, 2004).

MicroRNA and Gastric Cancer

Gastric cancer (GC) has a high incidence and ranks second in the leading causes of cancer mortality (Yin *et al.*, 2012, Jemal *et al.*, 2011, Jemal *et al.*, 2008). MiRNAs (miRNAs) could be a practical form of potential biomarkers in the diagnosis of human disease, and they are confirmed to be closely associated with GC. A number of miRNAs are closely associated with GC, suggesting a potential role of these miRNAs in the diagnosis of GC (Cho 2010). Meanwhile, other miRNAs such as mir-128b, mir-129 and mir-148 were reported to be down-regulated in undifferentiated GC tissue (Katada *et al.*, 2009). Elevated miR-21 expression was significantly correlated with size and depth (Motoyama *et al.*, 2010), and low expression levels of miR-451 (Bandres *et al.*, 2009) and miR-125a-5p was associated with enhanced malignant potential such as tumor size, tumor invasion, liver metastasis, and poor prognosis (Nishida *et al.*, 2011). The patients with down-regulated miR-409-3p (Zheng *et al.*, 2011) and miR-221 (Liu *et al.*, 2012) could be prone to suffer from lymph node metastasis. In a study on role of miRNAs in gastric cancer, Yao *et al.* (2009) reported that miRNAs are deregulated in gastric cancer, suggesting the involvement of few genes in the development and progression of gastric cancer.

In conclusion, GC-specific miRNAs may improve future cancer diagnosis and prognosis due to the close association of miRNAs with GC in several stages. Some important functions of GC-specific miRNAs during the processes of cancer development were found and several promising miRNAs as biomarkers were reported till date.

MicroRNA and Thyroid Cancer

A study investigated the expression patterns of miRNA in all major types of thyroid tumors, including tumors carrying distinct oncogenic mutations, and the utility of miRNA profiling for the preoperative diagnosis of thyroid nodules (Tai-You 2011, Nikiforova *et al.*, 2008). It was reported that a set of seven miRNAs (miR-187, miR-221, miR-222, miR-146b, miR-155, miR-224, and miR-197) were most differentially over-expressed in thyroid tumors. Moreover, it was demonstrated that various histopathological types of thyroid tumors have distinct miRNA profiles, which differ within the same tumor type, indicating specific oncogenic mutations. These results may suggest that a limited set of miRNAs can be used diagnostically with high accuracy to detect thyroid cancer in the surgical and preoperative samples (Tai-You 2011, Nikiforova *et al.*, 2008).

MicroRNA and Ovarian Cancer

Ovarian cancer is a leading cause of morbidity and mortality, with little change in survival rates over the past three decades (Guo *et al.*, 2009). A studies show that miRNA-9 (miR-9) is downregulated in human ovarian cancer relative to normal ovary, and overexpression of miR-9 suppresses cell growth in vitro. Furthermore, the 3′-UTR of nuclear factor of kappaB 1 (NF-kB1) mRNA is found to be regulated directly by miR-9, demonstrating that NF-kB1 is a functionally important target of miR-9 in ovarian cancer cells. When miR-9 is overexpressed in ovarian cancer cells, the mRNA and protein levels of NF-kB1 are both suppressed, whereas inhibition of miR-9 results in an increase in the NF-kB1 expression level. Ovarian cancer tissues display significantly low expression of miR-9 and a high level of NF-kB1 compared with normal tissues, indicating that regulation of NF-kB1 by miR-9 is an important mechanism for miR-9 to inhibit ovarian cancer proliferation (Guo *et al.*, 2009). Most ovarian cancer patients are diagnosed at an advanced stage (67 per cent) and prospects for significant improvement in survival reside in early diagnosis (Tai-You 2011, Taylor and Gercel-Taylor 2008). Tumors actively release exosomes into the peripheral circulation and the association of miRNA with circulating tumor-derived exosomes were demonstrated. These results suggest that miRNA profiling of circulating tumor exsomes could potentially be used as surrogate diagnostic markers for biopsy profiling, extending its utility to screening asymptomatic populations (Tai-You 2011, Taylor and Gercel-Taylor 2008).

MicroRNA and Prostate Cancer

Prostate cancer is the most common malignancy in men and one of the leading causes of cancer death (Jemal *et al.*, 2006). Early-stage prostate cancer is curable, whereas more advanced tumors can be successfully treated only before tumor metastasis has occurred (Loberg *et al.*, 2005). A recent study showed that miR-15a and miR-16-1 cluster targets encoding cyclin D1 (CCND1) and WNT3A, which promotes several tumorigenic features such as survival, proliferation and invasion. In cancer cells of advanced prostate tumors, the miR-15a and miR-16 level is significantly decreased, whereas the expression of BCL2, CCND1 and WNT3A is inversely up-regulated. Altogether, it was proposed that miR-15a and miR-16 act as tumor suppressor genes in prostate cancer through the control of cell survival, proliferation and invasion (Bonci *et al.*, 2008).

MicroRNA and Hepatocellular Carcinoma (HCC)

Development of chronic hepatitis (CH), cirrhosis, and in some instances hepatocellular carcinoma (HCC) is induced by infection of the human liver with hepatitis B virus (HBV) and hepatitis C virus (HCV) (Kiyosawa *et al.*, 1990). Ura and coworkers (2009) examined miRNA expression in liver tissue with HBV-related liver disease (CH-B and HCC-B) and HCV-related liver disease (CH-C and HCC-C) and in normal liver tissue via real-time detection polymerase chain reaction (RTD-PCR). They performed global analysis of messenger RNA expression in these tissues using complementary DNA (cDNA) microarray. These analyses allowed to find characteristic miRNAs associated with HBV or HCV infection as well as the progression of liver disease. The results suggest that common signaling pathways are involved in HCC development from CH, and that HBV and HCV-specific miRNAs participate in generating HCC-specific miRNA expressions (Figure 4.3). Therefore, these miRNAs might be good candidates for molecular targeting to prevent HCC occurrence, because they regulate a common signaling pathway underlying HCC-B and HCC-C development (Ura *et al.*, 2009).

MicroRNA and Hodgkin Lymphoma

The majority of miRNAs are found in cancer-associated genomic regions or in chromosome-fragile sites (Calin *et al.*, 2004), suggesting an important role for miRNAs in human tumorigenesis. There is also evidence that the influence of miRNAs in oncogenesis might be indirectly driven. For example, the presence of some viruses in a cell may change the host miRNA pattern (Yeung *et al.*, 2005) Viruses may participate in the origin of some tumors, such as the Epstein-Barr virus (EBV) in Hodgkin lymphoma (HL). Navarro *et al.*, 2008 analyzed miRNA expression in classic Hodgkin lymphoma (cHL) and the influence of Epstein-Barr virus (EBV) infection on the miRNA expression profiles. The expression of 157

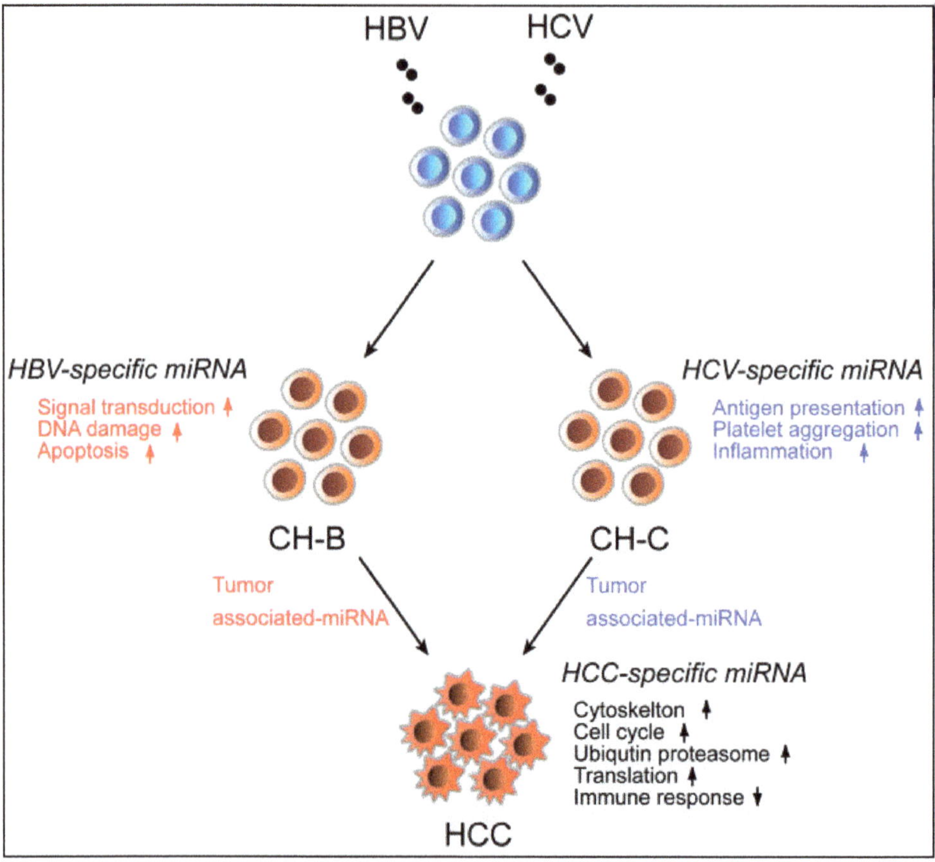

Figure 4.3: Infection-Associated and HCC-Specific miRNAs and Progression of Liver Disease.

miRNAs in lymph nodes from 49 cHL patients and 10 reactive lymph nodes (RLNs) was analyzed by real-time polymerase chain reaction (PCR). Hierarchic clustering revealed 3 well-defined groups: nodular sclerosis cHL, mixed cellularity cHL, and RLNs. A distinctive signature of 25 miRNAs differentiated cHL from RLNs, and 36 miRNAs were differentially expressed in the nodular sclerosis and mixed cellularity subtypes. These results were validated in a set of 30 cHLs and 5 RLNs, and in 3 cHL cell lines. miR-96, miR-128a, and miR- 128b were selectively down-regulated in cHL with EBV. The cHLs express a characteristic miRNA signature different from that of normal RLNs, with a small number of miRNAs differentially expressed in mixed cellularity and nodular sclerosis and one differentially expressed in early- and advanced stage disease. Some of these miRNAs were expressed in Hodgkin and Reed-Sternberg cells but not in reactive cells. In addition, EBV influences host miRNA expression in cHL. These findings suggest that miRNAs may play an important role in the biology of cHL, and they may be useful in the development of therapies targeting miRNAs in tumor cells in cHL patients (Navarro *et al.*, 2008, Si *et al.*, 2007). An understanding of these processes regulated by miRNAs suggests further avenues for research to uncover gene regulation and to design miRNA-based therapeutic approaches (Yendamuri and Calin 2009).

MicroRNA in Therapeutic Application in Cancer

MicroRNAs (miRNAs), in cancer studies, have increased exponentially over the last 10 years. Cancer is a frequent disease: at least one third of the population will develop cancer during their lifetimes. Despite progress in early detection, chemotherapy, immunotherapy, radiation and other treatments, most people with advanced cancer will ultimately die of the cancer. Overall, new treatments for cancer with fewer side effects are urgently needed. The discovery of miRNAs and other non-coding RNAs will lead to new biomarkers for determining the diagnosis, prognosis, and treatment response of cancer and may ultimately lead to new treatments for cancer.

Understanding of miRNA biogenesis may affect cancer in at least two ways. First, emerging data indicate that dysregulation of miRNAs by a variety of mechanisms including amplification, deletion, mutation, and epigenetic silencing is associated with certain types of cancer. Second, exploitation of the therapeutic potential of RNA interference may be achieved through the investigation of how endogenous miRNA and produced and exert their gene regulatory function (Gregory and Shiekhattar 2005). In addition, approximately 50 per cent of all annotated human miRNA genes are located at fragile sites or areas of the genome that are associated with cancer which are prone to breakage and rearrangement in cancer cells For example, miR-15a and miR-16-1, two tumor-suppressor microRNAs, are severely down-regulated in 70 per cent of patients with chronic lymphocytic leukemia (CLL) due to chromosomal deletions or mutations at the 13q13.4 loci where they are situated.

To date, there are a total of 6396 miRs (miRBase Release 11. http://microrna.sanger.ac.uk/sequences/), of which, 678 miRs are found in human beings.). The first human disease known to be associated with miRNA deregulation was chronic lymphocytic leukemia (Mraz *et al.*, 2012) and later many miRNAs have been found to have links with some types of cancer (Mraz *et al.*, 2012, He *et al.*, 2005, Mraz *et al.*, 2005) and are sometimes referred to as "oncomirs". MicroRNA-21 is involved in several cancer-types such as glioblastoma and astrocytoma was one of the first microRNAs to be identified as an oncomir (Moller *et al.*, 2013). However, numerous miR dysregulations have been described in glioblastoma, breast cancer, acute myeloid leukemia, melanoma, pancreatic cancer, lung cancer, ovarian cancer, hepato-cellular carcinoma, thyroid cancer, bladder and kidney cancer, gastric cancer, colorectal cancer, and others.

MicroRNAs are able to discriminate tumour origins, oncogenic mutations, subtypes and cancer predisposition, and regulating the most important cellular processes, therefore it can be predicted that miRNAs might be able to envisage cancer prognosis and/or response to specic therapies (Marilena *et al.*, 2009). Recently, several groups have reported success in utilizing miRNAs as prognostic markers to predict cancer outcome. After the first evidence in CLL, where a unique microRNA signature was associated with prognostic factors and disease progression in CLL (Calin *et al.*, 2005) and lung cancer, miR-155 overexpression and let-7a downregulation were able to predict poor disease outcome (Yanaihara *et al.*, 2006), several other reports have supported the signicance of microRNAs as prognostic biomarkers. MiRNA-based cancer diagnostic and therapeutic approaches are being established and tested in animal models. Evidence described up to date provides the experimental bases for the use of microRNAs as both targets and tools in anticancer therapy, but there are at least two primary issues to address to translate these fundamental research advances into medical practice: development of engineered animal models to study cancer-associated microRNAs, and improvement of miRNAs/anti-miRs *in vivo* delivery efficiency.

The two main strategies for miRNA-based therapeutic application in cancers:

1. Restoration of the expression of tumor suppressor miRNA. Two lines of evidence suggest miRNAs function as tumor suppressor rather than oncogenes. The global decrease of miRNA expression in cancer tissues compared to normal control (Lu *et al.*, 2005), and the enhanced cellular transformation and tumorigenesis by impaired miRNA processing (Kumar *et al.*, 2007). Synthetic miRNA mimics or miRNA expression vectors carrying either a pre-miRNA sequence or an artificial miRNA hairpin sequence have been widely used to perform the miRNA expression restoring *in vitro*. Recent publications demonstrated that miRNA reintroduction suppresses tumor growth in vivo (Trang *et al.*, 2010). Intranasal delivery of exogenous let-7 mimics to the lung tumors of mice (non-small-cell lung cancer) reduced the tumor burden. Intravenous delivery of miR-34a mimics using a lipid-based delivery vehicle accumulated miR-34a in the tumor tissue in mouse models of non-smallcell lung cancer, and blocked tumor growth. Furthermore, this approach did not induce an immune response. An adeno-associated virus (AAV)-mediated delivery of miR-26a to mouse liver resulted in reduced liver cancer cell proliferation, induction of tumor-specific apoptosis, and protection from disease progression without toxicity (Kota *et al.*, 2009).
2. Blocking the Function of Oncogenic miRNAs.

   Another strategy for cancer therapy is that, a small number of miRNAs show oncogenic function, such as miR-21, decreases the expression level or blocks the function of oncogenic miRNAs. To knock down miRNA in vitro, most frequently chemically modified antisense oligonucleotides (called anti-miRNA) are used to increase stability and specificity. The modification includes addition of 22-O-methyl, addition of 22-O-methoxyethyl and locked nucleic acid (LNA) with 22-O connecting to 42-C. The modified nucleic acid structure has high affinity and high specificity to bind with target miRNA. Moreover, the anti-miRNA–miRNA structure is highly stable. As such the delivery of a specific anti-miRNA into cells prevents the miRNA from binding to their cognate target genes thereby silencing miRNA function. Recently two more approaches were reported for blocking miRNAs. One is called the miRNA-sponge (Ebert *et al.*, 2007) which serves as a competitive inhibitor of miRNAs. An expression vector carrying multiple binding sites to a targeted miRNA is introduced into cells. Following the vector gene transcription, the over-expressed synthetic binding sequences occupy the endogenous miRNA in the cells with high affinity blocking miRNA regulation of its target genes. Another approach called the miRNA-mask (Choi *et al.,* 2007) which uses oligonucleotides perfectly complementary to miRNA binding sites of target mRNAs. The miRNA-mask blocks the access of the miRNA to the binding site on the target mRNAs thus blocking the miRNA-mRNA interaction. Tumor-targeted delivery and local administration are still major challenges to apply miRNA therapy to the clinic. The possibility of immune response, off-target effects and toxicity of exogenous miRNA mimics or antagonism to normal tissues will have to be taken into account and minimized to a safe level. miRNAs target a multitude of mRNAs involved in different signalling pathways that are often impaired in cancer. So miRNAs can be used to sensitize tumors to chemotherapy. Some examples are: miR-9 act as a negative regulator of SOX2, which indirectly induces ABCC3 and ABCC6 transporters. Thus when SOX2 is overexpressed, cancer cells are able to excrete drugs to the extracellular environment becoming resistant. The overexpression of mir-9 in a glioma stem cell line (chemotherapy-resistant) resulted in reduced ABC transporter expression and increased drug retention (Jeon *et al.,* 2011). These data provide hope that cancer cell drug reux can be reduced through manipulation of miRNAs. Therefore the potential of using miRNAs or antagomirs to make the tumors responsive to chemotherapy is of great promise. However, this is still a growing eld, and therefore in vivo data are not abundant. Nonetheless, recent in vitro experiments have shed light on what can become the new era of tumor sensitization drugs (Melo *et al.,* 2012). One of the most common reasons for acquisition of resistance to a broad range of anticancer drugs is expression of transporters that detect and eject anticancer drugs from cells. Despite all of the progress that has been made in the new era of miRNA therapeutics there is still a signicant gap between basic research on miRNAs and clinical application. Therefore, a better understanding of molecular mechanism underlying microRNA-mediated gene expression will help design better strategy for cancer treatment. Their immediate clinical implications will be very much dependent on how these microRNAs can be served as biomarkers or therapeutic targets.

Conclusion

It is hoped that research into the normal biochemical process will dovetail with better understanding of the pathological process that these molecules and pathway play. Within the past few years, studies on miRNA and cancer have burst onto the scene. Great discoveries and rapid progress in the past few years on miRNAs provide the hope that miRNAs will in the near future have a great potential in the diagnosis and treatment of many diseases (Tai-You, 2011).

References

Adai A, Johnson C, Mlotshwa S, Archer-Evans S *et al.*, Computational predictior of miRNAs in *Arabidopsis thaliana*. *Genome Res*. 15: 78–91. 2005.

Alexiou P, Vergoulis T, Gleditzsch M, Prekas G. miRGen 2.0: a database o microRNA genomic information and regulation. *Nucleic Acids Res*. 38 (Database issue): D137-41. 2010.

Allen E, Xie Z, Gustafson AM, Carrington JC. microRNAdirected phasing during trans-acting siRNA biogenesis in plants. *Cell* 12: 207–221. 2005.

Alvarez-Garcia I, Miska EA. MicroRNA functions in animal development anc human disease. *Developl. Compy. Biologists*. 132: 4653-4662. 2005.

Ambros V. Control of developmental timing in *Caenorhabditis elegans*. *Curr. Opin Genet. Dev*. 10: 428–433. 2000.

Ambros V. The functions of animal microRNAs. *Nature*. 431: 350-5. 2004.

Ambros V. MicroRNAs and developmental timing. *Curr Opin Genet Dev*. 21: 511–51 2011.

Ambros V, Horvitz HR. Heterochronic mutants of the nematode *Caenorhabditis elegans*. *Science*. 226: 409-416. 1984.

Aukerman MJ, Sakai H. Regulation of flowering time and floral organ identity by a microRNA and its *APETALA2-like* target genes. *Plant Cell*. 15: 2730–41. 2003

Baker CC, Sieber P, Wellmer F, Meyerowitz EM. The early extra petals1 mutant uncovers a role for microRNA miR164c in regulating petal number in *Arabidopsis*. *Curr. Biol*. 15: 303–15. 2005.

Bandres E, Bitarte N, Arias F, Agorreta J *et al.*, MicroRNA-451 regulates macrophage migration inhibitory factor production and proliferation of gastrointestinal cancer cells. *Clin. Cancer Res*. 15: 2281-2290. 2009.

Bartel DP. MicroRNAs: genomics, biogenesis, mechanism, and function. *Cell*. 116: 281–297. 2004.

Bazzini AA, Hopp HE, Beachy RN, Asurmendi S. Infection and coaccumulation of tobacco mosaic virus proteins alter microRNA levels, correlating with symptom and plant development. *Proc. Natl. Acad. Sci. USA*. 104: 12157–12162. 2007.

Bellingham SA, Coleman BM, Hill AF. Small RNA deep sequencing reveals a distinct miRNA signature released in exosomes from prion-infected neuronal cells *Nucleic Acids Res*. 40: 10937-10949. 2012.

Betel D, Wilson M, Gabow A, Marks DS, Sander C. The microRNA.org resource: targets and expression. *Nucleic Acids Res*. 36 (Database issue): D149-53. 2008.

Bonci D, Coppola V, Musumeci M, Addario A *et al.*, The miR-15a-miR-16-1 cluster controls prostate cancer by targeting multiple oncogenic activities. *Nat. Med*. 14: 1271-1277. 2008.

Bonnet E, Wuyts J, Rouze P, Van de Peer Y. Detection of 91 potential conserved plant microRNAs in *Arabidopsis thaliana* and *Oryza sativa* identifies important target genes. *Proc. Natl. Acad. Sci. USA*. 101: 11511–16. 2004.

Borchert GM, Lanier W, Davidson BL. RNA polymerase III transcribes human microRNAs. *Nat. Struct. Mol. Biol.* 13: 1097–1101. 2006.

Boyer JS. Plant productivity and environment. *Science*. 218: 443–448. 1982.

Brodersen P, Sakvarelidze-Achard L, Brunn-Rasmussen M, Dunoyer P *et al.*, Widespread translational inhibition by plant miRNAs and siRNAs. *Science*. 320: 1185–1190. 2008.

Butz H, Liko´ I, Czirja´k S, Igaz P *et al.*, Down-regulation of wee1 kinase by a specific subset of microRNA in human sporadic pituitary adenomas. *J. Clin. Endocrinol. Metab*. 95: E181-E191. 2010.

Calin GA, Croce CM. MicroRNA signatures in human cancers. *Nat. Rev. Cancer*. 6: 857-866. 2006.

Calin GA, Dumitru CD, Shimizu M, Bichi R *et al.*, Frequent deletions and down-regulation of micro-RNA genes miR15 and miR16 at 13q14 in chronic lymphocytic leukemia. *Proc. Natl. Acad. Sci. USA*. 99: 15524–15529. 2002.

Calin GA, Ferracin M, Cimmino A, Di Leva G *et al.*, A MicroRNA signature associated with prognosis and progression in chronic lymphocytic leukemia. *New Eng. J. Med.* 353: 1793-1801. 2005.

Calin GA, Sevignani C, Dumitru CD, Hyslop T. Human microRNA genes are frequently located at fragile sites and genomic regions involved in cancers. *Proc. Natl. Acad. Sci. USA*. 101: 2999- 3004. 2004b.

Chalfie M, Horvitz HR, Sulston JE. Mutations that lead to reiterations in the cell lineages of *C. elegans*. *Cell*. 24: 59-69. 1981.

Chen PS, Su JL, Hung MC. Dysregulation of MicroRNAs in cancer. *J. Biomed. Sci.* 19: 90. 2012.

Chen PY, Manninga H, Slanchev K, Chien M *et al.*, The developmental miRNA profiles of zebrafish as determined by small RNA cloning. *Genes Dev.* 19: 1288-1293. 2005.

Chen XM. microRNA biogenesis and function in plants. *FEBS Lett*. 579: 5923–5931. 2005.

Chendrimada TP, Gregory RI, Kumaraswamy E, Norman J, Cooch N. TRBP recruits the Dicer complex to Ago2 for microRNA processing and gene silencing. *Nature*. 436: 740–744. 2005.

Chiou TJ, Aung K, Lin SI, Wu CC, Chiang SF, Su CL. Regulation of phosphate homeostasis by MicroRNA in Arabidopsis. *Pl. Cell*. 18: 412–421. 2006.

Cho WC. MicroRNAs: Potential biomarkers for cancer diagnosis, prognosis and targets for therapy. *Intl. J. Biochem. Cell Biol.* 42: 1273-1281. 2010.

Choi WY, Giraldez AJ, Schier AF. Target protectors reveal dampening and balancing of Nodal agonist and antagonist by miR-430. *Science*. 318: 271–274. 2007.

Covarrubias AA, Reyes JL. Post-transcriptional gene regulation of salinity and drought responses by plant microRNAs. *Pl. Cell Environ*. 33: 481–489. 2010.

Croce CM. Causes and consequences of microRNA dysregulation in cancer. *Nat. Rev. Genet*. 10: 704-714. 2009.

Cross HS, Bareis P, Hofer H, Bischof MG *et al.*, 25-Hydroxyvitamin D3-1α-hydroxylase and vitamin D receptor gene expression in human colonic mucosa is elevated during early cancerogenesis. *Steroids*. 66: 287–92. 2001.

Cullen BR. Transcription and processing of human microRNA precursors. *Mol. Cell*. 16: 861-865. 2004.

Cuperus JT, Carbonell A, Fahlgren N, Garcia-Ruiz H *et al.*, Unique functionality of 22-nt miRNAs in triggering RDR6-dependent siRNA biogenesis from target transcripts in *Arabidopsis*. *Nat. Struct. Mol. Biol*. 17: 997–1003. 2010.

Davis BN, Hata A. Regulation of MicroRNA Biogenesis: A miRiad of mechanisms. *Cell Comm. Signal*. 7: 18-30. 2009.

Denli AM, Tops BB, Plasterk RH, Ketting RF, Hannon GJ. Processing of primary microRNAs by the microprocessor complex. *Nature*. 432: 231-235. 2004.

Dhandapani V, Ramchiary N, Paul P, Kim J, Choi SH, Lee J, Hur Y, Lim YP. Identification of potential microRNAs and their targets in *Brassica rapa* L. *Mol. Cell*. 32: 21-37. 2011.

Di LG, Calin GA, Croce CM. MicroRNAs: fundamental facts and involvement in human diseases. *Birth Defects Res. C. Embryo Today*. 78: 180-189. 2006.

Dusso AS, Brown AJ, Slatopolsky E. Vitamin D. *Amer. J. Physiol. Renal. Physiol*. 289: F8-F28. 2005.

Ebert MS, Neilson JR, Sharp PA. MicroRNA sponges: competitive inhibitors of small RNAs in mammalian cells. *Nat. Methods*. 4: 721–726. 2007.

Enright AJ, John B, Gaul U, Tuschl T *et al.*, MicroRNA targets in Drosophila. *Genome Biol*. 5: R1. Epub. 2003.

Esquela-Kerscher A, Slack FJ. Oncomirs- microRNAs with a role in cancer. *Nature Rev*. 6: 259-269. 2006.

Eva VR. The art of microRNA research. *Circulation Res*. 108: 219-234. 2011.

Fahlgren N, Howell MD, Kasschau KD, Chapman EJ *et al.*, High-throughput sequencing of Arabidopsis microRNAs: evidence for frequent birth and death of MIRNA genes. *PLoS ONE*. 2: 219. 2007.

Fazi F, Blandino G. MicroRNA: from development to human diseases: tentative outline. *Spel. Issue microRNA J*. 2013.

Fearon ER, Vogelstein B. A genetic model for colorectal tumorigenesis. *Cell*. 61: 759-767. 1990.

Feshani AM, Mohannadi S, Frazier TP, Abbasi A *et al.*, Identification and validation of Asteraceae miRNA by the expressed sequence tag analysis. *Gene*. 493: 253-259. 2012.

Fire A, Xu S, Montgomery MK, Kostas SA, Driver SE, Mello CC. Potent and specific genetic interference by double stranded RNA in *Caenorhabditis elegans*. *Nature*. 391: 806-811. 1998.

Friedman RC, Farh KK, Burge CB, Bartel DP. Most mammalian mRNAs are conserved targets of microRNAs. *Genome Res*. 19: 92-105. 2009.

Gaidatzis D, van Nimwegen E, Hausser J, Zavolan M. Inference of miRNA targets using evolutionary conservation and pathway analysis. *BMC Bioinform*. 8: 69. 2007.

Gao ZH, Wei JH, Yang Y, Zhang Z *et al.*, Identification of conserved and novel microRNAs in *Aquilaria sinensis* based on small RNA sequencing and transcriptome sequence data. *Gene*. 505: 167-175. 2012.

Garland CF, Garland FC, Gorham ED, Lipkin M, Newmark H, Mohr, SB, Holick MF. The role of vitamin D in cancer prevention. *Amer. J. Pub. Health*. 96: 252–61. 2006.

Garzon R, Marcucci G, Croce CM. Targeting microRNAs in cancer: Rationale, strategies and challenges. *Nat. Rev. Drug Discov*. 9: 775-789. 2010.

Gebeshuber CA, Zatloukal K, Martinez J. miR-29a suppresses tristetraprolin, which is a regulator of epithelial polarity and metastasis. *EMBO Rep*. 10: 400-405. 2009.

Gleave AP, Ampomah-Dwamena C, Berthold S, Dejnoprat S *et al.*, Identification and characterization of primary microRNAs from Apple (*Malus domestic acv.* Royal Gala) expressed sequence tags. *Tree Genet. Genomes*. 4: 343-358. 2008.

Gregory RI and Shiekhattar R. MicroRNA biogenesis and cancer. *Cancer Res*. 65: 3509-3512. 2005.

Gregory RI, Yan KP, Amuthan G, Chendrimada T *et al.*, The Microprocessor complex mediates the genesis of microRNAs. *Nature*. 432: 235-240. 2004.

Griffiths-Jones S. The microRNA registry. *Nucleic Acids Res*. 32: D109–11. 2004.

Griffiths-Jones S, Grocock RJ, van Dongen S, Bateman A, Enright AJ. miRNase: microRNA sequences, targets and gene nomenclature. *Nucleic Acids Res*. 34: D140–D144. 2006.

Grün D, Wang YL, Langenberger D, Gunsalus KC, Rajewsky N. microRNA target predictions across seven *Drosophila* species and comparison to mammalian targets. *PLoS Comput. Biol*. 1: e13. Epub. 2005.

Guo LM, Pu Y, Han Z, Liu T *et al.*, MicroRNA-9 inhibits ovarian cancer cell growth through regulation of NF-kappaB1. *FEBS J*. 276: 5537-5546. 2009.

Ha TY. The Role of microRNAs in regulatory T cells and in the immune response. *Immune Network*. 11: 11-41. 2011.

Hammell CM, Lubin I, Boag PR, Blackwell TK, Ambros V. nhl-2 modulates microRNA activity in *Caenorhabditis elegans*. *Cell*, 136: 926-938. 2009.

Han J, Lee Y, Yeom KH, Kim YK, Jin H, Kim VN. The Drosha-DGCR8 complex in primary microRNA processing. *Genes Dev*. 18: 3016-3027. 2004.

Han Y, Zhu B, Luan F, Zhu H *et al.*, Conserved miRNAs and their targets identified in lettuce (*Lactuca*) by EST analysis. *Gene*. 463: 1-7. 2010.

Hanahan D, Weinberg RA. Hallmarks of cancer. The next generation. *Cell*. 144: 646-674. 2011.

Hausser J, Berninger P, Rodak C, Jantscher Y *et al.*, MirZ: an integrated microRNA expression atlas and target prediction resource. *Nucleic Acids Res*. 37: W266-72. 2009.

He L, He X, Lowe SW, Hannon GJ. MicroRNAs join the p53 network—another piece in the tumour-suppression puzzle. *Nat. Rev. Cancer*. 7: 819-822. 2007.

He L, Thomson JM, Hemann MT, Hernando-Monge E *et al.*, A microRNA polycistron as a potential human oncogene. *Nature*. 435: 828-833. 2005.

He XF, Fang YY, Feng L, Guo HS. Characterization of conserved and novel microRNAs and their targets, including a TuMV-induced TIR-NBS-LRR class R gene-derived novel miRNA in Brassica. *FEBS Lett*. 582: 2445–2452. 2008.

Hermeking H. p53 enters the microRNA world. *Cancer Cell*. 12: 414-418. 2007.

Hill DA, Ivanovich J, Priest JR, Gurnett CA *et al.*, DICER1 mutations in familial pleuropulmonary blastoma. *Science*. 325: 965. 2009.

Hock J, Weinmann L, Ender C, Rudel S *et al.*, Proteomic and functional analysis of Argonaute containing mRNA-protein complexes in human cells. *EMBO Rep*. 8: 1052-1060. 2007.

Hofacker IL, Stadler PF. Memory efficient folding algorithms for circular RNA secondary structures. *Bioinformatics*. 22: 1172-6. 2006.

Horvitz HR, Sternberg PW, Greenwald IS, Fixsen W, Ellis HM. Mutations that affect neural cell lineages and cell fates during the development of the nematode Caenorhabditis elegans. *Cold Spring Harb. Symp. Quant Biol*. 48: 453-463. 1983.

Hsu SD, Chu CH, Tsou AP, Chen SJ *et al.*, miRNAMap 2.0: genomic maps of microRNAs in metazoan genomes. *Nucleic Acids Res*. 36: D165-9. 2008.

Hubbard T, Barker D, Birney E, Cameron G *et al.*, The Ensembl genome database project. *Nucleic Acids Res*. 30: 38-41.2002.

Iorio MV, Croce CM. MicroRNA dysregulation in cancer: diagnostics, monitoring and therapeutics. A comprehensive review. *EMBO Mol. Med*. 4: 143–159. 2011.

Iorio MV, Ferracin M, Liu CG, Veronese A *et al.*, MicroRNA gene expression deregulation in human breast cancer. *Cancer Res*. 65: 7065-7070. 2005.

Iorio MV, Visone R, Di Leva G, Donati V *et al.*, MicroRNA signatures in human ovarian cancer. *Cancer Res*. 67: 8699-8707. 2007.

agadeeswaran G, Saini A, Sunkar R. Biotic and abiotic stress down-regulate miR398 expression in Arabidopsis. *Planta*. 229: 1009–1014. 2009.

emal A, Bray F, Center MM, Ferlay J *et al.*, Global cancer statistics. *CA. Cancer J. Clin*. 61: 69-90. 2011.

emal A, Siegel R, Ward E, Hao Y *et al.*, Cancer statistics 2008. *CA. Cancer J. Clin*. 58: 71-96. 2008.

emal A, Siegel R, Ward E, Murray T *et al.*, Cancer statistics 2006. *CA. Cancer J. Clin*. 56: 106–130. 2006.

eon HM, Sohn YW, Oh SY, Kim SH *et al.*, ID4 imparts chemoresistance and cancer stemness to glioma cells by derepressing miR-9 -mediated suppression of SOX2. *Cancer Res*. 71: 3410–21. 2011.

i Z, Lee JY, Pan Z, Jiang B, Tian B. Progressive lengthening of 3′ untranslated regions of mRNAs by alternative polyadenylation during mouse embryonic development. *Proc. Natl. Acad. Sci. USA*. 106: 7028-7033. 2009.

iang J, Lee EJ, Gusev Y, Schmittgen TD. Real-time expression profiling of microRNA precursors in human cancer cell lines. *Nucleic Acids Res*. 33: 5394–5403. 2005.

in W, Li N, Zhang B, Wu F *et al.*, Identification and verification of microRNA in wheat. *J. Plant Res*. 121: 351-5. 2008.

ohn B, Enright AJ, Aravin A, Tuschl T *et al.*, Human MicroRNA Targets. *PLoS Biol*. 2: e363. 2004.

ohnson CD, Esquela-Kerscher A, Stefani G, Byrom M. The let-7 MicroRNA Represses Cell Proliferation Pathways in Human Cells. *Cancer Res*. 67: 7713-7722. 2007.

ones-Rhoades MW, Bartel DP. Computational identification of plant microRNAs and their targets, including a stress-induced miRNA. *Mol. Cell*. 14: 787–799. 2004.

ones-Rhoades MW, Bartel DP, Bartel B. Micro RNAs and their regulatory roles in plants. *Ann. Rev. Plant Biol*. 57: 19-53. 2006.

Karlin S, Altschul SF. Methods for assessing the statistical significance of molecular sequence features by using general scoring schemes. *Proc. Natl. Acad. Sci. USA*. 87: 2264-8. 1990.

Kasschau KD, Xie Z, Allen E, Llave C *et al.*, P1/HC-Pro, a viral suppressor of RNA silencing, interferes with Arabidopsis development and miRNA function. *Dev. Cell*. 4: 205–217. 2003.

Katada T, Ishiguro H, Kuwabara Y, Kimura M *et al.*, MicroRNA expression profile in undifferentiated gastric cancer. *Intl. J. Oncol*. 34: 537-542. 2009.

Kertesz M, Iovino N, Unnerstall U, Gaul U, Segal E. The role of site accessibility in microRNA target recognition. *Nat. Genet*. 39: 1278-84. 2007.

Kim HJ, Baek KH, Lee BW, Choi D, Hur CG. In silico identification and characterization of microRNAs and their putative target genes in Solanaceae plants. *Genome*. 54: 91-98. 2011.

Kim J, Jung JH, Reyes JL, Kim YS *et al.*, microRNA-directed cleavage of *ATHB15* mRNA regulates vascular development in *Arabidopsis* inflorescence stems. *Plant J.* 42: 84–94. 2005.

Kim VN, Nam JW. Genomics of microRNA. Trends *Genet.* 22: 165-73. 2006.

Kiriakidou M, Nelson PT, Kouranov A, Fitziev P *et al.*, A combined computational experimental approach predicts human microRNA targets. *Genes Dev.* 18: 1165-78. 2004.

Kiyosawa K, Sodeyama T, Tanaka E, Gibo Y *et al.*, Interrelationship of blood transfusion, non-A, non-B hepatitis and hepatocellular carcinoma: analysis by detection of antibody to hepatitis C virus. *Hepatology*. 12: 671-675. 1990.

Kloting N, Berthold K, Kovacs P, Schon MR *et al.*, MicroRNA expression in human omental and subcutaneous adipose tissue. *PLoS ONE*. 4: e4699. 2009.

Kota J, Chivukula RR, O'Donnell KA, Wentzel EA *et al.*, Therapeutic microRNA delivery suppresses tumorigenesis in a murine liver cancer model. *Cell.* 137: 1005–1017. 2009.

Kozomara A, Griffiths-Jones S. miRBase: integrating microRNA annotation and deep-sequencing data. *Nucleic Acids Res.* 39: D152-7. 2011.

Krek A, Grün D, Poy MN, Wolf R *et al.*, Combinatorial microRNA target predictions. *Nat. Genet.* 37: 495-500. 2005.

Krüger J, Rehmsmeier M. RNAhybrid: microRNA target prediction easy, fast and flexible. *Nucleic Acids Res.* 34: W451-4. 2006.

Lagos-Quintana M, Rauhut R, Lendeckel W, Tuschl T. Identification of novel genes coding for small expressed RNAs. *Science*. 294: 853–860. 2001.

Lai EC. Predicting and validating microRNA targets. *Genome Biol.* 5: 115. 2004.

Lai EC, Tomancak P, Williams R, Rubin GM. Computational identification of *Drosophila* microRNA genes. *Genome Biol.* 4: 1- 20. 2003.

Lall S, Grün D, Krek A, Chen K *et al.*, A genome-wide map of conserved microRNA targets in *C. elegans*. *Curr. Biol.* 16: 460-71. 2006.

Landgraf P, Rusu M, Sheridan R, Sewer A *et al.*, A mammalian microRNA expression atlas based on small RNA library sequencing. *Cell.* 129: 1401-14. 2007.

Landthaler M, Yalcin A, Tuschl T. The human DiGeorge syndrome critical region gene 8 and Its *D. melanogaster* homolog are required for miRNA biogenesis. *Curr. Bio.* 14: 2162-2167. 2004.

Lanet E, Delannoy E, Sormani R, Floris M *et al.*, Biochemical evidence for translational repression by Arabidopsis microRNAs. *Plant Cell.* 21: 1762–1768. 2009.

Lau NC, Lim LP, Weinstein EG, Bartel DP. An abundant class of tiny RNAs with probable regulatory roles in *Caenorhabditis elegans*. *Science*. 294: 858–62. 2001.

Lecellier CH, Dunoyer P, Arar K, Lehmann-Che J *et al.*, A cellular microRNA mediates antiviral defense in human cells. *Science*. 308: 557-560. 2005.

Lee EJ, Gusev Y, Jiang J, Nuovo GJ *et al.*, Expression profiling identifies microRNA signature in pancreatic cancer. *Intl. J. Cancer*. 120: 1046-1054. 2007.

Lee KH, Lotterman C, Karikari C, Omura N *et al.*, Epigenetic silencing of MicroRNA miR-107 regulates cyclin-dependent kinase 6 expression in pancreatic cancer. *Pancreatology*. 9: 293-301. 2009.

Lee RC, Ambros V. An extensive class of small RNAs in *Caenorhabditis elegans*. *Science*. 294: 862–864. 2001

Lee RC, Feinbaum RL, Ambros V. The C. elegans heterochronic gene lin-4 encodes small RNAs with antisense complementarity to lin-14. *Cell*. 75: 843–854. 1993.

Lee Y, Ahn C, Han J, Choi H *et al.*, The nuclear RNase III Drosha initiates microRNA processing. *Nature*. 425: 415-419. 2003.

Lee Y, Kim M, Han J, Yeom KH *et al.*, MicroRNA genes are transcribed by RNA polymerase II. *EMBO J*. 23: 4051–60. 2004.

Legrand S, Valot N, Niolé F, Moja S *et al.*, One-step identification of conserved miRNAs, their targets, potential transcription factors and effector genes of complete secondary metabolism pathways after 454 pyrosequencing of calyx cDNAs from the Labiate *Salvia sclarea* L. *Gene*. 450: 55-62. 2010.

Leidinger P, Backes C, Deutscher S, Schmitt K. A blood based 12-miRNA signature of Alzheimer disease patients. *Genome Biol*. 14: R78. 2013.

Lewis BP, Shih IH, Jones-Rhoades MW, Bartel DP, Burge CB. Prediction of mammalian microRNA targets. *Cell*. 115: 787- 798. 2003.

Li F, Pignatta D, Bendix C, Brunkard JO *et al.*, MicroRNA regulation of plant innate immune receptors. *Proc. Natl. Acad. Sci. USA*. 109: 1790–1795. 2012.

Li H, Dong Y, Sun Y, Zhu E *et al.*, Investigation of the microRNAs in safflower seed, leaf, and petal by high-throughput sequencing. *Planta*. 233: 611–619. 2010.

Li WX, Oono Y, Zhu J, He XJ *et al.*, The Arabidopsis NFYA5 transcription factor is regulated transcriptionally and posttranscriptionally to promote drought resistance. *Plant Cell*. 20: 2238–2251. 2008.

Lindsay EA. Chromosomal microdeletions: dissecting del22q11 syndrome. *Nat. Rev. Genet*. 2: 858-868. 2001.

Liston A, Linterman M, Lu LF. MicroRNA in the adaptive immune system, in sickness and in health. *J. Clin. Immunol*. 30: 339-346. 2010.

Liu K, Li G, Fan C, Diao Y, Wu B, Li J. Increased expression of microRNA-221 in gastric cancer and its clinical significance. *J. Intl. Med. Res*. 40: 467-474. 2012.

Llave C, Kasschau KD, Rector MA, Carrington JC. Endogenous and silencing associated small RNAs in plants. *Plant Cell*. 14: 1605–19. 2002.

Loberg RD, Logothetis CJ, Keller ET, Pienta KJ. Pathogenesis and treatment of prostate cancer bone metastases: targeting the lethal phenotype. *J. Clin. Oncol*. 23: 8232-8241. 2005.

Lu C, Tej SS, Luo S, Haudenschild CD, Meyers BC, Green PJ. Elucidation of the small RNA component of the transcriptome. *Science*. 309: 1567–1569. 2005a.

Lu J, Getz G, Miska EA, Alvarez-Saavedra E *et al.*, MicroRNA expression profiles classify human cancers. *Nature*. 435: 834-8. 2005.

Lu S, Sun YH, Amerson H, Chiang VL. MicroRNAs in loblolly pine (*Pinus taeda* L.) and their association with fusiform rust gall development. *Plant J*. 51: 1077–1098. 2007.

Lu S, Sun YH, Shi R, Clark C, Li L, Chiang VL. Novel and mechanical stress-responsive MicroRNAs in *Populus trichocarpa* that are absent from *Arabidopsis*. *Plant Cell*. 17: 2186–2203. 2005.

Lu Y, Okubo T, Rawlins E, Hogan BLM. Epithelial Progenitor Cells of the Embryonic Lung and the Role of MicroRNAs in their Proliferation. *Proc. Amer. Thorac. Soc.* 5: 300-304. 2008.

Lujambio A, Ropero S, Ballestar E, Fraga MF *et al.*, Genetic Unmasking of an Epigenetically Silenced microRNA in Human Cancer Cells. *Cancer Res*. 67: 1424-1429. 2007.

Majer A, Medina SJ, Niu Y, Abrenica B *et al.*, Early mechanisms of pathobiology are revealed by transcriptional temporal dynamics in hippocampal CA1 neurons of prion infected mice. *PLoS Pathog*. 8: e1003002. 2012.

Mallory AC, Elmayan T, Vaucheret H. MicroRNA maturation and action–the expanding roles of argonautes. *Curr. Opin. Plant Biol*. 11: 560–566. 2008.

Martin RC, Liu PP, Goloviznina NA, Nonogaki H. MicroRNA, seeds, and Darwin?: diverse function of miRNA in seed biology and plant responses to stress. *J. Expt. Bot*. 61: 2229–2234. 2010.

McManus MT. MicroRNAs and cancer. *Cancer Biol*. 13: 253-258. 2003.

Melo SA, Kalluri R. Molecular Pathways: MicroRNAs as Cancer Therapeutics. *Clin. Cancer Res*. 18: 4234-4239. 2012.

Melo SA, Moutinho C, Ropero S, Calin GA *et al.*, A genetic defect in exportin-5 traps precursor microRNAs in the nucleus of cancer cells. *Cancer Cell*. 18: 303–15. 2010.

Melo SA, Ropero S, Moutinho C, Aaltonen LA *et al.*, A TARBP2 mutation in human cancer impairs microRNA processing and DICER1 function. *Nat. Genet*. 41: 365–70. 2009.

Mette MF, van der Winden J, Matzke M, Matzke AJ. Short RNAs can identify new candidate transposable element families in *Arabidopsis*. *Plant Physiol*. 130: 6–9. 2002.

Michael MZ, O'Connor SM, van Holst Pellekaan NG, Young GP, James RJ. Reduced accumulation of specific microRNAs in colorectal neoplasia. *Mol. Cancer Res*. 1: 882–91. 2003.

Mohri T, Nakajima M, Takagi S, Komagata S, Yokoi T. MicroRNA regulates human vitamin D receptor. Intl. *J. Cancer*. 125: 1328–1333. 2009.

Moller HG, Rasmussen AP, Andersen HH, Johnsen KB *et al.*, A Systematic Review of MicroRNA in Glioblastoma Multiforme: Micro-modulators in the Mesenchymal Mode of Migration and Invasion. *Mol. Neurobiol.* 47: 131–144. 2013.

Motoyama K, Inoue H, Mimori K, Tanaka F *et al.*, Clinicopathological and prognostic significance of PDCD4 and microRNA-21 in human gastric cancer. *Intl. J. Oncol.* 36: 1089-1095. 2010.

Mraz M, Pospisilova S. MicroRNAs in chronic lymphocytic leukemia: From causality to associations and back. *Expert Rev. Hematol.* 5: 579–581. 2012.

Mraz M, Pospisilova S, Malinova K, Slapak I, Mayer J. MicroRNAs in chronic lymphocytic leukemia pathogenesis and disease subtypes. *Leuk. Lymphoma.* 50: 506–9. 2009.

Nagpal S, Na S, Rathnachalam R. Noncalcemic actions of vitamin D, receptor ligands. *Endocr. Rev.* 26: 662–87. 2005.

Nam S, Kim B, Shin S, Lee S. miRGator: an integrated system for functional annotation of microRNAs. *Nucleic Acids Res.* 36: D159-64. 2008.

Nam S, Li M, Choi K, Balch C *et al.*, MicroRNA and mRNA integrated analysis (MMIA): a web tool for examining biological functions of microRNA expression. *Nucleic Acids Res.* 37: W356-62. 2009.

Napoli C, Lemieux C, Jorgensen R. Introduction of a chimeric chalcone synthase gene into petunia results in reversible co-suppression of homologous genes in trans. *Plant Cell.* 2: 279–289. 1990.

Navarro A, Gaya A, Martinez A, Urbano-Ispizua A *et al.*, MicroRNA expression profiling in classic Hodgkin lymphoma. *Blood.* 111: 2825-2832. 2008.

Navarro L, Dunoyer P, Jay F, Arnold B *et al.*, A plant miRNA contributes to antibacterial resistance by repressing auxin signalling. *Science.* 312: 436–439. 2006.

Navarro L, Jay F, Nomura K, He SY, Voinnet O. Suppression of the microRNA pathway by bacterial effector proteins. *Science.* 321: 964–967. 2008.

Nikiforova MN, Tseng GC, Steward D, Diorio D, Nikiforov YE. MicroRNA expression profiling of thyroid tumors: biological significance and diagnostic utility. *J. Clin. Endocrinol. Metab.* 93: 1600-1608. 2008.

Nishida N, Mimori K, Fabbri M, Yokobori T *et al.*, MicroRNA-125a-5p is an independent prognostic factor in gastric cancer and inhibits the proliferation of human gastric cancer cells in combination with trastuzumab. *Clin. Cancer Res.* 17: 2725-2733. 2011.

Numnark S, Mhuantong W, Ingsriswang S, Wichadakul D. C-mii: a tool for plant miRNA and target identification. *BMC Genomics.* 7: S16. 2012.

O'Donnell KA, Wentzel EA, Zeller KI, Dang CV, Mendell JT. c-Myc-regulated microRNAs modulate E2F1 expression. *Nature.* 435: 839-843. 2005.

O'Neill LA, Sheedy FJ, McCoy CE. MicroRNAs. The fine-tuners of Toll-like receptor signalling. *Nat. Rev. Immunol.* 11: 163-175. 2011.

Osaki M, Takeshita F, Ochiya T. MicroRNAs as biomarkers and therapeutic drugs in human cancer. *Biomarkers*. 13: 658-670. 2008.

Palatnik JF, Allen E, Wu X, Schommer C *et al.*, Control of leaf morphogenesis by microRNAs. *Nature*. 425: 257–63. 2003.

Papadopoulos GL, Reczko M, Simossis VA, Sethupathy P, Hatzigeorgiou AG. The database of experimentally supported targets: a functional update of TarBase. *Nucleic Acids Res*. 37: D155-8. 2009.

Park W, Li J, Song R, Messing J, Chen X. Carpel Factory, a Dicer homolog, and HEN1, a novel protein, act in microRNA metabolism in *Arabidopsis thaliana*. *Curr. Biol*. 12: 1484–95. 2002.

Paul S. Molecule of the month: miRNA and Human Prion brain disease. *Bioinformation*. 9: 659-660. 2013.

Pfeffer S, Sewer A, Lagos-Quintana M, Sheridan R *et al.*, Identification of microRNAs of the herpesvirus family. *Nat. Methods*. 2: 269-276. 2005.

Pfeffer S, Zavolan M, Grässer FA, Chien M *et al.*, Identification of virus-encoded microRNAs. *Science*. 304: 734-736. 2004.

Qiu D, Pan X, Wilson IW, Li F *et al.*, High thoroughput sequencing technology reveals that the taxoid elicitor methyl jasmonate regulates microRNA expression in Chinese yew (*Taxus chinensis*). *Gene*. 436: 37-44. 2009.

Rajagopalan, R, Vaucheret H, Trejo J, Bartel DP. A diverse and evolutionarily fluid set of microRNAs in *Arabidopsis thaliana*. *Genes Dev*. 20: 3407. 2006.

Reinhart BJ, Weinstein EG, Rhoades MW, Bartel B, Bartel DP. MicroRNAs in plants. *Genes Dev*. 16: 1616–26. 2002.

Roubelakis MG, Zotos P, Papachristoudis G, Michalopoulos I *et al.* Human microRNA target analysis and gene ontology clustering by GOmir, a novel stand-alone application. *BMC Bioinformatics*. 6: S20. 2009. 2009.

Ruvkun, G. Molecular Biology: Glimpses of a Tiny RNA World. *Science*. 294: 797–799. 2001.

Saba R, Gushue S, Huzarewich RL, Manguiat K *et al.*, MicroRNA 146a (miR-146a) is over-expressed during prion disease and modulates the innate immune response and the microglial activation state. *PLoS ONE*. 7: e30832. 2012.

Sandberg R, Neilson J, Sarma A, Sharp P, Burge C. Proliferating cells express mRNAs with shortened 3′ untranslated regions and fewer microRNA target sites. *Science*. 320: 1643-1647. 2008.

Schetter AJ, Heegaard NH, Harris CC. Inflammation and cancer: interweaving microRNA, free radical, cytokine and p53 pathways. *Carcinogenesis*. 31: 37-49. 2010.

Schwamborn J, Berezikov E, Knoblich J. The TRIM-NHL protein TRIM32 activates microRNAs and prevents self-renewal in mouse neural progenitors. *Cell*. 136: 913-925. 2009.

Seki M, Narusaka M, Ishida J, Nanjo T *et al.*, Monitoring the expression profiles of 7000 Arabidopsis genes under drought, cold and high-salinity stresses using a full-length cDNA microarray. *Plant J.* 31: 279–292. 2002.

Selbach M, Schwanhausser B, Thierfelder N, Fang Z *et al.*, Widespread changes in protein synthesis induced by microRNAs. *Nature.* 455: 58-63. 2008.

Sempere LF, Freemantle S, Pitha-Rowe I, Moss E *et al.*, Expression profiling of mammalian MicroRNAs uncovers a subset of brain-expressed MicroRNAs with possible roles in murine and human neuronal differentiation. *Genome Biol.* 5: 1-13(R13). 2004.

Sethupathy P, Corda B, Hatzigeorgiou AG. TarBase: A comprehensive database of experimentally supported animal microRNA targets. *RNA.* 12: 192-7. 2006.

Shenouda SK, Alahari SK. MicroRNA function in cancer: Oncogene or a tumor suppressor? *Cancer Metastasis Rev.* 28: 369-378. 2009.

Shiohama A, Sasaki T, Noda S, Minoshima S, Shimizu N. Molecular cloning and expression analysis of a novel gene DGCR8 located in the DiGeorge syndrome chromosomal region. *Biochem. Biophys. Res.* Comm. 304: 184-190. 2003.

Shivaprasad PV, Chen H-M, Patel K, Bond DM *et al.*, A microRNA superfamily regulates nucleotide binding site–leucine-rich repeats and other mRNAs. *Plant Cell.* 24: 859–874. 2012.

Shuai P, Liang D, Zhang Z, Yin W, Xia X. Identification of drought-responsive and novel Populus trichocarpa microRNAs by high-throughput sequencing and their targets using degradome analysis. *BMC Genomics.* 14: 233. 2013.

Si ML, Zhu S, Wu H, Lu Z *et al.*, miR-21-mediated tumor growth. *Oncogene.* 26: 2799-2803. 2007.

Slaby O, Svoboda M, Michalek J, Vyzula R. MicroRNAs in colorectal cancer: Translation of molecular biology into clinical application. *Mol. Cancer.* 8: 102. 2009.

Soifer HS, Rossi JJ, Saetrom P. MicroRNAs in disease and potential therapeutic applications. *Mol Ther.* 15: 2070-2079. 2007.

Song C, Jia Q, Fang J, Li F *et al.*, Computational identification of citrus microRNAs and target analysis in citrus expressed sequence tags. *Plant Biol.* 12: 927–934. 2010.

Sullivan CS, Grundhoff AT, Tevethia S, Pipas JM, Ganem D. SV40-encoded microRNAs regulate viral gene expression and reduce susceptibility to cytotoxic T cells. *Nature.* 435: 682-686. 2005.

Sunkar R, Girke T, Jain PK, Zhu JK. Cloning and characterization of microRNAs from rice. *Plant Cell.* 17: 1397–411. 2005.

Sunkar R, Kapoor A, Zhu JK. Posttranscriptional induction of two Cu/Zn superoxide dismutase genes in *Arabidopsis* is mediated by downregulation of miR398 and important for oxidative stress tolerance. *Plant Cell.* 18: 2051–2065. 2006.

Sunkar R, Zhu JK. Novel and stress-regulated microRNAs and other small RNAs from Arabidopsis. *Plant Cell*. 16: 2001–19. 2004.

Tai-You H. MicroRNAs in Human Diseases: From Cancer to Cardiovascular Disease *Immune. Network*. 11: 135-154. 2011.

Tavazoie SF, Alarcón C, Oskarsson T, Padua D *et al.*, Endogenous human microRNAs that suppress breast cancer metastasis. *Nature*. 451: 147-152. 2008.

Taylor DD, Gercel-Taylor C. MicroRNA signatures of tumor- derived exosomes as diagnostic biomarkers of ovarian cancer. *Gynecol. Oncol*. 110: 13-21. 2008.

Tili E, Michaille JJ, Calin GA. Expression and function of micro-RNAs in immune cells during normal or disease state. *Intl. J. Med. Sci*. 5: 73-79. 2008.

Trang P, Medina PP, Wiggins JF, Ruffino L *et al.*, Regression of murine lung tumors by the let-7 microRNA. *Oncogene*. 29: 1580–1587. 2010.

Ura S, Honda M, Yamashita T, Ueda T *et al.*, Differential MicroRNA Expression Between Hepatitis B and Hepatitis C Leading Disease Progression to Hepatocellular Carcinoma. *Hepatology*. 49: 1098-1112. 2009.

Vasudevan S, Steitz J. AU-rich-element-mediated upregulation of translation by FXR1 and Argonaute 2. *Cell*. 128: 1105-1118. 2007.

Vasudevan S, Tong Y, Steitz J. Switching from repression to activation: microRNAs can up-regulate translation. *Science*. 318: 1931-1934. 2007b

Vazquez F. *Arabidopsis* endogenous small RNAs: highways and byways. *Trends Plant Sci*. 11: 460–468. 2006.

Vazquez F, Blevins T, Ailhas J, Boller T, Meins F. Evolution of Arabidopsis MIR genes generates novel microRNA classes. *Nucleic Acids Res*. 36: 6429–6438. 2008

Volinia S, Calin GA, Chang-Gong L, Ambs S *et al.*, A microRNA expression signature of human solid tumors defines cancer gene targets. *Proc. Natl. Acad. Sci. USA* 103: 2257–2261. 2006.

Volk N, Shomron N. Versatility of MicroRNA Biogenesis. *PLoS ONE*. 6: e19391. 2011.

Wang J, Hou X, Yang X. Identification of conserved microRNAs and their targets in Chinese cabbage (*Brassica rapa* subsp. pekinensis). *Genome*. 52: 1029–1040. 2011.

Wang J, Yang X, Xu H, Chi X *et al.*, Identification and characterization of micro RNAs and their target genes in *Brassica oleracea*. *Gene*. 505: 300-308. 2012.

Wang QZ, Xu W, Habib N, Xu R. Potential Uses of MicroRNA in Lung Cancer Diagnosis, Prognosis, and Therapy. *Curr. Cancer Drug Targt*. 9: 572-594. 2009.

Wang X. MiRDB: a microRNA target prediction and functional annotation database with a wiki interface. *RNA*. 14: 1012-7. 2008.

Wang X, El Naqa IM. Prediction of both conserved and nonconserved microRNA targets in animals. *Bioinformatics*. 24: 325-32. 2008.

Wang X, Zhang J, Li F, Gu J, He T *et al.*, MicroRNA identification based on sequence and structure alignment. *Bioinformatics*. 21: 3610-4. 2005.

Wang XJ, Reyes JL, Chua NH, Gaasterland T. Prediction and identification of *Arabidopsis thaliana* microRNAs and their mRNA targets. *Genome Biol.* 5: R65. 2004.

Watanabe Y, Tomita M, Kanai A. Computational methods for microRNA target prediction. *Methods Enzymol.* 427: 65-86. 2007.

Weber MJ New human and mouse microRNA genes found by homology search. *FEBS J.* 272: 59-73. 2005.

Williams L, Grigg SP, Xie M, Christensen S, Fletcher JC. Regulation of *Arabidopsis* shoot apical meristem and lateral organ formation by microRNA *miR166g* and its *AtHDZIP* target genes. *Development.* 132: 3657–68. 2005.

Xie F, Frazier TP, Zhang B. Identification and characterization of microRNAs and their targets in the bioenergy plant switchgrass (*Panicum virgatum*). *Planta.* 232: 417–434. 2010.

Xie F, Frazier TP, Zhang B. Identification, characterization and expression analysis of MicroRNAs and their targets in the potato (*Solanum tuberosum*). *Gene.* 473: 8-22. 2011.

Xin M, Wang Y, Yao Y, Xie C *et al.,* Diverse set of microRNAs are responsive to powdery mildew infection and heat stress in wheat (*Triticum aestivum* L.). *BMC Plant Biol.* 10: 123. 2010.

Yanaihara N, Caplen N, Bowman E, Seike M *et al.,* Unique microRNA molecular proles in lung cancer diagnosis and prognosis. *Cancer Cell.* 9: 189-198. 2006.

Yang JH, Qu LH. DeepBase: annotation and discovery of microRNAs and other noncoding RNAs from deep-sequencing data. *Methods Mol. Biol.* 822: 233-48. 2012.

Yang W, Liu X, Zhang J, Feng J *et al.,* Prediction and validation of conservative microRNAs of *Solanum tuberosum* L. *Mol. Biol. Rep.* 37: 3081-7. 2010.

Yao Y, Suo AL, Li ZF, Liu LY *et al.,* MicroRNA profiling of human gastric cancer. *Mol. Med. Rep.* 2: 963-970. 2009.

Yendamuri S, Calin GA. The role of microRNA in human leukemia: a review. *Leukemia.* 23: 1257-1263. 2009.

Yeung ML, Bennasser Y, Myers TG, Jiang G *et al.,* Changes in microRNA expression profiles in HIV- 1-transfected human cells. *Retrovirology.* 2: 81-88. 2005.

Yi R, Qin Y, Macara IG, Cullen BR. Exportin-5 mediates the nuclear export of pre-microRNAs and short hairpin RNAs. *Genes Dev.* 17: 3011–3016. 2003.

Yin Y, Li J, Chen S, Zhou T, Si J. MicroRNAs as diagnostic biomarkers in gastric cancer. *Intl. J. Mol. Sci.* 13: 12544-12555. 2012.

Yu B, Yang Z, Li J, Minakhina S, Yang M *et al.,* Methylation as a crucial step in plant microRNA biogenesis. *Science.* 307: 932–935. 2005.

Yu H, Song C, Jia Q, Wang C *et al.*, Computational identification of microRNAs in apple expressed sequence tags and validation of their precise sequences by miR-RAC. *Physiol. Plant.* 141: 56-70. 2011.

Zhai J, Jeong DH, Paoli ED, Park S *et al.*, MicroRNAs are master regulators of the plant NB-LRR defense gene family via the production of phased, trans-acting siRNAs. *Gene Dev.* 25: 2540-2553. 2011.

Zhang B, Wang Q, Wang K, Pan X *et al.*, Identification of cotton microRNAs and their targets. *Gene.* 397: 26-37. 2007.

Zhang BH, Pan XP, Anderson TA. Identification of 188 conserved maize microRNAs and their targets. *FEBS Lett.* 580: 3753–3762. 2006a.

Zhang BH, Pan XP, Cannon CH, Cobb GP, Anderson TA. Conservation and divergence of plant microRNA genes. *Plant J.* 46: 243–259. 2006b.

Zhang BH, Pan XP, Cobb GP, Anderson TA. Plant microRNA: a small regulatory molecule with big impact. *Dev. Biol.* 289: 3–16. 2006c.

Zhang BH, Pan XP, Stellwag EJ. Identification of soybean microRNAs and their targets. *Planta.* 229: 161–182. 2008a.

Zhang BH, Pan XP, Wang QL, Cobb GP, Anderson TA. Identification and characterization of new plant microRNAs using EST analysis. *Cell Res.* 15: 336–360. 2005.

Zhang J, Zeng R, Chen J, Liu X, Liao Q. Identification of conserved microRNAs and their targets from *Solanum lycopersicum* Mill. *Gene.* 423: 1-7. 2008b.

Zhang L, Huang J, Yang N, Greshock J *et al.*, MicroRNAs exhibit high frequency genomic alterations in human cancer. *Proc. Natl. Acad. Sci. USA.* 103: 9136–9141. 2006.

Zhang W, Luo Y, Gong X, Zeng W, Li S. Computational identification of 48 potato microRNAs and their targets. *Comput. Biol. Chem.* 33: 84–93. 2009.

Zhang Z, Wei L, Zou X, Tao Y *et al.*, Submergence-responsive microRNAs are potentially involved in the regulation of morphological and metabolic adaptations in maize root cells. *Ann. Bot.* 102: 509–519. 2008.

Zhang Z, Yu J, Li D, Zhang Z *et al.*, PMRD: plant microRNA database. Nucleic Acids Res. 38: D806-13. 2010.

Zhao B, Liang R, Ge L, Li W *et al.*, Identification of drought-induced microRNAs in rice. *Biochem. Biophys. Res. Comm.* 354: 585–590. 2007.

Zhao M, Ding H, Zhu JK, Zhang F, Li WX. Involvement of miR169 in the nitrogen-starvation responses in *Arabidopsis*. *New Phytol.* 190: 906–915. 2011.

Zheng B, Liang L, Huang S, Zha R *et al.*, MicroRNA-409 suppresses tumor cell invasion and metastasis by directly targeting radixin in gastric cancers. *Oncogene.* 31: 4509-4516. 2011.

Zhou X, Wang G, Zhang W. UV-B responsive microRNA genes in *Arabidopsis thaliana*. *Mol. Syst. Biol.* 3: 103. 2007.

Zhu JK. Salt and drought stress signal transduction in plants. *Ann. Rev. Plant Biol.* 53: 247–273. 2002.

Zuker M. Mfold web server for nucleic acid folding and hybridization prediction. *Nucleic Acids Res.* 31: 3406-15. 2003.

2016, Biotechnological Tools for Genetic Resources *Pages* 127–174
Editor: Pradip Chandra Deka
Published by: Daya Publishing House, NEW DELHI

Chapter 5

Plant Derived Vaccines: Progress, Innovations, Opportunities and Perspectives

Sharmistha Barthakur

National Research Center on Plant Biotechnology, Pusa Campus, New Delho – 110 012
E-mail: sbthakur@yahoo.com

ABSTRACT

Since the first report of development of plant based vaccine in the early nineties, plant derived vaccines and edible vaccines have come a long way. They are generally regarded as safe, act through different mechanism of action mainly stimulating the lymphoid system in the intestines. Unresolved problems faced by present day vaccinologists, the field of vaccine development are filled with enormous challenges today. There has been a shift from empirical to rational vaccine design. In early cases of vaccine development expression was less in plant systems, however with time, new technological innovations, optimum expression is being achieved with transient as well as stable expression systems. Plant vaccines can induce mucosal immunity and also cause cellular and humoral immunity. There is hope that plant vaccines may overcome some of the major problems encountered with traditional vaccination against infectious disease, autoimmune disorders and even bio-terrorism. In this article the evolution, progress and present day status in plant vaccine development with a few suitable examples will be discussed.

Keywords: *Plant derived vaccine, Edible vaccine, DNA vaccine, Immunology, Plant made antigen.*

Introduction

Prevention, protection and eradication are the three goals of immunization. Beginning with Edward Jenner's classic small pox intervention using a benign cowpox infection to Louis Pasteur's pioneering approach in vaccine development;

the basic attributes of successful vaccine had been established by the beginning o the 20th century. Traditionally live attenuated and killed whole pathogenic strain were used as effective vaccine candidates. With time an emphasis on safety led to a shift towards the development of subunit vaccines with increasing reliance on recombinant expression systems such as yeast, bacteria, animal and plant systems. Throughout the decade of the 90s, the concept of plant-based vaccines emerged as one of the applications of transgenic plants. Plants would be used as production platform of well-characterized immunoprotective antigens and also as delivered vehicles. Plant-based vaccines attracted the attention of many research groups as this approach offers the advantages of mucosal immunization, no requirement for fermentation, stability, pathogen free, low cost and a few side-effects. Additionally when the antigenic protein is produced in the edible parts of the plant, such as grain, fruit or even leaves, they may not require purification (Howard and Hood 2005). And plant produced and or delivered pharmaceuticals utilizing whole plants and plant cells have evolved over the past twenty four years with several purified plant based products advancing to phase II and phase III trials and beyond today

The excitement over plant-made pharmaceuticals began with the publication of a paper in 1989 in Nature showing that monoclonal antibodies could be produced in tobacco (Hiatt *et al.*, 1989). Curtiss and Cardineau (1990) reported expression of *Streptcoccus mutans* surface protein antigen, the causative epitope for dental caries in tobacco as a first step toward a potential plant-based mucosal vaccine. In the early 1990s, three main groups were working to prove the concept of plant-made vaccines. While the research of Arntzen's group resulted in the first peer reviewed paper (Mason *et al.*, 1992), research by the Curtiss's group resulted in the first patent (Curtiss and Cardineau, 1997). The third group (Charles Arntzen's group) initially worked on the expression of Hepatitis B surface antigen (HbsAg) in tobacco (Mason *et al.*, 1992). They found that if expressed as a transgene from the tobacco nuclear genome, the plant HbsAg was similar to yeast-derived HbsAg when used in immunization studies in mice. Their data showed that a plant-derived vaccine could be as effective as one produced by the conventional cell culture methods. At this early plant vaccine stage, it was proposed that antigen-producing fruit or vegetables would deliver vaccines in a safe and cost-effective manner, as well as increase the frequency of childhood vaccinations.

It was thought that edible vaccines would reduce the cost of vaccination by cutting down on costs associated with transport, production, purification and other downstream processes used by conventional vaccines. For instance, potatoes engineered to make a cholera protein worked as a vaccine when the spuds were fed to mice (Haq *et al.*, 1995). Thereafter, transgenic plant-derived vaccines comprise a new type of bioreactor that combines plant genetic engineering technology with an organism's immunological response. This combination can be considered as a bioreactor that is produced by introducing foreign genes into plants that elicit special immunogenicity when introduced into animals or human beings (Guan *et al.*, 2013).

Vaccination is considered to be the most efficient and cost-effective means for health intervention to combat infectious diseases. Approximately 15 million (>25 per cent) of 57 million deaths per year worldwide are estimated to be related directly to infectious diseases (Morens *et al.*, 2004). The majority of emerging and reemerging infectious pathogens, including *Vibrio cholerae*, *Escherichia coli*, HIV, influenza virus, or corona virus causing severe acute respiratory syndrome, invade and infect the host via the mucosal surfaces of the gastrointestinal, respiratory, and/or genitourinary tracts (Nochi *et al.*, 2007). Mucosal immunity forms a first line of defense by means of secretory IgA and cytotoxic T cells against epithelium transmitted pathogens. Therefore, so it would seem important to develop vaccines that induce effective immune responses at mucosal barriers. Most current vaccines are administered by needle and syringe, generating effective antibody and cell mediated responses in the systemic compartment, but not in mucosal sites (Czerkinsky *et al.*, 1999). In contrast, mucosal vaccines administered either orally or nasally have been shown to be effective in inducing antigen-specific immune responses in both systemic and mucosal compartments (Kiyono and Fukuyama, 2004, Holmgren and Czerkinsky 2005). Because it elicits this two-layered protective immunity, mucosal vaccination is thought to be an ideal strategy for combating both emerging and reemerging infectious diseases (Neutra and Kozlowski, 2006; Yuki and Kiyono, 2003). The Bill and Melinda Gates Foundation and the National Institutes of Health have proposed that mucosal vaccines be a focus of future vaccine development, a vision underlying the foundation of the Gates' research initiative, "Grand Challenges in Global Health" (Varmus *et al.*, 2003).

Plant Expression System

Plants can be used as a bioreactor or as an oral delivery system. Several attributes make plant based subunit vaccines practical and attractive for the propagation of mucosal vaccine on the global scale. First, it would be less expensive to produce vaccine antigens in plants than via industrial fermentation. Second, there is no need to take elaborate means to purify the vaccine if it is expressed in plant tissue. Third, the plant expression system minimizes risks arising from tissue or pathogen contamination. Collectively, these advantages make a plant-based subunit vaccine not only attractive, but also practical for the propagation of mucosal vaccine on the global scale (Streatfield and Howard 2003, Nochi *et al.*, 2007).

The list of vaccine antigen and many different plant systems used for transformation and vaccine development till December 2013 is shown in Table 5.1. Broadly there are two expression systems used to develop plant based vaccines; stable plant nuclear and chloroplast transformation and transient plant expression system. Stable transformation involves the production of true breeding lines of genetically transformed plants. Transient expression system can be achieved by either modified plant viruses, or with *Agrobacterium tumefaciens* carrying an expression plasmid through agroinfiltration.

A major hurdle for the oral delivery of any pharmaceutical is the digestive system degrading and digesting the protein before it can carry out its function. As a result, there can be significant variation in the quantity of antigen delivered to the immune system, necessitating administration of larger amounts of the vaccine formulation in order to offset the loss of antigens. The variability of responses between candidates, the large amount of antigen required, the concern regarding

Table 5.1: Selected Examples of Various Plant Derived Vaccines that Report Immunogenicity and Expression Level of Antigens

Antigen	*Pathogen*	*Plant Production System*	*Expression Level (per cent TSP)*	*Functional Evaluation*	*Reference*
			Bacterial antigens		
Heat-labiletoxin B subunit (LTB)	Enterotoxigenic *E. coli* (ETEC)	Carrots	0.3	Immunogenic and protective against CT challenge	Rosales-Mendoza *et al.*, 2007a
		Soybean	2.4	Immunogenic and partial protection against LT challenge in mice	Tomas *et al.*, 2007
		Maize seed	3.7	Immunogrnic and protective by oral delivery to mice	Chikwamba *et al.*, 2002b
		Tobacco, lettuce chloroplasts	4.1–12.3	Long term protection against CT challenge by both oral and subcutaneous immunization in mice	Davoodi-Semiromi *et al.*, 2009, Daniel *et al.*, 2009
Cholera toxin B subunit (CTB)	Cholera	Tomato	0.081	Gavage of mice induced both serum and mucosal CB specific antibpdies	Jiang *et al.*, 2007
		Rice	2.1	Immunogenic and protective against CT challenge to mice following oral administration	Nochi *et al.*, 2007
			Viral antigens		
Hepatitis B virus surface antigen (HBsAg)	Hepatitis B	Potato	8.5 mg/g FW	Immunogenic response in humans following oral administration	Thanavala *et al.*, 2005
Hepatitis EV E2	Hepatitis	Tobacco cp	0.63 -1.09 ng/ug	Immune response in mice	Zhou *et al.*, 2006
HBV S protein		Cherry tomatillo	2-10 ug/g FW	Elicited immediate high level antibody response	Gao *et al.*, 2003
Human group A rotavirus (VP6) protein	Rota virus	Alfalfa	0.06–0.28	Immunogenic in mice and offspring	Dong *et al.*, 2005
Rotavirus (VP7)		Potato tubers	0.3–0.4	Immunogenic in mice following oral Delivery. Neutralization activity against rotavirus	Li *et al.*, 2006

Contd...

Table 5.1–*Contd...*

Antigen	*Pathogen*	*Plant Production System*	*Expression Level (per cent TSP)*	*Functional Evaluation*	*Reference*
Norwalk virus capsid protein (NVCP)	Norwalk virus	Tomato fruit and potato	8 in tomato, 0.4 in potato	Elicit systemic and mucosal antibody responses in mice following oral administration	Zhang *et al.*, 2006
SARS–CoV S protein (S1)	SARS	Tomato and tobacco leaf	0.1	Immunogenic to mice following oral Administration	Pogrebnyak *et al.*, 2005
Japanese encephalitis virus (JEV) envelope protein (E)	Encephalitis virus	Rice	1.1–1.9	JEV specific neutralizing antibody detected in mice following intraperito-neal or oral administration	Wang *et al.*, 2009
Swine fever CSFV E2	Swine fever virus	Tobacco cp	1-2	Immune response in mice	Shao *et al.*, 2008
Human papilloma virus L1	Human papilloma virus	Tobacco cp	20-26	Systemic immune response in mice after intraperitoneal injection	Fernandez *et al.*, 2008
FMDV structural protein VP1 of FMDV	Foot and mouth disease virus	Stylosanthes guianensis	0.1 - 0.5	Immune response in mice	Wang *et al.*, 2008a
Rabies virus synthetic gene for surface glycoprotein	Rabies virus	Tobacco	0.38	Immune response in mice	Ashraf *et al.*, 2005
Full length nucleo protein of rabies virus		Tomato, Tobacco	1-5 in tomato, 45 in tobacco	Immune response in mice vide oral and ip administration	Perea Arango *et al.*, 2008
			Malaria asexual blood stage antigens		
P. falciparum MSP142 (PfMSP142)	Plasmodium parasite	*A. thaliana* seeds/nuclear transformation	5	Immunoreactivity to sera from malaria-infected patients; Immunogenic by i.p. and oral delivery toMice	Lau *et al.*, 2010
P. yoelii MSP4/5 (PyMSP4/5)		Tobacco/nuclear Tobacco/mag nICON	0.02–0.0410 (1-2mg/g FW)	Induction of specific antibodies by oral delivery or primed by a DNA vaccine to mice	Wang *et al.*, 2008, Webster *et al.*, 2009

Contd...

Table 5.1–*Contd...*

Antigen	*Pathogen*	*Plant Production System*	*Expression Level (per cent TSP)*	*Functional Evaluation*	*Reference*
P. yoelii MSP119 (PyMSP119)		Tobacco/mag nICON	23 (3-4mg/g FW)	Immunogenic by i.p. delivery with Freund's adjuvant or oral administration without any adjuvant	Ma *et al.*, 2011
P. falciparum AMA1 (PfAMA1)		Tobacco chloroplast Lettuce/ chloroplast	13.1 in tobacco, 7.3 in lettuce	Induction of specific antibodies in s.c. and orally immunized mice Immuno-reactivity to native parasite proteins	Davoodi-Semiromi 2010
P. falciparum MSP1 (PfMSP1)		Tobacco chloroplast Lettuce/ chloroplast	10.1 in tobacco, 6.1 in lettuce	Induction of specific antibodies in s.c. and orally immunized mice Immuno-reactivity to native parasite proteins	Davoodi-Semiromi 2010
			Malaria sexual stage antigens		
P. falciparum P230 (Pfs230)	Malaria	Tobacco/agro infiltration	800 mg/kg FW	Induction of transmission-blocking antibodies in s.c. and i.m. immunized mice Immunoreactivity to native parasite proteins	Farrance *et al.*, 2011a
P. falciparum P25 (Pfs25) 0.		Tobacco/agro infiltration	25 and 0.4 mg/g FW	Induction of transmission-blocking antibodies in i.m. immunized mice Immunoreactivity to native parasite proteins	Farrance *et al.*, 2011b

potentiating oral tolerance (Thomas *et al.*, 2011), and the continued concern of contamination of the food chain with pharmaceuticals led to the development of plant-based pharmaceuticals that are largely produced in non-food crops such as tobacco and are then highly purified for parenteral delivery. Presently there has been acceptance of recombinant, pharmaceutical proteins purified from plant sources for use in human clinical trials including Phase III (Faye and Gomord, 2010, Aviezer *et al.*, 2009, Biolex Therapeutics, 2009). Dosage and quality control of these plant-made pharmaceuticals are controlled in a manner similar to their traditional counterparts. Although several plants have currently been used for the creation of an "edible vaccine," seed crops such as rice, soybean, maize, wheat seem to be the most suitable plants for implementation of global vaccine production satisfying the following criteria: (i) produce sufficient quantities of inserted antigen for the immunization (Chargelegue *et al.*, 2001), (ii) preserve the expressed antigen for a long time at RT (Varmus *et al.*, 2003; Levine and Sztein, 2004), (iii) induce protective immunity (Yuki and Kiyono 2003, Levine and Sztein, 2004), (iv) protect from enzymatic digestion in gastrointestinal tract (Yuki and Kiyono, 2003) and (v) effectively deliver the inserted antigen to mucosal inductive tissues, including antigen-sampling M cells (Daniel *et al.*, 2001, Nochi *et al.*, 2007).

Advantages of Plant Vaccines

The world's first licensing of an (injectable) plant-made vaccine occurred in early 2006 (Sparrow *et al.*, 2007). With Dow AgroSciences LLC announcing that it had received the world's first regulatory approval for a plant-made vaccine from the United States Department of Agriculture Center for Veterinary Biologics' used to combat Newcastle Disease Virus (NDV) of poultry bird. The vaccine was made using a contained, suspension cell culture production system of transgenic tobacco in a conventional bioreactor system in large quantities in a relatively short period of a few weeks. The resulting cells were harvested and minimally processed to provide a partially purified antigen for formulation into the final vaccine. Birds vaccinated subcutaneously with the plant-made vaccine were protected against lethal challenge to NDV (Mihaliak *et al.*, 2005). Even though the product was not made commercially available, a proof of concept was established and demonstrated. Some of the advantages of producing recombinant proteins in plants are discussed.

Inbuilt Adjuvants

As potential delivery systems for oral vaccines plants has the added advantage of some phytochemicals and plant components such as unmethylated CpG motifs of DNA, carotenoids and immunogenic proteins that could synergistically affect the immunogenicity of plant-expressed antigens acting as endogenous adjuvants (Kapusta *et al.*, 1999, Jiang *et al.*, 2007, Guetard *et al.*, 2008, Thomas *et al.*, 2011). Plants are also known for their natural immune-stimulating or antimicrobial activity due to secondary metabolites such as lectins, saponins, alkaloids, phenolics and flavonoids (Granell *et al.*, 2010). Hence plants can be used in the short term as oral or injectable vaccine producers and as a source of endogenous adjuvants as well. Leaves also have a large number of heat shock proteins (HSPs), which have been demonstrated to have adjuvant properties in other organisms (Suze and Young, 1996, Echeverria *et al.*, 2006). Plants expressing HSP90 are able to induce *in vitro* B-cell proliferation from mice, suggesting that these proteins could be excellent *carriers* of interesting vaccine antigens and peptides expressed in plants (Corigliano *et al.*, 2011).

Eukaryotic Modifications

As with other eukaryotic systems, plant-produced vaccines enable the introduction of post-translational modifications. Proper folding and disulfide bond formation occur in chloroplasts (Davoodi-Semiromi *et al.*, 2009) or the endoplasmic reticulum (ER) (Moravec *et al.*, 2007). Proper lipid modifications of vaccine antigens have also been observed in chloroplasts (Glenz *et al.*, 2006). Therapeutic proteins are not glycosylated in chloroplasts but are glycosylated when targeted to the ER although glycosylation patterns are not identical to mammalian systems.

Room Temperature Friendly

Most traditional vaccines are not cost-effective because they cannot be stored at room temperature (RT), instead requiring that the "cold chain" en route from vaccine manufacturer to the field of vaccination. The cost of cold chain preservation for currently used vaccines is estimated at between $200 and $300 million a year (Giudice and Campbell, 2006). Further, if inappropriately processed or disposed of, the needles and syringes used for the vaccination can pose the threats of environmental contamination and secondhand spread of infectious disease. Plant derived vaccines has the potential to sidestep this step and to be practicable for global immunization, vide being storable at RT for long periods, be protected from the harsh environment of the gastrointestinal tract, and target mucosal inductive tissues, including Peyer's patches (PPs) (Walmsley and Arntzen, 2003).

Issues of Concerrn for Plant Vaccines

Efficiency and efficacy of the resulting proteins, safety and regulatory approval demonstrating the capacity for economical recombinant protein production at large scales in plants and time taken to produce them were the major perceived disadvantage of the plant-made recombinant protein platform in earlier days. Compared to other platforms such as bacteria or animal cells, plants produced at least 10-fold less protein of interest, and it could take up to 18 months to produce a stably transformed plant line. This situation has been tackled with the refinement of transient plant transformation systems. Agroinfiltration can be used to deliver minimal, deconstructed plant virus-based expression vectors, such as the system based on a disabled cowpea mosaic virus RNA-2 described by Sainsbury and colleagues (Sainsbury *et al.*, 2008) or the magnification system developed by Icon Genetics (Marillonnet *et al.*, 2004), resulting in recombinant protein accumulating up to 80 per cent of total soluble protein (TSP) in tobacco leaves (Marillonnet *et al.*, 2005). The transient expression systems have also drastically reduced the time to less than three weeks from release of viral sequence to purified vaccine product (D'Aoust *et al.*, 2008).

Recent advances in stable systems also have resulted in much higher levels of recombinant protein accumulation. Although transgene silencing in nuclear transgenic plants still requires further investigation and improvement, utilization of sub-cellular targeting and chloroplast transformation has resulted in levels of up to 46 per cent TSP being reported (Sharma and Sharma 2009). Stable expression of recombinant proteins such as vaccine antigens has also been actively pursued in seeds of crops such as rice and maize, as these platforms produce high yields and are easy to scale up. Another benefit of seeds is their inherently stable nature. For example, a rice-based cholera vaccine, MucoRice-CTB, was shown to be stable at room temperature for up to three years, as well as being resistant to pepsin digestion and protecting mice against both cholera and enterotoxigenic *Escherichia coli* (ETEC) (Tokuhara *et al.*, 2010). Likewise, an ETEC subunit vaccine produced in soybean seeds was found to be stable over four years, as well as when formulated into soymilk (Oakes *et al.*, 2009).

Specific examples of a few recent plant made vaccines categorized into various clinical conditions, caused by various pathogenic agents and plant transformation system are being discussed briefly.

Box 1: Immunology: A Primer

- ☆ **Active immunity:** Immunity that is induced by natural exposure to a pathogen or by vaccination
- ☆ **Adaptive or acquired immunity:** Host defenses that are mediated by B and T cells following exposure to antigen and that exhibit specificity, diversity, memory and self, non self recognition
- ☆ **Innate immunity:** Non specific host defenses that exist prior to exposure to an antigen and involve anatomic, physiologic, endocytic and phagocytic and inflammatory mechanisms.
- ☆ **Passive immunity:** Adaptive immunity conferred by the transfer of immune products, such as antibody or sensitized T cells, from an immune individual to a noninmmune one.
- ☆ **Cell mediated immune response:** Host defenses that are mediated by antigen specific T-cells and various non specific cells of the immune system.
- ☆ **Humoral immune response:** Host defenses that are mediated by antibody present in the plasma, lymph and tissue fluids.
- ☆ **Mucosal associated lymphoid tissue:** Lymphoid tissue situated along the mucous membrane that line the digestive, respiratory and urogenital tracts
- ☆ **Mucosal immunity:** The immune system which provides protection to an organism's various mucous membranes from invasion by potentially pathogenic microbes vide three main functions: protecting the mucus membrane against infection; preventing the uptake of antigens, microorganisms, and other foreign materials; and moderating the organism's immune response to that material.

Nuclear Transformed Vaccines against Human Diseases

Nuclear transformed vaccines developed against several human diseases are described in the following section.

Box 2: Traditional and modern vaccines

- ☆ **Killed inactivated:** Inactivation of the pathogen by heat or chemical means so that immunogenicity is retained but infectivity is lost
- ☆ **Live attenuated:** Attenuated or weakened microorganisms that have lost their ability to cause significant disease (pathogencity) but retain their capacity for transient growth within an inoculated host
- ☆ **Subunit vaccines:** Specific, purified macromolecules derived from pathogens *e.g.*: bacterial polysaccharide capsules, viral glycoproteins, synthetic peptides, pathogen proteins, toxoids
- ☆ **Multivalent subunit vaccines:** Solid matrix antibody-antigen complexes, liposomes, immune-stimulating complexes
- ☆ **DNA vaccines:** Plasmid DNA encoding antigenic proteins which is injected directly into the muscle of the recipient
- ☆ **Recombinant antigen vaccines: Antigen expressed in a heterologous system, purified**
- ☆ **Recombinant vector:** Genes encoding major antigens of especially virulent pathogens introduced into attenuated viruses or bacteria. The attenuated organisms serve as a vector, replicating within the host and expressing the gene product of the pathogen
- ☆ **Plant delivered/based/oral/edible vaccines:** Subunit vaccines produced by expression of heterologous proteins in plant through stable as well transient expression
- ☆ **RNA Vaccine:** mRNA encoding antigen injected intramuscularly; RNA replicon including the coding antigen
- ☆ **Cancer vaccines**

  Therapeutic: Stimulates immune system to recognize, attack human cancer cells (strengthen the body's natural defenses against cancers already developed)

  Prophylactic: Healthy individuals to attack cancer causing viruses and prevent viral infection

  Anti-Idiotype vaccines: Antibodies raised against the idiotype in the antibody by injecting the antibody into another animal and thereby raising an anti-idiotype antibody which mimics part of the three dimensional structure of the antigen and can be used as a vaccine.

Cholera Vaccine

Cholera and traveler's diarrhea, caused by *Vibrio cholera* and enterotoxigenic strains of *Eschericia coli* (ETEC), respectively, are two enteric diseases which are responsible for high mortality especially in young children in developing countries (Girard *et al.*, 2006). In 2011, the World Health Organization (WHO) reported 589,854 cholera cases and 7816 deaths, revealing a 85 per cent increase in the number of cases compared to 2010 (Hamorsky 2013). Thus there exists urgent need for effective vaccines for these diseases. The toxins, cholera toxin (CT) and heat labile enterotoxin from ETEC (LT), which are responsible for the harmful effects of these infections, are composed of pentameric non-toxic B subunit and toxic A subunit.

The B subunits bind to GM1ganglioside (galactosyl-N-acetylgalactosamyl-syalil-galactosylglucosylceramide) receptors on intestinal epithelial cells. This binding aids a portion of the toxic A subunit to be internalized into the cytosol, where it starts a series of cellular events leading to diarrhea (Williams *et al.*, 1999).

Currently, there are two WHO prequalified oral cholera vaccines, Dukoral (by Crucell) and Shanchol (by Shantha Biotechincs). Dukoral contains bacterially produced recombinant cholera toxin B subunit (CTB) plus killed whole-cells of *V. cholerae*, and has been found to be safe and effective over 25 years (Clamens *et al.*, 1986, Clemens *et al.*, 1988,Van Loon *et al.*, 1996, Jertborn *et al.*, 1992, Hashim *et al.*, 2012). CTB is the non-toxic subunit of cholera holotoxin. The protein forms stable homo pentamers with a molecular mass of about 55 kDa (Zhang *et al.*, 1995). The CTB component of the vaccine induces holotoxin neutralizing antibodies in the gut (Jelinek and Kollaritsch 2008), which act synergistically with the anti-bacterial immunity in protection against cholera (Clemens *et al.*, 2011). Several studies have reported various attempts at expressing vaccine antigens for these clinical conditions as evident from Table 5.1.

A rice-based oral vaccine expressing cholera toxin B subunit (CTB) was developed under the control of the endosperm-specific expression promoter 2.3-kb glutelin *GluB-1* with codon usage optimization and used for expression in rice seed (Nochi *et al.*, 2007). An average of 30 µg of CTB per seed was stored in the protein bodies, and induced CTB-specific serum IgG and mucosal IgA antibodies with neutralizing activity. CTB was protected from pepsin digestion *in vitro*, and also remained stable and maintained immunogenicity at room temperature for>1.5 years. Antigen-specific mucosal immune responses were induced at much lower doses than were necessary with purified recombinant CTB. The physically, chemically stable and immunologically effective vaccine antigen expressed in transgenic rice seed could withstand the harsh environment of the gastrointestinal tract and induce protective immunity against mucosal infections.

Tokuhara *et al.* (2010) reported another rice-based vaccine that expressed cholera toxin B subunit (MucoRice-CTB) to investigate whether the CTB-specific secretory IgA (SIgA) induced by MucoRice-CTB gives longstanding protection against diarrhea induced by *Vibrio cholerae* and LT-ETEC in mice. Oral immunization with MucoRice-CTB stored at room temperature for more than 3 years provided effective SIgA-mediated protection against cholera LT-induced diarrhea, but the protection was impaired in polymeric Ig receptor–deficient mice lacking SIgA. The vaccine gave longstanding protection against CT- or LT-induced diarrhea (for e"6 months after primary immunization), and a single booster immunization extended the duration of protective immunity by at least 4 months. Furthermore, MucoRice-CTB vaccination prevented diarrhea in the event of *V. cholerae* and LT-ETEC challenges showing that MucoRice-CTB is an effective long-term cold chain–free oral vaccine that induces CTB specific SIgA-mediated longstanding protection against *V. cholerae* or LT-ETEC–induced diarrhea.

A transgenic corn expressing a synthetic B subunit of cholera toxin (CT-B) from *Vibrio cholerae* was developed by Karaman *et al.* (2012) under the control of a Ý-zein promoter in maize seeds. While the mature CT-B in maize tissue was not processed for the removal of its signal peptide, the pentameric assembly of CT-B was demonstrated via ganglioside dependent ELISA. The study showed that maize derived CT-B can be immunogenic in mice. Ten micrograms of maize derived CT-B may be better at priming anti-CT-B IgG antibody production in comparison to 5 μg of maize derived CT-B. Since the maize does not process the bacterial native signal peptide effectively, anti-CT-B antibodies induced by maize derived CT-B may be different than that induced by bacterial CT-B. The initial intention of this study was to establish a combined vaccination system that can be effective for both CT-caused cholera and LT-caused traveler's diarrhea diseases. On certain days of sample collection, the antibody levels observed were higher in the mice from the CTB5- LTB5 combined treatment group than that of the CTB or LTB only groups. However, due to incomplete CT-B signal peptide processing in maize and other limitations, the data still requires further verification and improvement on production of a mature CT-B in maize by using a signal peptide from maize seed zein protein instead of its bacterial native signal peptide.

Cholera toxin B subunit (CTB) is a component of an internationally licensed oral cholera vaccine. The protein induces neutralizing antibodies against the holotoxin, the virulence factor responsible for severe diarrhea. A field clinical trial has suggested that the addition of CTB to killed whole-cell bacteria provides superior short-term protection to whole-cell only vaccines. However, challenges in CTB biomanufacturing (*i.e.*, cost and scale) hamper its implementation to mass vaccination in developing countries. To provide a potential solution to this issue, Hamorsky *et al.* (2013) developed a rapid, robust, and scalable CTB production system in plants. In a preliminary study of expressing original CTB in transgenic *Nicotiana benthamiana*, the protein was N-glycosylated with plant-specific glycans. Thus, an aglycosylated CTB variant (pCTB) was created and overexpressed via a plant virus vector. Upon additional transgene engineering for retention in the endoplasmic reticulum and optimization of a secretory signal, the yield of pCTB was dramatically improved, reaching >1 g per kg of fresh leaf material. The GM1-ganglioside binding capacity and conformational stability of pCTB were virtually identical to the bacteria-derived original B subunit, as demonstrated by competitive enzyme-linked immunosorbent assay, surface plasmon resonance, and fluorescence-based thermal shift assay. Mammalian cell surface-binding was corroborated by immunofluorescence and flow cytometry. pCTB exhibited strong oral immunogenicity in mice, inducing significant levels of CTB-specific intestinal antibodies that persisted over 6 months. Moreover, these antibodies effectively neutralized the cholera holotoxin *in vitro*. The results demonstrated that pCTB has robust producibility in *Nicotiana* plants and retains most of the major biological activities of the original protein.

Hepatitis Vaccine

Hepatitis B virus (HBV) is a major cause of acute and chronic hepatitis. HBV DNA was found in most of the newborns from hepatitis B surface antigen (HBsAg)-positive mothers (Wang *et al.*, 2000). HBV is mostly a double-stranded DNA virus in the *Hepadnaviridae* family. The HBV genome includes four genes: *pol*,*env*, *precore*, and X, which encode the viral DNA polymerase, envelope protein, precore protein which is processed to viral capsid), and protein X, respectively. The most recent vaccine is based on the cloned copies of the *env* gene in yeast, a biotechnology product that falls in the category of "subunit vaccines" and is made from yeast cells grown by fermentation. Studies of mRNA transcription suggest that this gene has the potential to code for three related proteins: i) a protein of 226 amino acids, identified as a major protein constituent of the HBV envelope, termed the S protein, ii) a protein with 55 additional amino acids at the N terminus, encoded by a portion of the *env* gene upstream of the *S* gene (*pre-S1*), and iii) a protein corresponding to the entire *env* gene (*pre-S2*). Three different proteins are produced by combining these proteins in different formations: large protein on the envelope (combination of the *pre-S1*, *pre-S2*, and *S* genes); middle-sized proteins on the envelope (*pre-S2* and *S* genes); and the major component of HBsAg, the S protein (Lou *et al.*, 2007). The vaccines have prevented numerous infections. However, administration of the vaccine intramuscularly causes some pain, and it is not widely accepted, especially for children, besides limitations of syringe-and-needle vaccination programs.

One of the earliest report on plant based vaccine showing promise of a low cost production system was reported by Mason *et al.* (1992), where tobacco plants were genetically transformed with the gene encoding hepatitis B surface antigen (HBsAg) linked to a nominally constitutive promoter. Enzyme-linked immunoassays using a monoclonal antibody directed against human serum-derived HBsAg revealed the presence of HBsAg in extracts of transformed leaves at levels that correlated with mRNA abundance. Recombinant HBsAg was purified from transgenic plants by immune affinity chromatography and examined by electron microscopy. Spherical particles with an average diameter of 22 nm were observed in negatively stained preparations. Sedimentation of transgenic plant extracts in sucrose and cesium chloride density gradients showed that the recombinant HBsAg and human serum-derived HBsAg had similar physical properties. The HBsAg produced in transgenic plants is antigenically and physically similar to the HBsAg particles derived from human serum and recombinant yeast.

Lou *et al.* (2007) synthesized the original hepatitis B virus (HBV) large surface antigen gene, fused the tobacco pathogenesis-related protein S signal peptide to the 5′ end of the modified gene and the sequence encoding amino acids S, E, K, D, E, and L was placed at the 3′ end. The gene encoding the modified HBV large surface antigen was placed under the control of a fruit-specific promoter and expressed in transgenic tomato plants. The expression of the antigen was confirmed by molecular techniques. Enzyme-linked immunoassays using a monoclonal antibody directed against human serum-derived HBsAg revealed that the maximal level of HBsAg was about 0.02 per cent of the soluble protein in transgenic tomato fruit. The amount of HBsAg in mature fruits was found to be 65- to 171-fold larger than in small or medium fruits and leaf tissues. Examination of transgenic plant samples by transmission electron microscopy proved that HBsAg had been expressed and had accumulated and the protein was capable of assembling into capsomers and virus-like particles. According to the authors, this was the first report on expression of the HBV large surface antigen in plants, suggesting the possibility of producing a new alternative vaccine for human HBV.

Rabies Vaccine

The rabies virus belongs to the Rhadoviridae family and causes the rabies disease in animals and humans (Rupprecht *et al.*, 2002). It is a disease that affects the central nervous system and it is fatal in humans and other mammals. The number of deaths from rabies worldwide is approximately 60,000 humans and millions of animals per year. Although rabies encephalitis remains untreatable, the disease is preventable by vaccination. However, the incidence of rabies in humans and animals still remains relatively high, particularly in poor areas of developing countries. Even though there are effective vaccines available, eradication of the rabies virus has remained problematic due to the high cost of production and administration of the vaccines. The increasing global incidence of rabies in wildlife (Nadin-Davis and Loza-Rubio 2006) and the recent discovery of new rabies-causing viruses are accelerating the development of safer, cheaper and effective vaccines against the disease.

The transmembrane glycoprotein (G) of rabies virus has been considered as the main antigen that induces neutralizing antibodies and many recombinant vaccines are based on this antigen to confer protection against lethal rabies infection (Nel *et al.*, 2003). Nevertheless, antigenic analysis of a wide variety of street rabies viruses and related lyssavirus has shown that there is considerable antigenic variation among the G protein, which may depend on the geographical location and on the host (Flamand *et al.*, 1980, Dietzschold *et al.*, 1987a, 1988). In addition, protection against rabies virus is not solely dependent on the levels of virus-neutralizing antibodies induced by the G protein (Dietzschold *et al.*, 1987b). An alternative candidate antigen for development of vaccines is the internal nucleoprotein (N), which is the major constituent of the internal ribonucleoprotein complex (RNP). The N protein is genetically and antigenically more conserved than the G protein across Lyssaviruses (Dietzschold *et al.*, 1988). Although it may not elicit virus-neutralizing antibodies when the protein is expressed in a recombinant virus vaccine or inoculated as purified protein, it has partially protected against peripheral challenge with rabies virus (Dietzschold *et al.*, 1987a, Fu *et al.*, 1991). The N protein can function as an immunomodulator for production of neutralizing antibodies induced by G protein and classical vaccines. Furthermore, the N protein has properties of super antigen and it can induce rabies virus-specific helper T cells that cross react between rabies and rabies-related viruses (Dietzschold *et al.*, 1987b, Fu *et al.*, 1991).The possibility of using plant systems for production of potential vaccine are described through the following examples.

An edible vaccine in maize was developed by Loza-Rubio *et al.* (2008) expressing the rabies virus glycoprotein (G) of the Vnukovo strain and its immunogenicity evaluated in mice, by the oral route. They used the ubiquitin maize promoter fused to the whole coding region of the rabies virus G gene along with the constitutive promoter from cauliflower mosaic virus and transformed maize embryogenic callus by the biolistic method. Regenerated maize plants were recovered and grown in a greenhouse. The presence of the G gene and its product was detected by PCR and western blot, respectively. The amount of G protein detected in the grains was approximately 1 per cent of the total soluble plant protein. Transformed kernels containing 50 µg of G protein were given once by the oral route to adult mice (BALB-C strain). Challenge was undertaken at 90-days post-vaccination using a lethal dose of a vampire bat rabies virus (100 LD 50 per cent in mice); which are one of the main reservoirs in Latin America. The edible vaccine induced viral neutralizing antibodies (VNA) which, protected mice 100 per cent against challenge whereas the control group did not survive. The G protein of the Vnukovo strain expressed in transgenic maize was demonstrated as an oral immunogen against rabies, conferring cross-protection.

Arango *et al.* (2008) reported expression of a full length nucleoprotein gene of rabies virus in transgenic tomato plants and transiently in *Nicotiana benthamiana* plants by agroinfiltration. In both cases, the nucleoprotein was expressed at high levels, 1–5 per cent of total soluble protein in tomato and 45 per cent in N. *benthamiana*. Previously, only epitopes of the nucleoprotein had been expressed in plants. The presence and expression of the transgene was verified by PCR, Southern, northern and western blots. Mice immunized both intraperitoneally (i.p.) and orally with tomato protein extracts containing the N protein induced the production of antibodies. The antibody titer of mice immunized i.p., was at least four times higher than that of mice immunized orally. These results were reflected in the challenge experiments where i.p.-immunized mice were partially protected against a peripheral virus challenge whereas orally immunized mice were not. This protection was also comparable to that obtained in previous experiments employing different expression systems.

Acquired Immune Deficiency Syndrome Vaccine

The acquired immune deficiency syndrome (AIDS) caused by the human immunodeficiency virus (HIV) is one of the most significant diseases worldwide. In 2008 the UNAIDS had estimated that 33.4 million people were HIV-positive and global spread of HIV-AIDS has reached pandemic proportions. The HIV belongs to the genus Lentivirus and the family Retroviridae. These enveloped RNA viruses produce characteristically slow, progressive infections. Lentivirus replication depends on the presence of an active reverse transcriptase responsible for the transformation of the viral RNA genome into a proviral DNA copy that integrates itself into the host cell chromosome. The provirus is eventually transcribed into a set of mRNAs that encode the viral proteins and progeny genomic RNA (Rosales-Mendoza *et al.*, 2012). Two types of HIV have been described: HIV-1 and HIV-2 (Rosales-Memndoza *et al.*, 2012). Based in part on genetic variation of the surface envelope glycoproteins, HIV-1 isolates fall into three groups–M (Major/Main), N (Non-M, Non-O/New) and O (Outlier)– of which group M is the most common. Group M is subdivided into several subtypes or clades (A–D, F–H, J and K), of which B is the most common in the Western world and subtype C is primarily found in India, China and sub-Saharan Africa. The remaining subtypes, as well as HIV-1 variants with characteristics of several different subtypes (circulating recombinant forms), and is mainly spread throughout Africa (Karlsson Hedestam *et al.*, 2008).

Antibody responses in HIV-1 infected individuals has revealed that antibodies are mainly directed against envelope glycoproteins gp120 and gp41 of the HIV-

1 virus that are responsible for both receptor binding and viral entry into host cells (Dalgleish *et al.*, 1984, Wyatt and Sodroski 1998), as well as for mediating virus neutralization. Among the most prominent neutralizing targets in HIV-1 neutralization scheme are the CD4 binding site and the co-receptor binding region, third variable (V3) loop, of gp120 (Zolla-Pazner *et al.*, 2008, Mascola and Montefiori 2010). In a recent HIV-1 vaccine trial (RV144) conducted in Thailand, it has been demonstrated, for the first time, protection in humans by a candidate vaccine (Rerks-Ngarm *et al.*, 2009). Individuals immunized with the RV144 vaccine elicited a humoral response that is well correlated with the observed protection. Thus, induction of broad cross neutralizing antibodies serves as a major goal in the field of HIV vaccine development (Haynes *et al.*, 2012).

In an effort to generate new candidate immunogens capable of eliciting broad humoral immune responses, Govea-Alonso *et al.* (2013) reported on the design of a protein C4(V3)6 carrying a T-helper epitope from the fourth conserved domain (C4) of gp120, as well as six tandem V3 loops corresponding to five different HIV isolates, including MN, IIIB, RF, CC and RU. This recombinant C4(V3)6 protein has been first expressed in a *Escherichia coli* platform and, subsequently, introduced into lettuce, obtaining yields of up to 240 µg/g of this protein per leaf dry weight. Overall, findings have demonstrated that both *E. coli* and lettuce-derived C4 (V3)6 are immunogenic via oral administration by inducing broad humoral responses in BALB/c test mice. More importantly, lettuce-derived C4(V3)6 has shown a higher immunogenic potential than that of *E.Coli* derived C4(V3)6. Moreover, when reactivity of sera from mice immunized with C4(V3)6 are compared with those elicited by a chimeric protein carrying a single V3 sequence, broader responses have been observed. The lettuce-derived C4(V3)6 has elicited antibodies with positive reactivity against V3 loops from isolates MN, RF, and CC. In addition, splenocyte proliferation assays indicate that significant T-helper responses are induced by the C4(V3)6 immunogen.

Rota Virus Mediated Infant Diarrhea Vaccine

Rotavirus is the leading cause of diarrhea in infants and young children worldwide, causing more than 114 million episodes of diarrhea annually in children under the age of 5, 80 per cent in developing countries (Parashar *et al.*, 2003). More than 600,000 children die annually from rotavirus (RV) infection worldwide. Although most RV-related deaths occur in low income countries, in developed countries, thousands of children under 5 years of age are hospitalized every year, including 50,000–80,000 in Japan and 60,000 in the US (Nakagomi *et al.*, 3005, Fischer *et al.*, 2007). Rotavirus is a double stranded RNA virus from the family Reoviridae. Currently, there are 2 licensed RV vaccines (Rotarix and RotaTeq) that have been reported to be highly effective (>85 per cent) in reducing severe RV-induced diarrhea in developed countries (Vesikari *et al.*, 2006, Ruiz-Palacios *et al.*, 2006, Glass and Parasharv 2006). More recent clinical trials in developing countries in Africa and Asia have also demonstrated a potential impact of these vaccines, but with a markedly lower efficacy, ranging from 39.3 per cent RotaTeq in Sub-Saharan Africa to 61.2 per cent Rotarix in Malawi and South Africa (Madhi *et al.*, 2010, Armah *et al.*, 2010, Zaman *et al.*, 2010). Both vaccines have proven to be safe in clinical trials and post-marketing studies, but presently, they are licensed for use only within a very narrow age window (>6 weeks and ≤26 weeks of age) to avoid the risk of intussusceptions. Vaccines are also often associated with poor efficacy in immune compromised individuals and such individuals may even acquire infections derived from the use of live vaccines. Cases of chronic diarrhea induced by the attenuated RotaTeq vaccine have indeed been recently reported, and the current RV vaccines are therefore not recommended for use in immunodeficient infants (Werther *et al.*, 2009, Patel *et al.*, 2010, Uygungil *et al.*, 2010).

Tokuhara *et al.* (2013) have developed a system for prophylaxis and therapy against rotavirus disease using transgenic rice expressing the neutralizing variable domain of a rotavirus-specific llama heavy-chain antibody fragment (MucoRice-ARP1). The variable domain of llama heavy chain antibodies (VHH) consists of a single domain and constitutes the smallest naturally occurring antigen-binding domain known to date. In addition to its high binding capacity, VHH has several attractive features, such as resistance to pepsin, acid environment, and heat. Furthermore, because of its small size and simple form, it is easy to produce VHH as a recombinant protein with an intact spatial structure.MucoRice-ARP1 was produced at high levels in rice seeds using an overexpression system and RNAi technology. To suppress the production of major rice endogenous storage proteins and to enhance accumulation of foreign proteins, an antisense genes specific for the 13-kDa prolamin and glutelin storage proteins was introduced to minimize the expression and expand space for ARP1 in the rice seeds. Orally administered MucoRice-ARP1 markedly decreased the viral load in immunocompetent and immunodeficient mice. The antibody retained *in vitro* neutralizing activity after long-term storage (>1 yr) and boiling and conferred protection in mice even after heat treatment at 94°C for 30 minutes. High-yield, water soluble, and purification-free MucoRice-ARP1 thus form the basis for orally administered prophylaxis and therapy against rotavirus infections.

In comparison with those plant-based antibodies (scFV, IgG, Fab, and VHH) described previously (Ismail *et al.*, 2007, Giritich *et al.*, 2006, Peeters *et al.*, 2001, Fiedler and Conrad 1996), the MucoRice system achieved an extremely high yield of soluble antibodies (8.5 g soluble ARP1 kg–1 of total weight or 11.9 per cent of total protein) in rice seeds. Most importantly, MucoRice-ARP1 is highly water soluble due to the localization of the ARP1 antibody fragment in the PB-II and cytoplasm fractions, which are the soluble components of rice. As MucoRice-ARP1 originates from edible rice seeds, it needs no purification and rice powder can be directly used as an ingredient for use in a broad range of nutraceuticals applied orally as rice powder or rice water by simply dissolving the MucoRice-ARP1 rice powder in water at room temperature. The authors showed that ARP1 produced in rice (MucoRice-A RP1) neutralizes RV strains in a range similar to that of the yeast produced ARP1. Thus it should be possible to use rice-based ARP1 treatment regardless of geographical differences in strain diversity.

Chloroplast Engineered Vaccines against Human Diseases

One method of increasing transgene expression level in plants is to express the transgene from the chloroplast genome through production of transplastomic plants. Initial immunological studies of chloroplast-derived vaccines have yielded promising results in animal models. Various vaccine antigens against several human and animal diseases have been successfully expressed in plastids, with an average expression level in the range of 4–31 per cent of TSP (Chebolu and Daniell 2009). The highest transgene expression in chloroplasts obtained to date is 70 per cent of TSP for an antibacterial lysin (Oey *et al.*, 2009). Transplastomic plants lack transgene silencing in spite of accumulating 100-fold higher transcripts than nuclear transgenic plants (Daniell *et al.*, 2009, Verma and Daniell 2007). High levels of expression (up to 72 per cent of total leaf protein) of several biopharmaceutical proteins and vaccine antigens have been attained via the chloroplast system (Ruhlman *et al.*, 2010). Plant chloroplasts facilitate formation of disulfide bonds and other post-translational modifications (Glenz *et al.*, 2006). The functionality of chloroplast-derived vaccine antigens has been validated by several assays including the macrophage lysis assay, GM1-ganglioside binding assay and immune response to challenge by pathogens or toxins (Davoodi-Semiromi *et al.*, 2010, Koya *et al.*, 2005). Additionally, chloroplast genomes facilitate transgene containment preventing escape through pollen because of maternal inheritance of the plastid genome (Daniell 2007). Further, total elimination of any reproductive structures is achieved when therapeutic proteins are harvested from leaves. For an effective oral plant vaccine, expressed from the chloroplast, the plant would need to be edible, plastid rich, be easy to manipulate genetically, have a sequenced chloroplast genome, be easy to grow where the vaccine is required, be edible raw and be non-perishable. Crop plants that seem to fit these requirements are tomatoes, spinach, maize, carrot, lettuce. A few examples of transplastomic vaccines are reviewed.

Tetanus Vaccine

The symptoms of tetanus are caused by tetanus toxin (tetanospasmin), a powerful protein toxin produced by the bacterium *Clostridium tetani*. Tetanus usually occurs after an acute injury, such as a puncture wound or laceration. Generalized tetanus, the most common form, is characterized by tetanic muscular contractions and an over-activity of the autonomic nervous system, which leads to spasms and a narrowing of the blood vessels, causing a rise in the blood pressure. Localized tetanus can occur in muscles near the wound, but it may progress to the generalized form. Tetanus can be prevented by immunization, which causes the production of anti-tetanus toxin antibodies, which block its action. Despite the availability of a parenteral vaccine, tetanus is still a common disease in many parts of the world, particularly in the African region, where neonatal tetanus (NT) remains an important public health problem, being responsible for 10–30 per cent of all infant deaths in many countries. The regional NT mortality rate is estimated at 5–10 per 1000 live births resulting in 120,000 deaths annually (WHO website). It is also a problem in pregnant mothers where *Clostridium tetani* may enter the uterine cavity through unclean instruments or hands, particularly during nonprofessional abortions or nonnstitutional deliveries. Globally 300,000 people die from tetanus each year. Current icensed tetanus vaccines are based on chemically inactivated tetanus toxin mixed vith an alum-based adjuvant delivered by injection. Tetanus toxin is composed of wo subunits (H and L chains) and has three functional domains. Domain HC, or he TetC fragment, consists of the 50-kDa carboxyl-terminal portion of the H chain. TetC has been widely used as a model vaccine antigen because of its non-toxicity and the potency of the response in both mucosal and parenteral systems (Stratford *et al.*, 2001, Tregoning *et al.*, 2004, Anderson *et al.*, 1996).

Tregoning *et al.* (2003) reported that TetC produced in tobacco chloroplasts is effective for mucosal immunization of mice when applied nasally and orally, and protects mice from a tetanus toxin challenge. They showed high-level TetC accumulation from both native bacterial high-AT (~25 per cent of TSP) and the synthetic high-GC (~10 per cent of TSP) *tetC* genes. TetC is a non-toxic 47 kDa polypeptide fragment of tetanus toxin that can be used as a subunit vaccine against tetanus. Expression of TetC in *Escherichia coli* and yeast was dependent on the availability of synthetic genes that were required to improve translation efficiency and stabilize the mRNA. To explore the feasibility of producing TetC in tobacco leaves, the authors attempted expression of both the bacterial high-AT (72.3 per cent AT) and the synthetic higher-GC genes (52.5 per cent AT) in tobacco chloroplasts. The results reported that the bacterial high-AT mRNA is stable in tobacco chloroplasts. Significant TetC accumulation was obtained from both genes, 25 and 10 per cent of total soluble cellular protein, respectively, proving the versatility of plastids for expression of unmodified high-AT and high-GC genes. Mucosal immunization of mice with the plastid- produced TetC induced protective levels of TetC antibodies. Thus, expression of TetC in chloroplasts provides a potential route towards the development of a safe, plant-based tetanus vaccine for nasal and oral applications.

Cervical Cancer Vaccine

Cervical cancer a global concern is caused by infection with human papillomaviruses (HPV) and is the second most common cancer in women worldwide, with approximately 493,000 new cases and 274,000 deaths occurring annually worldwide (Parkin and Bray 2006). Human papillomavirus (HPV) types 16 and 18 have been identified to be responsible for approximately 70 per cent of invasive cervical cancers, with HPV-16 being by far the most prevalent type and found in about 54 per cent of all cervical cancer cases (Smith *et al.*, 2007). L1 is the major capsid protein of HPV and self assembles into higher order molecular structures, such as capsomeres and virus-like particles (VLPs). Each VLP consists of 72 capsomeres, and each VLPs capsomere is a pentamer of the L1 protein arranged in an icosahedral surface lattice. VLPs are highly immunogenic as they can induce high titres of neutralizing antibodies (Rose *et al.*, 1998) that have been shown to successfully prevent HPV infections (Koutsky *et al.*, 2002, Villa *et al.*, 2006). The first two VLP-based vaccines using L1 protein as the selected antigen have been introduced onto the market (Harper *et al.*, 2004, Villa *et al.*, 2006, Muller and Gissmann 2007). However, their high cost has limited their application, and cytological screening programmes are still required to detect malignant lesions associated with the nonvaccine pathotypes. Thus, there is an urgent need for chea second-generation HPV vaccines that protect against multiple types.

Waheed *et al.* (2011) have expressed a mutated HPV-16 L1 (L1_2xCysM) gen that retained the ability to assemble L1 protein to capsomeres in tobacco chloroplast The recombinant protein yielded up to 1.5 per cent of total soluble protein. Th assembly of capsomeres was examined and verified by cesium chloride densit gradient centrifugation and sucrose sedimentation analysis. An antigen captur enzyme-linked immunosorbent assay confirmed the formation of capsomere by using a conformation specific monoclonal antibody which recognized th conformational epitopes. Transplastomic tobacco plants exhibited normal growt and morphology, but all such lines showed male sterility in the T0, T1 and T generations. However, taken together, these results indicate the possibility o producing a low-cost capsomere-based vaccine by plastids.

Pineo *et al.* (2013) used novel HPV-16 L1-based chimaeras, containing cross protective epitopes from the L2 minor capsid protein, in tobacco plants. These L1/L chimaeras contained epitope sequences derived from HPV-16 L2 amino acid 108-12 56-81 or 17-36 substituted into the C-terminal helix 4 (h4) region of L1 from amin acid 414. All chimaeras were expressed in *Nicotiana benthamiana* via an *Agrobacterium* mediated transient system and targeted to chloroplasts. The chimaeras were highl expressed with yields of ~1.2 g/kg plant tissue; however, they assembled differentl indicating that the length and nature of the L2 epitope affect VLP assembly. Th chimera containing L2 amino acids 108-120 was the most successful candidat vaccine. It assembled into small VLPs and elicited anti-L1 and anti-L2 response in mice, and antisera neutralized homologous HPV-16 and heterologous HPV-5 pseudovirions. The other chimaeras predominantly assembled into capsomeres an other aggregates and elicited weaker humoral immune responses, demonstratin the importance of VLP assembly for the immunogenicity of candidate vaccines.

Tuberculosis Vaccine

Tuberculosis (TB) caused by *Mycobacterium tuberculosis* (MTB), is one o the leading bacterial infections that is re-emerging due to drug resistant strain worldwide. The World Health Organization (WHO) estimated the global burde of TB in 2010 to be 8.8 million cases and 650,000 cases of multi drug resistant T (MDRTB) (WHO 2011). The development of TB vaccines has been recognized a a major public health priority by the World Health Organization. TB is also th leading cause of death in HIV-infected patients as immunosuppression amplifie the risk of reactivation of TB. Bacillus Calmette Guerin (BCG), an attenuated strai of *Mycobacterium bovis* is the only available licensed vaccine against TB. Many trial that evaluated BCG on the basis of protective immunity and age of vaccinatio have been inconsistent and variable, ranging from 0 to 80 per cent efficacy (Brewe and Colditz 1995, Colditz 1994, Xing and Lichty 2006, Tyagi *et al.*, 2011). In adult BCG blocks neither the development of latent TB nor revival of pulmonary T but prevents childhood TB (Anderson 2007). In mice, BCG vaccination provide protection up to 20 weeks post vaccination but the effectiveness gradually decline and was ultimately lost at 40 weeks post vaccination (Ozeki *et al.*, 2011). To confe protection, currently research groups are engaged in developing more efficient anti-TB vaccines which may have the potential to replace BCG as a primary TB vaccine or act as an effective boosting vaccine following BCG vaccination to augment protection ability (Lakshmi *et al.*, 2013).

In one of the first report of expression of TB vaccine antigens in chloroplasts, three candidate antigens, ESAT-6 (6kDa early secretory antigenic target) and Mtb72F (a fusion polyprotein from two TB antigens, Mtb32 and Mtb39) fused with cholera toxin B-subunit (CTB) and LipY (a cell wall protein) were expressed in tobacco and lettuce chloroplasts to facilitate bioencapsulation/oral delivery (Lakshmi *et al.*, 2013). Site-specific transgene integration into the chloroplast genome was confirmed by Southern blot analysis. In transplastomic leaves, CTB fusion proteins existed in soluble monomeric or multimeric forms of expected sizes and their expression levels varied depending upon the developmental stage and time of leaf harvest, with the highest-level of accumulation in mature leaves harvested at 6PM. The CTB-ESAT6 and CTB-Mtb72F expression levels reached up to 7.5 per cent and 1.2 per cent of total soluble protein respectively in mature tobacco leaves. Transplastomic CTB-ESAT6 lettuce plants accumulated up to 0.75 per cent of total leaf protein. Western blot analysis of lyophilized lettuce leaves stored at room temperature for up to six months showed that the CTB-ESAT6 fusion protein was stable and preserved proper folding, disulfide bonds and assembly into pentamers for prolonged periods. Antigen concentration per gram of leaf tissue was increased 22 fold after lyophilization. Hemolysis assay with purified CTB-ESAT6 protein showed partial hemolysis of red blood cells and confirmed functionality of the ESAT-6 antigen. GM1-binding assay demonstrated that the CTB-ESAT6 fusion protein formed pentamers to bind with the GM1-ganglioside receptor. The authors opined that expression of functional *Mycobacterium tuberculosis* antigens in transplastomic plants should facilitate development of a cost-effective and orally deliverable TB booster vaccine with potential for long-term storage at room temperature.

Transient Plant Expression System for Human Disease

Transient transformation implies the expression of a foreign DNA which is not inherited, but still transcribed within the host cell in a transiently manner. Transient expression systems are convenient tools that overcome the difficulties inherent to the stable transformation and they are used for many purposes taking advantage of the rapidity with which results can be obtained. There are two major approaches that are routinely used to achieve a transient expression of a heterologous protein in plants: via viral vectors or via *Agrobacterium* mediated transformation (Gomez *et al.*, 2009). The principle of plant virus approach relies on the fact that viruses can infect the plant by moving short and long distances, producing a systemic infection. Due to the high infection efficiency, tobacco mosaic virus (TMV)-based expression vectors were the most widely used systems, although other plus-sense single-stranded RNA viruses like cowpea mosaic virus (CPMV), alfalfa mosaic virus (AMV) and potato virus X (PVX) have also been modified to function as expression vectors, and have proven to be very useful for driving recombinant antigens expression (Grill *et al.*, 2005). The usual cloning strategy is to fuse the antigenic peptides to the viral capsid protein (CP) because of the high level of accumulation of this protein, its capability of self-assemble into particles and its ability to display the epitopes on the virus surface. However, the use of replicating RNA viruses has disadvantages in terms of the size and complexity of the proteins which can be expressed, potential problems of genetic drift and concerns regarding bio containment (Scholthof *et al.*, 1996). To address these issues, a non-replicating system based on Cowpea mosaic virus, the CPMV-HT (hyper translational) expression system, was developed which provides high yields of recombinant protein through extremely high translational efficiency without the need for viral replication. These vectors were subsequently refined to give the pEAQ series of transient expression vectors based on a deleted version of CPMV RNA-2 with a mutated 5'UTR which showed enhanced expression of candidate genes and antigens (Sainsbury and Lomonossoff, 2008).

The *Agrobacterium* based method involves the injection or vacuum infiltration of whole plants or parts of them with a suspension of bacteria harboring the expression construct of interest. Once the bacteria are in the tissue, the T-DNA is transferred into the host cell by bacterial proteins in a process that is equivalent to natural occurring infections. The T-DNA is further translocated into the nucleus where it can integrate or remain as an extra chromosomal form leading to a transient expression of the foreign gene. *Agrobacterium* transfers the T-DNA in such an efficient way that almost every cell of the patch is transformed. One important advantage of the "agroinfiltration" method relies on the fact that studies of multiple protein expression can be made concomitantly by infiltrating the plant with recombinant bacteria carrying different constructs. Agroinfiltration has been demonstrated as a powerful technique to study glycosylation, protein-protein interaction, conformation, folding and virus-like particles formation, and to evaluate the behavior of a certain construct prior to facing a stable transformation (Gomez *et al.*, 2009).

Another technology combining the agroinfiltration procedure and the viral replication in a TMV based transient expression system was demonstrated with the basic idea to amplify the foreign gene delivered by *Agrobacterium tumefaciens* to multiples areas of the plant (systemic delivery) allowing the virus to replicate and to cell-to-cell spread, rendering amplification and high level expression of the heterologous protein (mg to g quantities). In this process, the bacteria starts the initial infection delivering the T-DNA, encoding the viral replicon (TMV-based recombinant vector), to the nucleus of a large number of cells (Gomez *et al.*, 2009). Then, the transcripts are transported to the cytoplasm where the replication takes place rendering high yields of the desired protein (the yield is variable depending on the antigen expressed, but it is generally higher than the yield obtained when using other methodologies). This new platform for producing recombinant proteins was developed by Icon Genetics under the name of Magnification and permits the immediate possibility of scaling up the process with reduced production costs, reduced required time and reduced operational issues (Gleba *et al.*, 2005). Due to the fact that proteins obtained through agro infiltration plus viral replication based expression system can be evaluated just within a few days, and that the method is suitable for large scale production of vaccine proteins, this approach was employed to generate a plant-derived vaccine for influenza with potential human application

(Mett *et al.*, 2008). Two disease conditions where transient plant expression systems have been utilized for analyzing potential vaccines are discussed.

Non-Hodgkin's Lymphoma

Non-Hodgkin's lymphoma (NHL) has become the most common hematologic malignancy with an estimated 66,000 new cases reported in 2009 in the USA (Jemal *et al.*, 2009). Approximately 30 per cent of these cases are follicular B cell lymphoma, with a median survival of 8–10 years from diagnosis (Bendandi 2008). Most patients subjected to standard treatments, such as chemotherapy, radiation, or antibodies, still relapse. Newer approaches have focused on active immunotherapy through vaccination. For B cell lymphoma, the cell-surface Ig (Ig), or idiotype, is the unique tumor specific antigen (McCormick *et al.*, 2008). In contrast to passive therapy, an idiotype-induced immune response is (i) highly tumor specific, thus sparing normal cells; (ii) potentially more durable; and (iii) protective against tumor cell variants that might "escape" under selective pressure, because the response is polyclonal. There exists a 20-year history of idiotype vaccination for follicular lymphoma in animal models and clinical trials. The original vaccine manufacturing process, still used today in the majority of clinical research, used a patient's lymphoma B cells to derive a mouse/human heteromyeloma cell line for production of the tumor's monoclonal idiotype. Once purified, the idiotype antibody was chemically coupled to a highly immunogenic carrier protein, keyhole limpet haemocyanin (KLH), and administered with powerful colony stimulating factor (GM-CSF) (McCormick *et al.*, 2008).

The feasibility of using a plant viral expression system to produce personalized (patient-specific) recombinant idiotype vaccines against follicular B cell lymphoma and the results of administering these vaccines to lymphoma patients in a phase I safety and immunogenicity clinical trial was demonstrated (McCormick *et al.*, 2008). They expressed the single-chain form of the idiotype (scFv), which includes only the VH/VL domains and no constant regions, in a polypeptide of approx.30 KDa in *Nicotiana benthanania*. The system allowed rapid production and recovery of idiotypic single-chain antibodies (scFv) derived from each patient's tumor and immunization of patients with their own individual therapeutic antigen. Both low and high doses of vaccines, administered alone or co-administered with the adjuvant GM-CSF, were well tolerated with no serious adverse events. A majority (>70 per cent) of the patients developed cellular or humoral immune responses, and 47 per cent of the patients developed antigen specific responses. Because 15 of 16 vaccines were glycosylated in plants, this studies also shows that variation in patterns of antigen glycosylation does not impair the immunogenicity or affect the safety of the vaccines. Collectively, these findings support the conclusion that plant-produced idiotype vaccines are feasible to produce, safe to administer, and a viable option for idiotype specific immune therapy in follicular lymphoma patients.

The expression levels of plant-produced single-chain variable fragment lymphoma vaccines fragments were highly variable and required complex engineering of the linkers and the downstream processing could not be built around standard methods like protein A affinity capture. To tackle this limitation, Bendandi *et al.* (2010) reported a novel vaccine manufacturing process, magnifection, allowing consistent and efficient expression in plants of whole immunoglobulins (Igs). Full idiotype (Id)-containing IgG molecules of 20 lymphoma patients and 2 mouse lymphoma models were expressed at levels between 0.5 and 4.8 g/kg of leaf biomass. Protein A affinity capture purification yielded antigens of pharmaceutical purity. Several patient Igs produced in plants showed specific cross-reactivity with sera derived from the same patients immunized with hybridoma-produced Id vaccine. Mice vaccinated with plant- or hybridoma-produced Igs showed comparable protection levels in tumour challenge studies. A reliable and robust manufacturing process with the manufacturing time from biopsy to vaccine is <12 weeks and the expression and purification of antigens required only 2 weeks.

Influenza

Influenza is a serious respiratory disease caused by influenza viruses. During annual epidemics, three to five million cases of severe influenza illness are recorded worldwide, resulting in 250,000–500,000 deaths (WHO 2009). In addition to seasonal influenza out-breaks, occasional influenza pandemics can arise at any time when influenza A virus containing a novel hemagglutinin (HA) subtype is introduced and spreads efficiently among humans. In 2009, a novel, swine-origin influenza A H1N1 virus [A (H1N1) pdm09] emerged and infected humans. The virus, a triple reassortant with genes acquired from swine, avian and human influenza viruses, was first detected in the U.S. in April 2009 and spread rapidly across the globe, primarily in children and younger adult populations with little pre-existing serologic immunity to the novel HA, causing the World Health Organization to declare a pandemic on June, 2009 (Cummings *et al.*, 2013).

Currently licensed influenza vaccines are made in embryonated eggs (Mathews 2006). For the past four decades, these vaccines have been successfully used and proven to be safe and effective. Recently, safety and immunogenicity of several 2009 H1N1 influenza A vaccines in healthy volunteers have been demonstrated. However, the 2009 H1N1 pandemic demonstrated that egg-based technologies fall short of satisfying the global need for an emerging pandemic influenza vaccine in a timely manner. Therefore, developing alternative economic and scalable platforms for production of large amounts of safe and effective recombinant, or subunit, vaccines in a short timeframe was emphasized (Cunnigham *et al.*, 2013).

D'Aoust *et al.* (2008) made an important step with regards to utility of plant-based vaccines by transiently expressing protective antigens of multiple strains of influenza in *Nicotiana benthamiana* using an *Agrobacterium* mediated, transient expression system. The agro-infiltrated plants produced large amounts of protective antigen (50 mg/kg) from H5N1 (AIV) and H1N1 (human) strains. However most importantly this was performed in less than three weeks from release of viral sequence to purified vaccine product thereby proving potential value in protecting against disease outbreaks and in enabling expedient mobilisation of personnel. The plant-made influenza vaccine has completed Phase II human trials. More recently, safety and biological relevance of plant-produced therapeutic proteins and subunit vaccines, including H1N1 and H5N1 influenza vaccines, have been demonstrated in humans in Phase 1–3 clinical trials (Landry *et al.*, 2011).

The HAC1 vaccine, developed by Fraunhofer USA Center for Molecular Biotechnology (FhCMB), is a formulated recombinant HA monomer based on A/California/04/2009 (H1N1) influenza virus containing a poly-histidine (6 × His) affinity purification tag and the endoplasmic reticulum retention signal, KDEL,at the C-terminus. The HA antigen was cloned, expressed in *N. benthamiana*, purified and characterized (Shoji *et al.*, 2011). FhCMB engineered and produced HAC1 in less than one month and subsequently scaled it up for cGMP manufacturing in FhCMB's pilot facility. Pre-clinical studies demonstrated safety and protective immunogenicity of HAC1 in animals and prompted further investigation of this vaccine candidate in humans. Cummings *et al.* (2013) reported the first-in-human, Phase 1 clinical study which assessed safety and immunogenicity of HAC1. The experimental vaccine was fund to be safe and well tolerated, and comparable to placebo and the approved monovalent H1N1 vaccine. Nearly all adverse events were mild to moderate in severity. The HAC1 vaccine was also immunogenic, with the highest seroconversion rates, based on serum hemagglutination-inhibition and virus micro neutralization antibody titers, in the 90μg non-adjuvanted HAC1 vaccine group after the second vaccine dose (78 per cent and 100 per cent, respectively). This is the first study demonstrating the safety and immunogenicity of a plant-produced subunit H1N1 influenza vaccine in healthy adults. The results support further clinical investigation of the HAC1 vaccine as well as demonstrate the feasibility of the plant-based technology for quick vaccine antigen production.

Malaria

Malaria is unlike any infectious disease for which there is no successful vaccine. Mosquitoes carrying the deadly malaria parasite have flown along next to humans for thousands of years, and the disease appears in documented reports as early as 2700 B.C. and continues to plague humans today. According to the World Malaria Report (2012), about 219 million clinical cases of malaria were reported worldwide in 2010, predominantly in developing countries in sub-Saharan Africa and South-East Asia, causing approximately 660,000 deaths (Jones *et al.*, 2013). Moreover, children under the age of five, pregnant women, and people with HIV/AIDS are most at risk for severe illness and death. Quinine, a substance derived from the bark of the cinchona tree, has been known to be effective against malaria since 1600s. Malaria is caused by the parasite *Plasmodium*, a single-celled organism that has multiple life stages and requires more than one host for its survival. Five species of the parasite cause disease in humans – *Plasmodium falciparum, P. vivax, P. ovale, P. malariae,* and *P. knowlelsi.* Among these, *Plasmodium falciparum* is the most dangerous strain in humans and the target of most scientific research. Only the female Anopheles mosquito transmits the parasite (males do not feed on blood). The females of 60 different species of Anopheles mosquitoes can serve as malaria vectors (websites of CDC and History of vaccines). Sequencing the *P. falciparum* genome was reported in 2002, which allowed researchers to make great strides in better understanding ways to target it (Gardner *et al.*, 2002).

The Plasmodium Life Cycle

Most notable difference of malaria with other infectious diseases is that it is transmitted via a parasite that passes through multiple life stages, each of which presents a unique challenge to vaccine developers. The three stages in the *Plasmodium* life cycle can be divided into two distinct categories – in the first two, the parasite undergoes *asexual* reproduction in the host's body, and in the third it undergoes *sexual* reproduction in the mosquito vector gut. Because the parasite can reproduce both asexually and sexually, it has many advantages over the viruses and bacteria that are currently vaccinate against. The three stages of the *Plasmodium* life cycle are: the pre-erythrocytic stage or the liver stage (sporozite) before the parasite infects human red blood cells; the erythrocytic stage or the blood stage when the parasite is infecting the red blood cells (merozite) and the sexual stage, the stage when the parasite has been taken up by a mosquito and is sexually reproducing in the mosquito gut. One sporozoite can asexually reproduce to form up to 40,000 merozoites, large enough number to seriously challenge the ability of the immune system to control the parasite. Merozoite infects a red blood cell and begins asexually reproducing and releasing hundreds of new merozoites. In the third stage, or the sexual stage, a few merozoite-infected blood cells will stop asexually reproducing and instead mature into sexual forms of the parasites – known as male and female *gametocytes*. When an Anopheles mosquito bites a human who has malaria, it will take up the gametocytes along with the blood. These gametocytes are then able to further sexually reproduce in the mosquito gut, developing into mature sex cells or gametes, and finally fusing as they move up the mosquito gut wall to become an oocyst. The oocyst grows, divides, and eventually bursts and produces thousands of haploid *sporozoites*, which will travel to the mosquito's salivary glands to be injected into the next individual during the mosquito's next blood meal. Thus the parasite's life cycle comes full circle, allowing malaria to continue to spread and infect people across the globe.

Plant-made Antigen against the Asexual Blood Stage of Plasmodium

Pre-erythrocytic vaccines target the infectious phase aim either to prevent the sporozoites from getting into the liver cells or to destroy infected liver cells. The most significant challenge for a pre-erythrocytic vaccine is the time frame: sporozoites reach the liver less than an hour after being injected by the mosquito. The immune system has a limited amount of time to eliminate the parasite. Potential pre-erythrocytic vaccines are still in Phase I or Phase II trials, one vaccine, the RTS,S vaccine, is currently in Phase III trials and is showing promise. The RTS,S vaccine was engineered using genes from the repeat and T-cell epitope in the circumsporozoite protein (CSP) of *Plasmodium falciparum* malaria parasite and a viral envelope protein of the hepatitis B virus (HBsAg) and a chemical adjuvant to boost the immune system response Infection is prevented by inducing high antibody titers that block the parasite from infecting the liver (Foquet *et al.*, 2014)

A small number of merozoite surface proteins *viz.* apical membrane antigen-1 (AMA1), merozoite surface protein-1 (MSP1) and erythrocyte surface antigens have been analyzed as vaccines against the asexual bloodstage of *Plasmodium* that either blocks invasion of erythrocytes or inhibits its subsequent multiplication with few cases reaching clinical trials (Clemente and Corigliano 2012). The 19-kDa C-terminal fragment of *P. falciparum* merozoite surface protein 1 (PfMSP119) was the first malaria antigen expressed in plants by stable transformation, with a very low expression level (~0.0035 per cent of the total soluble protein (TSP) (Ghosh *et al.*, 2002). In another strategy a plant-codon-optimized version of the 42 kDa C-terminal fragment of PfMSP1 (PfMSP142) was designed and synthesized, and expressed in transgenic *Arabidopsis thaliana* seeds. For stable accumulation protein, the plant-optimized PfMSP142 gene was fused to the phaseolin peptide signal or the lysine rich protein resulting in a substantial improvement of approximately 5 per cent of TSP expression (Lau *et al.*, 2010). The *Plasmodium yoelii* merozoite surface protein 4/5 (PyMSP4/5), codon optimized and expressed in tobacco showed high effectiveness in protecting mice against a lethal challenge with expression level six-fold higher than that obtained with the native protein (Wang *et al.*, 2008). Webster *et al.* (2009) have expressed the plant codon-optimized PyMSP4/5 in *Nicotiana benthamiana* leaves, using the deconstructed TMV based transient expression system, magnICON, from ICON Genetics and reported expression levels of up to 10 per cent TSP. The use of magnICON has also been found to increase the expression level of the plant codon-optimized *P. yoelii* MSP119 (PyMSP119) to at least 23 per cent TSP (~3-4mg/g of fresh weight) (Ma *et al.*, 2011).

In tobacco transplastomic plants expressing *P. falciparum* PfAMA1 and PfMSP1, both fused to CTB, have been shown to accumulate CTB-PfAMA1 and CTB-PfMSP1 fusion proteins up to 13.1 per cent and 10.1 per cent of TSP in. Davoodi-Semiromi *et al.* (2010) expressed these same chimeric proteins in lettuce chloroplasts and found that the expression levels in lettuce were up to 7.3 per cent and 6.1 per cent of TSP, sufficient for oral delivery evaluation. They also found that subcutaneous and oral vaccination with candidate PfAMA1 and PfMSP1 genes fused to CTB are highly immunogenic in mice, showed a significant parasitic inhibition, providing evidence that the antibodies generated from immunized mice are effective in preventing parasite invasion of red blood cells. The levels of dual cholera-malaria vaccine antigens were ~50 fold higher in tobacco and ~30 fold higher in lettuce than other malaria antigens expressed in tobacco transgenic lines. The authors combined two attractive strategies to improve the level of expression: plastid expression and chimeric protein production. Besides transplastomic advantages, the *carrier* proteins contribute to a higher stability of the target protein in plants (Paul and Ma 2010).

Plant-made Antigens against Sexual Blood Stage of Plasmodium

Vaccines directed against proteins found in the sexual stages of *P. falciparum* parasites present in the *Anopheles* mosquito midgut are known as transmission-blocking vaccines (TBVs). They attack the parasite at a vulnerable stage of its life cycle, when it has to transfer from one host to another and when its numbers are very small (Clemente and Coriaglino 2012). Farrance *et al.* (2011) used the transient *N. benthamiana* expression system to express the *P. falciparum* gamete surface antigen P230 (Pfs230) and demonstrated that antibodies against this protein block the progression of the parasite's life cycle in the mosquito and thus block the transmission to the human host. The N terminal region of Pfs230 spanning aminoacids 444 to 730 was fused to the ER retention sequence (KDEL) and the recombinant protein was expressed in approximately 800 mg/kg in whole fresh leaf tissue, being 100 per cent soluble. This plant-made Pfs230 elicited high titers of anti-Pfs230 antibodies when administered to rabbits in the presence of complete/incomplete Freund's adjuvant. Furthermore, the antibodies generated combined with this adjuvant were shown to bind specifically to the native protein in *P. falciparum* on the surface of gametes/zygotes, resulting in significant TB activity. Farrance *et al.* (2011b) expressed an ookinete antigen present in the sexual form of the parasite–Pfs25–using the transient *N. benthamiana* expression system. Pf25 is able to induce TB antibodies and is present in the zygote and ookinete stages but is not expressed during human infection. Pfs25 expression levels were between 0.25 and 0.4mg/g of fresh leaf tissue and glycosylated versions determined that the non glycosylated antigens generated higher antibodies titers and enhanced TB activity. Since glycosylation does not occur in chloroplasts and the natural pathogen organism (*Plasmodium*) does not glycosylate the target proteins, these results support the idea that the chloroplast would be the best compartment to express this group of proteins, where the glycosylation may affect their antigenicity (Farrance *et al.*, 2011).

Veterinary Vaccines

Vaccination of animals decreases pharmaceutical treatment particularly use of antibiotic and prevents long-term suffering and death due to disease, decreases economic burden of disease through loss of livestock or well-being, and safeguards agricultural industries. Regulations associated with veterinary vaccines are significant yet still less burdensome than those associated with human pharmaceuticals. Therefore, crude or partially purified formulations and oral delivery are still possible (Ling *et al.*, 2010). A few plant derived vaccines for animals are described.

Foot-and-Mouth Disease Vaccine

Foot-and-mouth disease (FMD) is the most significant constraint to international trade in live animals and animal products today (Grubman and Baxt 2004). FMD affects all domesticated cloven-hoofed animals (such as cows, pigs, and sheep) as well as wild ruminants. The causative foot-and-mouth disease virus (FMDV), an aphthovirus of the Picornaviridae family, is highly contagious. The FMDV structural protein VP1 plays a key role in the immunogenicity of the virion, which can elicit the production of specific antibodies against a major immunogenic site located between amino acids 140 and 160 (Brown 1992). The VP1 protein has been overexpressed in *Arabidopsis thaliana*, alfalfa and potato (Dus Santos *et al.*, 2005).

Production of a highly immunogenic epitope containing amino acid residues 135–160 of the structural protein VP1 of the FMDV was reported (Das Santos *et al.*, 2005). The peptide was expressed as a fusion protein with the glucuronidase reporter gene (*uidA*). The recombinant protein represented the 51 per cent of the total soluble proteins in mature leaves. The FMDV epitope expressed in plants was highly immunogenic in mice and a strong anti-FMDV antibody response was detectable. Dus Santos *et al.* (2005) obtained the production of transgenic alfalfa plants containing the genes encoding the polyprotein P1 and the protease 3C of

FMDV. Parenterally immunized mice developed a strong antibody response and were completely protected when challenged with the virulent virus.

Lentz *et al.* (2010) used tobacco chloroplasts transformation for those of the Rubisco large subunit, the most abundant protein in the leaf of a wild-type plant. Despite high accumulation of heterologous protein, the transplastomic plants and wild-type tobacco were phenotypically indistinguishable and the FMDV epitope expressed in transplastomic plants was immunogenic in mice.

Porcine Viral Diarrhea Vaccine

Porcine viral diarrhea is a general term for some acute infectious diseases, which produce a water-like diarrhea in newborn piglets and are caused by porcine transmissible gastroenteritis virus (TGEV), porcine epidemic diarrhea virus (PEDV), or porcine rotavirus (RTV) and causes high mortality rates. Porcine epidemic diarrhea virus (PEDV) is an infectious, highly contagious virus of swine, which belongs to the Coronaviridae family (Pensaert and de Bouck 1978). Protective immunity against this disease has to be developed in pregnant sows in order to confer passive protection to the piglets through colostrum and milk. Neutralizing antibodies against the virus are directed mainly to glycoprotein S. Relevant epitopes in neutralization have been mapped into the N terminal domain of this protein (Correa *et al.*, 1988). Four major antigenic sites have been described in the globular part of glycoprotein S (gS), of which site A is considered to be immunodominant (De Diego *et al.*, 1994).

Transgenic potato plants were created to express the N-terminal domain of the glycoprotein S (N-gS) from TGEV. Extracts from transgenic tubers were inoculated intra peritoneally into mice, and the vaccinated mice developed serum IgG specific for TGEV (Gómez *et al.*, 2000). Tuboly *et al.* (2000) generated three transgenic tobacco plant lines expressing the spike (S) protein of TGEV. The results showed that antigens from all these lines induced TGEV-specific immune responses in pigs, and the resultant antibody titers for all three constructs were similar. Bae *et al.* (2003) developed transgenic tobacco plants that expressed the antigen protein corresponding to the neutralizing epitope of PEDV spike protein. Feeding the transgenic plants to mice induced both systemic and mucosal immune responses against the antigen.

By using a tobacco mosaic virus (TMV)-based vector, the coding sequence of a core neutralizing epitope of PEDV (COE) gene was expressed in tobacco and showed up to 5.0 per cent of the total soluble protein in the leaves of tobacco plants (Kang *et al.*, 2004a). A fusion gene encoding the synthetic LT-B subunit genetically fused with a synthetic neutralizing epitope of porcine epidemic diarrhea virus (sLTB-sCOE) was introduced into lettuce cells by *Agrobacterium*-mediated transformation methods. LTB-COE fusion protein comprised about 0.026–0.048 per cent of the total soluble protein in the transgenic lettuce leaf tissues (Huy *et al.*, 2009).

Newcastle Disease of Poultry Vaccine

Newcastle disease virus (NDV) infects a wide range of both domestic and wild birds in most countries and has a devastating effect on commercial poultry production (Alexander 1997, Seal *et al.*, 2000). NDV virions posses an envelope and contain a single molecule of linear, negative sense RNA coding for at least six proteins (Seal *et al.*, 2000). Two glycoproteins, the fusion protein (F) and the hemagglutinin-neuraminidase (HN), associated with the lipid envelope and forming spike-like structures on the surface of the particle (Morrison 2003). Protection against NDV is achieved by using live or inactivated vaccine strains. Guerrero-Andrade *et al.* (2006) expressed the fusion (F) gene of the Newcastle disease virus (NDV) in transgenic maize plants. The expression of the transgene, driven by the maize ubiquitin promoter, caused accumulation of the F protein in maize kernels. Feeding chickens with kernels containing the F protein induced the production of antibodies, conferring protection against a viral challenge comparable to that conferred by a commercial vaccine.

The world's first regulatory approval for a plant derived vaccine was against NDV in 2006. The HN protein from NDV was expressed in a tobacco cell system and found to retain the size and immuno reactivity of the native antigen. There was no degradation of the HN in the plant cells and it was bioactive in red blood cell hemagglutination assays. A master seed stock established from the cell line was used to produce a vaccine batch that was used in a disease challenge study in chickens. Non transgenic, negative controls plus four different formulations of the recombinant vaccine were prepared from plant cells. On days 0 and 14, specific pathogen-free chicks were vaccinated subcutaneously with the partially purified plant cell material. Individual blood samples were collected from each bird on day 24, and the chicks (except unchallenged controls) were challenged with NDV Texas GB strain on day 28. Birds vaccinated subcutaneously with the plant-made, subunit HN antigen from NDV proved to be protected against lethal challenge to NDV. The dose response capable of greater than 90 per cent protection ranged between 3 and 33 μg/dose with overall protection of 95 per cent. Thus, a plant cell-produced vaccine serologically converted birds and provided protective immunity against NDV. A formulation was advanced through the US Department of Agriculture Center for Veterinary Biologics' regulatory approval process in a feat that demonstrated that plant made vaccines could be developed within the existing regulatory framework (Ling *et al.*, 2010).

Fish Vaccine

Disease prevention is the key issue to maintain a sustainable development of aquaculture for sustainable protein based fish food production and also for the aquaculture industry and economy worldwide. Widespread use of antibiotics in aquaculture has led to the development of antibiotic-resistant bacteria and the accumulation of antibiotics in the environment. Vaccination is the most effective and environmentally-friendly approach to combat diseases in aquaculture to manage fish health. Compared to 760 vaccines against human diseases, there are only about 30 fish vaccines commercially available, suggesting the urgent need for development and cost-effective production of fish vaccines for managing fish health, in the fast growing fish farming worldwide.

Companjen *et al.* (2005) successfully expressed the non-toxic part of the *E. coli* heat-labile enterotoxin LTB fused with a viral peptide or GFP in potato tuber for oral immunization and induction of specific humoral immune response in carp upon feed-mediated administration. The study demonstrated the feasibility of producing fish vaccines for oral vaccination in an edible crop. To boost an efficient delivery of plant-made oral fish vaccine to immune-competent cells in the gut mucosa, a carrier molecule (LTB) was fused to the oral vaccine antigens to stimulate the uptake and immune response upon feed mediated oral immunization. Another approach is the production of a fish vaccine in tobacco chloroplasts against viral nervous necrosis (VNN) caused by Nodavirus (Clarke *et al.*, 2013). VNN affects farmed fish such as turbot, Atlantic halibut and Atlantic cod, as well as wild fish. In a study, transplastomic tobacco lines expressing RNA2 as the antigen candidate were produced and are currently being subjected to various molecular analyses (Clarke *et al.*, 2013).

Immunocontraceptive Vaccine

Fertility control may provide a non-lethal, more humane alternative for population control of vertebrate animals and one strategy is immune contraception and vaccination to induce antibodies against reproductive self-antigens, thereby resulting in reduced fertility (Ferro 2002). In most cases, the zona pellucida (ZP) has been used as the vaccine antigen, which is composed of three sulfated glycoproteins. One of the three glycoproteins, ZP3, is the primary binding site for the sperm and has been investigated as a target for immune contraception. As proof of concept, possums fed with potato-expressed LT-B had mucosal and systemic immune responses to the marsupial-specific reproductive antigens. Female possums vaccinated with immune contraceptive antigens showed reduced fertility, and demonstrated that immune contraception was effective in possums (Polkinghorne *et al.*, 2005, Guan *et al.*, 2013).

Conclusion

Plant derived subunit vaccines capable of inducing antigen-specific immune responses in both systemic and mucosal compartments without the use of syringe and needle or mucosal vaccination is considered ideal for the global control of infectious diseases. In recent times, several non-crop plants such as the duckweed *Lemna minor* and the moss *Physcomitrella patens* have been shown to be useful for the production of biopharmaceuticals (Büttner-Mainik *et al.*, 2011 and Gasdaska *et al.*, 2013). These frugal organisms can be cultivated in bioreactors (as opposed to being grown in fields), and thus secrete the transformed proteins into the medium. Thus, substantially reduce the burden of protein purification in preparing recombinant proteins for medical use. Both species can be engineered to cause secretion of proteins with human patterns of glycosylation, an improvement over conventional plant gene-expression systems (Cox *et al.*, 2006, Decker *et al.*, 2007). Biolex Therapeutics developed a duckweed-based expression platform which was later sold to Synthon in 2012 (Biolex website). Gregory *et al.* (2013) reported chloroplast engineering of the eukaryotic alga *Chlamydomonas reinhardtii* to produce a chimeric protein consisting of the 25kDa *Plasmodium falciparum* (Pfs25) fused to cholera toxin to investigate an alga based oral vaccine. Additionally, an Israel company, Protalix, has developed a method to produce therapeutics in culture transgenic carrot or tobacco cells (Protalix website). In 2012 Protalix and its partne Pfizer, received FDA approval to market its drug, a treatment for Gaucher's Diseas (Weinreb and Yeshayahou 2012).

Two plant-made antibody products have made it to human clinical trial undergoing Phase II U.S. clinical trials under a U.S. Food and Drug Administration approved Investigational New Drug application. Planet Biotechnology Inc produced the world's first clinically tested antibody, CaroRx™ in tobacco. CaroRx™ specifically binds to the bacteria that cause tooth decay thereby preventing adhesion of the bacteria to teeth (Plant Biotechnology website). Although, these product would still have to acquire regulatory approval before releasing for use. Initia products would likely have to go through more rigorous trials, however once the safety of the platform is confirmed there is no reason that regulatory approval would take longer for current technologies.

Antibody-producing tobacco leaves need storage under –20° C, and antibody-producing tomatoes need a temperature below 4 ° C. In contrast, antibody-producing cereals such as rice and wheat as well as pea seeds can be stored at room temperature (Tokuhara *et al.*, 2013). The problems associated with seed systems are largely down to regulatory issues, as containment can be problematic with wind dispersal and seeds can remain viable in the soil after the crop has been harvested. Also, especially with crops such as rice and maize that are a staple food source for many, the potentia for unwanted transgenes to enter the food supply could have major repercussions However, these risks can be managed through the spatial and temporal segregation of crops as well as other physical and biological segregation techniques (Naqvi *et al.*, 2011). Chloroplast transformation can address some of these concerns regarding foreign gene transfer via pollen, due to the maternal inheritance of transgenes (Daniell 2007). The potential for large-scale use of seed crops depends largely on the containment requirements decided on by regulatory agencies.

In general, rare codons, AU-rich destabilizing sequences and putative polyadenylation and splicing signals may contribute to rapid mRNA decay, thus limiting the expression of foreign genes in plants. In the plant codon-optimized PyMSP4/5 antigen, the A+T content is reduced from 67 per cent to 53 per cent and the AT-rich regions are disrupted, allowing the reduced A+T gene version to be more efficient in antigen production than the native version (Wang *et al.*, 2008) Plant codon optimization combined with the magnICON expression system has been shown to allow an increase of up to 100 fold with respect to the transgenic tobacco system (Webster *et al.*, 2009). These studies establish that not only codon optimization but also the viral provector system improves the expression level of plant-made malaria antigens (Ma *et al.*, 2011).

Three recent reviews by Floss *et al.* (2007), Joensuu *et al.* (2008) and Rybicki (2010) have provided an overview of production of veterinary vaccines in plants. However, plants as expression systems for production of fish vaccines are lagging behind compared with the plant-made veterinary vaccines for non-aquatic (land-based) animals.

Wirz *et al.* (2012) described a first of its kind automated plant based factory for production of vaccines and pharmaceuticals using tobacco plants. A collaboration between Fraunhofer CMI, USA and Boston University, the factory's custom-designed robotic machines uses plant seeds, nurture the growing plants, introduce a viral vector that directs the plant to produce a target protein, and harvest the biomass once the target protein has accumulated in the plants - all in compliance with Food and Drug Administration (FDA) guidelines (*e.g.* current Good Manufacturing Practices). The factory was designed to be time, cost, and space efficient. To quickly produce large quantities of protein-based medicines, they transformed a laboratory based biological process and scaled it into an industrial process. This enabled quick, safe, and cost-effective vaccine production that would be required in case of a pandemic.

A comprehensive analysis of the number of articles published every year on transgenic plant vaccines in various databases such as Science Direct, Springer link, Wiley Inter Science and Web of science was reported by Guan *et al.* (2013). There were 835 articles in Elsevier, 841 in Springer link, 808 in Wiley, and 313 in Web of Science in 2011. From 2000 to 2011, an increasing number of vaccine candidates have been successfully expressed in various transgenic plants. The day is not far when plant derived vaccines will be a proven clinical reality. Individualized plant made vaccines for clinical manifestations such as hypersensitivity and autoimmune disorder will be the order of the day.

References

Alexander DJ. Newcastle disease and other avian *Paramixoviridae* infections. In: Calnek BW, Barnes HJ, Beard CW, Reid WM, Yoder HW (eds) *Diseases of Poultry.* Iowa State University Press, Iowa. pp. 541–570. 1997.

Andersen P. Tuberculosis vaccines - an update. *Nat. Rev. Microbiol.* 5: 484–487. 2007.

Anderson R, Gao XM, Papakonstantinopoulou A, Roberts M, Dougan G. Immune response in mice following immunization with DNA encoding fragment C of tetanus toxin. *Infect. Immun.* 64: 3168–3173. 1996.

Arango PI, Elizabeth LR, Edith RA, Teresa O *et al.*, Expression of the rabies virus nucleoprotein in plants at high-levels and evaluation of immune responses in mice. *Plant Cell Rep.* 27: 677–685. 2008.

Arlen PA, Singleton M, Adamovicz JJ, Ding Y *et al.*, Effective plague vaccination via oral delivery of plant cells expressing F1-V antigens in chloroplasts. *Infect. Immun.* 76: 3640–3650. 2008.

Armah GE, Sow SO, Breiman RF, Dallas MJ *et al.*, Efficacy of pentavalent rotavirus vaccine against severe rotavirus gastroenteritis in infants in developing countries in sub-Saharan Africa: a randomised, double-blind, placebo-controlled trial. *Lancet.* 376(9741): 606–614. 2010.

Ashraf S, Singh PK, Yadav DK, Shahnawaz M, Mishra S, Sawant SV,Tuli R. High level expression of surface glycoprotein of rabies virus in tobacco leaves and its immunoprotective activity in mice. *J. Biotech.* 119: 1–14. 2005.

Aviezer D, Brill-Almon, E, Shaaltiel Y, Hashmueli S *et al.*, A plant-derived recombinant human glucocerebrosidase enzyme–a preclinical and phase I investigation. *PLoS One*. 4, e4792. 2009.

Bae JL, Lee JG, Kang TJ, Jang HS *et al.*, Induction of antigen-specific systemic and mucosal immune responses by feeding animals transgenic plants expressing the antigen. *Vaccine*. 21: 4052–4058. 2003.

Baur A, Reski, R, Gorr, G. Enhanced recovery of a secreted recombinant human growth factor using stabilizing additives and by co-expression of human serum albumin in the moss Physcomitrella patens. *Pl. Biotech. J.* 3 (3): 331–40. 2005. doi: 10.1111/j.1467-7652.2005. 00127.x. PMID 17129315

Bendandi M. Aiming at a curative strategy for follicular lymphoma. *CA Cancer J. Clin*. 58: 305–317. 2008.

Bendandi M, Marillonnet S, Kandzia R, Thieme F *et al.*, Rapid, high-yield production in plants of individualized idiotype vaccines for non-Hodgkin's lymphoma. *Ann. Oncol*. 21 (12): 2420-2427. 2010.

Bernstein DI. Rotavirus overview. *Pediatric Infect Dis J*. 28(suppl 3): S50–S53. 2009.

Bendandi M, Marillonnet S, Kandzia R, Thieme F *et al.*, Rapid, high-yield production in plants of individualized idiotype vaccines for non-Hodgkin's lymphoma. *Anal. Oncol*. 21: 2420–2427. 2010.

BiolexTherapeutics: OctoPlus Licensee Biolex Presents Locteron Phase IIa Results. *Proc. Intl. Liver Cong. Copenhagen, Denmark*. pp. 22–26. 2009.

Brewer TF, Colditz GA. Relationship between Bacille Calmette-Guerin (BCG) strains and the efficacy of BCG vaccine in the prevention of tuberculosis. *Clin. Infect. Dis*. 20: 126–135. 1995.

Brown F. Vaccination against foot-and-mouth disease. *Vaccine*. 10: 1022–1026. 1992.

Büttner-Mainik A, Parsons J, Jérôme, H, Hartmann A *et al.*, Production of biologically active recombinant human factor H in Physcomitrella. *Pl. Biotech. J.* 9 (3): 373–83. 2011. doi: 10.1111/j.1467-7652.2010. 00552.x. PMID 20723134

Chargelegue D, Obregon P, Drake PM. Transgenic plants for vaccine production: expectations and limitations. *Trends Pl. Sci*. 6: 495–496. 2001.

Chebolu S, Daniell H. Chloroplast-derived vaccine antigens and biopharmaceuticals: expression, folding,assembly and functionality. *Curr. Top Microbiol. Immunol*. 332: 33–54. 2009.

Chikwamba R, McMurray J, Shou H, Frame B *et al.*, Expression of a synthetic *E. coli* heat labile enterotoxin B sub-unit (LT-B) in maize. *Mol. Breed*. 10: 253–265. 2002.

Clemens J, Shin S, Sur D, Nair GB, Holmgren J. New-generation vaccines against cholera. *Natl. Rev. Gastroenterol. Hepatol*. 8: 701–710. 2011.

Clemens JD, Sack DA, Harris JR, Chakraborty J *et al.*, Field trial of oral cholera vaccines in Bangladesh. *Lancet*. 2: 124–127. 1986.

Clemens JD, Harris JR, Sack DA, Chakraborty J *et al.*, Field trial of oral cholera vaccines in Bangladesh: results of one year of follow-up. *J. Infect. Dis.* 158: 60–66. 1986.

Clemente M, Corigliano MG. Overview of Plant-Made Vaccine Antigens against Malaria. *J. Biomed. Biotech.* 8. 56- 64. 2012, doi: 10.1155/2012/206918

Colditz GA, Brewer TF, Berkey CS, Wilson ME *et al.*, Efficacy of BCG vaccine in the prevention of tuberculosis. *JAMA.* 271: 698–702. 1994.

Coler RN, Dillon DC, Skeiky YA, Kahn M *et al.*, Identification of *Mycobacterium tuberculosis* vaccine candidates using human CD4+ T-cells expression cloning. *Vaccine.* 27: 223–233. 2009.

Companjen AR, Florack DE, Bastiaans JH, Matos CI *et al.*, Development of a cost-effective oral vaccination method against viral disease in fish. *Dev. Biol. (Basel).* 121: 143–150. 2005.

Correa I, Jiménez G, Suñé C, Bullido MJ, Enjuanes L. Antigenic structure of E2-glycoprotein of transmissible gastroenteritis coronavirus. *Virus Res.* 10: 77–94. 1988.

Corigliano M G, A. Maglioco, M. L. Becher *et al.*, Plant Hsp90 proteins interact with B-cells and stimulate their proliferation. *PLoS ONE.* 6: 34-39. 2011

Cox KM, Sterling JD, Regan JT, Gasdaska, JR *et al.*, Glycan optimization of a human monoclonal antibody in the aquatic plant lemna minor. *Nature Biotech.* 24 (12): 1591–7. 2006.

Cummings JF, Guerrero ML, Moon JE, Waterman P *et al.*, Safety and immunogenicity of a plant-produced recombinant monomer hemagglutinin-based influenza vaccine derived from influenza A (H1N1) pdm09 virus: A Phase 1 dose-escalation study in healthy adults. *Vaccine.* 10: 17-21. 2013.

Curtiss RI, Cardineau CA. Oral immunisation by transgenic plants, *World Patent Application.* 1990.

Curtiss R, Cardineau GA. Oral immunization by transgenic plants. U.S. Patent. 5,679,880, 21. 1997.

Czerkinsky C, Anjuere F, McGhee JR, George-Chandy A. Mucosal immunity and tolerance: relevance to vaccine development. *Immunol. Rev.* 170: 197–222. 1999.

Dalgleish AG, Beverley PC, Clapham PR, Crawford DH *et al.*, The CD4 (T4) antigen is an essential component of the receptor for the AIDS retrovirus. *Nature.* 312: 763–767. 1984.

D'Aoust MA, Lavoie P-O, Couture MMJ, Trépanier S *et al.*, Influenza virus-like particles produced by transient expression in *Nicotiana benthamiana* induce a protective immune response against a lethal viral challenge in mice. *Pl. Biotech. J.* 6: 930–940. 2008.

D'Aoust MA, Couture MMJ, Charland, N, Trépanier S *et al.*, The production of hemagglutinin-based virus-like particles in plants: A rapid, efficient and safe response to pandemic influenza. *Pl. Biotech. J.* 8: 607–619. 2010.

Daniell H, Singh ND, Mason H, Streatfield SJ. Plant-made vaccine antigens and biopharmaceuti cals. *Trends Pl. Sci.* 14: 669–679. 2009.

Daniell H, Lee SB, Panchal T, Wiebe PO. Expression of the native cholera toxin B subunit gene and assembly as functional oligomers in transgenic tobacco chloroplasts. *J. Mol. Biol.* 311: 1001–1009. 2001.

Daniell H. Transgene containment by maternal inheritance: effective or elusive? *Proc. Natl. Acad. Sci. USA.* 104(17): 6879–6880. 2007.

Davoodi-Semiromi, A, Samson N, Daniel H. The green vaccine: a global strategy to combat infectious and autoimmune diseases. *Hum. Vaccin.* 5: 488–493. 2009.

Davoodi-Semiromi A, Schreiber M, Nalapalli S, Verma D *et al.*, Chloroplast-derived vaccine antigens confer dual immunity against cholera and malaria by oral or injectable delivery. *Pl. Biotech. J.* 8: 223–242. 2010.

Decker EL, Reski R. Current achievements in the production of complex biopharmaceuticals with moss bioreactors". *Bioproc. Biosyst. Engg.* 31 (1): 3–9. 2007.

Derrick SC, Yang AL, Morris SL. A polyvalent DNA vaccine expressing an ESAT6-Ag85B fusion protein protects mice against a primary infection with *Mycobacterium tuberculosis* and boosts BCG-induced protective immunity. *Vaccine.* 23: 780–788. 2007.

Dey B, Jain R, Gupta UD, Katoch VM, Ramanathan VD, *et al.*, A booster vaccine expressing a latency-associated antigen augments BCG induced immunity and confers enhanced protection against tuberculosis. *PLoS One.* 6(8): e23360. 2011.

Diego M, Rodríguez F, Alcaraz C, Gómez N *et al.*, Characterization of the IgA and subclass IgG responses to neutralizing epitopes after infection of pregnant sows with the transmissible gastroenteritis virus or the antigenically related porcine respiratory coronavirus. *J. Gen. Virol.* 75: 2585–2593. 1994.

Dietzschold B, Tollis M, Rupprecht CE, Celis E, Koprowski H. Antigenic variation in rabies and rabies-related viruses: cross-protection independent of glycoprotein-mediated virus neutralizing antibody. *J. Infect. Dis.* 156: 815–822. 1987a.

Dietzschold B, Wang HH, Rupprecht CE, Celis E. *et al.*, Induction of protective immunity against rabies by immunization with rabies virus ribonucleoprotein. *Proc. Natl. Acad. Sci. USA.* 84: 9165–9169. 1987b

Dietzschold B, Rupprecht CE, Tollis M, Lafon M, Mattei J, Wiktor TJ, Koprowski H. Antigenic diversity of the glycoprotein and nucleocapsid proteins of rabies and rabies-related viruses: implications for epidemiology and control of rabies. *Rev. Infect. Dis.* 10(Suppl. 4): S785–S798. 1988.

Doherty TM, Dietrich J, Billeskov R. Tuberculosis subunit vaccines: from basic science to clinical testing. *Expert Opin. Biol. Ther.* 7: 1539–1549. 2007.

Dong JL, Liang BG, Jin YS, Zhang WJ *et al.*, Oral immunization with pBsVP6-transgenic alfalfa protects mice against rotavirus infection. *Virology.* 339, 153–163. 2005.

Dus Santos MJ, Wigdorovitz A, Trono K, Ríos RD *et al.*, A novel methodology to develop a foot and mouth disease virus (FMDV) peptidebased vaccine in transgenic plants. *Vaccine*. 20: 1141–1147. 2002.

Dus Santos MJ, Carrillo C, Ardila F, Ríos RD *et al.*, Development of transgenic alfalfa plants containing the foot and mouth disease virus structural ployprotein gene P1 and its utilization as an experimental immunogen. *Vaccine*. 23: 1838–1843. 2005.

Echeverria P C, de Miguel N, Costas M, Angel SO. Potent antigen-specific immunity to *Toxoplasma gondii* in adjuvant-free vaccination system using Rop2-*Leishmaniainfantum* Hsp83 fusion protein. *Vaccine*. 24 (19): 4102–4110. 2006.

Farrance CE, Rhee A, Jones RM *et al.*, A plant-produced Pfs230 vaccine candidate blocks transmission of *Plasmodium falciparum*. Clinl. *Vaccine Immunol.* 18: 1351–1357. 2011a.

Farrance CE, Chichester JA, Musiychuk K *et al.*, Antibodies to plant-produced *Plasmodium falciparum* sexual stage protein Pfs25 exhibit transmission blocking activity. *Human Vaccines*. 7: 191–198. 2011b.

Faye L, Gomord, R. Editorial: Success stories in molecular farming-a brief overview. *Pl. Biotech. J.* 8, 525–528. 2010.

Ferro VA. Current advances in antifertility vaccines for fertility control and noncontraceptive applications. *Expert Rev. Anti Vaccine*. 1: 443–452. 2002.

Fernandez-SanMillan A, Ortigosa SM, Herves-Stubbs S, Corral-Martinez P *et al.*, Human papillomavirusL1 protein expressed in tobacco chloroplasts self-assembles into virus-like particles that are highly immunogenic. *Pl. Biotech. J.* 6, 427–441. 2008.

Fischer TK, Viboud C, Parashar U, Malek M *et al.*, Hospitalizations and deaths from diarrhea and rotavirus among children < 5 years of age in the United States, 1993–2003. *J. Infect. Dis.*, 195(8): 1117–1125. 2007.

Fiedler U, Conrad U. High-level production and long-term storage of engineered antibodies in transgenic tobacco seeds. *Biotech*. 13(10): 1090–1093. 1995.

Floss DM, Falkenburg D, Conrad U. Production of vaccines and therapeutic antibodies for veterinary applications in transgenic plants: an overview. *Trans Res*. 16: 315–332. 2007.

Fu ZF, Dietzschold B, Schumacher CL, Wunner WH *et al.*, Rabies virus nucleoprotein expressed in and purified from insect cells is efficacious as a vaccine. *Proc. Natl. Acad. Sci. USA*. 88: 2001–2005. 1991.

Foquet, L, Hermsen C, van Gemert, GJ, Van B *et al.*, Vaccine-induced monoclonal antibodies targeting circumsporozoite protein prevent *Plasmodium falciparum* infection". *J. Clinic. Invest*. 124 (1): 140. 2014.

Flamand A, Wiktor TJ, Koprowski H. Use of hybridoma monoclonal antibodies in the detection of antigenic differences between rabies and rabies-related virus proteins II. The glycoprotein. *J. Gen. Virol*. 48: 105–109. 1980.

Gali W, Koby Y. FDA approves Protalix Gaucher treatment. *Globes*. May 2, 2012.

Gao Y, Ma Y, Li M, Cheng T *et al.*, Oral immunization of animals with transgeni cherry tomatillo expressing HBsAg. *World J. Gastroenterol*. 9: 996–1002. 2003.

Gardner MJ, Hall N, Fung E, White O *et al.*, Genome sequence of the human malari parasite *Plasmodium falciparum*. *Nature*. 419: 498-511. 2002.

Gasdaska JR, Spencer D, Dickey L. Advantages of therapeutic protein productio in the aquatic plant lemna. *BioProcessing. J*. 2 (2): 49–56. 2003.

Giudice EL, Campbell JD. Needle-free vaccine delivery. *Adv. Drug Deliv. Rev*. 58 68–89. 2006.

Gisby MF, Mellors P, Madesis P, Ellin M *et al.*, A synthetic gene increases TGFb accumulation by 75-fold in tobacco chloroplasts enabling rapid purificatio and folding into a biologically active molecule. *Pl. Biotech. J*. 9: 618–628. 2011.

Glass RI, Parashar UD. The promise of new rotavirus vaccines. *New Eng. J. Med* 354(1): 75–77. 2006.

Guan ZJ, Bin G, Yan-lin H, Zheng-ping G *et al.*, Recent advances and safety issues o transgenic plant-derived vaccines. *Appl. Microbiol. Biotech*. 97: 2817-2840. 2013

Guetard D, Greco R, Gonzalez MC, Celli S *et al.*, Immunogenicity and toleranc following HIV-1/HBV plant-based oral vaccine administration. *Vaccine*. 26(35) 4477– 4485, 2008.

Granell A, Fern´andezdel-Carmen A, Orz´aez D. In planta production of plant derived and non-plant-derived adjuvants. Expert Rev. *Vaccines*. 9(8): 843-858 2010

Gregory JA , Aaron BT, David Z D, Mayfield S. Algae-produced cholera toxin-Pfs2 fusion proteins as oral vaccines. *Appl. Env. Microbiol*. 79(13): 3917-3925. 2013.

Glenz K, Bouchon B, Stehle T, Wallich R, Simon MM, *et al.*, Production of recombinant bacterial lipoprotein in higher plant chloroplasts. *Nature Biotech* 24: 76–77. 2006.

Girard MP, Steele D, Chaignat CL, Kieny MP. A review of vaccine research and development: human enteric infections. *Vaccine*. 24: 2732–2750. 2006.

GoveaAlonso D, Néstor Rubio I, GarciaHernandez AL, Javier T *et al.*, Immunogenic properties of a lettucederived C4(V3)6 multiepitopic HIV protein. *Planta*. 238 785-792. 2013.

Grill LK, Palmer KE, Pogue GP. Use of plant viruses for production of plant-derived vaccines. *Critical Rev. Pl. Sci*. 24: 309-23. 2005.

Gomez E, Zoth SC, Berinstein A. Plant-based vaccines for potential human application: A review. *Human Vaccines*. 5: 11, 738-744. 2009

Gleba Y, Klimyuk V, Marillonnet S. Magnifection - a new platform for expressing recombinant vaccines in plants. *Vaccine*. 23: 2042-8. 2005.

Ghosh S, Malhotra P, Lalitha PV, Guha-Mukherjee S, Chauhan VS. Expression of *Plasmodium falciparum* C terminal region of merozoite surface protein (PfMSP1 19), a potential malaria vaccine candidate, in tobacco. *Pl. Sci.* 162: 335–343. 2002.

Grubman MJ. Baxt B. Foot-and-mouth disease. *Clin. Microbiol. Rev.* 17: 465–493. 2004.

Gómez N, Wigdorovitz A, Castañón S, Gill F *et al.*, Oral immunogenicity of the plant derived spike protein from swine-transmissible gastroenteritis coronavirus. *Arch. Virol.* 145: 1725–1732. 2000.

Giritch A, Marillonnet S, Engler C, Eldik G *et al.*, Rapid high-yield expression of full-size IgG antibodies in plants coinfected with noncompeting viral vectors. *Proc. Natl. Acad. Sci. USA.* 103(40): 14701–14706. 2006.

Guerrero-Andrade O, Loza-Rubio E, Olivera-Flores AET, Fehe´rva´ri-Bone T. Expression of the Newcastle disease virus fusion protein in transgenic maize and immunological studies. *Transgenic Res.* 15: 455–463. 2006.

Haq TA, Mason HS, Clements, JD, Arntzen, CJ. Oral immunization with a recombinant bacterial antigen produced in transgenic plants. *Science.* 268, 714-716. 1995.

Harper DM, Franco EL, Wheeler C, Ferris DG *et al.*, Efficacy of a bivalent L1 virus-like particle vaccine in prevention of infection with human papillomavirus types 16 and 18 in young women: a randomized controlled trial. *Lancet.* 364: 1757-1765. 2004.

Holmgren J, Czerkinsky C. Mucosal immunity and vaccines. *Nat. Med.* 11: S45–S53. 2005.

Hiatt A, Caffferkey R, Bowdish K. Production of antibodies in transgenic plants. *Nature.* 342, 76 - 78. 1989.

Heermann, KU, Goldmann U, Schwartz W, Seyffarth T *et al.*, Large surface proteins of hepatitis B virus containing the pre-*s* sequence. *J. Virol.* 2: 396–402.1984.

Howard AH, Hood E. Bioindustrial and biopharmaceutical products produced in plants. *Adv. Agronomy.* 85, 91–124. 2005.

Hamorsky KT, Kouokam JC, Bennett LJ, Baldauf KJ *et al.*, Rapid and calable plant-based production of a cholera toxin B subunit variant to mid in mass vaccination against cholera outbreaks. *PLoS. Negl. Trop. Dis.* 7(3): e2046. 2013. doi: 10.1371/journal.pntd.0002046

Hashim R, Khatib AM, Enwere G, Park JK *et al.*, Safety of the recombinant cholera toxin B subunit, killed whole-cell (rBS-WC) oral cholera vaccine in pregnancy. *PLoS. Negl. Trop. Dis.* 6: e1743. 2012.

Haynes BF, Gilbert PB, McElrath MJ, Zolla-Pazner S *et al.*, Immune-correlates analysis of an HIV-1 vaccine efficacy trial. *New Eng. J. Med.* 366: 1275–1286. 2012.

Huy NX, Kim YS, Jun SC, Jin ZW *et al.*, Production of a heat-labile enterotoxin B subunit-porcine epidemic diarrhea virus-neutralizing epitope fusion protein in transgenic lettuce (*Lactuca sativa*). *Biotech. Bioproc. Engg.* 14: 731–737. 2009.

Ismaili A, Jalali-Javaran M, Rasaee MJ, Rahbarizadeh F *et al.*, Production and characterization of anti-(mucin MUC1) single-domain antibody in tobacco (*Nicotiana tabacum* cultivar Xanthi). *Biotech. Appl. Biochem.* 47(1): 11–19. 2007.

Jiang XL,He ZM, Peng ZQ, Qi Y *et al.*, Cholera toxin B protein in transgenic tomato fruit induces systemic immune response in mice. *Transgenic Res.* 16(2): 169–175. 2007.

Jemal A, Siegel R, Ward E, Hao Y *et al.*, Cancer statistics. *CA Cancer J. Clin.* 59: 225–249. 2009.

Jones RM, Chichester JA, Mett V, Jaje J *et al.*, A plant-produced Pfs25 VLP malaria vaccine candidate induces persistent transmission blocking antibodies against *Plasmodium falciparum* in immunized mice. *PLoS ONE.* 8(11): e79538. 2013. doi: 10.1371/journal.pone.00795

Jelinek T, Kollaritsch H. Vaccination with Dukoral against travelers' diarrhea (ETEC) and cholera. *Expert Rev. Vaccines.* 7: 561–567. 2008.

Jertborn M, Svennerholm AM, Holmgren J. Safety and immunogenicity of an oral recombinant cholera B subunit-whole cell vaccine in Swedish volunteers. *Vaccine.* 10: 130–132. 1992.

Jihong LC, Mohammad TW, Andreas G, Lo¨ssl G *et al.*, How can plant genetic engineering contribute to cost-effective fish vaccine development for promoting sustainable aquaculture? *Pl. Mol. Biol.* 83: 33–40. 2013.

Joensuu JJ, Niklander-Teeri V, Brandle JE. Transgenic plants for animal health: plant-made vaccine antigens for animal infectious disease control. *Phytochem. Rev.* 7: 553–577. 2008.

Kostrzak A, M. Cervantes Gonzalez, D. Guetard *et al.*, Oral administration of low doses of plant-based HBsAg induced antigen-specific IgAs and IgGs in mice, without increasing levels of regulatory T cells. *Vaccine.* 27(35): 4798–4807. 2009.

Kapusta J, A.Modelska, M. Figlerowicz, Pniewski T *et al.*, A plant-derived edible vaccine against hepatitis B virus. *FASEB J.* 13 (13): 1796–1799. 1999

Kiyono H, Fukuyama S. NALT- versus Peyer's-patch-mediated mucosal immunity. *Natl. Rev. Immunol.* 4: 699–710. 2004.

Karaman S, Cunnick J, Wang K. Expression of the cholera toxin B subunit (CT-B) in maize seeds and a combined mucosal treatment against cholera and traveler's diarrhea. *Plant Cell Rep.* 31: 527–537. 2012.

Karlsson Hedestam GB, Fouchier RA, Phogat S, Burton DR *et al.*, The challenges of eliciting neutralizing antibodies to HIV-1 and to influenza virus. *Natl. Rev. Microbiol.* 6: 143–155. 2008.

Kang TJ, Kang KH, Kim JA, Kwon TH *et al.*, High-level expression of the neutralizing epitope of porcine epidemic diarrhea virus by a tobacco mosaic virus-based vector. *Protein Exp. Purific.* 38: 129–135. 2004a.

Koya V, Moayeri M, Leppla SH, Daniell H. Plant-based vaccine: mice immunized with chloroplast-derived anthrax protective antigen survive anthrax lethal toxin challenge. *Infect. Immun*. 73: 8266–8274. 2005.

Koutsky LA, Ault KA, Wheeler CM, Brown DR *et al.*, A controlled trial of a human papillomavirus type 16 vaccine. *New Eng. J. Med*. 347: 1645–1651. 2002.

Lakshmi PS, Verma D, Yang X, Lloyd B, Daniell H. Low cost tuberculosis vaccine antigens in capsules: expression in chloroplasts, bio-encapsulation, stability and functional evaluation in vitro. *PLoS ONE*. 8(1). 2013. e54708. doi: 10.1371/journal.pone.0054708

Levine MM, Sztein MB. Vaccine development strategies for improving immunization: the role of modern immunology. *Nat. Immunol*. 5: 460–464. 2004.

Landry N, Ward BJ, Trépanier S, Montomoli E *et al.*, Preclin-ical and clinical development of plant-made virus-like particle vaccine against avian H5N1 influenza. *PLoS ONE*. 5(12): e15559. 2011.

Li JT, Fei L, Mou ZR, Wei J *et al.*, Immunogenicity of a plant-derived edible rotavirus subunit vaccine transformed over fifty generations. *Virology*. 356: 171–178. 2006.

Lou M, Yao QH, Zhang Z, Peng RH *et al.*, Expression of the human hepatitis B virus large surface antigen gene in transgenic tomato plants. *Clinl. Vaccine Immunol*. 44: 464-469. 2007.

Lau OS, Ng DWK, Chan WW, Chang SP, Sun SS, Production of the 42-kDa fragment of *Plasmodium falciparum* merozoite surface protein 1, a leading malaria vaccine antigen, in *Arabidopsis thaliana* seeds. *Pl. Biotech. J*. 8(9) 994–1004, 2010

Loza-Rubio E, Rojas E, Gomez L, Olivera MT *et al.*, Development of an edible rabies vaccine in maize using the Vnukovo strain. *Dev. Biol. Basel*. 131: 477-82. 2008.

Ma C, Wang L, Webster DE, Campbell AE, Coppel RL. Production, characterisation and immunogenicity of a plant-made *Plasmodium* antigen-the 19 kDa C-terminal fragment of *Plasmodium yoelii* merozoite surface protein 1. *Appl. Microbiol. Biotech*. 94 (1): 151–161. 2011

Morens D.M, Folkers GK, Fauci AS. The challenge of emerging and re-emerging infectious diseases. *Nature*. 430: 242–249. 2004.

Mason HS, Lam DM, Arntzen, CJ. Expression of hepatitis B surface antigen in transgenic plants. *Proc. Natl. Acad. Sci. USA*. 89: 11745–11749. 1992.

Mihaliak CA, Webb S, Miller T, Fanton M *et al.*, Development of plant cell produced vaccines for animal health applications. *Proc. 108th Annl. Meeting US Anim. Health Assoc. Greensboro, NC*, 158-163. 2005.

Marina C, Mariana C G. Overview of plant-made vaccine antigens against malaria. *J. Biomed. Biotech*. 43: 34-43. 2012. doi: 10.1155/2012/206918

Moravec T, Schmidth MA, Herman EM, Woodfound-Thomas T. Production of *Escherichia coli* heat labile toxin (LT) B subunit in soybean seed and analysis of its immunogenicity as an oral vaccine. *Vaccine*. 25: 1647–1657. 2007.

Marillonnet S, Giritch A, Gils M, Kandzia R *et al.*, In planta engineering of viral RNA replicons: Efficient assembly by recombination of DNA modules delivered by *Agrobacterium*. *Proc. Natl. Acad. Sci. USA*. 101: 6852–6857. 2004.

Marillonnet S, Thoeringer C, Kandzia R, Klimyuk V, Gleba Y. Systemic *Agrobacterium tumefaciens*-mediated transfection of viral replicons for efficient transient expression in plants. *Nat. Biotech*. 23: 718–723. 2005.

Madhi SA, Nigel MD, Cunliffe NA, Steel D, *et al.*, Effect of human rotavirus vaccine on severe diarrhea in African infants. *New Eng. J. Med*. 362(4): 289–298. 2010.

Mascola JR, Montefiori DC. The role of antibodies in HIV vaccines. *Ann. Rev. Immunol*. 28: 413–444. 2010.

Mett V, Musiychuk K, Bi H, Farrance CE *et al.*, A plant-produced influenza subunit vaccine protects ferrets against virus challenge. *Influenza Other Respiratory Viruses*. 2: 33-40. 2008.

Musiychuk K, Stephenson N, Bi H, Farrance C *et al.*, A launch vector for the production of vaccine antigens in plants. *Influenza Other Respiratory Viruses*. 1: 19-25. 2007.

Matthews JT. Egg-based production of influenza vaccine: 30 years of commercial experience. *The Bridge, Natl. Acad. Engg*. 36(3): 17–24. 2006.

McCormick A, Reddy AS, Reinl SJ, Cameron TI *et al.*, Plant-produced idiotype vaccines for the treatment of non-Hodgkin's lymphoma: Safety and immunogenicity in a phase I clinical study. *Proc. Natl. Acad. Sci. USA* 105 (29): 10131–10136. 2008.

Muller M, Gissmann L. A long way: history of the prophylactic papillomavirus vaccine. *Dis. Markers*. 23: 331–336. 2007.

Morrison TG. Structure and function of a paramyxovirus fusion protein. *Biochem. Biophys. Acta*. 1614: 73–84. 2003.

Nakagomi T, Nakagomi O, Takahashi Y, Enoki M *et al.*, Incidence and burden of rotavirus gastroenteritis in Japan, as estimated from a prospective sentinel hospital study. *J. Infect. Dis*. 192 (Suppl. 1): S106–S110. 2005.

Nadin-Davis SA, Loza-Rubio E. The molecular epidemiology of rabies associated with chiropteran hosts in Mexico. *Virus Res*. 117(2): 215–226. 2006.

Naqvi S, Ranessar K, Farre G, Sabalza M *et al.*, High-value products from transgenic maize. *Biotech. Adv*. 29: 40–53. 2011.

Nochi T, Takagi H, Yuki Y, Yang L *et al.*, Rice-based mucosal vaccine as a global strategy for cold-chain and needle-free vaccination. *Proc. Natl. Acad. Sci. USA*. 104: 10986–1099. 2007.

Neutra MR, Kozlowski PA. Mucosal vaccines: the promise and the challenge. *Nat. Rev. Immunol*. 6: 148–158. 2006.

Nel LH, Niezgoda M, Hanlon CA, Morril PA *et al.*, A comparison of DNA vaccines for the rabies-related virus, Mokola. *Vaccine*. 21: 2598–2606. 2003.

Oey M, Lohse M, Kreikemeyer B, Bock R. Exhaustion of the chloroplast protein synthesis capacity by massive expression of a highly stable protein antibiotic. *Plant J*. 57: 436–445. 2009.

Oakes JL, Bost, K.L, Piller, KJ. Stability of a soybean seed-derived vaccine antigen following long-term storage, processing and transport in the absence of a cold chain. *J. Sci. Food Agric*. 89: 2191–2199. 2009.

Ozeki Y, Hirayama Y, Takii T, Yamamoto S *et al.*, Loss of anti-mycobacterial efficacy in mice over time following vaccination with *Mycobacterium bovis* bacillus Calmette-Gue´rin. *Vaccine*. 29: 6881–6887. 2011.

Parashar UD, Hummelman EG, Bresee JS, Miller MA, Glass RI. Global illness and deaths caused by rotavirus disease in children. *Emerg. Infect. Dis*. 9(5): 565–572. 2003.

Parkin DM, Bray F. The burden of HPV related cancers. *Vaccine*. 24S3: S11–S25. 2006.

Patel NC, Hertel PM, Estes MK *et al.*, Vaccine-acquired rotavirus in infants with severe combined immunodeficiency. *New Eng. J. Med*. 362(4): 314–319. 2010.

Peeters K, De Wilde C, Depicker A. Highly efficient targeting and accumulation of a F_{ab} fragment within the secretory pathway and apoplast of *Arabidopsis thaliana*. *Euro. J. Biochem*. 268: 4251–4260. 2001. doi: 10.1046/j.1432-1327.2001.02340.x

Pensaert MB, de Bouck P. A new coronavirus-like particle associated with diarrhea in swine. *Arch Virol*. 58: 243–247. 1978.

Paul M, Ma JKC. Plant-made immunogens and effective delivery strategies. *Expert Rev. Vaccines*. 9 (8): 821–833. 2010.

Polkinghorne I, Hamerli D, Cowan P, Duckworth J. Plant-based imtel-munocontraceptive control of wildlife-potentials, limitations, and possums. *Vaccine*. 23: 1847–1850. 2005.

Pasquevich KA, Iba˜nez AE, Coria LM *et al.*, An oral vaccine based on U-Omp19 induces protection against *B. abortus* mucosal challenge by inducing an adaptive IL-17 immune response in mice. *PLoS ONE*. 6: e16203. 2011.

Perea AI, Loza RE, Rojas AE, Olivera FT *et al.*, Expression of the rabies virus nucleoprotein in plants at high-levels and evaluation of immune responses in mice. *Plant Cell Rep*. 27: 677–685. 2008.

Pineo CB, Hitzeroth II, Rybicki EP. Immunogenic assessment of plant-produced human papillomavirus type 16 L1/L2 chimaeras. *Pl. Biotech. J*. 11(8): 964-75. 2013.

Pniewski T, J. Kapusta, P. Bociag *et al.*, Low-dose oral immunization with lyophilized tissue of herbicide-resistant lettuce expressing hepatitis B surface antigen for prototype plant-derived vaccine tablet formulation. *J. Appl. Genet*. 52: 125–136, 2011.

Pogrebnyak, N, Golovkin M, Andrianov V, Soitsin S *et al.*, Severe acute respiratory syndrome (SARS) S protein production in plants: development of recombinant vaccine. *Proc. Natl. Acad. Sci. USA*. 102, 9062–9067. 2005.

Qian, B, Shen H, Liang W, Guo X *et al.*, Immunogenicity of recombinant hepatitis B virus surface antigen fused with preS1 epitopes expressed in rice seeds. *Transgenic Res.* 17, 621–631. 2008.

Rupprecht CE, Hanlon CA, Hemachudha T. Rabies reexamined. *Lancet Infect. Dis.* 2: 327–343. 2002.

Rosales-Mendoza S, Soria-Guerra RE, Olivera-Flores MT, López-Revilla R *et al.* Expression of Escherichia coli heat-labile enterotoxin b subunit (LTB) in carrot (*Daucus carota* L.). *Plant Cell Rep.* 26: 969–976. 2007a

Rosales-Mendoza S, Ne´stor Rubio I, Dania O, Govea A *et al.*, Current status and perspectives of plant-based candidate vaccines against the human immunodeficiency virus (HIV). *Plant Cell Rep.* 31: 495–511. 2012.

Rerks-Ngarm S, Pitisuttithum P, Nitayaphan S, Kaewkungwal J *et al.*, Vaccination with ALVAC and AIDSVAX to prevent HIV-1 infection in Thailand. *New Eng J. Med.* 361: 2209–222. 2009.

Ruiz-Palacios GM, Perez-Schael I, Velazquez FR, Abate H *et al.*, Human rotavirus vaccine study group. Safety and efficacy of an attenuated vaccine against severe rotavirus gastroenteritis. *New Eng. J. Med.* 354(1): 11–22. 2006.

Ruhlman T, Verma D, Samson N, Daniell H. The role of heterologous chloroplast sequence elements in transgene integration and expression. *Plant Physiol.* 152 2088–2104. 2010.

Ruhlman T, Ahangari R, Devine A, Samsam M, Daniell H. Expression of cholera toxin B-proinsulin fusion protein in lettuce and tobacco chloroplasts - oral administration protects against development of insulitis in non-obese diabetic mice. *Pl. Biotech. J.* 5: 495–510. 2007.

Rybicki EP. Plant-made vaccines for humans and animals. *Pl. Biotech. J.* 8: 620–637 2010.

Streatfield SJ, Howard JA. Plant based vaccines. *Intl. J. Parasitol.* 33: 479–493. 2003

Sparrow PAC, Irwin J.A, Dale PJ, Twyman RM, Ma JKC. Pharma-Planta: Road testing the developing regulatiory guidelines for plant-made pharmaceuticals *Transgenic Res.* 16: 147–161. 2007.

Soria-Guerra RE, Moreno-Fierros L, Rosales-Mendoza S. Two decades of plant-based candidate vaccines: a review of the chimeric protein approaches. *Plant Cell Rep.* 30: 1367–1382. 2011.

Suzue K, Young RA. Adjuvant-free hsp70 fusion protein system elicits humoral and cellular immune responses to HIV- 1 p24. *J. Immunol.* 156: 873–879. 1996.

Scholthof HB, Scholthof KB, Jackson AO. Plant virus gene vectors for transient expression of foreign proteins in plants. *Ann. Rev. Phytopathol.* 34: 299-323. 1996

Sainsbury F, Lomonossoff GP. Extremely high-level and rapid transient protein production in plants without the use of viral replication. *Plant Physiol.* 148: 1212–1218. 2008.

Shao HB, Qian KX, Shen GF, Su ZL *et al.*, The expression of classical swine fever virus structural protein E2 gene in tobacco chloroplasts for applying chloroplasts as bioreactors. *C. R. Biol.* 331: 179–184. 2008.

Shoji Y, Chichester JA, Jones M, Manceva SD *et al.*, Plant-based rapid production of recombinant subunit hemagglutinin vaccines targeting H1N1and H5N1 influenza in human. *Vaccine.* 7(Suppl.): 41–50. 2011.

Sainsbury F, Lavoie P-O, D'Aoust MA, Vezina, LP, Lomonossoff GP. Expression of multiple proteins using full-length and deleted versions of cowpea mosaic virus RNA-2. *Pl. Biotech. J.* 6: 82–92. 2008.

Sharma AK, Sharma MK. Plants as bioreactors: Recent developments and emerging opportunities. *Biotech. Adv.* 27: 811–832. 2009.

Sagara FA, Marcotte H, Frenken LGJ, Iturriza-Gómara M *et al.*, Rice-based oral antibody fragment prophylaxis and therapy against rotavirus infection. *J. Clinl. Invest.* 123: 3829-3838. 2013. doi: 10.1172/JCI70266

Seal BS, King DJ, Sellers HL. The avian response to newcastle disease virus. *Dev. Comp. Immunol.* 24: 257–268. 2000.

Stratford R, Douce, G, Bowe F, Dougan, GA. Vaccination strategy incorporating DNA priming and mucosal boosting using tetanus toxin fragment C (TetC). *Vaccine.* 20: 516–525. 2001.

Smith JS, Lindsay L, Hoots B, Keys J *et al.*, Human papillomavirus type distribution in invasive cervical cancer and high-grade cervical lesions: a meta-analysis update. *Intl. J. Cancer.* 121: 621–632. 2007.

Thomas DR, Penney CA, Majumder A, Walmsley AM. Evolution of plant-made pharmaceuticals. *Intl. J. Mol. Sci.* 12: 3220-3236. 2011.

Thanavala Y, Yang YF, Lyons P. Immunogenicity of transgenic plant-derived hepatitis B surface antigen. *Proc. Natl. Acad. Sci. USA.* 92: 3358–3361. 1995.

Tomas M, Monica AS, Eliot MH, Terry WT. Production of *Escherichia coli* heat labile toxin (LT) B subunit in soybean seed and analysis of its immunogenicity as an oral vaccine. *Vaccine.* 25: 1647–1657. 2007.

Tokuhara D, Yuki Y, Nochi T, Kodama T *et al.*, Secretory IgA-mediated protection against *V. cholerae* and heat-labile enterotoxin producing enterotoxigenic *Escherichia coli* by rice-based vaccine. *Proc. Natl. Acad. Sci. USA.* 107: 8794–8799. 2010.

Tregoning JS, Nixon P, Kuroda H, Svab Z *et al.*, Expression of tetanus toxin Fragment C in tobacco chloroplasts. *Nucleic Acids Res.* 31: 1174–1179. 2003.

Tyagi AK, Nangpal P, Satchidanandam V. Development of vaccines against tuberculosis. *Tuberculosis.* 91: 469–478. 2011.

Tokuhara D, Álvarez B, Mejima M, Hiroiwa T *et al.*, Human papillomavirus type 11 recombinant L1 capsomeres induce virus neutralizing antibodies. *J. Virol.* 72: 6151–6154. 1998.

Tuboly T, Yub W, Bailey A, Degrandisc S *et al.*, Immunogenicity of porcine transmissible gastroenteritis virus spike protein expressed in plants. *Vaccine.* 18: 2023–2028. 2000.

Uygungil B, Bleesing JJ, Risma KA, McNeal MM, Rothenberg ME. Persistent rotavirus vaccine shedding in a new case of severe combined immunodeficiency: A reason to screen. *J. Allergy Clinl. Immunol.* 125(1): 270–271. 2010.

Verma D, Daniell H. Chloroplast vector systems for biotechnology applications. *Pl. Physiol.* 145: 1129–1143. 2007.

Van Loon FP, Clemens JD, Chakraborty J, Rao MR *et al.*, Field trial of inactivated oral cholera vaccines in Bangladesh: results from 5 years of follow-up. *Vaccine.* 14: 162–166. 1996.

Varmus H, Klausner R, Zerhouni E, Acharya T *et al.*, Grand challenges in global health. *Science.* 302: 398–399. 2003.

Vesikari T, Matson DO, Dennehy P, Vam Damme P *et al.*, Rotavirus efficacy and safety trial (REST) study team. Safety and efficacy of a pentavalent human-bovine (WC3) reassortant rotavirus vaccine. *New Eng. J. Med.* 354(1): 23–33. 2006.

Wang, SP, Xu DZ, Yan YP, Shi MY *et al.*, Hepatitis B virus infection status in the PBMC of newborns of HBsAg positive mothers. *World J. Gastroenterol.* 6 (Suppl. 3): 58. 2000.

Villa LL, Costa RLR, Petta CA, Andrade RP *et al.*, High sustained efficacy of a prophylactic quadrivalent human papillomavirus types 6/11/16/18 L1 virus-like particle vaccine through 5 years of follow-up. *Brit. J. Cancer.* 95: 1459–1466. 2006.

Wyatt R, Sodroski J. The HIV-1 envelope glycoproteins: fusogens, antigens, and immunogens. *Science.* 280: 1884-1888. 1998.

Williams NA, Hirst TR, Nashar TO. Immune modulation by the cholera-like enterotoxins: from adjuvant to therapeutic. *Immunol. Today.* 20: 95–101. 1999.

Werther RL, Crawford NW, Boniface K, Kirkwood CD, Smart JM. Rotavirus vaccine induced diarrheain a child with severe combined immune deficiency. *J. Allergy Clinl. Immunol.* 124(3): 600. 2009.

Walmsley AM, Arntzen CJ. Plant cell factories and mucosal vaccines. *Curr. Opin. Biotech.* 14: 145–150. 2003.

Wang DM, Zhu JB, Peng M, Zhou P. Induction of a protective antibody response to FMDV in mice following oral immunization with transgenic *Stylosanthes* spp. as a feedstuff additive. *Transgenic Res.* 17: 1163–1170. 2008a.

Wang L, Webster DE, Campbell AE, Dry IB *et al.*, Immunogenicity of *Plasmodium yoelii* merozoite surface protein 4/5 produced in transgenic plants. *Intl. J. Parasitol.* 38: 103-110, 2008

Wang Y, Deng H, Zhang X, Xiao H *et al.*, Generation and immunogenicity of Japanese encephalitis virus envelope protein expressed in transgenic rice. *Biochem. Biophys. Res. Comm.* 380: 292–297. 2009.

Waheed MT, Thones N, Muller MS, Hassan W *et al.*, Transplastomic expression of a modified human papillomavirus L1 protein leading to the assembly of capsomeres in tobacco: a step towards cost-effective second-generation vaccines. *Transgenic Res.* 20: 271–282. 2011.

Webster DE, Wang L, Mulcair M *et al.*, Production and characterization of an orally immunogenic *Plasmodium* antigen in plants using a virus-based expression system. *Pl. Biotech. J.* 7: 846–855, 2009

Wigdorovitz A, Carrillo C, Dus Santos MJ, Trono K *et al.*, Induction of a protective antibody response to foot and mouth disease virus in mice following oral or parenteral immunization with alfalfa transgenic plants expressing the viral structural protein VP1. *Virology.* 255: 347–53. 1999.

Wirz H, Sauer-Budge AF, Briggs J, Sharpe A *et al.*, Automated production of plant-based vaccines and pharmaceuticals. *J. Lab. Automation.* 17: 449-457. 2012. DOI: 10.1177/22110 68212460037

Xing Z, Lichty BD. Use of recombinant virus-vectored tuberculosis vaccines for respiratory mucosal immunization. *Tuberculosis.* 86: 211–217. 2006.

Yuki Y, Kiyono H. New generation of mucosal adjuvants for the induction of protective immunity. *Rev. Med. Virol.* 13: 293–310. 2003.

Yusibov V, Rabindran S. Recent progress in the development of plant derived vaccines. *Expert Rev. Vaccines.* 7: 1173-83. 2008.

Zhang RG, Westbrook ML, Westbrook EM, Scott DL *et al.*, The 2.4 A crystal structure of cholera toxin B subunit pentamer: choleragenoid. *J. Mol. Biol.* 251: 550–562. 1995.

Zolla-Pazner S, Cohen SS, Krachmarov C, Wang S *et al.*, Focussing the immune response on the V3 loop, a neutralizing epitope of the HIV-1 gp120 envelope. *Virology.* 372: 233–246. 2008.

Zaman K, *et al.*, Efficacy of pentavalent rotavirus vaccine against severe rotavirus gastroenteritis in infants in developing countries in Asia: a randomised, double-blind, placebo-controlled trial. *Lancet.* 376: : 615–623. 2010.

Zhu JG, Wei YH, Guo ZG. The transformation and expression of HBsAg gene in *Arachis hypogaea. China Bull. Bot.* 23L: 665–669. 2006.

Zhang X, Buehner NA, Hutson AM, Estes MK *et al.*, Tomato is a highly effective vehicle for expression and oral immunization with Norwalk virus capsid protein. *Pl. Biotech. J.* 4: 419–432. 2006.

Websites

http: //www.who.int/mediacentre/factsheets/fs094/en/

http: //www.cdc.gov/malaria/about/history/

http: //www.malariavaccine.org/malvac-lifecycle.php

http: / /www.niaid.nih.gov / topics / malaria / pages / lifecycle.aspx

http: / /www.who.int/ mediacentre / factsheets / fs211 / en / index.html

http: / /www.dowagro.com / animalhealth/ resources / firstlic.htm

http: / /www.who.int/ tb / publications / global_report / en/ WHO (2011) Global Tuberculosis Control

http: / /www.biolex.com

http: / /www.protalix.com

http: / /www.plant biotechnology.com

2016, Biotechnological Tools for Genetic Resources Pages 175–200
Editor: Pradip Chandra Deka
Published by: Daya Publishing House, NEW DELHI

Chapter 6

Functional Foods and Realities of Personalized Nutrition

Bojlul Bahar[1]* and Albin M. Ahmed[2]

[1]Institute of Food and Health, School of Agriculture and Food Science, University College Dublin, Belfield, Dublin 4, Ireland
[2]School of Veterinary Medicine, University College Dublin, Belfield, Dublin 4, Ireland
**E-mail: bojlul.bahar@gmail.com*

ABSTRACT

Diseases within the metabolic syndrome spectrum are growing at an alarming rate throughout the world. Genetic make-up and diet and lifestyle habits are perceived to be among the major underlying factors which predispose the risk of metabolic diseases. Careful selection food ingredients rich in bioactive compounds which can impart additional health benefits can be a safe, effective and sustainable way of preventing metabolic diseases. Because of the fact that every individual is unique in terms of the genetic make-up, biomarkers need to be identified and techniques need to be developed to diagnose and predict the risk of developing metabolic diseases. An approach of nutritional recommendation based on nutritional need as determined by the genetic make-up of an individual or a genetic sub-group could be an effective way of harnessing the health benefit of bioactive food ingredients.

Keywords: *Metabolic syndrome, Metabolic disease, Biomarkers, Nutritional need, Bioactive food ingredients.*

Introduction

In recent years, there has been a rapid increase in incidences of diseases within the metabolic spectrum that include obesity, insulin resistance, dyslipidaemia and hypertension. Metabolic diseases are associated with an increased risk of mortality and morbidity such as those caused by type-2-diabetes (T2D) and cardiovascular disease (CVD) (Moller and Kaufman, 2005). It is necessary that today's global consumers are aware of the dire consequence of metabolic diseases and hence the need for healthy eating and adopting a healthy lifestyle (Hasler 2002, Brown *et al.*, 2011, Kim *et al.*, 2012). Extensive spread of internet and popularity of social media have been playing a role in creating mass awareness on healthy foods and the need of preventing common metabolic diseases. Metabolic diseases such as obesity, T2D and cardiovascular diseases are increasing at an alarming rate and are not too far from reaching a global epidemic level affecting millions of people of the developed and developing nations (Flier, 2004; Misra and Khurana, 2008). Therapeutic treatment of many of the metabolic diseases with the available drugs can be effective. However these treatments are highly expensive often ineffective in completely cure of the disease, and associated with adverse side effects (Grundy, 2006, Israili *et al.*, 2007) This failure is partly due to the fact that the diagnoses of most metabolic diseases are performed only at an advance stage of disease development (Khan and Awan 2012). Therefore, diagnostic procedures enable detection of major metabolic diseases at an earliest possible stage of disease development and subsequent adaption of therapeutic, diet and lifestyle measures are important to minimize the mortality associated with metabolic diseases (Yang and Pratt, 2008).

Table 6.1: Food as a Source of Bioactive Compounds and their Associated Health Benefits

Food Ingredients	*Bioactive(s)*	*Health Benefit*
Cereal grains (barley, oat, wheat)	β-glucan, fibre	Strong immune system, lowering blood glucose, reduce colon cancer
Tomatoes, Guava, Papaya, Watermelon	Lycopene	Anti-cancer
Broccoli	Lutein, vitamin C, diindolylmethane, glucoraphanin, indol-3-carbinol, selenium, dietary fibre	Boost immune system, anti-cancer
Avocado	Monounsaturated fatty acids, potassium, folic acid	Lowering of blood cholesterol and triglycerides
Citrus	Vitamin C, flavanones	Anti-oxidant, anti-cancer and strong immune system
Fish	Omega-3 fatty acids	Reduced risk of cardiovascular disease
Milk	Bioactive proteins and peptides	Anti-microbial and immune modulation

Functional foods include those foods and food ingredients which provide additional health benefits beyond supply of regular nutrients (carbohydrate, protein, fat, vitamins, minerals and water). These additional health benefits are generally exhibited due to the presence biologically active chemical compounds (bioactives) naturally present in the food ingredients. Functional foods have been a part of human diet probably since the begining of the human civilization. However, their roles in health and prevention of diseases have only recently acknowledged (Siró *et al.*, 2008). In the last few decades, a numbers of bioactives from plant and animal sources have been characterized and their specific health benefits established (Table 6.1). Functional food can be classified into two main categories: 1) naturally occurring foodstuffs containing the bioactive ingredients, and 2) processed foodstuffs but fortified with ingredients to provide additional health benefits. Few examples of fortified functional foods which are enriched artificially with one or more bioactive compounds are presented in Table 6.2.

Table 6.2: Foods Fortified with Bioactive Ingredients and their Associated Health Benefits

Functional Food	*Functional Ingredient*	*Potential Benefit*
Orange juice with added vitamin D	Vitamin D	Reduced risk of bone diseases
Yogurt with probiotics	Probiotics	Improved health of gastrointestinal tract
Breads and cereals with added fiber	Fiber	Alleviates constipation and reduced risk of certain cancers
Margarine fortified with plant sterols	Plant sterols and phytosterols	Reduces blood cholesterol

The latest scientific research on functional foods and neutraceuticals have provided convincing evidences that functional foods can contribute to the health and wellbeing of the consumer and help in prevention of diseases relating to diet (Hasler 2002; Fenech *et al.*, 2011). The present functional foods and neutraceuticals market globally is worth $167 billion with an annual growth of about 14 per cent. The leading countries producing and consuming functional foods and neutraceuticals include Japan, USA, Canada and EU. This review will attempt to highlight different functional foods and bioactive ingredients present in common foodstuffs and their role in prevention of metabolic diseases in human followed by a brief overview and realities of a personalized nutrition approach.

Growing Incidences of Metabolic Diseases in India

Globally, there has been a decreasing trend of infectious diseases while a rapid and conspicuous increase in the incidences metabolic diseases (Borch-Johnsen 2007). A rapid industrialization and economic boom in developing countries including India led to a major shift in the food and lifestyle habits, especially in the larger cities (Misra and Khurana 2008). A westernized dietary habit characterized by consumption of calorie intense diets coupled with a sedentary lifestyle contributed to the booming of the metabolic diseases including T2D, obesity and CVD (Drewnowski and Popkin 1997, Sawant *et al.*, 2011). Among the major metabolic diseases in India, CVD is the major killer with about 2 million casualties per year and it is projected that by 2020 this figure will be doubled (Gupta *et al.*, 2011). India has a T2D population of 63 millions where 1 million peoples die of T2D, annually. Considering the rapid surge of metabolic diseases in India and the fact that access to affordable health care to a staggering mass of 1.2 billion Indian remains a big challenge, it may be cautioned that India is yet to face the worst ever causalities due to metabolic diseases (Shetty 2012). Because of the fact that Asian Indian are genetically ill adapted to handle high calorie diet and are genetically more susceptible to develop metabolic diseases than other human races, there is an urgent need of developing highly effective, safe and sustainable measures to check the growing incidences of major metabolic diseases (Marinangeli and Jones 2010).

India has a unique historical reputation to be a home of highly diverse food ingredients with varieties of cereals, fruits, vegetables, herbs and spices. Many of these food ingredients remain a part of rural Indian society and are used as a part of traditional food habits in India (Lobo 2010). The health benefits associated with the consumption of many of these foods were well recognized and the knowledge of their uses has been passed on from generation to generation as a part of cultural tradition and religious taboos. However, extensive scientific basis on most of the traditional functional foods is lacking and information relating to their potential use in preventing metabolic diseases was limited to the general masses. Based on the chemical nature of the bioactive ingredients present in the food, few major classes of functional foods are discussed in the following section.

Bioactive Carbohydrates

Role of bioactive carbohydrates in maintaining good health and their mode of action are described in the following sections.

Dietary Fibre

Dietary fibre was originally described to include cellulose, hemi-cellulose and lignin derived from plant those can resist the action of digestive enzyme inside the stomach (Trowell *et al.*, 1976). Currently, a universal definition of dietary fibre which is acceptable to the wider scientific communities is lacking (Buttriss and Stock 2008). From a functional food perspective, dietary fibre should generally fulfill the criteria of: i) resistant to digestion by the digestive enzyme and absorption in the small intestine, ii) undergo complete or partial fermentation in the large intestine, and iii) promote beneficial physiological effects such as laxation, reduction in blood cholesterol and modulation of the blood glucose status (Brennan 2005). Dietary fibre can be soluble or insoluble in water and may often include artificially added fibre which was previously isolated and purified from a variety of sources. Dietary fibre generally includes a wide range of non-digestible carbohydrates (Table 6.3) and can be broadly classified as follows (Buttriss and Stock 2008):

1. Non-starch polysaccharides (NSP): cellulose, hemi-cellulose, pectins, hydrocolloids (gums, mucilage)
2. Resistant oligosaccharides: fructo-oligosaccharides, galacto-oligosaccharides
3. Resistant starch: modified starch
4. Lignin

Mechanism of Action

Although dietary fibre remains an integral part of human diet during the process of human evolution, the health benefit associated with the consumption of dietary fibre and the underlying mechanisms are only recently understood. Solubility in water is one of the important physical characteristics of dietary fibre which determine its potential as functional food. Soluble dietary fibre generally swells and forms gel when come in contact with water. Formation of gel inside the stomach alters the viscosity of the food material and this makes the content gummy. An increase in

Table 6.3: Major Sources of Common Dietary Fibre

Fibre Component	*Description*	*Dietary Source*
Cellulose	Linear polymer of D-glucose linked with $\beta(1 \rightarrow 4)$ glycosidic linkage. Abundantly found in the cell wall of green plants and algae. Cellulose constitutes about 33 per cent of plant biomass.	Cereal grains, fruits, vegetables and nuts
Hemi-cellulose	Complex polymer of monosaccharides such as glucose, xylose, mannose, galactose, rhamnose and arabinose. Hemicellulose constitutes about 20 per cent of the plant biomass.	Cereal grain, legumes, nuts, fruits and vegetables
Pectin	A heteropolysaccharide made up of galacturonic acid and monosaccharides found in the cell wall of plant.	Fruits, vegetables, legumes and nuts

the viscosity and gumminess make the food material less accessible to the digestive enzymes (Brennan 2005). This results in lesser digestion and release of nutrients from the food material which is often beneficial for weight management purposes. The insoluble dietary fibre increases bulkiness of the content and reduces the transit time within the small intestine.

Another important mechanism underlying the health benefit of dietary fibre includes the inhibition of starch digestion and subsequent release of glucose which is highly beneficial for lowering the glucose burden in T2D patients. Soluble dietary fibre can effectively reduce starch digestion through alteration of viscosity and accessibility of the starch granule to amylase enzyme. The undigested starch supports the growth of micro-organism in the large intestine and often undergoes microbial fermentation resulting in production of short chain volatile fatty acids such as acetic acid, butyric acid and propanoic acid (Gibson and Roberfroid, 1995). These fatty acids are readily absorbed and are reported to be associated with a number health benefits (Wong *et al.*, 2006). Dietary fibre often contains bioactive compounds such as beta-glucan (see below) as present in cereal grains such as oat which can directly alter cellular processes and associated with numerous health benefits (Brennan 2005).

Dietary Fibre and Human Health

A number of human epidemiological and clinical studies have established the health benefits associated with an optimal consumption of dietary fibre (Brown *et al.*, 1999; Streppel *et al.*, 2008). There are three major physiological implications of dietary fibre in human health (Buttriss and Stoke 2008) which include: i) prevention of constipation, ii) lowering of blood cholesterol, and iii) increasing satiety. Water insoluble fibre such as cellulose and hemicellulose are highly effective in reducing constipation as they increase bulkiness and have laxative effect. However, excessive intake of cellulose and hemi-cellulose can inhibit the release of digestive enzymes resulting inhibition of the release of vitamin and mineral from food materials and their subsequent bioavailability. A recommended allowance of 25-50 g of total dietary fibre per day is approved in many countries and this level was found to have no adverse affect on human health. Vegetarians, frequently consuming about

40-50 gm of dietary fibre on a daily basis were reported to have no adverse affect on the health. Hence, a daily intake of 25-50 g dietary fibre can be easily achievable through careful selection of food consumed on a daily basis through inclusion of whole cereals, fruits and vegetables in the daily menu.

In order to calculate the total intake of dietary fibre from a variety of foods we consume on a daily basis, it is necessary to know the fibre content of individual food ingredients. Fibre content of various cereal food ingredients are presented in Table 6.4. Currently, analytical methods for accurate quantification of dietary fibre in a wide range of food ingredients are lacking which limits the assertion that the recommended allowance have been reached. In addition, processing and preparation of foods may also result in an unpredictable chemical alteration of dietary fibre. It is quite reasonable that accurate monitoring of the dietary fibre intake on a daily basis is often difficult but consumer should be well aware of the fact that failure to reach the minimal dietary requirements of fibre for long may make them vulnerable to develop metabolic diseases. Few relevant heath promoting effect associated with consumption of dietary fibre is highlighted in the following section.

Table 6.4: Some Major Cereals with their Total Carbohydrate and Fibre Content

Cereals	*Carbohydrate Content (Per cent)*	*Fibre Content (Per cent)*
White rice	70.0	1.3
Brown rice	76.2	3.4
Glutinous rice	81.7	2.8
Oats	66.3	10.6
Wheat flour (white refined)	78.0	1.7
Wheat flour (whole grain)	72.0	10.7
Millet flour	73.0	3.5
Sorghum flour	74.6	6.3
Corn	74.3	7.3

Dietary Fiber and Type-2 Diabetes

Type-2 diabetes constitutes more than 90 per cent of the diabetes mellitus cases diagnosed globally. With a rapid change in dietary habits and lifestyle due to the recent economic boom, there has been a rapid increase in the incidences of T2D in India (Shetty 2012). A number of epidemiological studies have investigated the role of dietary fibre in management of T2D and the results till date are promising (Meyer *et al.*, 2000; Tabatabai and Li 2000). In T2D patients, dietary fibre increases satiety and lower food intake. In addition, a reduction in the activity of digestive enzymes due to the action of dietary fibre can effectively prevent release of large quantity of glucose from the dietary carbohydrate and developing insulin resistance. Glycemic index (GI) of the food ingredient is a measure of the speed at which the available carbohydrate from the food reaches the blood of the consumer. GI is a measure of the available carbohydrate (excluding the dietary fibre) which is available n the form of blood glucose relative to the consumption of pure glucose. Foods with high GI indicated that the glucose is released immediately after consumption and digestion of the food. Foods can be classified as a) high GI- >70 or more (pure Glucose has GI 100), b) medium GI- 55 to 70 and c) low GI- <55 (Brennan 2005). Since dietary fibre contains little or no digestible carbohydrates, hence they have a considerably low GI.

For the purpose of knowing the exposure of human body to dietary glucose, a biochemical marker of T2D, the GI of the foods consumed alone is not sufficient. This is because a person may consume very small quantity of carbohydrate with a high GI, which may not adversely elevate the level of blood glucose. For example, watermelon has a GI of 72 but the carbohydrate content is just 5 per cent while highly polished rice grain (white rice) has a GI of 73 and the carbohydrate content is about 80 per cent. Therefore, an individual consuming 100 gm of watermelon is expected to have lower blood glucose compared to consuming equivalent quantity of rice. In order to determine the extent of carbohydrate consumption and its adverse consequence in elevation of the blood glucose level, the concept of glycemic load (GL) was introduced (Salmeron *et al.*, 1997). GL is the measurement of the total load of the carbohydrate, which the body receives following consumption of a food in terms of the production of glucose. GL can be defined as GI of the food ingredient multiplied by its carbohydrate content. One unit of GL corresponds to the effect of consuming one gram of glucose. Therefore, from the measurement of GL, it is quite apparent that consumption of 100 gm portion of a watermelon is associated with a glycemic load of 3.6 while equivalent weight of polish rice is associated with a GL of 58.4. GL are classified as a) high >20, b) medium 11-19 and c) low <10. Glycemic index of some common foodstuffs are presented in Table 6.5. Dietary fibre, particularly those from cereals are associated with a low GL are highly effective in reducing the incidences of T2D (Schulze *et al.*, 2004).

Table 6.5: Glycemic Index of some Major Food Ingredients

Food	*Glycemic Index*
White rice (boiled)	73
Brown rice (boiled)	68
Barley	28
Wheat bread (white)	75
Wheat bread (whole)	74
Wheat roti	62
Sweet corn	52
Chickpeas	28
Lentil	32
Soybean	15
Potato (boiled)	78

Dietary Fiber and Obesity

Obesity is characterized by deposition of excessive body fat in human and is considered to be a global threat to human health. Development of obesity is a complex phenomenon, where a number of factors including genetic, nutritional and environmental factors are involved. In general, excessive deposition of body fat occurs when the level of food energy assimilated exceeds the overall energy consumption of the body. A sedentary lifestyle characterized by a lack of physical activities and frequent consumption of energy dense foods are thought to be among the major causes of deposition of excessive body fat common in the populations of most westernized cities (Ebbeling *et al.*, 2002). An interesting Mexican study demonstrated that while one hour intense physical activity daily reduces the chance of getting overweight by 10 per cent, chances of getting overweight increases by 12 per cent per hours of watching television (Hernández *et al.*, 1999).

Diets containing good balance of fibre provide low calorie to the body and increase satiety, which is beneficial for maintaining optimum body weight and health. Dietary fibers are generally bulky in nature and hence, reduce the amount of energy present in per gm of the food material consumed. Another vital role dietary fibre can play in weight reduction is through formation of gels and increases the viscosity of the food material inside the intestine which makes energy rich nutrients such as carbohydrates and lipids less accessible to digestive enzymes (Slavin and Green 2007). More refine food ingredients generally lack fibrous materials otherwise naturally present and hence consumption of such foods provides only the nutrients present which generally results in a lower satiety effect. Regular consumption of dietary fibre also supports a healthy gut micro-flora, which also contributes to a healthy body weight.

Role of β-glucan

Beta-glucan is a complex polysaccharide made of D-glucose molecules linked with beta 1→3, 1→4 glycosidic linkages. Beta-glucan can be soluble when the glucose molecules are linked with β (1→ 3) and β(1→ 4) glycosidic linkages or insoluble when the linkages are β (1→ 4) and β(1→ 4). Cereal grains are a rich source of β-glucan particularly barley (5-11 per cent), oats (3-7 per cent) and wheat (1 per cent) (Skendi *et al.*, 2003). In the cereal grains, β-glucan is predominantly present as the cell wall component, which is generally removed during milling and polishing of grains using mechanical means. Soluble β-glucan is found in the cereal grains including oat, barley while the insoluble β-glucan is mostly present in yeast and mushrooms.

Beta glucans are highly potent bioactives and can act as soluble dietary fibre. The β-glucan mediated beneficial health effect mostly occurs at the upper gastro-intestinal tract. Like most other dietary fibre, β-glucan can increase the viscosity of food material inside the stomach that results in lesser accessibility of food ingredients to digestive enzymes, promoting gelatinization of dietary starch and keeping intact the physical integrity of the food material. Dietary β-glucan also contributes to a reduction in the GL associated with consumption of food rich in carbohydrate with high GI and thereby β-glucan help in keeping the blood glucose level checked and managing metabolic diseases. Another mechanism of β-glucan mediated health promoting bioactivity is through promotion of the growth of healthy gut-microbiota. Due to the presence of β-glucan in the diet, a substantial proportion of polysaccharides including starch in the small intestine resist enzymatic degradation resulting in reaching of higher quantity of fermentable carbohydrate in the large intestine. These carbohydrates in the large intestine support the growth of healthy microbiota which utilize and ferment these complex carbohydrates and produce numerous by product such as the short chain volatile fatty acids. Many of these short chain fatty acids have health promoting activities. In addition, β-glucans were found to lowering of the bowel transit time and prevention of constipation, reduction in blood cholesterol (Brennan and Clearly, 2005).

In animal husbandry, β-glucans are found to have anti-microbial and immune stimulatory properties. However, excessive intake of β-glucan in the animal feedstuffs may have detrimental health consequence relating to productivity, as β-glucan can reduce feed digestibility and metabolizable energy as well as sticky consistency of the droppings (Bergh *et al.*, 1999). To eliminate this problem in animal husbandry, β-glucan hydrolyzing enzymes were included in the animal feed.

Bioactive Proteins, Peptides and Amino Acids

Bioactive proteins of the human diet and their component constituents such as polypeptides and the amino acids play important role in the in growth and development. These aspects are discussed in the following section.

Bioactive Proteins

Proteins are a vital component of human diet as they supply amino acids required for building of tissues. Dietary proteins play a variety of role affecting nutritional, functional and biological activities within the host (Korhonen and Pihlanto 2003). Bioactive proteins present in dietary ingredients can alter physiological processes of the host (Lönnerdal 2013). However, some foods may contain harmful bioactive proteins which may cause adverse heath consequence such as toxicity and allergy. These groups of proteins are not included in the bioactive proteins to be used as functional food.

There are a number of vital physiological processes which may be altered by the bioactive proteins present in the diet. These may include: improvement in the nutrient uptake by binding and transportation of specific nutrients such as vitamins and minerals, promotion or inhibition of enzymatic activity, enzymatic activities involving digestion and absorption of nutrients from food, stimulation of growth, modulation of immune system and defense against harmful micro-organisms (Lönnerdal 2013). Moreover, dietary proteins serve as an important precursor of bioactive peptides and amino acids those are released following a partial or complete digestion of the dietary protein within the host.

Among the naturally abundant sources of bioactive proteins in human diet include milk, eggs, soybean and edible seaweeds (Lönnerdal, 2013). Few examples of commonly occurring bioactive proteins present in the food ingredients are listed in Table 6.6. Mammalian milk is a classical example of a rich source of dietary bioactive proteins (lactoferrin, lysozyme, immunoglobulins, haptocorrin and α-lactalbumin), precursor of bioactive peptides (Lönnerdal 2013). Recently, marine plant and animals are recognized as rich sources of novel bioactive proteins, peptides and amino acids which can be explored as functional foods for human and animal consumption (Harnedy and FitzGerald 2011). Two major bioactive proteins found in seaweeds include macro-algal lectins and phycobiliproteins. These bioactive proteins were reported to have numerous health benefits in humans and animals (Giri and Ohshima 2012). The physiological processes altered by the dietary bioactive proteins in the host and their specific mode of action leading to the promotion of health in the consumer are elaborately discussed in a number of recent reviews (Walther and Sieber 2011, Ricci-Cabello *et al.*, 2012, Lönnerdal 2013).

Table 6.6: Bioactive Proteins Present in Food and their Health Promoting Effect in Human

Foods	*Bioactive Protein*	*Bioactivity*	*Reference*
Milk	Casein	Precursor of bioactive peptides	Silva and Malcata 2005, Boutrou *et al.*, 2013
	Whey protein	Anti-cancer, immunomodulatory	Xiao *et al.*, 2006
	Immunoglobulins	Immune stimulation, cholesterol lowering	Earnest *et al.*, 2005
	Lactoferrin	Anti-microbial, immune stimulation	García-Montoya *et al.*, 2012, Lönnerdal 2013
	Lysozyme	Anti-microbial	Lönnerdal 2013
Egg	Egg white Immunoglobulins	Wound healingImmune stimulation	Adham *et al.*, 2013, Lee *et al.*, 2013
Soybean	Genistein and daidzein	Lowering blood cholesterol	Sacks *et al.*, 2006
Seaweed	Phycobiliproteins	Anti-oxidant	Pumas *et al.*, 2011

Bioactive Peptides and Amino Acids

Peptides are short sequences of amino acids and are often produced as a product of enzymatic breakdown of the intact protein. In many instances, the intact protein and the individual amino acids that make-up the protein may not have any bioactivity, while the short sequences of amino acids of the same protein may have a conspicuous biological activity. Bioactive peptides generally remain in a latent state and are released in its active form following a process of proteolysis (Gobbetti *et al.*, 2004). Following the enzymatic digestion of proteins present in milk in the stomach and microbial fermentation in the large intestine a number of bioactive peptides are released and absorbed in the body. These bioactive peptides have direct health promoting effect in the host (Meisel, 1998) including prevention of metabolic diseases.

Bioactive peptides obtained from milk are widely commercialized and are generally considered safe for human consumption (Mills *et al.*, 2011). Bioactive peptides present in milk and their associated health benefit is presented in Table 6.7. The most common type of bioactive peptides generated from milk are the antihypertensive peptides which can inhibit ACE, a key enzyme involve in the regulation of blood pressure in human. A number of ACE inhibitory peptides are characterized in dairy products, which have the potential therapeutic use against high blood pressure and CVD. Bioactive peptides such as carnosine and glutathione are found in marine algae. For bioactive amino acids, some amino acids abundantly found in marine sources including taurine, laminine, kainoids, mycosporine have potential health promoting effect in humans and animals (Harnedy *et al.*, 2011, Suarez-Jimenez *et al.*, 2012). Following characterization, many of these novel amino acids can be utilized for developing safe functional foods effective for prevention or cure of metabolic diseases.

Table 6.7: Bioactive Peptides Present in Milk and Associated Health Benefit

Bioactive Peptides	*Protein-source*	*Bioactivity*
Casomorphins	α-, β-Casein	Opioid agonist
α-Lactorphin	α-Lactalbumin	Opioid agonist
β-Lactorphin	β-Lactoglobulin	Opioid agonist
Lactoferroxins	Lactoferrin	Opioid antagonist
Casoxins	k-Casein	Opioid antagonist
Casokinins	α-, β-Casein	ACE-inhibitory
Immunopeptides	α-, β-Casein	Immunomodulatory
Lactoferricin	Lactoferrin	Antimicrobial
Casoplatelins	k-Casein, transferrin	Antithrombotic
Phosphopeptides	α-, β-Casein	Mineral binding

Bioactive Lipids

Lipids include a large number of chemically heterogeneous compounds which are soluble in organic solvents. Lipids such as fatty acids, phospholipids, carotenoids, phytosterols are present as an integral part of foods we consume on a daily basis (Lands, 2012). A number of lipids are bioactive and have health promoting effect in humans and animals (Nagao and Yanagita, 2008; McClements *et al.*, 2009). Among the major groups of bioactive fatty acids with dietary relevance includes short chain fatty acids and poly-unsaturated fatty acids (PUFA). Short chain fatty acids are generally produced due to microbial fermentation in the large intestine (Topping and Clifton, 2001) while the PUFA are abundantly found in meat, milk, eggs and plant seed oils (Woods and Fearon, 2009). Carotenoids and phytosterols are two other groups of lipid compounds generally obtained from plant sources and have importance in promoting health (Kritchevsky and Chen, 2002; Ntanios and Duchateau, 2002; Trautwein and Dmonty, 2007). Bioactive lipids are essentially involved in the biosynthesis of cellular hormones and other signaling molecules, which can alter biochemical reactions within the cells, and cause alteration of the cell membrane fluidity. Few examples of bioactive lipids present in foods are presented in Table 6.8 and major groups of bioactive lipids are discussed in the following section.

Table 6.8: Common Bioactive Lipids Present in Foods and their Potential Health Benefits

Name	*Types*	*Potential Health Benefit*
Fatty Acids	dinu123 - 3 Fatty Acids, Conjugated Linoleic Acid, Butyric Acid	Coronary Heart Disease, Bone Health, Immune Response Disorders, Weight Gain, Stroke Prevention, Mental Health, Cancer, and Visual Acuity
Carotenoids	β - Carotene, Lycopene, Lutein, and Zeaxanthin	Cancer, Coronary Heart Disease, Macular Degeneration, and Cataracts
Antioxidants	Tocopherols, Flavonoids, Polyphenols	Coronary Heart Disease, Cancer, and Urinary Tract Disease
Phytosterols	Stigmasterol, β -Sitosterol, and Campesterol	Coronary Heart Disease

Bioactive Fatty Acids

Role of bioactive fatty acids in maintain good health and their mode of action are described in the following section.

Short Chain Fatty Acids

Short chain fatty acids are generally produced through a process of microbial fermentation of the undigested polysaccharides and dietary fibre in the large intestine (Topping and Clifton, 2001). The major short chain fatty acids include butyric acid, propionic acid and acetic acid. Based on the dietary composition and developmental stage of the host which can alter the microbial population in the large intestine, the proportion of the short chain fatty acids produced vary (Topping and Clifton, 2001). For example, breast fed infants generally have high fecal levels of acetic acid and low propionic acid and almost absence of butyric acid, while fed formula have relatively low level of acetic acid and high levels of propionic and butyric acids (Edward *et al.*, 1994, Siigur *et al.*, 1993). Few short chain fatty acids such as butyrate are also present as a component of food such as the milk. The bioactivity of many of the short chain fatty acids occurs firstly, through lowering the pH in the colonic micro-environment due to inhibition of the growth of harmful micro-organism by the short chain fatty acids (Cherrington *et al.*, 1991), and thereby reducing the load of microbial toxic metabolite in the colon. Secondly, short chain fatty acids create a gut environment which supports the growth of beneficial microbes such as lactobacillus and bifidobacteria (Pan *et al.*, 2009). Thirdly, the epithelical cells of large intestine (colonocyte) can utilize short chain fatty acids as substrate which support growth and regeneration of cells within large intestine and prevents the growth of cancerous cell (Vanhoutvin *et al.*, 2009). Fourthly, short chain fatty acids can be absorbed into the portal blood circulation of the host and participate in the intracellular metabolic processes systemically which effect physiological processes (Topping and Clifton, 2001).

Long Chain Polyunsaturated Fatty Acids (PUFA)

Long carbon chain (generally 18 or more C), polyunsaturated (>1 double bond in the carbon chain) fatty acids are an important group of lipids which have drawn considerable attention in recent days. The long chain PUFA includes two classes of fatty acids: omega-3 and omega-6 fatty acids (Simopoulos 1991). The omega-3 fatty acids are a group of long chain PUFA which contain a double bond between the 3rd and 4th C atoms (counted from the CH3 end). Three major omega-3 fatty acids are alpha linolenic acid (ALA, 18:3), eicosapentaenoic acid (EPA, 20:5) and docosahexaenoic acid (DHA, 22:6). The omega-6 fatty acids have a carbon-carbon double bond between the 6th and 7th C atoms (counted from the CH3 end). The major omega-6 fatty acid includes linoleic acid (LA, 18:2) which is converted to produce arachidonic acid (20:4). Both omega-3 and omega-6 fatty acids are considered as essential fatty acids since human and other mammals cannot synthesize these within the body and hence rely on the dietary sources (Simopoulos 1991). Within the human body, both omega-3 and omega-6 PUFA are involved in the production of a number of key signaling molecules including eicosanoids and prostaglandins. The metabolism of omega-3 PUFA generally lead to the production of eicosanoids which are of anti-inflammatory in nature, while that of omega-6 PUFA lead to eicosanoids of pro-inflammatory in nature. Therefore, a balanced intake of omega-3 and omega-6 PUFA is essential for optimal health (Simopoulos, 2002). Ideally, the ratio of omega-3 and omega-6 PUFA in the diet should be at 1:1 ratio.

Dietary consumption of omega-3 and omega-6 fatty acids has a number of associated health implications. Western diets generally containing high proportion of omega-6 PUFA over omega-3 PUFA which predispose the risk of metabolic diseases (Simopoulos 2002). In contrast, higher proportion of omega-3 PUFA over omega-6 PUFA in diet have health benefits which include lower incidence of coronary heart disease and lowering of blood cholesterol, lipid induced insulin resistance. Some of the underlying mechanism of omega-3 PUFA include: i) inhibition of the activity of ApoB, a lipoprotein carrier involve in trafficking of cholesterol in the blood, ii) increase in insulin sensitivity, iii) increase in the leptin level, iv) inhibition of angiotensin-converting enzyme (ACE), a major enzyme involve in vasoconstriction and blood pressure, e) lowering the level of inflammatory cytokines such as C-reactive protein (CRP), interleukin 6 (IL-6) and prostaglandins, and e) enhance production of vasodilatory prostaglandins.

Conjugated Fatty Acids Isomers

Conjugated linoleic acids (CLA) represent a heterogeneous mixture of different isomers of linoleic acid mostly found in meat and dairy products of ruminant origin (Reynolds and Roche 2010). A group of naturally occurring CLA also includes conjugated α-linoleinic acids (CLNA) isomers. CLNA isomers contain the conjugated double bond along with the octadecatrienoic fatty acid (C18:3) structure of α-linolenic acid. Both CLA and CLNA are naturally present in a number of food ingredients and are reported to have bioactivity (Hennessy *et al.*, 2011). In ruminants such as cattle, sheep, buffalo and deer, CLA are produced by the microbial action as well as through the biotransformation of the forage-derived unsaturated fatty acids (Crumb, 2011). Milk and milk products contain a rich diversity of linoleic acid isomers that provides a range of health benefits mediated by the CLA. Few of the CLA isomers are also produced in small quantity by the intestinal gut microbiota of human. The naturally abundant food sources of CLNA isomers include pomegranate seeds and seeds of many plants of Cucurbitaceae family (Hennessy *et al.*, 2011).

CLA isomers have been found to be effective against a number of human diseases including cancer, atherosclerosis, obesity and diabetes (Hennessay *et al.* 2011). Due to the fact that CLA isomers include a heterogeneous mixture of different isomers of linoleic acid, the molecular mode of action of the individual isomers are not yet well understood. One of the most well characterized mode of action of CLA includes the activation of peroxisome proliferator- activated receptors (PPARs) which ultimately lead to the activation/deactivation of the expression of a cascades of gene (Benjamin and Spener 2009). The CLA bind with the PPARs and form a transcription activation complex that eventually binds in the PPAR responsive elements present in the promoter regions of a wide variety of genes. Many of these genes are involved in signaling pathways affecting a number of physiological functions including the energy homeostasis and immune response. CLA induce fatty acid oxidation and lipolysis, thereby increase the over all energy expenditure while inhibiting pre-adipose tissue proliferation and lipid synthesis. These bioactivities make CLA a potential functional ingredient for obesity and type-2 diabetes. CLA can also inhibit the growth of malignant cells quite effectively and stimulate the immune system and hence can be explored as bioactive ingredients against cancer and inflammation related metabolic diseases (Hennessay *et al.*, 2011).

Bioactive Carotenoids

Carotenoids are tetraterpenoid compounds and are organic pigments present in the chloroplasts and chromoplasts of photosynthetic plants, algae, selected species of bacteria and fungi (Rao and Rao 2007). Carotinoids are present many in naturally occurring food stuffs of plant origin (carrot, tomato, maize), animal origin (egg yolk, meat, fish). Carotinoids cannot be produced by animals, and hence they need to rely on a constant supply through foods. Major carotenes present in food ingredients include β-carotene, α-carotene, lycopene, β-cryptoxanthine and lutein (Rao and Rao, 2007).

Fruits and vegetables are among the common sources of carotinoids in human diet (Table 6.9). Carotinoids are strong anti-oxidant those help in minimizing the adverse health effect caused by the reactive oxygen species (ROS). Reactive oxygen species are generated by with the cells as a result of metabolic processes. Although ROS are produces as a result of normal metabolic processes, they can damage to the cell in numerous ways. Being chemically highly reactive compounds, ROS can react with cellular biomolecules such as protein, lipid and DNA and can cause damage to cell organelles. Such an oxidative stress is closely related to a number of metabolic diseases and hence, food ingredients with anti-oxidant bioactivity are found to have beneficial health effects. In general, cooking of food materials by heating, microweaving or steaming does not break down carotenoids substantially. However, excessive heating, boiling for frying causes damage to carotenoids (Thane and Reddy, 1997). Carotenoids are essential for human health. However, currently there is no dietary reference value recommended for carotenoids intake and there is no report of adverse health effect associated with excessive dietary intake of carotenoids.

Table 6.9: Carotenoids Content in Various Dietary Ingredients

Carotenoid	*Food Source*	*Amount*
β-Carotene	Apricot	17600
	Carrots	9771
	Spinach	5300
	Beet Green	2560
	Broccoli	1300
	Tomato	520
α-Carotene	Carrots	3723
Lycopene	Tomatoes	3100
	Tomato juice	10000
	Tomato paste	36500
	Tomato ketchup	12390
	Tomato sauce	13060
β-Cryptoxanthin	Tangerine	1060
	Papaya	470
Lutein	Spinach	12475
	Beet	7700
	Broccoli	1839
	Green peas	1690

Nutrition and Health

Scientific evidences convincingly support the fact that dietary and lifestyle habits play critical roles in the overall health of an individual (Pitsavos *et al.*, 2006, Shrestha and Ghimire, 2012). Growing evidences also support that nutritional excess or deficiency is detrimental to the health and if such condition persistent for long, can cause alteration in physiological processes leading to metabolic diseases (Pitsavos *et al.*, 2006). Bioactive ingredients present in foods have potential to prevent or cure many of the diseases caused due to nutritional excess. However, individual's response to the bioactive compound(s) present in food ingredients may vary and such response is likely to be determined by the genetic make-up of the individual. Therefore, a generalized nutritional recommendation which is often designed to target large population groups may not be effective in every individuals especially those are genetically susceptible to develop metabolic diseases. Recently, a number of genome wide association studies have identified genetic mutations having association with the risk of developing metabolic diseases (Ridker *et al.*, 2008, Kooner *et al.*, 2011). These studies provide scientific basis for the need of individualized dietary and lifestyle recommendations.

Interaction of dietary nutrients with the genetic material of the host which affects the health of an individual is investigated through the approaches of nutrigenomics and nutrigenetics. Nutrigenomics is the study of the interaction of a particular nutrient with the genome of an individual (Mariman, 2006). Such an interaction is often manifested in terms of expression of a subset of genes and production of proteins, which subsequently alters biochemical processes and physiological status of the individual. On the other hand, nutrigenetics is the study of genetic variations present in an individual which lead to a differential response to a particular nutrient (Mariman, 2006). Due to the presence of a specific genetic mutation in the genome of an individual, he/she may respond differently to a particular dietary nutrient and bioactives. Such a genotype specific interaction of nutrient often results in development of diseases due to failure of utilization of a particular nutrient and its associated biochemical processes. Hence, nutrigenetic approaches particularly deal with identification of the genetic susceptibility to any nutrient related disease. Nutrigenomics and nutrigenetics are two rapidly expanding fields of nutrition research and are promising in the context of understanding the interaction of gene and specific dietary nutrient leading to prevention of metabolic diseases (Vandeberg and Boon 2009, Fenech *et al.*, 2011).

Personalized Nutrition

Sequencing of the human genome is considered as a landmark scientific discovery. Since the first publication of human genome sequence in 2001 (McPherson *et al.*, 2001, Venter *et al.*, 2001), two distinct areas of genomics; the structural genomics- deal with the genetic variations present in the human genome and the functional genomics- deal with the expression of various genes, have made substantial progress. These two specialized areas of genomics immensely contributed to our understanding of the role of different genes in overall functioning of the human body and their contribution in health and disease.

In the last few decades, considerable progresses have been made on establishing the role of gene in various genetic diseases. The concept of one gene underlying one disease is valid for a number of genetic diseases (Table 6.10). One classical example of genetic disease controlled by single gene and liked to nutritional requirement is phenylketonuria (PKU). Individuals with PKU carry mutation for the gene coding phenylalanine hydroxylase, an enzyme required to metabolize phenylalanine. Such individuals when consume food rich in phenylalanine, an incomplete metabolism of excessive dietary phenylalanine result in excessive accumulation of phenylpyruvic acid which is toxic to the brain. Therefore, individual susceptible to PKU should eat diets low in phenylalanine (Phillips 2013). Therapeutic approaches are often effective in curing many of the monogenic diseases (Weatherall 2003). However, the most killer metabolic diseases such as T2D, obesity and CVD are highly complex in nature and are controlled by a large number of individual genes with small effect (Song *et al.*, 2006, Terán-García and Bouchard 2007). Metabolic diseases involve a complex interaction of large number of genes various environmental factors such as diet, living style and emotional status of an individual. Development of diseases takes place in more slowly and silently during pre-clinical phases. Because of the fact that metabolic diseases are controlled by a large number of genes and expression of each individual gene are highly susceptible to environmental factors, identification of candidate gene/genes and associated genetic variants underlying the disease risk is challenging. Genes underlying metabolic diseases are presented in Table 6.11.

Table 6.10: Human Diseases of Monogenic Nature

Disease	*Gene Responsible*
Phenylketonuria (PKU)	Phenylalanine hydroxylase (*PAH*)
Cystic fibrosis	Cystic fibrosis conductance transmembrane regulator (*CFTR*)
Sickle-cell anemia	Beta hemoglobin (*HBB*)
Huntington's disease	Huntingtin (*HTT*)
Hemophilia A	Coagulation factor VIII (*F8*)
Muscular dystrophy, Duchenne type	Dystrophin (*DMD*)
Albinism, oculocutaneous, type II	Oculocutaneous albinism II (*OCA2*)

Table 6.11: Candidate Genes Associated with Metabolic Diseases in Human

Disease	*Gene Responsible*
Obesity	Leptin
	Leptin receptor
	Melanocortin receptor
Lipid/fatty acid metabolism	Adiponectin
	Lipases
	Fatty Acid Binding Protein 2
	Uncoupling protein
	CD36
	Apolipoprotein E
	β-Hydroxysteroid dehydrogenase type 1
	Upstream transcription factor 1
Insulin sensitivity	Peroxisome proliferator activated receptor γ
	Glycoprotein PC-1
	Insulin receptor substrates
	Skeletal muscle glycogen synthase 1
	Calpain-10
	Tumor necrosis factor α
Inflammation	Tumor necrosis factor α
	C-reactive protein
	Interleukin 6 (IL6), IL8

Scientific evidences have convincingly suggested the fact that dietary nutrients, through a complex interaction with the genome of the host play important roles in prevention of metabolic diseases (Fenech *et al.*, 2011). Hence, careful selection and inclusion of food ingredients rich in bioactive ingredients in daily menu can potentially prevent or delay the onset of metabolic diseases in otherwise genetically susceptible individuals (Phillips 2013). Since every individual is genetically unique, it is expected that individual's risk to develop metabolic disease can vary as does his response to the dietary bioactives and functional foods (Ferguson 2009, Phillips 2013). This could be one of the underlying reasons as to why the same bioactive promote health in one individual while it may fail in another individual. For the purpose of identification of any genetic risk associated with the development of metabolic disease, there is a need of screening of the genome of an individual. But genome screening and providing personalized nutritional recommendations for a large population is technically challenging. Moreover, the biological role of every genetic mutation present in the genome of an individual and their potential interaction with nutritional and environmental factors are yet to be known. Hence, the dietary recommendations should atleast be designed to specifically target otherwise manageable genetic sub-groups of the population (Fenech *et al.,* 2011). With a rapid advancement of genomic technologies, it is believed that a personalized nutritional recommendation tailored to the genetic make-up of an individual may be feasible in the future. Some issues relevant to realization of a personalized nutritional approach are highlighted in the following section.

Biomarkers for Diagnosis of Individual Risk

Discovery of novel biomarker(s) for diagnosis of the risk of developing metabolic disease(s) is currently one of the hot topics of research. Methodologies for diagnosis of individual for prediction of the risk of metabolic disease based on the genetic make-up and individualized nutritional guideline are yet to be developed. Interestingly, current diagnostic procedure enable detection of metabolic diseases such as T2D and CVD only when they reach an advanced stage of diseases development, which makes it difficult to cure even after following the best available treatment and disease management procedures (Khan and Awan 2012). Hence, there is an immediate need of developing procedure for detection of the onset of metabolic disease in an early stage.

Candidate Gene and SNP Markers

Through genome wide association studies in distinct population sub-groups, a number of SNP markers were identified and many of these markers were found to have association with the metabolic diseases. One study in South Asian population identified *MC4R* genes to be associated with waist circumference, a phenotypic marker of obesity and T2D (Chambers *et al.,* 2008). Another study identified common genetic variants at *GRB14, ST6GAL1, VPS26A, AP3S2* and *HNF4A* genes have genetic association with T2D in the South Asian population (Kooner *et al.,* 2011). A recent study (Tabassum *et al.,* 2012) also identified locus 2q21 with SNP rs6723108 being associated with the risk of T2D in an Indian population.

The major advantage of developing a SNP based tools of screening for metabolic disease is that the genetic risk can be predicted at an early stage of development. However, these interesting candidate genes and SNP markers are yet to be explored in developing any diagnostic test for predicting the genetic risk of metabolic diseases. Technical difficulties are still associated with the development of methodologies for large scale DNA preparation followed by rapid screening of patient's DNA samples for the presence of mutation(s) pre-disposing genetic risk to metabolic diseases. These diagnostic procedures should be simple enough to use and reasonably affordable.

Proteome Markers

A number of serum proteins including insulin, adiponectin, C-reactive protein (CRP), ferritin and interleukin-2 receptor agonist (IL-2RA) were found promising in predicting the risk of metabolic disease in human (Kolberg *et al.*, 2009). For T2D, serum levels of adiponectin, aplolipptoeint-B (apoB), CRP, interleukin-1 receptor agonist (IL-RA) and ferritin was reported to be among the strong predictors of T2D (Salomaa *et al.*, 2010). Wu *et al.* (2011) suggested the levels of adiponectin, plasma-angiotensin-1 (PA-1), IL-6 and ferritin present in blood serum are strongly associated with T2D. For CVD, a number of proteome markers including lipoproteins, adipokines, leptin, adiponectin and a range of peptides are found to have close association with the disease development (Kim *et al.*, 2010).

Gut-Microbiome Markers

Gut microbiota plays an important role in development of metabolic diseases. Qin *et al.* (2012) identified about 60,000 T2D associated microbiota in 345 Chinese individuals through metagenome sequencing and association. They further demonstrated that patients with T2D have a lower level of butyrate-producing bacteria and a higher population of various opportunistic pathogens and those involve in sulphate reduction and oxidative stress. This study also demonstrated that different species of gut microbes have association with the incidences of metabolic diseases and hence presence of a particular microbial species in the gut can be explored in predicting the risk of developing metabolic diseases in the host.

Target Tissue

Complex metabolic disease often involves a number of organs including brain, gut, pancreas, liver, muscle, adipose tissue and heart which makes it difficult to identify biomarker based on targeting a single tissue (Herder *et al.*, 2011). Moreover, collection of biopsy samples from a range of internal organs for routine diagnosis or large-scale screening is technically challenging and hence unlikely to be practically feasible. Hence, analysis of blood is a practical way, as blood represents the secretion from different tissues and organs at a systemic level. Blood is considered as the ideal tissue for obtaining DNA, metabolite and protein biomarkers which are involve in communication between various types of organs within the body (Khan and Awan, 2012).

The blood peripheral cells can be harvested for genomic DNA and RNA extraction and the transcriptome of these cells may represent the systemic transcriptome profile of an individual (Zampetaki *et al.*, 2010). Analysis of urine is another alternate approach for identification of metabolite which can effectively predict the incidence of metabolic disease in human. In fact, a number of major metabolites linked to metabolic diseases including those related to sugar and amino acid metabolisms are recently identified (Wei *et al.*, 2012). However, most of these protein or metabolite markers are yet to be practically used for diagnosis of metabolic disease and subsequent nutritional recommendations.

Conclusion

Food ingredient contains numerous bioactive ingredients which have potential to prevent metabolic diseases. However, every individual is unique in terms of his/her genetic composition and response to particular dietary nutrients. Therefore nutritional recommendation tailored to a generalized target population may not be highly effective for every individual. Identification of reliable genetic risk factors to metabolic diseases for the purpose of nutritional recommendation is a highly challenging task. A practical approach of achieving this could be through population stratification based on familial history, race and ethnic origin and dividing the entire population into a manageable sub-group.

With the advancement of 'omics' technologies and their application in metabolic disease research and generation of high quality association data, effective biomarker(s) that can be used for diagnosis of metabolic disease at an early stage of disease development is yet to be developed. Currently, there is a lack of integration of data generated from different population specific 'omics' studies, which could be an underlying reason as to why a robust biomarker for predicting the risk of major metabolic disease has not yet developed. Strength of integrating the data from different 'omics' studies in discovery of novel biomarker has been demonstrated in mice model (Connor *et al.*, 2010). Biomarkers, which can effectively diagnose metabolic diseases at pre-clinical stage and diagnostic test, which can be easily performed for large number of individuals, are urgently needed. Because of the facts that these markers are highly specific to a particular human population and genetic make-up of the human population differs in different geographical habitat, biomarkers identified for a Caucasian population may not be effective in predicting the risk of metabolic disease in a South East Asian population. Hence, every population and sub-populations within each large population should be investigated.

References

Adham AM, Mujo K, Kenji S. Functional proteins and peptides of hen's egg origin, bioactive blood peptides in health and disease, Blanca Hernández-Ledesma (Ed.), 2013, doi: 10.5772/54030.

Atkinson FS, Foster-Powell K, Brand-Miller JC. International tables of glycemic index and glycemic load values: 2008. *Diabetes Care* 31: 2281-2283. 2008.

Benjamin S, Spener F. Conjugated linoleic acids as functional food: an insight into their health benefits. *Nutri. Metabol.* 6: 36. 2009.

Bergh MO, Razdan A, Aman P. Nutritional influence of broiler chicken diets based on covered normal, waxy and high amylase barleys with or without enzyme supplementation. *Animal. Feed Sci. Tech.* 78: 215-226. 1999.

Borch-Johnsen K (2007). The metabolic syndrome in a global perspective. The public health impact. *Danish Med. Bull.* 54: 157–159. 2007.

Boutrou R, Gaudichon C, Dupont D, Jardin J, *et al.*, Sequential release of milk protein–derived bioactive peptides in the jejunum in healthy humans. *Amer. J. Clinical Nutri.* 2013. doi: 10.3945/ajcn.112.055202

Brennan CS. Dietary fibre, glycemic response, and diabetes. *Mol. Nutri. Food Res.* 49: 560 - 570. 2005.

Brennan CS, Cleary LJ. The potential use of cereal (1→3, 1→4)-β-D-glucans as functional food ingredients. *J. Cereal Sci.* 42: 1-13. 2005.

Brown KA, Timotijevic L, Barnett J, Shepherd R, *et al.*, A review of consumer awareness, understanding and use of food-based dietary guidelines. *British J. Nutri.* 106: 15-26. 2011.

Brown L, Rosner B, Willett WW and Sacks FM. Cholesterol-lowering effects of dietary fiber: a meta-analysis. *Amer. J. Clinical Nutri.* 69: 30-42. 1999.

Buttriss JL, Stokes CS. Dietary fibre and health: an overview. *Nutri. Bull.* 33: 186-200. 2008.

Chambers JC, Elliott P, Zabaneh D, Zhang W *et al.*, Common genetic variation near MC4R is associated with waist circumference and insulin resistance. *Nature Genet.* 40: 716-718. 2008.

Cherrington CA, Hinton M, Pearson GR, Chopra I. Short-chain organic acids at pH 5.0 kill *Escherichia coli* and *Salmonella spp* without causing membrane perturbation. *J. Appl. Bacteriol.* 70: 161-165. 1991.

Chial H. Rare genetic disorders: learning about genetic disease through gene mapping, SNPs, and microarray data. *Nature Edu.* 1 (1). 2008.

Connor SC, Hansen MK, Corner A, Smith RF Ryan TE. Integration of metabolomics and transcriptomics data to aid biomarker discovery in type 2 diabetes. *Mol. Biosyst.* 6: 909-921. 2010.

Crumb DJ. Conjugated Linolenic Acids (CLA)- an overview. *Intl. J. Appl Res. Natural Prod.* 4: 12-18. 2011.

Dixit AA, Azar KM, Gardner CD, Palaniappan LP. Incorporation of whole, ancient grains into a modern Asian Indian diet to reduce the burden of chronic disease. *Nutrition Res.* 69: 479-488. 2011.

Drewnowski A, Popkin BM. The nutrition transition: new trends in the global diet. *Nutrition Rev.* 55: 31-43. 1997.

Earnest CP, Jordan AN, Safir M, Weaver E, Church TS. Cholesterol-lowering effects of bovine serum immunoglobulin in participants with mild hypercholesterolemia. *Amer. J. Clinical Nutrition.* 81: 792-798. 2005.

Ebbeling CB, Pawlak DB, Ludwig DS. Childhood obesity: public health crisis, common sense cure. *Lancet.* 360: 473-482. 2003.

Edwards CA, Parrett AM, Balmer SE, Wharton BA. Faecal short chain fatty acids in breast-fed and formula-fed infants. *Acta Paedatrica.* 83: 459-462. 1994.

Fenech M, El-Sohemy A, Cahill L, Ferguson LR *et al.*, Nutrigenetics and nutrigenomics: viewpoints on the current status and applications in nutrition research and practice. *J. Nutrigenet. Nutrigenomics.* 4: 69-89. 2011.

Ferguson LR. Nutrigenomics approaches to functional foods. *J. Amer. Dietetic Assoc.* 109: 452-458. 2009.

Flier JS. Obesity wars: molecular progress confronts and expanding epidemic. *Cell.* 116: 337-350. 2004.

García-Montoya IA, Cendón TS, Arévalo-Gallegos S, Rascón-Cruz Q. Lactoferrin a multiple bioactive protein: an overview. *Biochim. et Biophys. Acta.* 1820: 226-236. 2012.

Gibson GR, Roberfroid MB. Dietary modulation of the human colonic microbiota: introducing the concept of prebiotics. *J. Nutrition.* 125: 1401-1412. 1995.

Giri A and Ohshima. Bioactive marine peptides: nutraceutical value and novel approaches. *Adv. Food Nutrition Res.* 65: 73-105. 2012.

Gobbetti M, Minervini F, Rizzello CG. Angiotensin I-convertingenzyme inhibitory and antimicrobial bioactive peptides. *Intl. J. Dairy Tech.* 57: 173-188. 2004.

Grundy SM. Drug therapy of the metabolic syndrome: minimizing the emerging crisis in polypharmacy. *Nature Rev. Drug Discov.* 5: 295-309. 2006.

Gupta R, Guptha S, Joshi R, Xavier D. Translating evidence into policy for cardiovascular disease control in India. *Heal. Res. Poly. Syst.* 9: 2011.: doi: 10.1186/1478-4505-9-8

Harnedy PA, FitzGerald RJ. Bioactive proteins, peptides and amino acids from macroalgae. *J. Phycol.* 47: 218-232. 2011.

Hasler CM. Functional foods: benefits, concerns and challenges- a position paper. *Amer. Coun. Sci. Heal. J. Nutri.* 132: 3772-3781. 2002.

Hennessy AA, Ross RP, Devery R, Stanton C. The health promoting properties of the conjugated isomers of a-linoenic acid. *Lipids.* 46: 105-119. 2011.

Herder C, Karakas M, Koenig W. Biomarkers for the prediction of type 2 diabetes and cardiovascular disease. *Clinil. Pharmacol. Therap.* 90: 52-66. 2011.

Hernández B, Gortmaker SL, Colditz GA, Peterson KE, *et al.*, Association of obesity with physical activity, television programs and other forms of video viewing among children in Mexico city. *Intl. J. Obesity Relat. Metabol. Disord.* 23: 854-845. 1999.

Israili ZH, Lyoussi B, Hernandez-Hernandez R and Velasco M. (2007). Metabolic syndrome: treatment of hypertensive patients. *Amer. J. Therap.* 14: 386-402. 2007.

Khan AR and Awan FR. Mining of protein based biomarkers for type 2 diabetes mellitus. *Pakistan J. Pharmacul. Sci.* 25: 889-901. 2012.

Kim CX, Bailey KR, Klee GG, Ellington AA *et al.*, Sex and ethnic differences in 47 candidate proteomic markers of cardiovascular disease: the mayo clinic proteomic markers of arteriosclerosis study. *PLoS ONE*. 5: e9065. 2010.

Kim MK, Lopetcharat K, Gerard PD, Drake MA. Consumer awareness of salt and sodium reduction and sodium labeling. *J. Food Sci.* 77: S307-S313. 2012.

Kolberg JA, Jorgensen T, Gerwien RW, Hamren S *et al.*, Development of a type 2 diabetes risk model from a panel of serum biomarkers from the Inter99 cohort. *Diabetes Care*. 32: 1207-1212. 2009.

Kooner JS, Danish Saleheen D, Sim X, Sehmi J *et al.*, Genome-wide association study in individuals of South Asian ancestry identifies six new type 2 diabetes susceptibility loci. *Nature Genet*. 43: 984-991. 2011.

Kooner JS, Saleheen D, Sim X, Sehmi J *et al.*, Genome-wide association study in individuals of South Asian ancestry identifies six new type 2 diabetes susceptibility loci. *Nature*. 43: 984-1000. 2011.

Korhonen H, Pihlanto A. Food derived bioactive peptides- opportunities for designing future foods. *Curr. Pharmacel. Design*. 9: 1297-1308. 2003.

Kritchevsky D, Chen SC. Phytosterols- health benefits and potential concerns: a review. *Nutri. Res*. 25: 413-428. 2002.

Lands B. Consequences of essential fatty acids. *Nutrients*. 4: 1338-1357. 2012.

Lee A, Molloy MP, Baker MS, Kapur A. Tandem ion exchange fractionation of chicken egg white reveals the presence of proliferative bioactivity. *J. Agril. Food Chem*. 61: 4079-4088. 2013.

Lobo V, Patil A, Phatak A, Chandra N. Free radicals, antioxidants and functional foods: Impact on human health. *Pharmacognosy Rev*. 4: 118-126. 2010.

Lönnerdal B. Bioactive proteins in breast milk. *J. Pediatrics Child Health* 49: 1-7. 2003.

Mariman EC. Nutrigenomics and nutrigenetics: the 'omics' revolution in nutritional science. *Biotech. Appl. Biochem*. 44: 119-128. 2006.

Marinangeli CP, Jones PJ. Functional food ingredients as adjunctive therapies to pharmacotherapy for treating disorders of metabolic syndrome. *Annul. Medicine*. 42: 317-333. 2010.

McClements DJ, Decker EA, Park Y, Weiss J. Structural design principles for delivery of bioactive components in nutraceuticals and functional foods. *Critl. Rev. Food Sci. Nutri*. 49: 577-606. 2009.

McPherson JD, Marra M, Hillier L, Waterston RH *et al.*, A physical map of the human genome. *Nature*. 409: 934-941. 2001.

Meisel H. Overview on milk protein- derived peptides. *Intl. Dairy J*. 8: 363-373. 1998.

Meyer KA, Kushi LH, Jacobs DR, Slavin J *et al.*, Carbohydrates, dietary fiber, and incident type 2 diabetes in older women. *Amer. J. Clinil. Nutri*. 71: 921-930. 2000.

Mills S, Ross RP, Hill C, Fitzgerald GF, Stanton C. Milk intelligence: mining milk for bioactive substances associated with human health. *Intl. Dairy. J.* 21: 377-401. 2011.

Misra A, Khurana L. Obesity and the metabolic syndrome in developing countries. *J. Clinil. Endocrinol. Metabol.* 93: s9-s30. 2008.

Moller DE, Kaufman KD. Metabolic syndrome: a clinical and molecular perspective. *Annl. Rev. Medie.* 56: 45-62. 2005.

Nagao K, Yanagita T. Bioactive lipids in metabolic syndrome. *Prog. Lipids Res.* 47: 127-146. 2008.

Ntanios FY, Duchateau GS. A healthy diet rich in carotenoids is effective in maintaining normal blood carotenoid levels during the daily use of plant sterol-enriched spreads. *Intl. J. Vitn. Nutri. Res.* 72: 32-39. 2002.

Pan XD, Chen FG, Wu TX, Tang HG, Zhao ZY. Prebiotic oligosaccharides change the concentrations of short-chain fatty acids and the microbial population of mouse bowel. *J. Zhejiang Univ. Sci.* B 10: 258-263. 2009.

Phillips CM. Nutrigenetics and metabolic disease: current status and implications for personalized nutrition. *Nutrients.* 5: 32-57. 2013.

Pitsavos C, Panagiotakos D, Weinem M, Stefanadis C. Diet, exercise and the metabolic syndrome. *Rev. Diabetic Stud.* 3: 118-126. 2006.

Pumas C, Vacharapiyasophon P, Peerapornpisal Y, Leelapornpisid P *et al.*, Thermostablility of phycobiliproteins and antioxidant activity from four thermotolerant cyanobacteria. *Psychol. Res.* 59: 166-174. 2011.

Qin J, Li Y, Cai Z, Li S *et al.*, A metagenome-wide association study of gut microbiota in type 2 diabetes. *Nature.* 490: 55-60. 2012.

Rao AV, Rao LG. Carotenoids and human health. *Pharma. Res.* 55: 207-216. 2007.

Reynolds CM, Roche HM. Conjugated linoleic acids and inflammatory cell signaling. *Prostaglandins, Leukotrienes Essential Fatty Acids.* 82: 199-204. 2010.

Ricci-Cabello I, Olalla Herrera M and Artacho R. Possible role of milk-derived bioactive peptides in the treatment and prevention of metabolic syndrome. *Nutril. Rev.* 70: 241–255. 2012.

Ridker PM, Pare G, Parker A, Zee RYL *et al.*, Loci related to metabolic-syndrome pathways including *LEPR, HNF1A, IL6R,* and *GCKR* association with plasma C-reactive protein: the women's genome health study. *Amer. J. Human Genet.* 82: 1185-1192. 2008.

Sacks FM, Lichtenstein A, Van Horn L, Harris W *et al.*, Soy protein, isoflavones and cardiovascular health: an American heart association science advisory for professionals from the nutrition committee. *Circulation.* 113: 1034-1044. 2006.

Salmeron J, Ascherio A, Rimm EB, Colditz GA *et al.*, Dietary fibre, glycemic load, and risk of NIDDM in men. *Diabètes Care.* 20: 545-550. 1997.

Salomaa V, Havulinna A, Saarela O, Zeller T *et al.*, Thirty-one novel biomarkers as predictor for clinically incident diabetes. *PLoS One.* 5: e10100. 2010.

Salvin J, Green H. Dietary fibre and satiety. *Nutri. Bull.* 32: S32-S42. 2007

Sawant A, Mankeshwar R, Shah S, Raghavan R *et al.*, Prevalence of metabolic syndrome in urban India. *Cholesterol.* 2011: doi: 10.1155/2011/920983

Schulze MB, Liu S, Runn EB, Manson JAE *et al.*, Glycemic index, glycemic load, and dietary fibre intake and incidence of type 2 diabetes in younger and middle-aged women. *Amer. J. Clinical Nutri.* 80: 348-356. 2004.

Shetty P. Public health: India's diabetes time bomb. *Nature.* 485: S14-S16. 2012.

Shrestha P, Ghimire L. A review about the effect of life style modification on diabetes and quality of life. *Global J. Health Sci.* 4: 185-190. 2012.

Siigur U, Ormisson A, Tamm A. Faecal short-chain fatty acids in breast-fed and bottle-fed infants. *Acta Paediatrica.* 82: 536-568. 1993.

Silva SV, Malcata FX. Caseins as source of bioactive peptides. *Intl. Dairy. J.* 15: 1-15. 2005.

Simopoulos AP. Omega-3 fatty acids in health and disease and in growth and development. *Amer. J. Clinical Nutrition.* 54: 438-463. 2002.

Simppoulos AP. The importance of the ratio of omega-6/omega-3 essential fatty acids. *Biomed. Pharmacotherapy.* 56: 865-879. 2002.

Siró I, Kápolna E, Kápolna B, Lugasi A. Functional food. Product development, marketing and consumer acceptance- a review. *Appetite.* 51: 456-467. 2008.

Skendi A, Biliaderis CG, Lazaridou A and Izydorczyk MS. Structure and rheological properties of water soluble β-glucans from oat cultivars of *Avena sativa* and *Avena bysantia. J. Cereal Sci.* 38: 15-31. 2003.

Song Q, Wang SS, Zafari AM. Genetics of the metabolic syndrome. *Hospital Physician.* 42: 51-61. 2006.

Streppel MT, Ocké MC, Boshuizen HC, Kok FJ, Kromhout D. Dietary fiber intake in relation to coronary heart disease and all-cause mortality over 40 y: the Zutphen Study. *Amer. J. Clinical Nutri.* 88: 1119-1125. 2008.

Suarez-Jimenez GM, Burgos-Hernandez A, Ezquerra-Brauer JM. Bioactive peptides and depsipeptides with anticancer potential: sources from marine animals. *Marine Drugs.* 10: 963-986. 2012.

Tabassum R, Chauhan G, Dwivedi OP, Mahajan A *et al.*, Genome-wide association study for Type 2 Diabetes in Indians identifies a new susceptibility locus at 2q21. *Diabetes.* 62: 977-986. 2012.

Tabatabai A, Li S. Dietary fiber and type 2 diabetes. *Clin. Excel. Nurse Practir.* 4: 172-176. 2000.

Terán-García M, Bouchard C. Genetics of the metabolic syndrome. *Appl Physiol. Nutri. Metabol.* 32: 89-114. 2007.

Thane C, Reddy S. Processing of fruits and vegetables: effects on carotenoids. *Nutri. Food Sci.* 97: 58-65. 1997.

Topping DL, Clifton PM. Short-chain fatty acids and human colonic function: roles o resistant starch and non-starch polysaccharides. *Physiol. Rev.* 81: 1031-1064. 2001

Trautwein EA, Demonty I. Phytosterols: natural compounds with established and emerging health benefits. *OCL*. 14: 259-265. 2007.

Trowell H, Southgate DAT, Wolever TMS *et al.*, Dietary fibre redefined. *Lancet*. 1 967. 1976.

US Department Agriculture. Nutrient Data Laboratory. 2013 http: //www.nal usda.gov/ fnic/foodcomp/search/.

Vandeberg RLJ, Boon WPC. Anticipating emerging genomics technologies: the role of patents and publication for research and policy strategies. *Genomics Soc. Policy*. 5: 1-21. 2009.

Vanhoutvin SALW, Troost FJ, Hamer HM, Lindsey PJ *et al.*, Butyrate-induced transcriptional changes in human colonic mucosa. *PLoS ONE*. 4: e6759. 2009.

Venter JC, Adams MD, Myers EW, Li PW *et al.*, The sequence of the human genome *Science*. 291: 1304-1351. 2001.

Walther B, Sieber R. Bioactive proteins and peptides in foods. *Intl. J. Vitan. Nutri. Res*. 81: 181-192. 2011.

Weatherall DJ. Pharmacological treatment of monogenic disease. *Pharmacogenomics* J. 3: 264-266. 2003.

Wei H, Pasman W, Rubingh C, Wopereis S *et al.*, Urine metabolomics combined with the personalized diagnosis guided by Chinese medicine reveals subtypes of pre-diabetes. *Mol. Biosyst*. 8: 1482-1491. 2012.

Wong JMW, de Souza R, Kendall CWC, Emam A, Jenkins DJA. Colonic health: fermentation and short chain fatty acids. *J. Clinical Gastroenterol*. 40: 235-243. 2006.

Woods VB, Fearon AM. Dietary sources of unsaturated fatty acids for animals and their transfer into meat, milk and eggs: a review. *Livestock Sci*. 126: 1-20. 2009.

Wu H, Yu Z, Qi Q, Li H *et al.*, Joint analysis of multiple biomarkers for identifying type 2 diabetes in middle-aged and older Chinese: a cross sectional study. *BMJ Open*. 1: e000191. 2011.

Xiao R, Carter JA, Linz AL, Ferguson M *et al.*, Dietary whey protein lowers serum C-peptide concentration and duodenal SREBP-1c mRNA abundance, and reduces occurrence of duodenal tumors and colon aberrant crypt foci in azoxymethane-treated male rats. *J. Nutriti. Biochem*. 17: 626-634. 2006.

Yang P, Pratt CA. Metabolic syndrome and its association with diet and physical activity in USA adolescents. *J. Amer. Dietetic Assoc*. 108: 276-286. 2008.

Zampetaki A, Kiechl S, Drozdov I, Willeit P *et al.*, Plasma micro RNA profiling reveals loss of endothelial MiR-126 and other micro RNAs in type 2 diabetes. *Circulation Res*. 107: 810-817. 2010.

2016, Biotechnological Tools for Genetic Resources Pages 201–231
Editor: Pradip Chandra Deka
Published by: Daya Publishing House, NEW DELHI

Chapter 7

Associating the Genes to Functions, Involved in Secondary Metabolism of Plants

Shubhra Rastogi, Amita Misra and Ajit Kumar Shasany*

Biotechnology Division,
CSIR-Central Institute of Medicinal and Aromatic Plants,
P.O. CIMAP, Lucknow – 226 015, U.P.
**E-mail: akshasany@yahoo.com*

ABSTRACT

Secondary metabolites are the natural products that are believed to be not essential for normal growth and development of plants and have multiple functions throughout the plant's life cycle. Plant secondary metabolites represent an enormous value from economical point of view as they are used as specialty chemicals, such as drugs, flavors, fragrances, insecticides and dyes. There is a diverse array of secondary metabolites synthesized in the plant. However, information about the enzymes involved in secondary metabolism is scarce. In the high-throughput era of functional genome analysis now it has become easier to broadly assign functions to unknown genes. Despite the high-throughput clues associating a gene to a specific function can exclusively be not inferred by using a single approach. Rather, there is requirement of collecting all the information using different methods which may help in unambiguously assigning functions to unknown plant genes. Such methods involve analysis of the important cell constituents that may help deducing the gene function and these are mainly the transcripts and proteins. Metabolomics is another method which aims to identify gene function on the basis of analyzing the full complement of metabolites of an organism. Unlike transcriptomic and proteomic strategies quantifying changes in mRNA and protein levels, metabolic profile allows the closer identification of the specific role that a certain gene performs in a biochemical process. Additionally, links leading to the novel products arising from the side-reactions could also be identified. Plant genomics research has also stepped into the stage of fast functional characterization of plant genes. From a multitude methods in the plant functional genomics toolbox researchers can make a choice for competent gene function analysis. The functional genomics pertains in bringing together various complementary approaches such that one can get the full benefit of the available genomic information on plant genes by applying multidisciplinary integrated approach. In order to broadly assign functions to unknown genes, different fast and multiparallel approaches are effortlessly being developed. This chapter provides some example for assigning function to genes of particular secondary metabolic pathway in plants.

Keywords: *Secondary metabolites, Metabolic pathways, Biosynthetic pathways, Functional genomics, Metabolomics, Metabolic profile, Plant genome.*

Introduction

A large number of genes in plants are responsible for the biosynthesis of plant secondary metabolites. The evolution of new genes to make novel secondary compounds in plants is an ongoing process and might account for most of the differences in gene function among plant genomes (Pichersky and Gang 2000). In most cases, it has been found that secondary metabolite biosynthesis does not occur in all cells of plant but is organ or tissue specific. Even, the site of biosynthesis and site of accumulation of secondary metabolites may also differ (Wink 1989). Knowledge of genes involved in secondary metabolite biosynthetic pathway allowed the genetic engineering tools to be utilized for production of altered contents of metabolites in plants (Siebert *et al.*, 1996), for example the accumulation of stilbenes was observed when stilbene synthase from *Vitis vinifera* was expressed in tobacco (*Nicotiana tabacum*) and hence an increased resistance to *Botrytis cinerea* (Hain *et al.*, 1993). Secondary metabolites are produced by plants to carry out diverse type of functions like production of floral scent volatiles and pigments to attract insect pollinators and thus enhance fertilization rates, toxic chemicals to ward off pathogens and herbivores or to suppress the growth of neighboring plants etc. (Pichersky and Gang 2000). Genomes of different plants are estimated to contain 20,000 to 60,000 genes, and around 15–25 per cent of these genes are supposed to encode enzymes for secondary metabolism (Bevan *et al.*, 1998, Somerville and Somerville 1999). Medicinal and aromatic plants (MAPs) are important sources for plant secondary metabolites, which are important for human healthcare. Raising the yield and quality of these natural phytomolecules through conventional breeding is still a challenge. However, recent advances in plant genomics research has generated knowledge leading to a better understanding of the complex genetics and biochemistry involved in biosynthesis of these plant secondary metabolites (Kumar and Gupta 2008). Genomics research is also concerned with identication and isolation of genes involved in different steps of a number of metabolic pathways. For associating a function to a particular gene of plant, various types of approaches are used. These include knocking down or silencing of gene in the plant by using RNAi or similar approach, complementing gene in its respective mutant, overexpression of gene in heterologous system for *in vitro* functional analysis by providing different substrates based on their homology with other genes *etc*. Some example for assigning function to genes of particular secondary metabolic pathway in medicinal and aerometric plants (MAPs) is discussed in the following section.

Association of Genes in Seconadary Metabolism of Plants

A wide range of secondary metabolites are being produced by different plants *viz.* terpenes, phenylpropanoids, flavonoids, alkaloids *etc.* Key steps involved in the biosynthesis of these metabolites are catalyzed by different enzymes encoded by various types of genes. Genes responsible for biosynthesis of some important compounds for human health and welfare are described in details in following section.

Genes Involved in Menthol Biosynthesis of *Mentha* spp.

Mints are cultivated for their essential oils having a large variety of aromatic chemicals in varying composition. The oils and their fractions are of great demand world-wide and used in chewing gum, mouthwash, toothpaste, shaving cream, vaporub, cough syrup and several other products. (-)-Menthol is the most abundant and characteristic component of the essential oil of mature peppermint plants. A superior oil is defined as rich in menthol with moderate amounts of (-)-menthone and low levels of (+)-pulegone and (+)-menthofuran (Mahmoud *et al.*, 2003). The menthol along with other components such as (-)-limonene, carvone, linalool *etc.* finds various uses in the pharmaceutical, food and confectionery industries. In mints, peltate glandular trichomes are the site for biosynthesis and accumulation of essential oil, and the essential oil components are composed of different types of terpenes and their derivatives. It is now well established that in plants, isopentenyl diphosphate (IPP) the precursor for terpenes, is synthesized in the plastids through 1-deoxy-D-xylulose-5-phosphate (DXP) pathway and in the cytosol through the mevalonic acid (MVA) pathway (McCaskill and Croteau 1995). The DXP pathway (Lichtenthaler 1999, Rohmer 1999) generates IPP as well as its isomer dimethylallyl diphosphate (DMAPP), whereas only IPP is released from the MVA pathways which further isomerize into DMAPP.

In plastids, a head-to-tail condensation of one IPP molecule and one DMAPP molecule catalyzed by geranyl diphosphate synthase (GPPS) forms GPP (C10), the universal precursor of all monoterpenes (Ogura and Koyama 1998, Poulter and Rilling 1981). In the cytosol, the condensation of two IPP molecules and one DMAPP molecule catalyzed by the enzyme farnesyl diphosphate synthase (FPPS) results in FPP formation (C15), the natural precursor of sesquiterpenes (McGarvey and Croteau 1995). Condensation of one DMAPP molecule with three IPP molecules by the action of geranyl geranyl diphosphate synthase (GGPPS) yields GGPP, the C20 diphosphate precursor of diterpenes (Koyama and Ogura 1999). After the formation of the acyclic precursors GPP, FPP and GGPP, a wide range of structurally diverse cyclic and acyclic monoterpenes, sesquiterpenes and diterpenes are generated through the action of a large family of terpene synthases/cyclases (Cane 1999, Wise and Croteau, 1999).

The (–)-menthol pathway consisted of eight-step from primary metabolism was defined by the combination of feeding studies and cell-free enzymology (Figure 7.1). The first committed step towards the menthol biosynthetic pathway, the conversion of geranyl diphosphate to (-)-limonene, is catalyzed by (-)-limonene synthase (Alonso *et al.*, 1992, Colby *et al.*, 1993), which is localized in leucoplasts (Turner *et al.*, 1999).

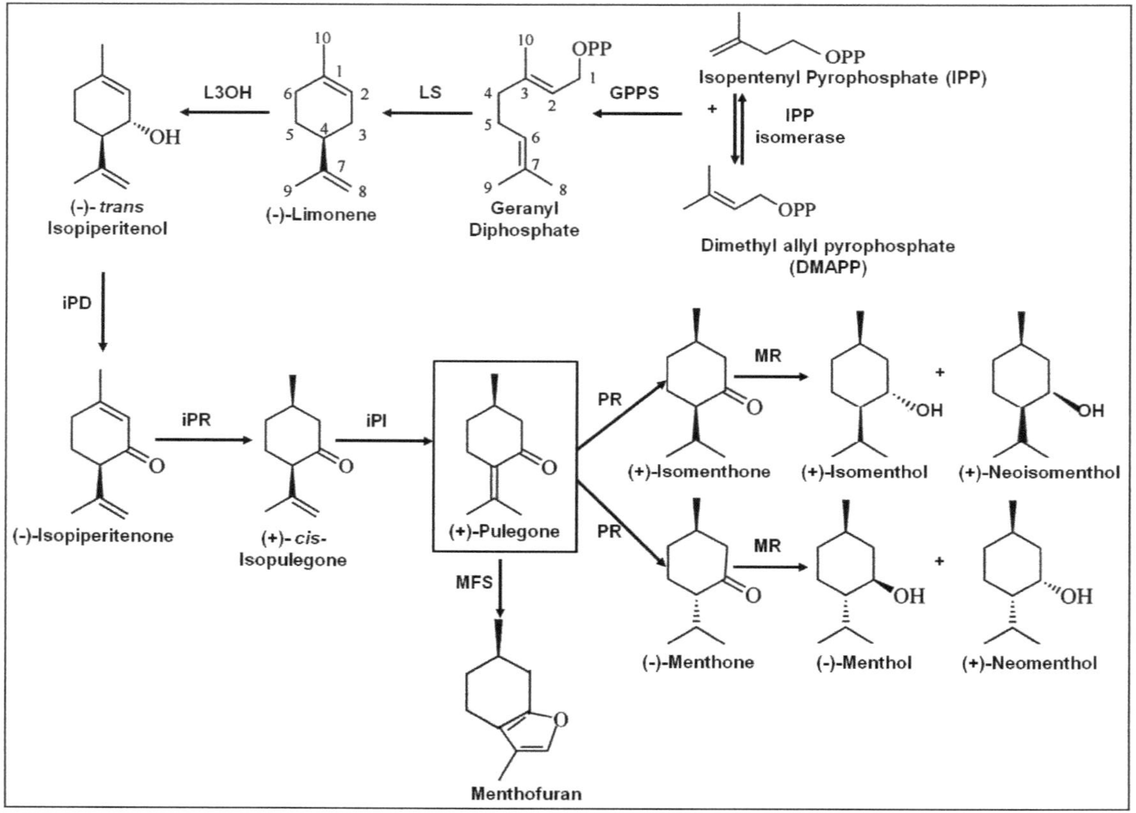

Figure 7.1: Menthol Biosynthestic Pathway in the Secretory Glands of Peppermint.

The enzymatic steps are catalyzed by geranyl diphosphate synthase (GPPS), (-)-limonene synthase (LS), (-)-limonene-3-hydroxylase (L3OH), (-)-*trans*-isopiperitenol dehydrogenase (iPD), (-)-isopiperitone reductase (iPR), (+)-*cis*-isopulegone isomerase (iPI), (+)-pulegone reductase (PR), (-)-menthone reductase (MR), and menthofuran synthase (MFS).

(–)-(4S)-Limonene synthase was first purified from extracts of isolated spearmint oil glands. The enzyme require divalent metal ion for activity and encodes a large N-terminal plastidial transit peptide (Colby *et al.*, 1993) which directs the newly synthesized enzyme to the leucoplasts of the oil gland secretory cells for proteolytic processing into mature form (Turner *et al.*, 1999). The next step takes place in the endoplasmic reticulum where (-)-limonene undergoes a cytochrome P450-dependent hydroxylation, catalyzed by (-)-limonene 3-hydroxylase (Lupien *et al.*, 1999), to form (-)-transisopiperitenol. A very similar enzyme mediates the regioselective C6-hydroxylation of (–)-limonene to (–)- trans-carveol *en route* to (–)-carvone in spearmint. After entry into mitochondria, (-)-transisopiperitenol is oxidized to (-)-isopiperitenone by a specific NAD+-dependent short-chain isopiperitenol dehydrogenase (Ringer *et al.*, 2005, Turner and Croteau 2004). Further isopiperitenol is converted into isopiperitenone by (-)-isopiperitenone reductase which introduces double bond in the structure (Ringer *et al.*, 2003). Isopiperitenone then isomerizes into (-)-cis-isopulegone by cis-isopulegone isomerase (Kjonass *et al.*, 1985) which leads to the generation of the branch point intermediate (-)-pulegone in cytosol. (-)-Pulegone reductase (PR) present in cytosol synthesizes both (-) - menthone and (-)-isomenthone from (-)-pulegone (Ringer *et al.*, 2003). Further conversions in the main monoterpene pathway are catalyzed by the bifunctional cytosolic activities of (-)-menthone:(-)- (3R)-menthol reductase and (-)-menthone:(-)-(3S)-neomenthol reductase (Davis *et al.*, 2005). The byproduct (-)-menthofuran can be formed from (-)-pulegone by the action of (-)-menthofuran synthase (MFS), an endoplasmic reticulum-localized cytochrome P450-dependent monooxygenase (Bertea *et al.*, 2001). In spearmint (*M. spicata*), limonene is oxygenated by (-)-4S-limonene-6-hydroxylase to form (-)-trans-carveol (Karp *et al.*, 1990) followed by oxidation into (-)-carvone, which is the principal component of spearmint oil (Lawrence 1981).

Several of the genes encoding early pathway enzymes have been cloned by reverse genetic methods and characterized. These include geranyl diphosphate synthase (Burke *et al.*, 1999), limonene synthase (LS) (Colby *et al.*, 1993) and cytochrome P450 limonene-3-and limonene-6-hydroxylases (Lupien *et al.*, 1999). Limonene synthase of peppermint and spearmint share 93 per cent identity at amino acid level (Colby *et al.*, 1993). Similarly, the hydroxylases, *i.e.* (-)-4S-limonene-3-hydroxylase in peppermint and (-)-4S-limonene-6-hydroxylase in spearmint convert common precursor (-)-limonene to (-)-trans-isopiperitenol or (-)-trans-carveol, respectively (Karp *et al.*, 1990), share only 70 per cent deduced identity with most of the sequence differences localized to the presumptive active sites (Lupien *et al.*, 1999). The other cytochrome P450 involved in monoterpene metabolism of peppermint is menthofuran synthase (Lange *et al.*, 2000). At amino acid level, (+)-menthofuran synthase exhibits 35 per cent and 38 per cent sequence identity with peppermint (-)-limonene-3-hydroxylase and spearmint limonene-6-hydroxylase, respectively (Bertea *et al.*, 2001). The (-)-trans-carveol dehydrogenase of spearmint and (-)-trans-isopiperitenol dehydrogenase of peppermint show 99 per cent amino acid similarity and are capable of utilizing both (-)-trans-isopiperitenol and (-)-trans-carveol (Tucker 1992). These isopiperitenol/carveol dehydrogenases are members of the short-chain dehydrogenase superfamily which are involved in secondary metabolism (lignin biosynthesis), stress responses, and phytosteroid biosynthesis

(Ringer *et al.*, 2005). The double bond reductases of pippermint (-)-isopiperitenone reductase and (+)-pulegone reductase are highly substrate specific and shows less than 12 per cent identity. (-)-Isopiperitenone reductase is a member of short chain reductase superfamily and (+)-pulegone reductase is a member of medium chain reductase superfamily. The two NADPH dependent keto-reductases which convert (-)-menthone to (-)-(3R)-menthol and (+)-3S-neomenthol are menthone: (-)-(3R)-menthol reductase (MMR) and menthone: (+)-(3S)-neomenthol reductase (MNR). These two reductases shares 73 per cent identity and belong to short-chain reductase family of enzymes (Kallberg *et al.*, 2002, Ringer *et al.*, 2003). In contrast pulegone reductase, mechanistically similar to isopieritenone reductase belongs to medium-chain reductase (Ringer *et al.*, 2003) and share little sequence identity with peppermint SDRs and contains no characteristics of SDR motifs. Deduced sequence comparison from peppermint revealed that these two (pulegone reductase and isopiperitenone reductase) highly substrate specific double-bond reductases show less than 12 per cent identity. (–)-Isopiperitenone reductase is a member of the short-chain dehydrogenase/reductase superfamily and (+)-pulegone reductase is a member of the medium-chain dehydrogenase/reductase superfamily, implying very different evolutionary origins in spite of the similarity in substrates utilized and reactions catalyzed. This implies that origin of these enzymes cannot be related to the reaction types they catalyze. Probably they have evolved from distant ancestral redox genes that encoded enzymes with shared binding determinants for these structurally similar monoterpenoid substrates (Davis *et al.*, 2005). The way the plant regulates its metabolism to account to a reduction in menthol and menthone concentration under adverse conditions, is still a matter of debate.

Artemisinin Biosynthetic Pathway in *Artemisia annua*

Artemisia species shows substantial medicinal properties, which include their use as antibiotic (*A. capillis*), anti-malarial (*A. annua*), anti-helmintic (*A. cina*), anti-feedent and insecticidal (*A. absinthium*) (Wagner 1977, Facknath and Kawol 1993). *Artemisia annua*, a member of family Asteraceae, produces antimalarial artemisinin. Terpenoids (especially sesquiterpene lactones) and flavonoids are the main constituents responsible for medicinal properties of plant. The essential oil of several *Artemisia* species has been found to exert different biological activities against microbes (Janssen *et al.*, 1987). Artemisinin, found mainly in *A. annua*, and to some extent in *A. apiacea* and *A. lancea* also (Hsu 2006), is a sesquiterpene lactone with an endoperoxide bridge. Artemisinin and some of its synthetic derivatives, for example artesunate, arteether, artemether *etc.* are highly effective against the malaria caused by *Plasmodium falciparum*. Drugs derived from these derivatives have pharmacological properties superior to those of the parent compound (Begue and Bonnet 2005) and exhibit greater potency than artemisinin itself, as well as improved solubility, and favourable metabolic and hydrolytic stabilities. Artemisinin-based combination therapies (ACTs) are now considered as the best current treatment for uncomplicated *Plasmodium falciparum* malaria (He *et al.*, 2009). Artemisinin has been detected in leaves, small green stems, buds, flowers and seeds of *A. annua* (Acton *et al.*, 1985, Zhao and Zeng 1985, Liersch *et al.*, 1986, Martinez and Staba 1988, Singh *et al.*, 1988, Madhusudanan 1989, Ferreira *et al.*, 1995). Recent investigations have shown that artemisinin have possible uses in cancer therapy (Efferth 2006, Nakase *et al.*, 2007, Withers and Keasling 2007), tryptanosomiasis (Kaiser *et al.*, 2002, Stephenson and Wiselka 2000), hepatitis (Paeshuyse *et al.*, 2006, Romero *et al.*, 2005), and as an herbicide (Lee, 2007).

The basic structure of artemisinin is derived from the sesquiterpene backbone which is synthesized by the same pathway described in the previous section of menthol biosynthesis in *Mentha piperita*. Sesquiterpenes are C15 isoprene units

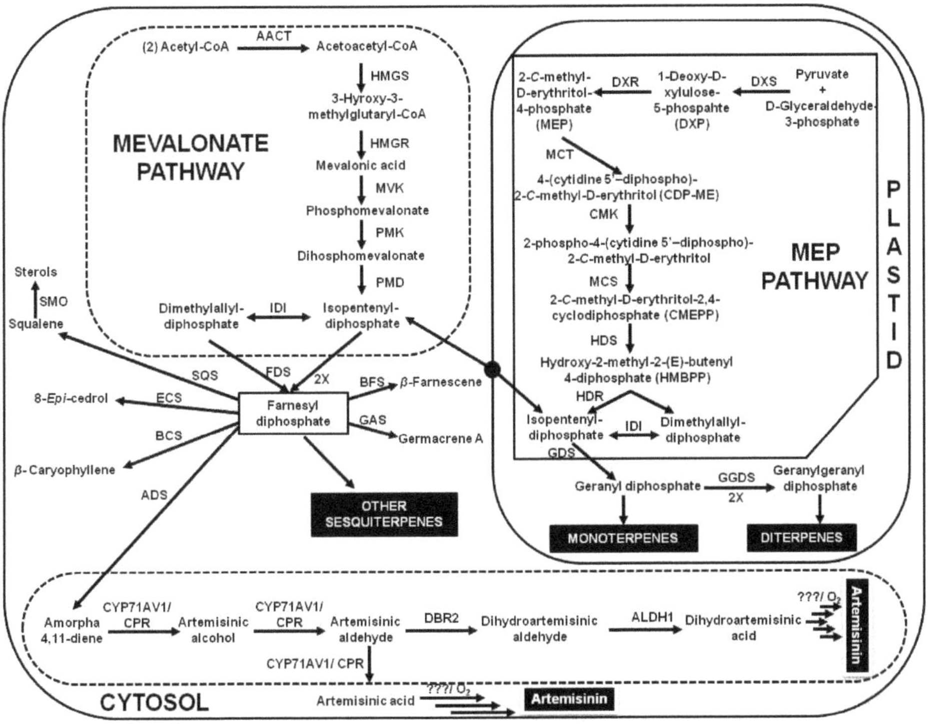

Figure 7.2: Artemisinin Biosynthetic Pathway in *Artemisia annua*.

Cytosol: **AACT: acetoacetyl-CoA thiolase; ADS: amorpha-4,11-diene synthase; ALDH1: aldehyde dehydrogenase 1; BFS: β-farnesene synthase; CPR: cytochrome P450 reductase; CPS: β-caryophyllene synthase; CYP71AV1: amorphadiene-12-hydroxylase; DBR2: artemisinic aldehyde Δ11(13) reductase; ECS: *epi*-cedrol synthase; FDS: farnesyl diphosphate synthase; GAS: germacrene A synthase; HMGR: 3-hydroxy-3-methyl-glutaryl coenzyme A reductase; HMGS: 3-hydroxy-3-methyl-glutaryl coenzyme A synthase; IDI: isopentenyl diphosphate isomerase; MVK: mevalonate kinase; PMD: diphosphomevalonate decarboxylase; PMK: phosphomevalonate kinase; SMO: squalene monooxygenase; SQS: squalene synthase. *Plastid:* CMK: 4-cytidine 5´-diphospho-2-C-methyl-Derythritol kinase; DXR: 1-deoxy-D-xylulose-5-phosphate reductoisomerase; DXS: 1-deoxy-D-xylulose-5-phosphate synthase; GGDS: geranylgeranyl diphosphate synthase; GDS: geranyl diphosphate synthase; HDR: hydroxy-2-methyl-2-(*E*)-butenyl 4-diphosphate reductase; HDS; hydroxy-2-methyl-2-(*E*)-butenyl 4-diphosphate synthase; IDI: isopentenyl diphosphate isomerase; MCT: 2-*C*-methyl-D-erythritol-4-(cytidyl-5-diphosphate) transferase; MCS: 2-C-methyl-D-erythritol-2,4-cyclodiphosphate synthase.**

synthesized by mevalonate pathway operated in cytosol. Although whole pathway of artemisinin biosynthesis is still not known, enzymes involved in major steps of the pathway have been cloned and functionally characterized. Carbon skeleton of artemisinin is derived from farnesyl diphosphate, a common precursor in the plant cell, which is formed by the condensation of 3 isoprene (C5) units. The first committed step towards the conversion of farnesyl diphosphate (FPP) to artemisinin is catalysed by amorpha-4, 11-diene synthase (ADS) which converts FPP to amorpha 4, 11 diene (Bouwmeester *et al.*, 1999, Mercke *et al.*, 2000) as shown in Figure 7.2. Bouwmeester *et al.* (1999) first reported the partial purification of natural ADS protein from *A. annua*. This enzyme has a pH optimum around 6.5–7.0, a Km of 0.6 µM for FPP, and a molecular weight of 56 kDa. Since ADS catalyses the commit step of artemisinin biosynthesis so it has been proved to be a reasonable target for artemisinin metabolic engineering. Several groups have identified and cloned *ads* independently (Mercke *et al.*, 2000, Chang *et al.*, 2000, Wallaart *et al.*, 2001). Alam and Abdin (2011) while studying the effect of overexpression of *ads* gene from *A. annua* L. and HMG-Co A reductase gene (*hmgr*) introduced from *Catharanthus roseus* (L) G. Don on artemisinin yields in *A. annua* L. plants, observed the increased levels of artemisinin in the transgenic plants. Thus the increased artemisinin levels were found to be correlated with HMG-Co A reductase and amorpha- 4, 11-diene synthase enzymatic activities in the biochemical analyses. In the next step, amorpha-4, 11-diene is hydroxylated to form artemisinic alcohol. This reaction is catalyzed by a cytochrome P450 dependent amorpha-4,11-diene hydroxylase (CYP71AV1) (Teoh *et al.*, 2006). This enzyme can covert the amorpha-4,11-diene all the way to artemisinic acid in an *in vitro* assay (Ro *et al.*, 2006) which is the final enzymatic intermediate and precursor of arteannuin B (Brown and Sy 2004). Alternatively, the artemisinic alcohol can be oxidized to the corresponding aldehyde by alcohol dehydrogenase 1 (ADH1) (Polichuk *et al.*, 2010). In the next step, the aldehyde is reduced to dihydroartemisinic aldehyde by artemisinic aldehyde D11(13) reductase (DBR2) (Zhang *et al.*, 2008). The final enzymatic step known in artemisinin biosynthesis is catalyzed by aldehyde dehydrogenase 1 (ALDH1) (Teoh *et al.*, 2009). After this step many possible intermediates have been identified through metabolic fingerprinting of *A. annua* (Zeng *et al.*, 2008). Radio active isotop labeling has shown that artemisinic acid is a common precursor of arteannuin B and artemisinin (Wang *et al.*, 1988, Sangwan *et al.*, 1993). Nair and Basile (1993) proposed that arteannuin B may be an intermediate in the conversion of artemisinic acid to artemisinin, which was supported by Bharel *et al.* (1998). An enzyme involved in bioconversion of arteannuin B to artemisinin was purified and characterized from *A. annua* (Dhingra *et al.*, 2000 and Dhingra and Narasu 2001). Some workers showed the evidence that the main route for artemisinin biosynthesis is through dihydroartemisinic acid (Wallaart *et al.*, 1999, Sy and Brown 2002). Brown and Sy (2004) fed C^{13} labelled artemisinic acid to intact plantlets through cut shoots and observed no conversion to artemisinin but a large enrichment of arteannuin B occurred, suggesting this may be the end product in the artemisinic acid pathway and not artemisinin as had been previously hypothesized. Role of non-enzymatic or spontaneous photo-oxidative reactions in conversion of artemisinin from its precursors has also been reported. Feeding isotope-labelled dihydroartemisinic acid to intact *A. annua* plant through roots led to production of many labelled sesquiterpene metabolites in shoot tissue but no enrichment of labelled artemisinin was observed. This suggested that artemisinin is not produced by dihydroartemisinic acid (Brown and Sy 2004). However, a variety of other labelled sesquiterpenes were observed but no conversion to artemisininc acid. Included in these metabolites was a carboxyenol derivative of dihydroartemisinic acid that when incubated in chloroform will convert spontaneously to artemisinin. Brown and Sy (2004) hypothesized that this conversion may only happen in a lipophilic environment capable of stabilizing the hydroxyl groups and that *in planta* this could explain the observed enrichment of artemisinin in the lipophilic glandular trichomes. Almost all the genes encoding known enzymes of artemisinin biosynthetic pathway have been cloned and characterized in the form of recombinant enzyme in heterologous system. When the amplification of three main enzymes of artemisinin biosynthesis was performed from the different types of trichome cells, a very interesting finding was that only three enzymes were amplified from the apical cells. No detectable amplification was observed in the sub-apical cells (Olsson *et al.*, 2009). This indicated that the initial steps of artemisinin biosynthesis are taking place exclusively in the apical cells and possibilities of whole pathway starting from FPP to be operated in trichomes cannot be overruled. No amplification of the above three genes was observed in mesophyll cells whereas FPP was found to be expressed in these cells, which is in agreement of the fact that the artemisinin is only produced in trichomes of *A. annua* (Duke *et al.*, 1994).

Liu *et al.* (2011) showed that regulating artemisinin biosynthesis at the gene level is possible. However, overexpressing a single gene is insufficient to increase the nal artemisinin content. Genes for artemisinic aldehyde reductase (Dbr2) might be a good candidate as its overexpression will lead to an increase in artemisinin production. Furthermore, there are still unknown enzymatic (or non-enzymatic) steps between dihydroartemisinic acid and artemisinin in the artemisinin biosynthesis. Elucidation of these steps will be helpful in precise metabolic engineering strategies to improve artemisinin production.

Phenylpropanoid Pathway of *Ocimum* spp.

The genus *Ocimum* belonging to the family Lamiaceae, collectively known as basil, has long been acclaimed for the genetic diversity of the species. The major constituents of plant essential oils fall into two entirely distinct chemical classes, terpenoids and phenylpropanoids. Although terpenes represent the predominant components, occurring much more frequently and abundantly, whenever phenylpropanoids are present they provide indispensable and significant flavour and odour to the oil (Chappell 1995). However, essential oils found in different basil cultivars may vary (Labra *et al.*, 2004). Sweet basil (*O. basilicum*), contains primarily phenol derivatives, such as eugenol, methyl eugenol, chavicol, estragole, and methyl cinnamate, often combined with various amounts of linalool (Miele *et al.*, 2001, Werker *et al.*, 1993). Indian 'sacred basil' (*O. sanctum* = *O. tenuiflorum*) owes a stronger, somewhat pungent taste than other basils due to the presence of sesquiterpenoid, beta-caryophyllene, and a phenylpropanoid, methyl eugenol. The magnificent diversity of phenylpropanoids, in principle, is the result of efficient modification and amplification of a limited set of core structures, derived from the shikimate pathway (Herrmann, 1995).

The largest class of plant volatiles (PVs) is derived from isoprenoid pathways. The second largest class of PVs consists of compounds containing an aromatic ring. Although not all reactions leading to the synthesis of the basic skeletons have been determined, most are derived from intermediates in the pathway that leads from shikimate to phenylalanine and then to an array of primary (such as lignin) and secondary non-volatile compounds (Dudareva *et al.*, 2004). Eugenol (clove essence) is a reduced version of coniferyl alcohol, a lignin precursor (Gang *et al.*, 2001). A large body of literature exists describing the biosynthesis of terpenoid constituents of herb essential oils, with many of the proteins and genes involved in this latter pathway having been purified and cloned (Chappell 1995, Bohlmann *et al.*, 1998, Wise *et al.*, 1998). However, surprisingly little is known about the biosynthesis of eugenol and chavicol, the simplest phenylpropenes and their derivatives. Labelling experiments of leaf segments with radioactive Phenylalanine (Phe) indicated that Phenylalanine is their initial precursor (Manitto *et al.*, 1974, Klischies *et al.*, 1975, Manitto *et al.*, 1975, Senanayake *et al.*, 1977). Based on these results, two proposed biosynthetic pathways to these and related phenylpropenes are proposed. The first committed step to the phenylpropenes, the de-amination of Phe to generate cinnamic acid, is catalysed by the well-known and widely distributed enzyme Phe ammonia lyase (PAL). The next steps are likely to be the formation of *p*-coumaric and ferulic acids from cinnamic acid (addition of 4-hydroxyl and 3-methoxyl functionalities). These reactions may involve the prior formation of the coenzyme A (CoA) esters, or they may proceed directly, with the substrates in the free acid form. Both pathways have been proposed to be involved in the formation of the monolignols required for lignification (Boudet *et al.*, 1998). Confirmation of the last step in the formation of methylchavicol and methyleugenol, the addition of the methyl group to the 4-OH, has been reported (Wang *et al.*, 1997, Wang and Pichersky, 1999, Lewinsohn *et al.*, 2001). Thus, the critical intermediary steps in chavicol and eugenol biosynthesis are still an open question.

The initial three steps of the pathway catalysed by PAL, cinnamate 4-hydroxylase, and 4-coumaroyl CoA- ligase are mandatory and provide the basis for all subsequent branches and resulting metabolites. Three enzymes of phenylpropanoid metabolism, including phenylalanine ammonia-lyase (PAL), 4-coumarate:CoA ligase (4CL) and NADPH:cytochrome P450 oxidoreductase (CPR) form tight regulatory. The first step in the pathway consists of a deamination of phenylalanine by the phenylalanine ammonia-lyase (PAL) that produces cinnamic acid. Subsequent steps downstream of PAL, leading to phenylpropanoid monomers (with exception of cinnamate 4-hydroxylase), are encoded by small gene families (Hamberger *et al.*, 2007). With respect to its impact on the phenylpropanoid metabolism, it seems surprising that among nearly 300 functional genes encoding cytochrome P450s in *Arabidopsis*, 4-hydroxylation of trans-cinnamate to 4-coumarate is encoded by a single gene that is CYP73A5 or cinnamate 4-hydroxylase (C4H). CYP73A5 catalyses the 4-hydroxylation of cinnamic acid to form *p*-coumaric acid. C4H is the type of cytochrome P450 enzymes which are membrane-bound, heme iron containing monooxygenases and in most of the cases use NADPH+H+ as a co-substrate by forming a complex with a cytochrome P450 reductase (Fischer *et al.*, 2001). Mutations in CYP73A5 severely affect the growth and development of plants and result in the accumulation of the quite unusual cinnamoylmalate in leaves (Schilmiller *et al.*, 2009). Until this step the pathways for general phenylpropanoid and lignin biosynthetic pathway are similar. But in the subsequent steps different enzymes were involved in two pathways. The main genes encoding enzymes for general phenylpropenes like eugenol, isoeugenol, or chavicol is shown in Figure 7.3.

The subsequent step, encoded by the small gene family of 4-CL ligases, channels the resulting aromatic CoA-esters to different biosynthetic pathways. 4-coumaroyl CoA probably represents the most important branch point within the central phenylpropanoid biosynthesis in plants.

4CL plays an important role in plant defence reactions because of its position, joining the phenylpropanoid pathway with lignin and flavonoid branch pathways. Different isoforms of 4CL direct carbon flow to the diverse pathways of phenylpropanoid metabolism according to different substrate preferences (Singh *et al.*, 2010). Multiple isoforms of *4CLs* have been identified and cloned in many plant species (Lee *et al.*, 1995, Allina *et al.*, 1998, Hu *et al.*, 1998, Ehlting *et al.*, 1999, Cukovic *et al.*, 2001, Costa *et al.*, 2005, Shi *et al.*, 2010). Phylogenetic reconstruction studies from several plants indicate two large, evolutionary ancient classes of *4CLs* (Class I and Class II) (Ehlting *et al.*, 1999). Class I *4CLs* are more closely associated with the biosynthesis of lignin as demonstrated by antisense or RNAi suppression studies (Kajita *et al.*, 1997, Lee *et al.*, 1997, Li *et al.*, 2003, Wagner *et al.*, 2009, Gui *et al.*, 2011). Likely involvement of Class II *4CLs* is predicted for other phenolic compounds biosynthesis on the basis of compartmentalized expression in various plant organs and tissues (Hu *et al.*, 1998, Ehlting *et al.*, 1999) but this has never been demonstrated biochemically. Rastogi *et al.* (2013) have reported a class II 4CL isolated from the glandular trichomes of *Ocimum sanctum* diverging the flux towards eugenol biosynthesis. The study involved the RNAi suppression of the 4CL gene *in planta* and the effect of suppression was the reduced eugenol content as compared to the control. This was the first report of 4CL gene involvement in the eugenol biosynthesis as its role was reported in lignin, flavonoid and other phenolic compounds biosynthesis (Hamada *et al.*, 2004, Kumar and Ellis 2003, Costa *et al.*, 2005, Hu *et al.*, 1998, Weitzel and Petersen 2010, Yamauchi *et al.*, 2003, Hamberger and Hahlbrock 2004, Ehlting *et al.*, 1999, Endler *et al.*, 2008).

In the next step, cinnamoyl CoA reductase (CCR) catalyses the conversion of hydroxyl cinnamic acid CoA esters to the corresponding hydroxyl cinnamaldehydes (Van der Rest *et al.*, 2006) which belongs to oxido-reductase family (Lauvergeat *et al.*, 2001). Cinnamoyl CoA reductase is the rst committed enzyme of the lignin branch biosynthetic pathway. Cloning, expression and phylogenetic relationships have shown the role of this enzyme in controlling the carbon ux into lignins (Piquemal *et al.*, 1998). Lauvergeat *et al.* (2001) reported the characterisation of two functionally and structurally distinct cDNA clones, AtCCR1 and AtCCR2 (81.6 per cent protein sequence identity) in *Arabidopsis thaliana,* where AtCCR1 was found to be ve times more efficient with feruloyl-CoA and sinapoyl-CoA than AtCCR2.

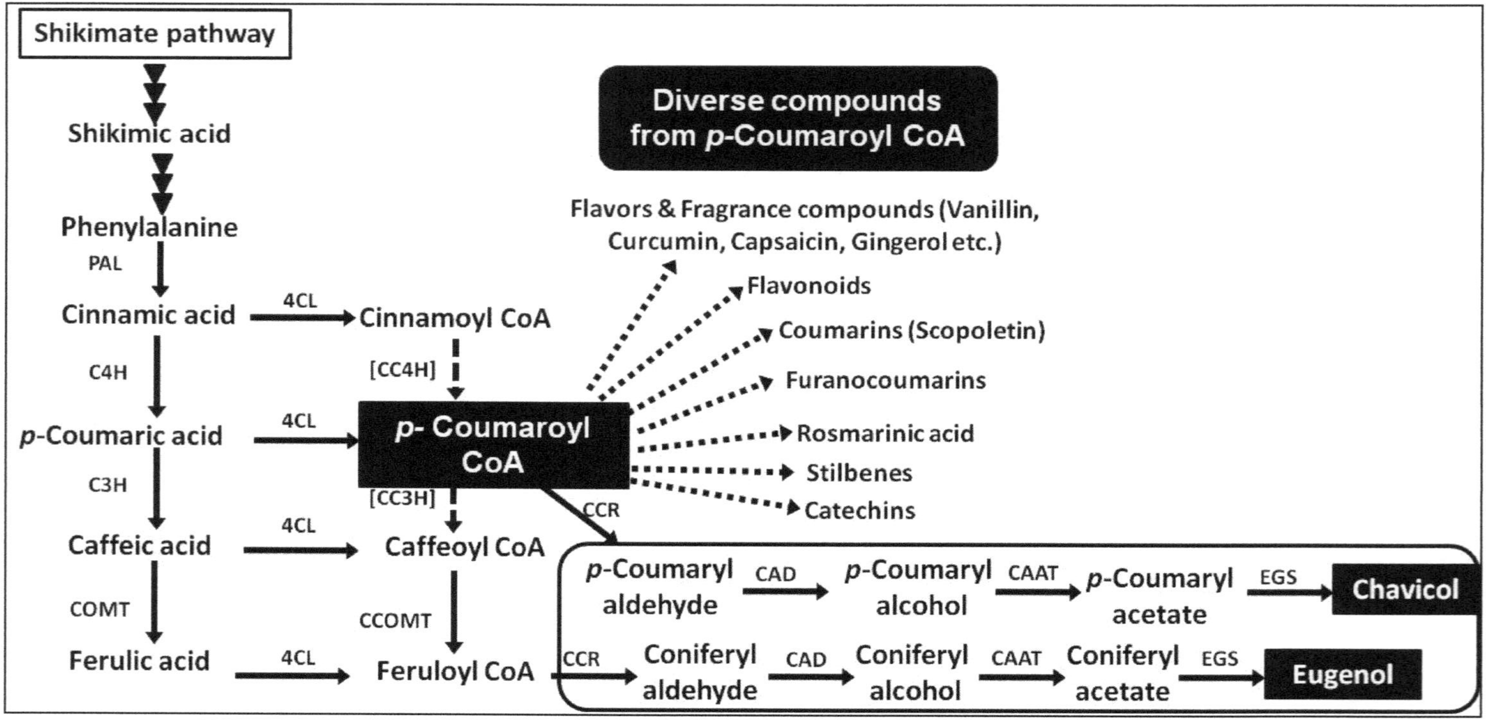

Figure 7.3: Proposed Biosynthetic Pathway of Eugenol/Chavicol Synthesis in *Ocimum sanctum.*

(C4H, cinnamate 4-hydroxylase; C3H, p-coumarate 3-hydroxylase; COMT, caffeoyl O-methyl transferase; CC4H, cinnamoyl-CoA 4-hydroxylase; CC3H, p-coumaroyl-CoA 3-hydroxylase; CCOMT, caffeoyl-CoA O-methyl transferase; CCR, cinnamoyl-CoA reductase; and CAD, cinnamyl alcohol dehydrogenase; CAAT, coniferyl alcohol acetyl transferase; EGS, eugenol (and chavicol) synthase). The enzymes for 4- and 3-hydroxylation of CoA esters have not been demonstrated yet and hence [CC4H] and [CC3H] are indicated in parenthesis to indicate their probable role.

In addition, dierential expression of the two genes during development and in response to infection was studied and AtCCR1 was observed to be preferentially expressed in tissues undergoing lignication. In contrast, AtCCR2, poorly expressed during development, but strongly and transiently induced during the incompatible interaction with *Xanthomonas campestris* pv. *campestris* leading to a hypersensitive response. Altogether, the work of Lauvergeat *et al.* (2001) suggested that AtCCR1 is involved in constitutive lignication whereas AtCCR2 is involved in the biosynthesis of phenolics whose accumulation may lead to resistance. Derikvand *et al.* (2008) identified and characterized two new knockout mutants for CCR1. Both mutants had a dwarf phenotype with delayed senescence. At complete maturity, their inflorescence stems displayed decreased lignin levels with some alterations in lignin structure and a higher content in cell wall- bound ferulic esters. Ferulic acid-coniferyl alcohol ether dimers were found for the first time in dicot cell walls and at similar levels in wild-type and mutant plants. The expression of CCR2, a CCR gene usually involved in plant defense, was increased in the mutants and could account for the biosynthesis of lignins in the CCR1-knockout plants. Derikvand *et al.* (2008) demonstrated the redirection of the phenylpropanoid pathway to feruloyl malate in *Arabidopsis* mutants deficient for cinnamoyl-CoA reductase 1 emphasizing the remarkable plasticity of *Arabidopsis* phenylpropanoid metabolism. After the synthesis of coniferaldehyde from *p*-coumaroyl-CoA by cinnamoyl-CoA reductase (CCR) comes into play the enzyme, cinnamyl alcohol dehydrogenase (CAD). The cinnamyl alcohol dehydrogenase (CAD) multigene family *in planta* depicts a class of NADPH dependent enzymes catalysing reduction of various phenylpropenyl aldehyde derivatives and whose metabolic products are the precursors of structural lignins, health-related lignans, and various other metabolites (Kim *et al.*, 2004, Youn *et al.*, 2006). CAD catalyses the reduction of coniferaldehyde to coniferyl alcohol in the biosynthesis of eugenol. Barakat *et al.* (2009) while describing the cinnamyl alcohol dehydrogenase gene family in *Populus* based on the phylogeny, organization, and expression showed that CAD genes fall into three main classes (clades): one represented by CAD sequences from both gymnosperms and angiosperms whereas the other two clades represented sequences from the angiosperms only. A total of 16 CAD genes were reported from *Populus* out of which all CAD genes, except PoptrCAD 4, got distributed in Class II and Class III. CAD genes associated with xylem development (PoptrCAD 4 and PoptrCAD 10) belong to Class I and Class II. Phylogenetic analyses associated with expression profiling and results from previous studies suggested that CAD genes involved in wood development belong to Class I and Class II. The other CAD genes from Class II and Class III may function in plant tissues under biotic stresses. In *Arabidopsis*, CAD exists as a multigene family consisting of nine genes (AtCAD1 to AtCAD9) (Tavares *et al.*, 2000, Sibout *et al.*, 2003). Although all nine have been classified as CAD genes based on their predicted protein sequences, only CAD-C (AtCAD5) and CAD-D (AtCAD4) have been shown to have major roles in lignin synthesis in *Arabidopsis* (Sibout *et al.*, 2003, Kim *et al.*, 2007). AtCAD7 and AtCAD8 may also be involved to some extent in lignin biosynthesis (Kim *et al.*, 2007). AtCAD2, AtCAD3, AtCAD6, and AtCAD9 appear to encode mannitol dehydrogenases. A double mutation of AtCAD2 and AtCAD6 led to an over-expression of AtCAD1 (AtCAD7) suggesting a compensation between some CAD genes (Sibout *et al.*, 2005). In *Oryza*, 12 CAD genes have been reported (Zhang *et al.*, 2006). Damiani *et al.* (2005) reported the functional characterization of CAD1 in tobacco by generating transgenic tobacco plants with reduced CAD1 expression through an RNAi strategy to support a signicant contribution of CAD1 to the synthesis of coniferyl alcohol *in planta*, along with the previously characterized CAD2 enzymes.

It was reported that coniferyl alcohol is converted into coniferyl acetate by a member of BAHD family- coniferyl alcohol acetyltransferase to produce coniferyl acetate (Dexter *et al.*, 2007, Koeduka *et al.*, 2006). BADH family is named for the first four biochemically characterized enzymes of this family, BEAT (acetyl- CoA:benzyl alcohol acetyltransferase), AHCT (anthocyanin *O*- hydroxy-cinnamoyltransferase), HCBT (anthranilate *N*-hydroxycinnamoyl/benzoyltransferase) and DAT (deacetylvindoline 4-*O*-acetyltransferase) (Osbourn and Lanzotti 2009). Subsequently, NADPH-dependent reduction of the coniferyl acetate by eugenol synthase (EGS) and/isoeugenol synthase (IGS) results in eugenol/isoeugenol synthesis. Eugenol and isoeugenol differ exclusively at the position of the double bond in propene side chain. In petunia their formation is mediated by two different and highly divergent NADPH-dependent reductases (Osbourn and Lanzotti 2009). To substantiate coniferyl acetate as the substrate of isoeugenol synthase Dexter *et al.* (2006) identied and characterized a novel petunia gene (PhIGS1) encoding an enzyme belonging to the BAHD acyltransferase family whose expression correlated with isoeugenol biosynthesis. RNAi suppression of PhIGS1 gene resulted in the inhibition of isoeugenol biosynthesis rendering the direct correlation of coniferyl acetate being the substrate of PhIGS1 (Dexter *et al.*, 2006). Koeduka *et al.* (2008) reported presence of CbIGS1 and CbEGS1 genes in *Clarkia breweri*, which catalyze the formation of isoeugenol and eugenol, respectively.

The structure of EGS, catalysing the reductive replacement of the propenyl side chain has been resolved by X-ray crystallography. EGS is the main enzyme involved in regulation of eugenol in *Ocimum* (Louie *et al.*, 2007). Other enzymes which catalyse important steps in other phenylpropenes, lignin etc. were also characterized. Coumarate 3-Hydroxylase (C3H) was originally named after its suspected function of C3-hydroxylation of *p* -coumaric acid and production of caffeic acid. In *Arabidopsis* CYP98A3 (C3H1) was shown to preferentially convert the shikimate and quinate esters of *p*-coumaric acid into the corresponding caffeic acid conjugates, whereas *p*-coumaric acid and *p*-coumaroyl- CoA were not substrates of this enzyme (Raes *et al.*, 2003). Schoch *et al.* (2006) observed that meta-hydroxylation is not catalyzed on the free *p*-coumaric acid as anticipated, but on its conjugates with shikimic, quinic, or phenyllactic acids. All CYP98s show phenol meta-hydroxylase activity but *p*-coumaroylshikimate remains the preferred substrate. Since the disruption of CYP98A3 gene in *Arabidopsis thaliana* leads to a drastic inhibition of lignin synthesis, cell growth, and plant development it was suggested that meta-hydroxylation of phenolic precursors is essential for higher plant development (Schoch *et al.*, 2006). Most importantly, the occurrence of the meta-hydroxylation on esters of shikimic or quinic acids introduces a new biochemical regulation mechanism in the phenylpropanoid pathway. A bifunctional

O- Methyl transferase (OMT) appears to be involved in catalysing the methylation of both caffeic and 5-hydroxyferulic acids, although it is generally referred to as COMT. Plant *O*-methyltransferases (OMTs) have important roles in secondary metabolite biosynthesis and use S-adenosyl-l-methionine (SAM) as methyl source, yielding S-adenosyl- homocysteine and the methyl ether derivative as product (Schwab 2003). Some basil varieties are able to convert the phenylpropenes chavicol and eugenol to methylchavicol and methyleugenol, respectively. Gang *et al.* (2002) isolated Chavicol *O*-methyltransferase (CVOMT) and eugenol *O*-methyltransferase (EOMT). Both CVOMT1 and EOMT1 catalyzes the *O*-methylation of chavicol, with equal efficiency, but EOMT1 was much more efficient in *O*-methylating eugenol. Molecular modelling, based on the crystal structure of IOMT, suggested that a single amino acid difference was responsible for the difference in substrate discrimination between CVOMT1 and EOMT1, as confirmed by site-directed mutagenesis with appropriate mutants of both the genes exhibiting the opposite substrate preference relative to the respective native enzyme (Gang *et al.*, 2002).

Withanolides Biosynthesis in *Withania* sp.

Withania somnifera (family Solanaceae), commonly known as "Ashwagandha" or Indian ginseng, is an important medicinal plant of Indian origin and has been used for centuries in Ayurvedic medicine to increase longevity and vitality. The roots are the main portions of the plant used therapeutically. *W. somnifera* has been used as an antioxidant, adaptogen, aphrodisiac, liver tonic, antiinflammatory agent, astringent and more recently to treat ulcers, bacterial infection, venom toxins and senile dementia. Clinical trials and animal research support the use of plant for anxiety, cognitive and neurological disorders, inflammation, hyperlipidemia and Parkinson's disease (Gupta and Rana 2007). In view of its varied therapeutic potential, it has also been the subject of considerable modern scientific attention. The biologically active constituents of the *Withania* genus are withanolides which are a group of naturally occurring C28 -steroidal lactone triterpenoids built on an intact or rearranged ergostane framework, in which C-22 and C-26 are appropriately oxidized to form a six-membered lactone ring (Mirjalili *et al.*, 2009).

Though *W. somnifera* constituents have been extensively explored for the pharmacological importance and metabolic proling (Gupta *et al.*, 2011) very little information is available on biosynthetic pathways of these steroidal bioactive molecules. In recent years, biochemical and molecular studies have been initiated for elucidation of biosynthetic pathways of various withanolides in *W. somnifera* (Sharma *et al.*, 2007, Madina *et al.*, 2007, Senthil *et al.*, 2010). These signature secondary metabolites of *W. somnifera* may diverge from sterol pathway at the level of 24-methylene cholesterol (Sangwan *et al.*, 2008). Thus, 24-methylene cholesterol through classical cytosolic mevalonate (MVA) and plastid localized 2-C-methyl-D-erythritol-4-phosphate (MEP) pathways (Figure 7.4) are the probable sources of synthesis of major bioactive molecules of *Withania* (Gupta *et al.*, 2011). It has been demonstrated that there is only 30 per cent of plant contribution for withanolides production *via* MEP pathway in biosynthesis of precursor isoprenoids (Tuli and Sangwan, 2010).

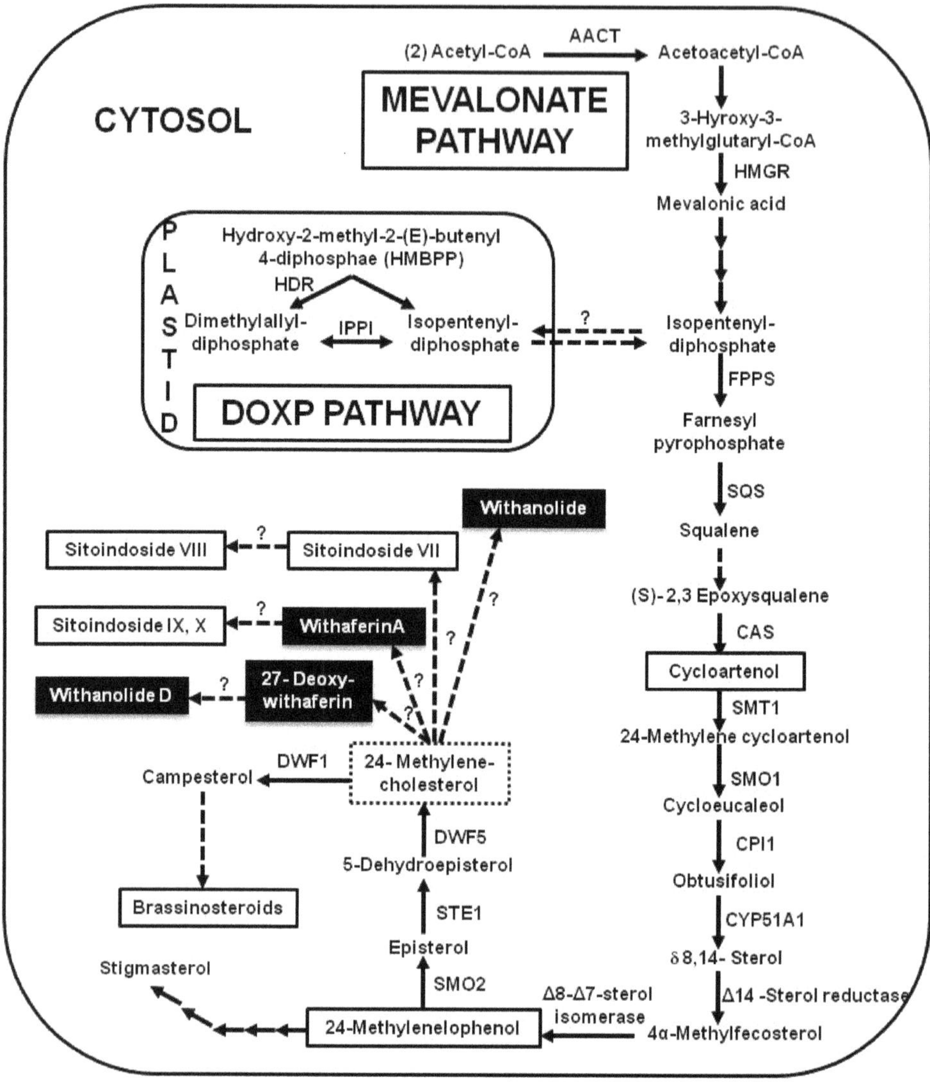

Figure 7.4: An Overview of Putative Withanolide Biosynthesic Pathway. HMBPP: 1-hydroxy-2-methyl-2- (E)-butenyl 4-diphosphate, IPPI:Isopentylpyrophosphate isomerase, FPPS: farnesyldiphosphate synthase, SQS: Squalene synthase, CAS: Cycloartinol synthase, SMT-1: Sterol methyl transferase/cytochrome P450 reductase, CPL1: cycloeucalenol cycloisomerase, CYP51A1: Obtusifoliol-14-demethylase/ cytochrome P450 reductase, SMO2: methylsterol monooxygenase, STE1: Delta7-sterol-C5-desaturase, DWF5: Sterol-delta7-reductase and DWF1: Delta24-reductase. Single dark arrows represent one step, two or more dark arrows represent multiple steps and dashed arrow represents unknown steps.

First step in the MEP pathway is condensation of pyruvate with D-glyceraldehyde-3-phosphate to form 1-deoxy-D-xylulose-5-phosphate (DXP), catalyzed by DXP synthase (DXS). DXP not only serves as a precursor for isopentanyl diphosphate

IPP) and dimethylallyl diphosphate (DMAPP) biosynthesis but is also involved as an intermediate for thiamine and pyridoxal biosynthesis (Julliard and Douce 1991, Julliard 1992, Himmeldirk *et al.*, 1996). The subsequent step of MEP pathway involves conversion of DXP to MEP, catalyzed by DXP reductoisomerase (DXR). Gupta *et al.* (2012) characterized two genes encoding 1-deoxy-D-xylulose-5-phosphate synthase (DXS; EC 2.2.1.7) and 1-deoxy-D-xylulose-5-phosphate reductase (DXR; EC 1.1.1.267) enzymes from *W. somnifera*, *WsDXS* and *WsDXR*. The expression analysis suggests that *WsDXS* and *WsDXR* are differentially expressed in different tissues (with maximal expression in flower and young leaf). Expression of WsDXS and WsDXR also vary in chemotypes of *Withania*, and in response to salicylic acid, methyl jasmonate, as well as in mechanical injury. Analysis of genomic organization of *WsDXS* shows close similarity with tomato DXS in terms of exon–intron arrangements. Gupta *et al.* (2012) characterized isoprenoid biosynthesis pathway genes from *Withania*. In MEP/MVA pathways, farnesyl diphosphate (FPP), which is synthesized by catalytic action of the enzyme farnesyl diphosphate synthase (FPPS), serves as a substrate for rst committed reaction of several branched pathways (Chappell 1995). This leads to synthesis of compounds that are essential for plant growth including metabolites like sterols, dolichols, ubiquinones and carotenoids as well as substrates for farnesylation and geranylgeranylation of proteins (Gupta *et al.*, 2011). FPPS and squalene synthase (SqS) constitute key steps en route to production of the progenitor(s) of withanolide biosynthesis (Figure 7.4). Gupta *et al.* (2011) have characterized a gene (WsFPPS), encoding farnesyl diphosphate synthase (FPPS; EC 2.5.1.10), a key enzyme in the pathway of biosynthesis of isoprenoids, from *W. somnifera*. The amino acid sequence homology and phylogenetic analysis suggested the close similarity of *WsFPPS* to its counterparts from tomato (*SlFPPS*) and capsicum (*CaaFPPS*) (Gupta *et al.*, 2011). Expression pattern of the *WsFPPS* gene differs in tissues of *Withania* chemotypes, as well as in response to elicitors (salicylic acid and methyl jasmonate) and mechanical wounding. Thus expression of *WsFPPS* varies in different tissues (with maximal expression in ower and young leaf) and chemotypes. There was a signicant elevation in response to salicylic acid, methyl jasmonate and mechanical injury (Gupta *et al.*, 2011).

For the perspective of biochemical, molecular and pathway engineering, it is important to characterize key pathway genes and to have the understanding of regulatory role in the biosynthesis of bioactive metabolites. Cytochrome P450 enzymes are one of the largest and most functionally diverse protein super-families which have a crucial role in various metabolic molecular reactions like- hydroxylations, dealkylations, sulphoxidations, epoxidations, reductive dehalogenations, peroxidations and various types of isomerization for the synthesis of a group of primary and secondary metabolites essential for plant growth and development (Guengerich 2001, Hrycay and Bandiera 2012). Different paralogs of CPR were found to possess diverse physiological roles particularly in secondary metabolism, plant adaptation and defence mechanism by maintaining electron supply to different P450 monooxygenases (Schuler and Reichhart 2003). Rana *et al.* (2013) reported cloning and characterization of two paralogs of CPR (*WsCPR1*and *WsCPR2*). Quantitative real-time PCR analysis indicated that both genes were widely expressed in leaves, stalks, roots, flowers and berries with higher expression level of *WsCPR2* as compared to *WsCPR1*. Similar to CPRs of other plant species *WsCPR1* was un-inducible while *WsCPR2* transcript level increased in a time dependent manner after elicitor treatments. The investigation was also inclusive of comparative tissue-specific expression analysis of *WsCPR1* and *WsCPR2* and changes in three key withanolides namely withanolide A (WS-1), withanone (WS-2) and withaferin A (WS-3) in response to elicitor stimuli methyl jasmonate (MeJA) and salicylic acid (SA). High performance liquid chromatography of withanolides extracted from elicitor-treated samples showed a significant increase in two of the key withanolides, withanolide A and withaferin A, possibly indicating the role of *WsCPR2* in withanolide biosynthesis.

Since expressed sequence tags (ESTs) are robustly proven for gene prospection, Pal *et al.* (2011) used an EST-based approach to analyse gene expression profiles in *W. somnifera* plants by generating separate leaf and root cDNA libraries which yielded 495 leaf and 76 root ESTs. Two of the leaf ESTs *viz.* sterol methyl transferase (*SMT1*) and obtusifoliol-14-demethylase (*ODM*) were then converted into full-length gene sequences as their products claimed to be involved in the biosynthetic pathway leading to withanolide biosynthesis. Since there is no detailed description about the withanolide biosynthesis pathway, we have tried to recollect and provide concise information about this pathway referring to the KEGG PATHWAY Database (http://www.genome.jp/kegg/pathway.html). Isoprenyl pyrophosphate (IPP) from the plastidial MEP pathway and cytosolic MVA pathway gets converted to geranyl pyrophosphate (GPP) which acts as substrate for FPPS, leading to the formation of FPP. Then comes into play squalene synthase (SqS) which converts FPP to squalene. Further squalene gets converted to (s)-2, 3-epoxysqualene by yet unknown enzyme. (s)-2, 3-Epoxysqualene is not only the precursor to sterols biosynthesis but also contributes to α- amyrin, lupeol and saponin biosynthesis. (s)-2, 3-Epoxysqualene upon reaction catalysed by cycloartenol synthase results in the formation of cycloartenol. This cycloartenol is then converted to 24- methylenecycloartenol with the help on enzymes sterol methyl transferase 1(SMT1). 24- methylenecycloartenol in the presence of methylsterol mono-oxygenase (SMO1) enzyme gets converted to cycloeucaleol, which is the substrate for the enzyme cycloeucaleol cycloisomerase, resulting in the formation of obtusifoliol. Obtusifoliol is then converted to δ 8,14-sterol by a cytochrome P450, family 51 (CYP51A1) enzyme, obtusifoliol-14α-demethylase. The next step involves the enzyme Δ14 -Sterol reductase which takes up δ 8,14-sterol as a substrate and converts it to 4α-methylfecosterol, which gets acted upon by Δ8-Δ7-sterol isomerase to form 24-methylenelophenol. This diverging step is the decisive step for the carbon flux towards the synthesis of 24-methylenecholesterol (precursor for withanolide biosynthesis) and stigmasterol. 24-methylenelophenol. They can be acted upon by C4-demethylase, as well as sterol methyl transferase2 (SMT2) to form episterol and 24-ethylidenelophenol, respectively. Episterol branch leads to 24-methylenecholesterol while 24-ethylidenelophenol leads to stigmasterol synthesis. The enzyme Δ^7-sterol C5-desaturase, which catalyses episterol to form 5-dehydro episterol, finally converted to 24-methylenecholesterol in the presence of the enzyme sterol Δ^7 reductase. The level of 24-methylene cholesterol formation is imperative because the signature secondary metabolites (withanolides, withaferin and sitoinosides) of *W. somnifera* diverge from sterol pathway at this level.

Approaches for Associating Functions to a Gene

There are various approaches to associate a function to a particular gene of plant but one of the most revolutionary is RNA interference technology (RNAi). RNAi technology has also been used to accelerate breeding of aromatic and medicinal plants, where a conventional mutation breeding approach fails as in case of opium poppy (Allen *et al.*, 2004). Medicinal and aromatic plants have always been intimately linked with human health and culture. Despite of immense uses secondary metabolites produced from medicinal and aromatic plants, identification and characterization of species specific genes involved in the following possible reasons associated with medicinal plants: (i) low concentration of desired phytomolecules, (ii) medicinal crops being low priority crops, (iii) technical difculty in cultivation of these crops, (iv) over-harvesting of naturally occurring herbal plants, (v) destructive collection techniques, and (vi) conversion of habitats of medicinal plants to crop-based agriculture (Kumar and Gupta, 2008).

Transgenic approach for improvement of yield and quality of a secondary metabolite can be applied in order to target a rate- limiting steps through manipulation of the expression of individual structural genes, which in turn would increase the ux rate towards the downstream reactions either by overexpression of genes encoding enzymes or by blocking the competitive pathways using anti-sense genes or RNAi (Verpoorte *et al.*, 1999, Gomez-Galera *et al.*, 2007). Maeda *et al.* (2010) using RNAi suppression of arogenate dehydratase1 (ADT1) revealed that phenylalanine is synthesized predominantly via the arogenate pathway in *Petunia* petals. This provided genetic evidence to uncover a novel posttranscriptional regulation of the shikimate pathway. Klempien *et al.* (2012) in order to explore the contribution of CoA Ligases to benzenoid biosynthesis in *Petunia* flowers, performed RNA interference suppression of Ph-4CL1 and observed no effect on the petunia benzenoid scent prole. Whereas downregulation of Ph-CNL resulted in a decrease in emission of benzylbenzoate, phenylethylbenzoate, and methylbenzoate, thereby associating Ph-CNL in aromatic compounds synthesis. Rastogi *et al.* (2013) reported a 4CL gene isoform (Os4CL) isolated from the peltate glandular trichomes of *Ocimum sanctum*, to be directly involved in the synthesis of aromatic compound eugenol, as the RNAi construct infiltrated leaves of the gene (pART/*Os4CLi*) *in planta* showed reduced eugenol content. Hence RNAi has the potential to be used as a fruitful technology in associating functions to the genes involved in the complex secondary metabolites synthesis network.

Conclusion

The genomics and post-genomics developments in plant biology have enhanced our knowledge on the genetics and biochemistry of the production of secondary metabolites in MAPs. In the past, more emphasis has been given on the development of transgenic plants in order to improve yield and quality of pharmaceutically important secondary metabolites in simple and model plant species. However, use of genetic engineering in medicinal plant species for improving yield of pharmaceutical products has been a challenge because of several limitations such as gene silencing, unpredictable results due to the complex network of genes, and no increment in the concentration of desirable secondary metabolites up to the level of commercialization. New strategies of genetic manipulation of metabolic pathways that have been developed are proving useful. The use of regulatory genes can be an alternative to overcome the limitation of the structural gene approach for manipulation of entire or a part of a metabolic pathway, but the progress in identication of regulatory genes is slow. For developing the full potential of metabolic engineering it is necessary to increase our knowledge about plant secondary metabolism, at the level of the intermediates, the enzymes and the genes. The silencing of genes by RNA interference has become the technology of choice for investigation of gene functions in different organisms including MAPs. RNAi in recent years has been tested successfully for improving secondary metabolite production in MAPs. The tremendous potential with RNAi technology is expected to revolutionize the secondary metabolites production for meeting the growing requirements.

References

Acton N, Klayman DL, Rollman IJ. Reductive electrochemical HPLC assay for artemisinin (Qinghaosu). *Planta Medica*. 47: 445-446. 1985.

Alam P, Abdin MZ. Over-expression of HMG-CoA reductase and amorpha-4, 11-diene synthase genes in *Artemisia annua* L. and its inuence on artemisinin content. *Pl. Cell Rep*. 30: 1919–1928. 2011.

Allen RS, Millgate AM, Chitty JA, Thistleton J *et al.*, RNAi-mediated replacement of morphine with the non-narcotic alkaloid reticuline in opium poppy. *Nat. Biotech*. 22: 1559–1566. 2004.

Alonso WR, Rajaonarivony JIM, Gershenzon J, Croteau R. Purification of 4-S limonene synthase, a monoterpene cyclase from glandular trichomes of peppermint (*Mentha* x *piperita*) and spearmint (*M. spicata*). *J. Biologl. Chem*. 267: 7582-7587. 1992.

Begue JP, Bonnet-Delpon D. The future of antimalarials: Artemisinins and synthetic endoperoxides. *Drugs Future*. 30: 509-518. 2005.

Bertea C M, Schalk M, Karp F, Maffei M, Croteau R. Demonstration that menthofuran synthase of mint (*Mentha*) is a cytochrome P450 monooxygenase: cloning, functional expression and characterization of the responsible gene. *Arch. Biochem. Biophys*. 390: 279-286. 2001.

Bevan, M. Bancroft I, Bent E, Love K *et al.*, Analysis of 1.9 Mb of contiguous sequence from chromosome 4 of *Arabidopsis thaliana*. *Nature*. 391: 485–488. 1998.

Bharel S, Gulati A, Abdin MZ, Srivastava PS *et al.*, Enzymic synthesis of artemisinin from natural and synthetic precursors. *J. Natl. Prod*. 61: 633-636. 1998.

Bohlmann J, Meyer-Gauen G and Croteau R. Plant terpenoid synthases: molecular biology and phylogenetic analysis. *Proc. Natl. Acad. Sci. USA*. 95: 4126. 1998.

Boudet AM, Goffner D, Marque C, Grima PJ. Genes involved in the final steps of monolignol biosynthesis and their manipulation for tailoring new lignins. *Amer. Chem. Soc*. 697: 65–75. 1998.

Bouwmeester HJ, Wallaart TE, Janssen MH, van Loo B, Jansen BJ *et al.*, Amorpha-4, 11-diene synthase catalyses the first probable step in artemisinin biosynthesis. *Phytochem.* 52: 843–854. 1999.

Brown GD, Sy LK. In vivo transformations of dihydroartemisinic acid in *Artemisia annua* plants. *Tetrahedron.* 60: 1139-1159. 2004.

Burke CC, Wildung MR, Croteau R. Geranyl diphosphate synthase: cloning, expression and characterization of this prenyl transferase as heterodimer. *Proc. Natl. Acad. Sci.* USA. 96: 13062-13067. 1999.

Cane DE. Sesquiterpene biosynthesis: cyclization mechanisms. In: *Comprehensive Natural Products Chemistry: Isoprenoids Including Steroids and Carotenoids* (ed: Cane DE) Pergamon, Oxford. P. 1-13.1999.

Chang YJ, Song SH, Park SH, Kim SU. Amorpha-4,11-diene Synthase of *Artemisia annua*: cDNA Isolation and Bacterial Expression of a Terpene Synthase Involved in Artemisinin Biosynthesis. *Arch. Biochem. Biophy.* 383: 178-184. 2000.

Chappell J. The biochemistry and molecular biology of isoprenoid metabolism. *Plant Physiol.* 107: 1–6.1995.

Chapple C, Carpita N. Plant cell walls as targets for biotechnology. *Curr. Op. Plant Biol.* 1: 179–85. 1998.

Colby SM, Alonso WR, Katahira EJ, McGarvey DJ, Croteau R. 4S-Limonene synthase from the oil glands of spearmint (*Mentha spicata*): cDNA isolation, characterization and bacterial expression of the catalytically active monoterpene cyclase. *J. Biologl. Chem.* 268: 23016–23024. 1993.

Costa MA, Bedgar DL, Moinuddin SGA, Kim K *et al.*, Characterization in vitro and in vivo of the putative multigene 4-coumarate: CoA ligase network in *Arabidopsis*: syringyl lignin and sinapate/sinapyl alcohol derivative formation. *Phytochem.* 66: 2072–2091. 2005.

Cukovic D, Ehlting J, VanZiffle JA, Douglas CJ. Structure and evolution of 4-coumarate: coenzyme A ligase (*4CL*) gene families. *Biol. Chem.* 382: 645–654. 2001.

Damiani I, Morreel K, Danoun S, Goeminne G *et al.*, Metabolite proling reveals a role for atypical cinnamyl alcohol dehydrogenase CAD1 in the synthesis of coniferyl alcohol in tobacco xylem. *Pl. Mol. Biol.* 59: 753–769. 2005.

Davis EM, Ringer KL, McConkey ME, Croteau R. Monoterpene metabolism. Cloning, expression, and characterization of menthone reductases from peppermint. *Plant Physiol.* 137: 873-881. 2005.

Derikvand MM, Sierra JB, Ruel K, Pollet B, Do C *et al.*, Redirection of the phenylpropanoid pathway to feruloyl malate in *Arabidopsis* mutants de W cient for cinnamoyl-CoA reductase 1. *Planta.* 227: 943–956. 2008.

Dexter R, Qualley A, Kish CM, Ma CJ *et al.*, Characterization of a Petunia acetyltransferase involved in the biosynthesis of the floral volatile isoeugenol. *Plant J.* 49: 265–275. 2007.

Dhingra V, Narasu ML. Purification and characterization of an enzyme involved in biochemical transformation of arteannuin B to artemisinin from *Artemisia annua*. *Biochem. Biophys. Res. Comm.* 281: 558–561. 2001.

Dhingra V, Rao KV, Narasu ML. Current status of artemisinin and its derivatives as antimalarial drugs. *Life Sci.* 66: 279-300. 2000.

Dudareva N, Pichersky E, Gershenzon J. Biochemistry of plant volatiles. *Pl. Physiol.* 135: 1893–1902. 2004.

Duke MV, Paul RN, Elsohly HN, Sturtz G, Duke SO. Localization of artemisinin and artemisitene in foliar tissues of glanded and glandless biotypes of *Artemisia annua* L. *Intl. J. Pl. Sci.* 155: 365–372. 1994.

Efferth T. Molecular pharmacology and pharmacogenomics of artemisinin and its derivatives in cancer cells. *Curr. Drug Targets.* 7: 407-421. 2006.

Ehlting J, Buttner D, Wang Q, Douglas CJ *et al.*, Three 4-coumarate: coenzyme A ligases in *Arabidopsis thaliana* represent two evolutionarily divergent classes in angiosperms. *Pl. J.* 19: 9–20. 1999.

Endler A, Martens S, Wellmann F, Matern U. Unusually divergent 4-coumarate: CoA-ligases from *Ruta graveolens* L. *Pl. Mol. Biol.* 67: 335–346. 2008.

Facknath S, Kawol D. Antifeedant and insecticidal effects of some plant extracts on *Crocidolomia binotalis*. *Insect Sci. Appl.* 14: 571-574. 1993.

Ferreira JFS, Simon JE and Janick J. Developmental studies of *Artemisia annua*: flowering and artemisinin production under greenhouse and field conditions. *Planta Medica.* 61: 167-170. 1995.

Fischer TC, Klattig JT, Gierl A. A general cloning strategy for divergent plant cytochrome P450 genes and its application in *Lolium rigidum* and *Ocimum basilicum*. *Theo. Appl. Genet.* 103: 1014–1021. 2001.

Gang DR, Lavid N, Zubieta C, Chen F *et al.*, Characterization of Phenylpropene *O*-Methyltransferases from Sweet Basil: Facile Change of Substrate Specificity and Convergent Evolution within a Plant *O*-Methyltransferase Family. *Pl. Cell.* 14: 505–519. 2002.

Gang DR, Wang J, Dudareva N, Nam KH *et al.*, An investigation of the storage and biosynthesis of phenylpropenes in sweet basil. *Pl. Physiol.* 125: 539-555. 2001.

Gomez-Galera S, Pelacho AM, Gene A, Capell T, Christou P. The genetic manipulation of medicinal and aromatic plants. *Pl. Cell Rep.* 26: 1689–1715. 2007.

Guengerich FP. Common and uncommon cytochrome P450 reactions related to metabolism and chemical toxicity. *Chem. Res. Toxicol.* 14: 611–650. 2001.

Gui J, Shen J, Li L. Functional characterization of evolutionarily divergent 4-coumarate coenzyme: a ligases in rice. *Pl. Physiol.* 157: 574–586. 2011.

Gupta GL, Rana AC. *Withania somnifera* (Ashwagandha): A Review. *Pharmaco. Rev.* 1(1): 129- 136. 2007.

Gupta P, Agarwal AV, Akhtar N, Sangwan RS *et al.*, Cloning and characterization of 2-C-methyl-D-erythritol-4-phosphate pathway genes for isoprenoid biosynthesis from Indian ginseng, *Withania somnifera*. *Protoplasma*. 250(1): 285-295. 2012.

Gupta P, Akhtar N, Tewari SK, Sangwan RS, Trivedi PK. Differential expression of farnesyl diphosphate synthase gene from *Withania somnifera* in different Chemotypes and in response to elicitors. *Pl. Grow. Reguln*. 65(1): 93- 100. 2011.

Hain R, Reif HJ, Krause E, Langebartels R *et al.*, Disease resistance results from foreign phytoalexin expression in a novel plant. *Nature*. 361: 153-156. 1993.

Hamada K, Nishida T, Yamauchi K, Fukushima K *et al.*, 4-Coumarate: coenzyme A ligase in black locust (*Robinia pseudoacacia*) catalyses the conversion of sinapate to sinapoyl-CoA. *J. Pl. Res*. 117: 303–310. 2004.

Hamberger B, Hahlbrock K. The 4-coumarate: CoA ligase gene family in Arabidopsis thaliana comprises one rare, sinapate activating and three commonly occurring isoenzymes. *Proc. Natl. Acad. Sci. USA*. 101(7): 2209-2214. 2004.

Hamberger B, Ellis M, Friedmann M, de Azevedo Sousa C *et al.*, Genome-wide analyses of phenylpropanoid-related genes in *Populus trichocarpa, Arabidopsis thaliana,* and *Oryza sativa*: the *Populus* lignin toolbox and conservation and diversification of angiosperm gene families. *Can. J. Bot*. 85: 1182–1201. 2007.

He SP, Tan GY, Li G, Tan WM *et al.*, Development of a sensitive monoclonal antibody-based enzyme linked immunosorbent assay for the antimalaria active ingredient artemisinin in the Chinese herb *Artemisia annua*. *Analyl. Bioanalyl. Chem*. 393: 1297–1303. 2009.

Herrmann K. The shikimate pathway as an entry to aromatic secondary metabolism. *Pl. Physiol*. 107: 7–12. 1995.

Himmeldirk K, Kennedy IA, Hill RE, Sayer BG, Spenser ID. Biosynthesis of vitamins B1 and B6 in *Escherichia coli*: concurrent incorporation of 1-deoxy-D-xylulose into thiamin and pyridoxol. *J. Chem. Soci. Chem. Comm*. 27: 1187–1188. 1996.

Hrycay EG, Bandiera SM. The monooxygenase, peroxidase, and peroxygenase properties of cytochrome P450. *Arch. Biochem. Biophys*. 522: 71–89. 2012.

Hsu E. The history of qing hao in the Chinese materia medica. *Roy. Soc. Tropl. Med. Hyg*. 100: 505-508. 2006.

Hu WJ, Kawaoka A, Tsai CJ, Lung J *et al.*, Compartmentalized expression of two structurally and functionally distinct 4-coumarate: CoA ligase genes in aspen (*Populus tremuloides*). *Proc. Natl. Acad. Sci. USA*. 95: 5407–5412. 1998.

Janssen AM, Scheffer JJC, Svendsen AB. Antimicrobial activity of essential oils–a 1976–86 literature review-aspects of the test methods. *Planta Medica*. 5: 395-398. 1987.

Julliard JH, Douce R. Biosynthesis of the thiazole moiety of thiamin (vitamin B1) in higher plant chloroplasts. *Proc. Natl. Acad. Sci. USA*. 88: 2042–2045. 1991.

Julliard JH. Biosynthesis of the pyridoxal ring (vitamin B6) in higher plan chloroplasts and its relationship with the biosynthesis of the thiazole ring (vitamin B1). *Comp Rendus de l'Académie des Sci - Series III*. 314: 285–290. 1992.

Kaiser A, Gottwald A, Wiersch C, Maier W, Seitz HM. The necessity to develop drugs against parasitic diseases. *Pharmazie*. 57: 723-728. 2002.

Kajita S, Hishiyama S, Tomimura Y, Katayama Y, Omori S. Structural characterization of modified lignin in transgenic tobacco plants in which the activity of 4-coumarate: coenzyme A ligase is depressed. *Pl. Physiol*. 114: 871–879. 1997.

Kallberg Y, Oppermann U, Jornvall H, Persson B. Short-chain dehydrogenases/reductases (SDRs) Coenzyme-based functional assignments in completed genomes. *Euro. J. Biochem*. 269: 4409-4417. 2002.

Karp F, Mihaliak CA, Harris JL, Croteau R. Monoterpene biosynthesis: specificity of the hydroxylations of (–)-limonene by enzyme preparations from peppermint (*Mentha piperita*), spearmint (*Mentha spicata*), and perilla (*Perilla frutescens*) leaves. *Arch. Biochem. Biophy*. 276: 219–226. 1990.

Kim SJ, Kim KW, Cho MH, Franceschi VR *et al.*, Expression of cinnamyl alcohol dehydrogenases and their putative homologues during Arabidopsis thaliana growth and development: lessons for database annotations? *Phytochem*. 68(14) 1957-1974. 2007.

Kim SJ, Kim MR, Bedgar DL, Moinuddin SGA *et al.*, Functional reclassification of the putative cinnamyl alcohol dehydrogenase multigene family in *Arabidopsis* *Proc. Natl. Acad. Sci. USA*. 101: 1455–1460. 2004.

Kjonaas R, Venkatachalam KV, Croteau R. Metabolism of monoterpenes: oxidation of isopiperitenol to isopiperitenone, and subsequent isomerization to piperitenone by soluble enzyme preparations from peppermint (*Mentha piperita*) leaves. *Arch Biochem. Biophy*. 238: 49-60. 1985.

Klempien A, Kaminaga Y, Qualley A, Nagegowda DA *et al.*, Contribution of CoA Ligases to Benzenoid Biosynthesis in Petunia Flowers. *Plant Cell*. 24: 2015–2030

Koeduka, T., Fridman, E., Gang, D.R., Vassao, D.G., Jackson, B.L., Kish, C.M. *et al* (2006) Eugenol and isoeugenol, characteristic aromatic constitutents of spices are biosynthesized via reduction of a coniferyl alcohol ester. *Proc. Natl. Acad Sci. USA*. 103: 10128- 10133. 2012.

Klischies M, Stockigt J, Zenk MH. Biosynthesis of the allylphenols eugenol and methyleugenol in *Ocimum basilicum* L. *J. Chem. Soc. Chem. Comm*. 21: 879–880. 1975.

Koeduka T, Fridman E, Gang DR, Vassao DG *et al.*, Eugenol and isoeugenol, characteristic aromatic constitutents of spices, are biosynthesized via reduction of a coniferyl alcohol ester. *Proc. Natl. Acad. Sci. USA*. 103: 10128–10133. 2006.

Koyama T, Ogura K. Isopentenyl diphosphate isomerase and prenyltransferases. In: *Comprehensive Natural Product Chemistry: Isoprenoids Including Carotenoids and Steroids*. (ed: Cane DE). Pergamon, Oxford Press. pp. 69-96.1999.

Kumar A, Ellis BE. 4-Coumarate: CoA ligase gene family in *Rubus idaeus*: cDNA structures, evolution, and expression. *Pl. Mol. Biol.* 31: 327–340. 2003.

Kumar J, Gupta PK. Molecular approaches for improvement of medicinal and aromatic plants. *Pl. Biotech. Rep.* 2: 93–112. 2008.

Lange BM, Wildung MR, Stauber EJ, Sanchez C *et al.*, Probing essential oil biosynthesis and secretion by functional evaluation of expressed sequence tags from mint glandular trichomes. *Proc. Natl. Acad. Sci. USA.* 97: 2934–2939. 2000.

Lauvergeat V, Lacomme C, Lacombe E, Lasserre E *et al.*, Two cinnamoyl-CoA reductase (CCR) genes from *Arabidopsis thaliana* are differentially expressed during development and in response to infection with pathogenic bacteria. *Phytochem.* 57: 1187–1195. 2001.

Lawrence BM. Monoterpene interrelationships in the *Mentha* genus: a biosynthetic discussion. In: *Essential oils.* (eds: Mookherjee BD and Mussinan CJ) Allured, Wheaton, Illinois. pp. 1-81.1981.

Lee D, Ellard M, Wanner LA, Davis KR, Douglas CJ. The *Arabidopsis* 4-coumarate: CoA ligase (*4CL*) gene, stress and developmentally regulated expression and nucleotide sequence of its cDNA. *Pl. Mol. Bi*ol. 28: 871-884. 1995.

Lee D, Meyer K, Chapple C, Douglas CJ. Antisense suppression of 4- coumarate: coenzyme A ligase activity in *Arabidopsis* leads to altered lignin subunit composition. *Pl. Cell,* 9: 1985-1998. 1997.

Lee S. Artemisinin, promising lead natural product for various drug developments. *Mini Rev. Medl. Chem.* 7: 411-422. 2007.

Lewinsohn E, Ziv-Raz I, Dudai N, Tadmor Y *et al.*, Biosynthesis of estragole and methyl-eugenol in sweet basil (*Ocimum basilicum* L.): developmental and chemotypic association of allylphenol *O*-methyltransferase activities. *Pl. Sci.* 160: 27–35. 2001.

Li L, ZhouY, Cheng X, Sun J *et al.*, Combinatorial modification of multiple lignin traits in trees through multigene cotransformation. *Proc. Natl. Acad. Sci. USA.* 100: 4939–4944. 2003.

Lichtenthaler HK. The 1-deoxy-D- xylulose-5-phosphate pathway of isoprenoid biosynthesis in plants. *Annl. Rev. Pl. Physiol. Pl. Mol. Biol.* 50: 47-65. 1999.

Liersch R, Soicke H, Stehr C, Tullner HU. Formation of artemisinin in *Artemisia annua* during one vegetation period. *Planta Medica.* 52: 387-390. 1986.

Liu B, Wang H, Du Z, Li G, Ye H. Metabolic engineering of artemisinin biosynthesis in *Artemisia annua* L. *Pl. Cell Rep.* 30: 689–694. 2011.

Louie GV, Baiga TJ, Bowman ME, Koeduka T *et al.*, Structure and reaction mechanism of basil eugenol synthase. *PLoS ONE.* 2(10): e993. 2007. doi: 10.1371/journal. pone.0000993.

Lupien S, Karp F, Wildung M, Croteau R. Regiospecific cytochrome P450 limonene hydroxylases from mint (*Mentha*) species: cDNA isolation, characterization, and functional expression of (–)-4S-limonene-3-hydroxylase and (–)-4S-limonene-6-hydroxylase. *Arch. Biochem. Biophys.* 368: 181–192. 1999.

Madhusudanan KP. Mass spectral studies on artemisinin, dihydroartemisinin and arteether. *Ind. J. Chem.* 28: 751–754. 1989.

Madina BR, Sharma LK, Chaturvedi P, Sangwan RS, Tuli R. Purication and characterization of a novel glucosyltransferase specic to 27b-hydroxy steroidal lactones from *Withania somnifera* and its role in stress responses. *Biochim. et Biophys. Acta.* 1774: 1199–1207. 2007.

Maeda H, Shasany AK, Schnepp *et al.*, RNAi suppression of arogenate dehydratase1 reveals that phenylalanine is synthesized predominantly via the arogenate pathway in petunia petals. *Pl. Cell.* 22: 832–849. 2010.

Mahmoud SS, Croteau R. Menthofuran regulates essential oil biosynthesis in peppermint by controlling a downstream monoterpene reductase. *Proc. Natl. Acad. Sci. USA.* 100: 14481–14486. 2003.

Manitto P, Granatica P, Monti D. Biosynthesis of phenylpropanoid compounds: II. Incorporation of specifically labeled cinnamic acids into eugenol (*Ocimum basilicum*). *J. Chem. Soc. Perkin.Trans. I.* 16: 1549–1551. 1975.

Manitto P, Monti D, Gramatica P. Biosynthesis of phenylpropanoid compounds: I. biosynthesis of eugenol in *Ocimum basilicum* L. *J Chem Soc, Perkin Trans I,* 14: 1727–1731. 1974.

Martinez BC and Staba J. The production of artemisinin in *Artemisia annua* L. tissue cultures. *Adv. Cell Cul.* 6: 69–87. 1988.

McCaskill D, Croteau DR. Monoterpene and sesquiterpene biosynthesis in glandular trichomes of peppermint (Mentha x piperita) rely exclusively on plastid-derived isopentenyl diphosphate. *Planta.* 197: 49–56. 1995.

McGarvey DJ, Croteau R. Terpenoid metabolism. *Pl Cell,* 7: 1015-1026. 1995.

Mercke P, Bengtsson M, Bouwmeester HJ, Posthumus MA, Brodelius PE. Molecular cloning, expression, and characterization of amorpha-4,11-diene synthase, a key enzyme of artemisinin biosynthesis in *Artemisia annua* L. *Arch. Biochem. Biophy.* 381: 173–180. 2000.

Miele M, Pondero R, Ciarallo G, Mazzei M. Methyl-eugenol in *Ocimum basilicum* L. cv Genovese gigante. *J. Agril. Food Chem.* 49: 517-521. 2001.

Mirjalili MH, Moyano E, Bonfill M, Cusido RM, Palazón J. Steroidal lactones from *Withania somnifera,* an ancient plant for novel medicine. *Molecules.* 14: 2373-2392. 2009.

Nair MSR, Basile DV. Bioconversion of arteannuin B to artemisinin. *J. Natl. Prodt.* 56: 1559–1566. 1993.

Nakase I, Lai H, Singh NP and Sasaki T. Anticancer properties of artemisinin derivatives and their targeted delivery by transferrin conjugation. *Intl. J. Pharmaceut.* 341: 1-19. 2007.

Ogura K, Koyama T. Enzymatic aspects of isoprenoid chain elongation. *Chem. Rev.* 98: 1263-1276. 1998.

Olofsson L, Engström A, Lundgren A, Brodelius PE. Relative expression of genes of terpene metabolism in different tissues of *Artemisia annua* L. *BMC Pl. Biol.* 11: 45. 2011.

Olsson ME, Olofsson LM, Lindah AN, Lundgren A *et al.*, Localization of enzymes of artemisinin biosynthesis to the apical cells of glandular secretory trichomes of *Artemisia annua* L. *Phytochem.* 70: 1123–1128. 2009.

Osbourn AE, Lanzotti V. *Plant-derived natural products. synthesis, function and application.* Springer Dodrecht Heidelberg London New York. pp. 413-428. 2009.

Paeshuyse J, Coelmont L, Vliegen I, Van hemel J *et al.*, Hemin potentiates the anti-hepatitis C virus activity of the antimalarial drug artemisinin. *Biochem. Biophy. Res. Comm.* 348: 139-144. 2006.

Pal S, Singh S, Shukla AK, Gupta MM *et al.*, Comparative withanolide profiles, gene isolation, and differential gene expression in the leaves and roots of *Withania somnifera. J. Hort. Sci. Biotech.* 86(4): 391–397. 2011.

Pichersky E, Gang DR. Genetics and biochemistry of secondary metabolites in plants: an evolutionary perspective. *Trends Pl. Sci.* 5: 439-445. 2000.

Piquemal J, Lapierre C, Myton K, O'Connell A *et al.*, Down-regulation of cinnamoyl-CoA reductase induces signicant changes of lignin proles in transgenic tobacco plants. *Pl. J.* 13: 71–83. 1998.

Polichuk DR, Zhang Y, Reed DW, Schmidt JF, Covello PS. A glandular trichome-specific monoterpene alcohol dehydrogenase from *Artemisia annua. Phytochem.* 71: 1264–1269. 2010.

Poulter CD, Riling HC. *Prenyl transferases and isomerase. In: Biosynthesis of Isoprenoid Compounds.* (eds: Porter JW and Spurgeon SL). John Wiley and Sons, New York. pp. 162–209. 1981.

Raes J, Rohde A, Christensen JH, de Peer YV, Boerjan W. Genome-Wide Characterization of the Lignification Toolbox in *Arabidopsis. Pl. Physiol.* 133: 1051–1071. 2003.

Rana S, Lattoo SK, Dhar N, Razdan S *et al.*, NADPH-Cytochrome P450 Reductase: Molecular Cloning and Functional Characterization of Two Paralogs from *Withania somnifera* (L.) Dunal. *PLoS One.* 8(2): 1-16. 2013.

Rastogi S, Kumar R, Chanotiya CS, Shanker K *et al.*, 4-Coumarate: CoA Ligase Partitions Metabolites for Eugenol Biosynthesis. *Pl. Cell Physiol.* 2013. doi: 10.1093/pcp/pct073.

Ringer KL, Davis EM, Croteau R. Monoterpene metabolism: Cloning, Expression, and Characterization of (-)-Isopiperitenol/(-)-Carveol dehyrogenase of peppemint and spearmint. *Pl. Physiol.* 137: 863-872. 2005.

Ringer KL, McConkey ME, Davis EM, Rushing GW, Croteau R. Monoterpene double- bond reductases of the (-)-menthol biosynthesis pathway: isolation and characterization of cDNAs encoding (-)-isopiperitenone reductase and (+) pulegone reductase of peppermint. *Arch. Biochem. Biophy*. 418: 80-92. 2003.

Ro DK, Paradise EM, Ouellet M, Fisher KJ *et al.*, Production of the antimalarial drug precursor artemisinic acid in engineered yeast. *Nature*. 440: 940–943. 2006.

Rohmer M. The discovery of a mevalonate-independent pathway for isoprenoid biosynthesis in bacteria, algae and higher plants. *Nat. Product Rep*. 16: 565–574. 1999.

Romero MR, Efferth T, Serrano MA, Castano B *et al.*, Effect of artemisinin/artesunate as inhibitors of hepatitis B virus production in an "*in vitro*" replicative system. *Antiviral Res*. 68: 75-83. 2005.

Sangwan RS, Agarwal K, Luthra R, Thakur RS, Singh-Sangwan N. Biotransformation of arteannuic acid into arteannuin-B and artemisinin in *Artemisia annua*. *Phytochem*. 34: 1301–1302. 1993.

Schilmiller AL, Stout J, Weng JK, Humphreys J *et al.*, Mutations in the cinnamate 4-hydroxylase gene impact metabolism, growth and development in *Arabidopsis*. *Pl. J*. 60 (5): 771- 782. 2009.

Schoch GA, Morant M, Abdulrazzak N, Asnaghi C *et al.*, Functional genomics of P450s. *Annl. Rev. Pl. Biol*. 54: 629–667. 2003.

Schwab W, Rikanati RD, Lewinsohn E. Biosynthesis of plant-derived flavor compounds. *Pl J*, 54: 712-732. 2008.

Senanayake UM, Wills RBH, Lee TH. Biosynthesis of eugenol and cinnamic aldehyde in *Cinnamomum zeylanicum*. *Phytochem*. 16: 2032–2033. 1977.

Senthil K, Wasnik NG, Kim YJ, Yang DC.Generation and analysis of expressed sequence tags from leaf and root of *Withania somnifera* (Ashwgandha). *Mol. Biol. Rep*. 37: 893–902. 2010.

Sharma LK, Madina BR, Chaturvedi P, Sangwan RS, Tuli R. Molecular cloning and characterization of one member of 3beta-hydroxy sterol glucosyltransferase gene family in *Withania somnifera*. *Arch. Biochem. Biophy*. 460: 48–55. 2007.

Shi R, Sun YH, Li Q, Heber S, Sederoff R, Chiang VL. Towards a Systems Approach for Lignin Biosynthesis in *Populus trichocarpa*: Transcript Abundance and Specicity of the Monolignol Biosynthetic Genes. *Pl. Cell Physiol*. 51(1): 144–163. 2010.

Sibout R, Eudes A, Mouille G, Pollet B *et al.*, Cinnamyl alcohol dehydrogenase-C and -D are the primary genes involved in lignin biosynthesis in the floral stem of *Arabidopsis*. *Pl. Cell*. 17(7): 2059-2076. 2005.

Sibout R, Eudes A, Pollet B, Goujon T *et al.*, Expression pattern of two paralogs encoding cinnamyl alcohol dehydrogenases in *Arabidopsis*. Isolation and characterization of the corresponding mutants. *Pl. Physiol*. 132(2): 848-860. 2003.

Siebert M, Sommer S, Li S, Wang Z *et al.*, Genetic engineering of plant secondary metabolism. *Pl Physiol,* 112: 811-819. 1996.

Singh A, Vishwakarma RA, Husain A. Evaluation of *Artemisia annua* strains for higher artemisinin production. *Planta Medica.* 7: 475–476. 1988.

Singh R, Rastogi S, Dwivedi UN. Phenylpropanoid metabolism in ripening fruits. comprehensive rev. *Food Sci. Food Safety.* 9: 398-416. 2010.

Somerville C, Somerville S. Plant functional genomics. *Science,* 285: 380–383. 1999.

Stephenson I, Wiselka M. Drug treatment of tropical parasitic infections: recent achievements and developments. *Drugs.* 60: 985-995. 2000.

Sy LK, Brown GD. The mechanism of the spontaneous autoxidation of dihydroartemisinic acid. *Tetrahedron.* 58: 897-908. 2002.

Tavares R, Aubourg S, Lecharny A, Kreis M. Organization and structural evolution of four multigene families in *Arabidopsis thaliana*: AtLCAD, AtLGT, AtMYST and AtHD-GL2. Pl. *Mol. Biol.* 42(5): 703-17. 2000.

Teoh KH, Polichuk DR, Reed DW, Covello PS. Molecular cloning of an aldehyde dehydrogenase implicated in artemisinin biosynthesis in *Artemsia annua. Botany.* 87: 635–642. 2009.

Teoh KH, Polichuk DR, Reed DW, Nowak G, Covello PS. *Artemisia annua* L. (Asteraceae) trichome-specific cDNAs reveal CYP71AV1, a cytochrome P450 with a key role in the biosynthesis of the antimalarial sesquiterpene lactone artemisinin. *FEBS Lett.* 580: 1411–1416. 2006.

Tucker AO. The truth about mints. *Herb Companion.* 4: 51–52. 1992.

Tuli R, Sangwan RS. Ashwagandha (*Withania somnifera*): a model Indian medicinal plant. In: Tuli R, Sangwan (ed) Army Printing Press, Lucknow, India. 2010.

Turner GW, Croteau R. Organization of monoterpene biosynthesis in Mentha: immunocytochemical localization of geranyl diphosphate synthase, limonene-6-hydroxylase, isopiperitenol dehydrogenase, and pulegone reductase. *Pl. Physiol.* 136: 4215-4227. 2004.

Turner GW, Gershenzon J, Neilson EE, Froelich JE, Croteau R. Limonene synthase, the enzyme responsible for monoterpene biosynthesisin peppermint, is localized in leucoplasts of oil gland secretory cells. *Pl. Physiol.* 120: 879-886. 1999.

Van Der Rest B, Danoun S, Boudet AM, Rochange SF. Down-regulation of cinnamoyl-CoA reductase in tomato (*Solanum lycopersicum*) induces dramatic changes in soluble phenolic pools. *J. Exptl. Bot.* 57: 1399–1411.

Verpoorte R, van der Heijden R, ten Hoopen HJG, Memelink J. Metabolic engineering of plant secondary metabolic pathways for the production of ne chemicals. *Biotech. Lett.* 21: 467–479. 1999.

Wagner A, Donaldson L, Kim H, Phillips L *et al.*, Suppression of 4-coumarate-CoA ligase in the coniferous gymnosperm *Pinus radiata. Pl. Physiol.* 149: 370–383. 2009.

Wagner WL. Floristic affinities of animas mountains, southwestern New Mexico *M.S. thesis*. University of New Mexico, Albuquerque. 1999.

Wallaart TE, Bouwmeester HJ, Hille J, Poppinga L, Maijers NC. Amorpha-4,11-diene synthase: cloning and functional expression of a key enzyme in the biosynthetic pathway of the novel antimalarial drug artemisinin. *Planta*. 212: 460-465. 2001

Wallaart TE, van Uden W, Lubberink HGM, Woerdenbag HJ *et al.*, Isolation and identification of dihydroartemisinic acid from *Artemisia annua* and its role in the biosynthesis of artemisinin. *J. Nat. Prod*. 62: 430-433. 1999.

Wang J, Pichersky E. Only a few amino acid changes can interconvert two *O*-methyltransferases with different substrate specificities. *Arch. Biochem Biophy*. 368: 172. 1999.

Wang J, Dudareva N, Bhakta S, Raguso R, Pichersky E. Floral scent production in *Clarkia breweri* (Onagraceae): II. Localization and developmental modulation of the enzyme *S*-adenosyl-l-methionine: (iso) eugenol *O*-methyltransferase and phenylpropanoid emission. *Plant Physiology*. 114: 213–221. 1997.

Wang Y, Xia Z, Zhou F, Wu Y and Huang J. Xuaxue Xueabo. *Chem Abstracts*. 46 1152. 1988.

Weitzel C and Petersen M. Enzymes of phenylpropanoid metabolism in the important medicinal plant *Melissa ofcinalis* L. *Planta*. 232(3): 731- 743. 2010.

Werck-Reichhart D. The meta-hydroxylation step in the phenylpropanoid pathway a new level of complexity in the pathway and its regulation. *Envtl. Chem. Lett* 4: 127–136. 2006.

Werker E, Putievsky E, Ravid U, Dudai N, Katzir I. Glandular hairs and essential oil in developing leaves of *Ocimum basilicum* L. (Lamiaceae). *Ann Bot*. 71: 43–50 1993.

Wink M. Genes of secondary metabolism: differential expression in plant and In vitro cultures and functional expression in genetically transformed microorganisms In: *Primary and secondary metabolism of plant cell cultures*. (ed: Kurz WGW) Springer-Verlag, Berlin Heidelberg. pp. 239-251.1989.

Wise MI, Savage TJ, Katahira E, Croteau R. Monoterpene synthases from common sage (*Salvia officinalis*): cDNA isolation, characterization, and functional expression of (1)-sabinene synthase, 1: 8-cineole synthase, and (1)-bornyl diphosphate synthase. *J. Biol. Chem*. 273: 14891–14899. 1998.

Wise ML, Croteau R. Monoterpene biosynthesis. In: *Isoprenoids Including Carotenoids and Steroids, Comprehensive Natural Products Chemistry*. (ed: Cane DE). Elsevier Science, Oxford. pp. 97–153. 1999.

Withers ST, Keasling JD. Biosynthesis and engineering of isoprenoid small molecules. *Appl. Microbiol. Biotech*. 73: 980-990. 2007.

Yamauchi K,Yasuda S, Hamada K, Tsutsumi Y, Fukushima K. Multiform biosynthetic pathway of syringyl lignin in angiosperms. *Planta*. 216: 496–501. 2003.

Youn B, Camacho R, Moinuddin SGA, Lee C *et al.*, Crystal structures and catalytic mechanism of the *Arabidopsis* cinnamyl alcohol dehydrogenases AtCAD5 and AtCAD4. *Org. Biomol. Chem.* 4: 1687–1697. 2006.

Zeng Q, Qiu F, Yuan L. Production of artemisinin by genetically-modified microbes. *Biotech. Lett*. 30: 581–592. 2008.

Zhang K, Qian Q, Huang Z, Wang Y *et al.*, Gold Hull and Internode2 encodes a primarily multifunctional cinnamyl-alcohol dehydrogenase in rice. *Pl. Physiol.* 140(3): 972-983. 2006.

Zhang Y, Teoh KH, Reed DW, Maes L *et al.*, The molecular cloning of artemisinic aldehyde D11(13) reductase and its role in glandular trichome-dependent biosynthesis of artemisinin in *Artemisia annua*. *J. Biol. Chem.* 283: 21501–21508. 2008.

Zhao SS, Zeng M. Spectrometric high pressure liquid chromatography studies on the analysis of Qinghaosu. *Planta Medica*. 3: 233-237. 1985.

2016, Biotechnological Tools for Genetic Resources Pages 233–274
Editor: **Pradip Chandra Deka**
Published by: **Daya Publishing House, NEW DELHI**

Chapter 8

Advances in Molecular Breeding of Capsicum Species

Sushil Chhapekar, Mechuselie Kehie and Nirala Ramchiary*

School of Life Sciences, Jawaharlal Nehru University, New Delhi – 110 067

****E-mail: nrudsc@gmail.com***

ABSTRACT

Capsicum species commonly known as Chilli pepper is one of the world's most important vegetable and spice crop. India is the world's largest producer, consumer and exporter of chilli pepper. Despite comprising 38 species, only six species of Capsicum namely, Capsicum annuum, C. assamicum, C. baccatum, C. frutescence, C. chinense and C. pubescens are cultivated. They are used as vegetables, spices, coloring agent and folk remedies (for diseases), proving their diverse role in human's life. Chilli pepper in mainly known for its pungency characteristics. The presence of capsaicinoids, a pungency character classifies pepper into sweet peppers and hot peppers. The molecular markers, quantitative trait loci developed by conventional breeding and classical genetic analysis have revealed number of genes for major and important traits. While, the newly developed next generation sequencing and genotyping technologies have been able to generate large scale genomic resources and to find the molecular basis of economically important traits in Capsicum genome. This chapter summarizes the advances in genomics and their applications in the form of generation of resources, comparative mapping, and identification of candidate genes for fruit trait, pungency, male sterility, disease resistance, viral resistance, nematode resistance and abiotic stress tolerance. In summary, we propose the integrated use of genomics and breeding approach in Capsicum translational research to enhance the crop productivity.

Keywords: *Capsicum, Biotic stress, Abiotic stress, Genomics, Transcriptome, Molecular markers.*

Introduction

Chilli or Capsicum is one of the world's most important vegetable and spice crop which have been a part of the human diet as a Chilli pepper in the America since 7500 BC. *Capsicum* is derived from the Greek word "Kapsimo", which means "to bite" (Basu and De 2003). Chilli pepper was domesticated more than 6000 years ago and is considered to be first spice used by human. *Capsicum* species is a member of Solanaceae family and is believed to have ancestral origins in the Central and South America (Bosland 1996, Perry *et al.*, 2007). Chilli pepper plants are grown throughout the tropical, sub tropical and temperate regions of the world. In 2011, the world's annual production was 3.4 million tons for dry chilli and 29.6 million tons for fresh green chilli (FAOSTAT 2013). India is the world's largest producer, consumer and exporter of chilli pepper. The diploid *Capsicum* genome consists of n = 12 chromosomes with an estimated haploid genome size of 3.3–3.6 GB (Arumuganathan *et al.*, 1991, Moscone *et al.*, 2003). The *Capsicum* species were characterized into two groups based on chromosome numbers, 2n = 24 and 2n = 26. However, only one species, *C. annuum* var. glabriusculum, is tetrapoid (2n = 4x = 48). *Capsicum chacoense* appeared to be the most primitive taxa, and the species with chromosome number 26 were likely to be more advanced than the species with 2n = 24 (Pickersgill, 1977).

Importance of *Capsicum*

The *Capsicum* is having rich diversity, constitutes of about 38 species (USDA-ARS, 2011) but only 6 species, namely *Capsicum annuum*, *C. baccatum*, *C. chinense*, *C. frutescens*, *C. pubescens*, and *C. assamicum* are cultivated. The *C. assamicum* has been recently identified as a distinct domesticated species from the North Eastern part of India (Purukayastha *et al.*, 2012); which is closely related to *C. frutescencs* and *C.chinense* but can be distinguished by its distinct morphological features. Globally, *C. annuum* is the most extensively cultivated species, while the most pungent one is *C. chinense.* Chilli fruits contain rich metabolites that are beneficial for human health, such as carotenoids (pro-vitamin A), vitamins C, vitamin A (which destroy free radicals), vitamin E, flavonoids and capsaicinoids (Maga 1975 and Simonne *et al.*, 1997). Although these compounds functions as antioxidants and nutrients; they are also used in traditional medicine due to their enormous medicinal properties. Several studies have found that capsaicin can be used as pain-relieving agent in chemotherapy or radiation therapy (Berger *et al.*, 1996), diabetic neuropathy and nerve pain (also called neuropathic pain). The plants have also been used as folk remedies for dropsy, colic, diarrhea, asthma, arthritis, muscle cramps and toothache (Ravishankar *et al.*, 2003). *Capsicum* is also found to be very helpful in preventing cancers of the pancreas, cervix, prostrate and bladder by inducing apoptosis (Surh 2002). Capsaicinoids cause the spicy flavor (pungency) of chilli pepper fruit. This pungency is due to capsaicinoid complex of the capsaicin (unsaturated and saturated amides) and dihydrocapsaicin (Kosuge *et al.*, 1965 and Pruthi 1980), which distinguishes pepper as hot pepper and sweet peppers based on the presence or absence of pungency traits in the fruits. In nature, only chilli pepper fruits synthesize capsaicinoids and suggested that it might provide protection against some pathogens (Tewksbury *et al.*, 2008).

Quantitative trait loci (QTL) developed by conventional breeding and classical genetic analysis have revealed number of genes for major and important traits. While, the newly developed next generation sequencing and genotyping technologies have been able to generate large scale genomic resources and to find the molecular basis of economically important traits in capsicum genome. However, traditional breeding tools with the help of molecular markers analyzed several QTLs/genes responsible for desired agronomically and economically important traits. The most vital and core component of chilli pepper is capsaicinoid biosynthetic pathway which largely remain unexplored. Some of the reports have helped to suggest the possible roles of different candidate genes in capsaicinoid biosynthesis pathway. In *Capsicum*, several genetic maps/linkage maps have been constructed using different populations. The productivity of capsicum is hampered by different abiotic and biotic stresses. To overcome this many QTLs/candidate genes have been identified. This chapter emphasizes the agronomic and economic challenges of *Capsicum* crop and how recent developments in the field of molecular breeding including genomics can be utilize for *Capsicum* improvement.

Conservation Initiatives

The Asian Vegetable Research and Development Center (AVRDC, Taiwan) has the largest collection of Capsicum germplasm, with a total of 8170 accessions belonging to wild and cultivated *Capsicum* species from around the world. Several institutes/organizations are engaged in collecting and maintaining important genetic resources (in the form of germplasm) of different *Capsicum* species for their use in the applied and basic research. For example, the United Sates Department of Agriculture (USDA) has 6067 accessations while the National Bureau of Plant Genetic Resources (NBPGR), New Delhi, India has collections of 2774 accessions. Babu *et al.* (2011) reviewed a vast number of capsicum germplasm showing resistances against pathogens arthropods, nematodes and virus. A notable genetic resource centers in the world engaged in collection, maintenance and development of genetic resources/varieties of different capsicum species are listed in Table 8.1.

Genetic Mapping

The availability of large-scale genomic resources has accelerated the development of high density genetic linkage maps in *Capsicum*. Analysis of these genetic maps with phenotypic information of the respective segregating mapping population has facilitated the identification of molecular markers linked to the important QTLs/genes controlling several agronomic characters. Mapping populations used to construct the pepper genetic maps were mostly F2, recombinant inbred line (RIL), double haploid (DH) or backcross mapping populations, with anonymous markers such as genomic DNA based restriction fragment length polymorphic (RFLP), amplified fragment length polymorphism (AFLP), random amplified length polymorphic DNA (RAPD) and isozyme markers (Livingstone *et al.*, 1999, Kang *et al.*, 2001, Rao *et al.*, 2003, Lee *et al.*, 2004, Ben-Chaim *et al.*, 2006).

Using an inter-specific cross of *C. annuum* and *C. chinense*, Tanksley *et al.* (1988) constructed one of the first genetic map with wide genome coverage that contained 85 RFLP markers. Thereafter, Prince *et al.* (1993) constructed a more detailed map with 192 markers using cross of same chinense parent with different

Table 8.1: List of Resources and Germplasm Databases of *Capsicum*

Institute	*Country*	*Description*	*Website*
Banco de Germoplasma de Hortaliças (BGH)	Brazil	The BGH varieties collections in the Chileman database can be found by entering BGH text into the name box.	http://www.thechileman.org/search.php
The Centre for Genetic Resources, the Netherlands (CGN)	Netherland	A total of 1009 accessations of improved disease resistance and harvesting characteristics are available with institute. The CGN varieties are also listed in the Chileman database and can be found by entering CGN text in the database	http://applicaties.wageningenur.nl/applications/cgngenis/ZoekGewas.aspx?ID=pzlo0t45 and Cropnumber =38 ORhttp://www.thechileman.org/search.php
The Chile Pepper Institute (New Mexican State University)	Mexico	An elite institute having maximum genetic resources, germplasm collection of different Capsicum species	http://www.chilepepperinstitute.org ORhttp://www.thechileman.org/search.php
The German Research Centre for Biotechnology (CAP)	Germany	Many of the varieties used by the institution can be found in the Chileman database by entering the CAP in the name box	http://www.thechileman.org/search.php
United States Department of Agriculture Research Service (USDA)	United States of America	They are having most extensive Capsicum genotype collections, resistant to different diseases.	http://www.ars-grin.gov/npgs/acc/acc_queries.html ORhttp://www.thechileman.org/search.php
The Asian Vegetable Research and Development Center (ARVDC)	Taiwan	A collection of several Capsicum species resistant to different diseases specially viral with accessation number, characterization and evaluation data.	http://www.avrdc.org
National Bureau of Plant Genetic Resources	India	A collection of germplasm of different Capsicum species with accessation number, characterization and evaluation data	www.nbpgr.ernet.in/pgrportal
ECPGR Pepper Database, Aegean Agricultural Research Institute, AARI	Turkey	A collection of germplasm of different Capsicum	http://www.etae.gov.tr/eng/Default.aspx#
The Chile variety database		A collection of large number of cultivars and hybrids resistant to most diseases and nematodes	http://www.g6csy.net/chile/database.html

C. annuum (NuMex RNaky) parent. Later, with same population, Livingstone *et al.* (1999) constructed the pepper-tomato comparative map using AFLP, RFLP and RAPD markers covering a total of 1245.7 cM distance. In another study, a genetic map based on RFLP markers was developed by Kang *et al.* (2001). This map was subsequently expanded by Lee *et al.* (2004) which included 46 SSR markers. Using F_2 population of *C. annuum* (NuMex RNaky) x *C. frutescence* cross, Ben-Chaim *et al.* (2006) developed a most comprehensive genetic map with a total of 728 molecular markers (489 SSRs, 195 AFLPs, 8 specific PCR based and 36 RFLP markers) covering a total length of 1358.7 cM. Some of the candidate genes of proposed model of capsaicinoid biosynthesis pathway such as *pAMT, COMT,* and *Bcat* genes are included in this map (Blum *et al.*, 2003, Stewart *et al.*, 2005). Using *C. annuum* derived genomic DNA library, Minamiyama *et al.* (2005) developed genetic linkage map comprising 374 markers, including 106 new SSR markers which covered 1042 cM of pepper genome. Lee *et al.* (2008) used several markers such as RFLP, SSR, CAPS, AFLP, WRKY, rRAMP, and BAC end sequences derived markers to construct an integrated pepper map.

C. frutescens played a small role in mapping, while most interspecic maps were derived from *C. chinense* due to higher compatibility and fertility of the hybrid progeny. Yi *et al.* (2006) mapped a total of 180 EST-SSRs in addition of 63 RFLP markers, spanning 2,201.5 cM. Portis *et al.* (2007) screened a total of total of 204 EST-SSRs for polymorphism between parental set of four *C. annuum* inbred lines and one *C. frutescens* accession and observed 49 polymorphic SSRs which could be used for assessing genetic diversity within an extended *Capsicum* species. Another wide range genetic map was constructed comprising 587 conserved orthologous set II markers (COSII) between the pepper and tomato genomes (Wu *et al.*, 2009a). This map revealed a total of 35 conserved syntenic segments (CSSs) within which gene/marker order are well preserved. Kumar *et al.* (2011) reviewed several genetic maps which have been constructed and published.

Lu *et al.* (2012) developed 41 SNP markers through comparative transcriptomics and integrated those markers by mapping in previous genetic map of *C. annuum.* This new map comprises a total of 458 molecular markers. A linkage map using a doubled haploid population has been reported by Mimura *et al.* (2012) with 253 markers covering 1,336 cM of *Capsicum* genome. Recently, using intraspecific cross of *C. annuum,* Sugita *et al.* (2013) constructed the EST-SSR based map (designated as KL-DH map) spanning a total distance of 2,028 cM pepper genome. An updated genetic map used in pepper breeding is shown in Table 8.2.

Marker-Assisted Breeding for Useful Agronomic and Economic Traits

A number of QTLs/candidate genes in peppers for fruit size, shape and color, male sterility system and fertility restorer genes, metabolites such as pungency and disease resistances have been identified. Some of the major QTLs/genes are listed in Table 8.3.

Table 8.2: List of Genetic Maps in Pepper Translational Research

Population	*Population Type*	*Marker Type*	*No. of Markers*	*No. of Linkage Groups*	*Length (cM)*	*References*
Doux des lands (*C. annuum*) X PI159234 (*C. chinense*)	BC_1	RFLP	85	14	—	Tanksley *et al.*, 1988
NuMex RNaky (*C. annuum*) X PI159234 (*C. chinense*)	F_2	RFLP	192	19	720	Prince *et al.*, 1993
NuMex RNaky (*C. annuum*) X PI159234 (*C. chinense*)	F_2	RAPD, AFLP, RFLP	1007	13	1246	Livingston *et al.*, 1999
Maor (*C. annuum*) X	F_2	RAPD, RFLP	177	12	1740	Ben-Chaim *et al.*, 2001
Perennial (*C. annuum*)						
TF68 (*C. annuum*) X Habanero (*C. chinense*)	F_2	RFLP, AFLP	580	16	1320	Kang *et al.*, 2001
H3 (*C. annuum*) X Vania (*C. annuum*)	DH	RAPD, AFLP, RFLP	543	20	1513	Lefebvre *et al.*, 2002
Perennial (*C. annuum*) X Yo lo Wonder (*C. annuum*)	DH	RAPD, AFLP, RFLP	630	26	1668	Lefebvre *et al.*, 2002
Yo lo Wonder (*C. annuum*) X Criollo de Morelos334 (*C. annuum*)	F_2	RAPD, AFLP, RFLP	208	18	685	Lefebvre *et al.*, 2002
Maor (*C. annuum*) X BG 2816 (*C. frutescens*)	BC_2	RFLP	92	12	1100	Rao *et al.*, 2003
Integrated Map:4 [*C.annuum* X *C. annuum*] +[*C. annuum* X *C. chinense*] + 1[*C. annuum* X *C. chinense*] X *C. annumm*	F2	RAPD, AFLP, RFLP	2262	81	1832	Paran *et al.*, 2004
NuMex RNaky (*C. annuum*) X BG 2816 (*C. frutescens*)	F_2	RFLP, AFLP	728	16	1358	Ben-Chaim *et al.*, 2006

Contd...

Table 8.2–*Contd...*

Population	*Population Type*	*Marker Type*	*No. of Markers*	*No. of Linkage Groups*	*Length (cM)*	*References*
Manganji (*C. annuum*) X Tongari (*C. annuum*)	DH	SSR	374	13	1042	Minamiyama *et al.*, 2006
TF68 (*C. annuum*) X Habanero (*C. chinense*)	F_2	SSR, RFLP	180 (SSR), 63 (RFLP)	14	2201.5	Yi *et al.*, 2006
Integrated Maps: Two inter-specific TF68 X Habanero (*C. annuum*) and Two intra-specific CM334 (*C. annuum*) X Chilsungcho (*C. annuum*)	F2	SSR, RFLP, CAPS, AFLP, WRKY, rRAMP	805 (inter-specific), 745 (intra-specific)	—	1858 (inter-specific), 1892 (intra-specific)	Lee *et al.*, 2008
NuMex RNaky (*C. annuum*) X BG 2816 (*C. frutescens*)	F_2	COSII	587	12	—	Wu *et al.*, 2009a
California Wonder (*C. annuum*) X LS2341 (JP187992) (*C. annuum*)	DH	SSR, AFLP, CAPS, STS	253	12	1336	Mimura *et al.*, 2012
K9-11 (*C. annuum*) XMZC-180 (*C. annuum*)	DH	SSR, AFLP, CAPS	597	12	2028	Sugita *et al.*, 2013

—: Not determined.

Table 8.3: List of Major Genes/QTLs which Could be used in *Capsicum* Breeding

Genes/Qtls	*Population*	*References*
	Capsaicinoid Biosynthesis	
Pun 1 (locus C), *At3*	NMCA-30036 (*C. chinense*)	Blum *et al.*, 2002
Pal, Ca4h, Comt, 3-ketoacyl-ACP synthase (*Kas*), putative amino-transferase (*pAmt*), *Acl, Fat*, SB2-149 and SB1-158 clones (Similarity to *pAmt* and *Kas*). SB2-66, SB2-115, SB2-115	*Capsicum* sp.	Curry *et al.*, 1999, Kim *et al.*, 2001, Aluru *et al.*, 2003
BCAT and *3A2*	BG2814-6 (*C. frutescens*) X NuMexRNaky (*C. annuum*)	Ben-Chaim *et al.*, 2006
pun1[2]	*C. chinense and C. annuum*	Stewart *et al.*, 2007
3.1, 4.2, 4.13, 4.14, 4.15, 4.16, 5.4, 6.8, 7.3, 10.2, 10.3, 11.8 (12 QTLs)	2814-6 (*C. frutescens*) X NuMexRNaky (*C. annuum*)	Yarnes *et al.*, 2013
	Fruit Characteristics (*weight, size, shape, length, colors*)	
cl, c2 and *y*	*C. annuum*	Hurtado-Hernandez and Smith 1985
cl, c2, y	PI 152225 (*C. chinense*) X Kelvin- 4751 (*C. annuum*)	Popovsky and Paran 2000
Yld8.1 and *yld1.1*	Maor (*C. annuum*) X BG 2816 (*C. frutescens*)	Rao *et al.*, 2003
Phytoene synthase (*PSy*), phytoene desaturase, and capsanthin, capsorubin synthase (*Ccs*) genes, *LcyB, CrtZ*-2	*Capsicum* sp.	Ha *et al.*, 2007, Rodriguez-Uribe *et al.*, 2012
fw2.1, *fw4.1* and *fw4.2*	*C. chinense* X *C. frutescens*	Zygier *et al.*, 2005
fs10.1	*C. annum* X *C. chinense*	Ben Chaim *et al.*, 2003
CaOvate	*Capsicum annuum*	Tsaballa *et al.*, 2011
fs10.1	Yolo Wonder (*C. annum*) X CM334 (*C. annum*)	Barchi *et al.*, 2009
2.6, 2.7, 2.9, 6.4, 9.3, 9.4, 9.6, 9.8 (QTLs for fruit lobedness)	2814-6 (*C. frutescens*) X NuMexRNaky (*C. annuum*)	Yarnes *et al.*, 2013
3.6, 3.13, 4.3, 4.4, 4.5, 4.6, 4.9, 4.10, 4.11, 9.8, 9.9, 11.4, 11.5, 11.7 (QTLs for pericarpthickness and area)	2814-6 (*C. frutescens*) X NuMexRNaky (*C. annuum*)	Yarnes *et al.*, 2013
2.1, 4.5, 4.6, and 4.9 (QTLs for latitudinal fruit traits and branching density)	2814-6 (*C. frutescens*) X NuMexRNaky (*C. annuum*)	Yarnes *et al.*, 2013
Ofw.iivr-2.1, Otfw.iivr-2.1,Otofw.iivr-2.1, Onfp.iivr-2.1, Opt.iivr-2.1, Otofw.iivr-3.1 and *Ofl.iivr.3.4*	*C. annuum*	Dwiwedi *et al.*, 2013
	Leaf characteristics	
1.2, 1.3, 1.5, 2.2, 3.1, 3.3, 3.7, 4.12, 5.3, 6.7, 7.2, 7.5, 9.1, 9.5, 11.9, 12.1	2814-6 (*C. frutescens*) X NuMexRNaky (*C. annuum*)	Yarnes *et al.*, 2013

Contd...

Table 8.3–Contd...

Genes/Qtls	Population	References
Whole Plant (*for Early habit, vigour, height, branching and leaf density*)		
2.1, 3.1, 3.2, 4.1, 4.5, 4.6, 4.7, 4.8, 4.9, 5.2, 5.3, 5.4, 5.5,10.1, 10.4, 11.3, 11.10	2814-6 (*C. frutescens*) X NuMexRNaky (*C. annuum*)	Yarnes *et al.*, 2013
Plant Defence		
Methionine sulfoxide reductase (*B2*)	*C. annuum*	Oh *et al.*, 2010
CaBtf3	*C. annuum*	Huh *et al.*, 2012
Genetic/Cytoplasmic male sterility		
orf456	*C. annuum*	Kim *et al.*, 2007
PmsM1-CAPS	*C. annuum*	Lee *et al.*, 2010a
ms1, ms3	*C. annuum*	Lee *et al.*, 2010b,c
CaMF2	*C. annuum*	Chen *et al.*, 2011
Resistance genes		
CaWRKYb	*C. annuum*	Lim *et al.*, 2011
pvr1, pvr2[1], pvr22, pvr3, pvr4, pvr5, pvr6, Pvr7	*Capsicum sps.*	Caranta *et al.*, 1996, Kyle and Palloix 1997, Grube *et al.*, 2000
Cmr1	*C. annuum* cv 'Bukang'	Kang *et al.*, 2010
L1, L3, L4	*Capsicum sps.*	Lefebvre *et al.*, 1995, Ben-Cham *et al.*, 2001, Matsunaga *et al.*, 2003, Tomita *et al.*, 2008
Tsw	*Capsicum chinense*	Moury *et al.*, 2000
CaWRKYb, CaPR-10, CaPR-1, CaPR-5	*C. annuum*	Lim *et al.*, 2011
***Phytopthora* resistance**		
Phyto.5.2	*C. annuum* and *C. chinense*	Quirin *et al.*, 2005
Ipcr	*C. annuum*	Reeves *et al.*, 2013
CaRGA2	CM33 (*C. annuum*)	Zhang *et al.*, 2013
***Ralstonia solanacearum* resistance**		
caWRKY40	*Capsicum sps.*	Dang *et al.*, 2013
***Xanthomonas* resistance**		
Bs1, Bs4, bs5, bs6, gdr	*Capsicum sps.*	Jones *et al.*, 2002, 2004, Csillery *et al.*, 2004
CaPO2	*C annuum*	Choi *et al.*, 2007
CaMLO2	*C. annuum*	Kim *et al.*, 2012
Root-Knot Nematode resistance gene		
Me4, Mech1, Mech2	*C. annuum*	Djian-Caporalino *et al.*, 2001, 2007
CaMsrB2	*C. annuum*	Oh *et al.*, 2010

Contd...

Table 8.3–*Contd...*

Genes/Qtls	*Population*	*References*
	Delayed Senescence	
CaSD1	*C. annuum*	Seo *et al.*, 2013
	Trichome Enhancement	
Ptel1 and *Ptel2*	CM334 (*C. annuum*) X Chilsungcho (*C. annuum*)	Kim *et al.*, 2011
	Abiotic stress resistance	
CaPF1	*C. annuum*	Yi *et al.*, 2004
CAZFP1	*C. annuum*	Kim *et al.*, 2004
Ca-DREBLP1	*C. annuum*	Hong *et al.*, 2005
CaXTH3	*C. annuum*	Cho *et al.*, 2006
CaBI-1	*C. annuum*	Isbat *et al.*, 2009
Sod	*C. annuum*	Chatzidimitriadou *et al.*, 2009
CaELIP	*C. annuum*	Tao *et al.*, 2011

Capsaicinoids (Pungency)

Capsaicinoids, found only in peeper fruits, is a special and economically important quality trait, have been studied extensively for many years. This characteristic of *Capsicum* is due to the presence of capsaicinoid complex (formed by combination of capsaicin and dihydrocapsaicin). In pepper fruits, over 22 different capsaicinoids are found, which is synthesized and accumulated in the placenta of fruits (Bosland and Walker 2010). The major ones being Capsaicin and Dihydrocapsacin, which occurs in comparatively higher concentration. Capsaicin is an amide derivative of vanillylamine and 8-methylnon-*trans*-6-enoic acid (Bennett and Kirby 1968). In capsaicin biosynthesis two pathways are involved (i) fatty acid metabolism, which determines the molecule's fatty acids, and (ii) phenylpropanoid, which determines phenolic structure (Ochoa-Alejo and Gomez-Peralta 1993).

Despite extensive studies on capsaicinoid pathway, the most mysterious element remain in the pathway is capsaicinoid synthase, which catalyzes the final condensation of vanillylamine and the branched-chain fatty acid. Initially, three genes namely, *Pal*, *Ca4h*, and *Comt* were successfully isolated from a cDNA library of Habanero (*C. chinense*) placenta, which were found to be co-segregated with pungency (Curry *et al.*, 1999). The isolated genes encodes 3-ketoacyl-ACP synthase (*Kas*) and the putative aminotransferase (*pAmt*), which expressed only in the placental tissues. Kim *et al.* (2001) constructed a subtractive cDNA library from placental tissues of *C. chinense* cv. Habanero. They found two clones, SB2-149 and SB1-158 which showed high similarity to the *pAmt* and *Kas* genes indicating their involvement in capsaicinoid pathway. Aluru *et al.* (2003) characterized and mapped three candidate genes *Kas*, *Acl*, and *Fat* which was found to be placental-specific and was positively correlated with degree of pungency. Stewart *et al.* (2005) found that the SB2-66 clone, previously isolated by Kim *et al.* (2001), co-segregated with the pungency trait, and it was mapped to a locus in close proximity to *Pun 1* (locus C), which modifies the pungency level (Blum *et al.*, 2002). The allele was named *pun1*, and labeled as *At3*. The *At3* gene was found to be related to capsaicinoid production.

Based on sequence of Capsaicinoid Synthase, SCAR markers have been developed and their usefulness in early detection of pungent genotype has been demonstrated (Lee *et al.*, 2005). Ben-Chaim *et al.* (2006) identified 6 QTLs for three capsaicinoids: capsaicin, dihydrocapsaicin and nordihydrocapsaicin. Stewart *et al.* (2007) analyzed the *At3* gene in a non-pungent *C. chinense* NMCA 30036 chilli pepper, where the *At3* gene sequence revealed a 4-bp deletion in the first exon and this allele was named *pun*[2]. For Solanaceae family, the SolCyc database was developed at the SOL Genomics Network (http://www.sgn.cornell.edu) which describes the role of over 30 putative genes in capsaicinoid biosynthesis pathway (*CapCyc*) of pepper (Mazourek *et al.*, 2009; Aza-González *et al.*, 2011). Yarnes *et al.* (2013) identified 96 QTLs for different traits of which 12 QTLs have been mapped for capsaicinoids which could be used for *Capsicum* breeding.

Fruit Characteristic

A large variation in capsicum fruit traits such as fruit size, shape, texture and their chemical composition exist (Figure 8.1). Several QTLs have been identified that are associated with fruit size and shape in pepper (Ben Chaim *et al.*, 2001, Rao *et al.*, 2003, Zygier *et al.*, 2005, Barchi *et al.*, 2009, Borovsky and Paran 2011, Tsaballa *et al.*, 2011). In one of the early studies, Ben Chaim *et al.* (2001) identified a total of 55 QTLs for fruit weight, fruit diameter, fruit weight, fruit length, fruit shape, pericarp thickness and for soluble solid concentration.

Rao *et al.* (2003) detected two QTLs for yield, while one QTL namely *yld8.1* was also associated with fruit weight and the other *yld1.1* with flowering and fruit setting. Ben Chaim *et al.* (2003) using population derived from *C. annum* and *C. chinense* detected an anthocyanin QTL and mapped a major fruit shape QTL *fs10.1* on chromosome 10. The major QTL affecting fruit shape was *fs3.1*. The same QTL previously found by Ben Chaim *et al.* (2001). Zygier *et al.* (2005) identified a major QTL *fw2.1* for fruit weight (mapped on chromosome 2), in addition with that *fw4.1* and *fw4.2* (mapped on chromosome 4) using a cross of *C. annuum* and *C. frutescense*. These QTLs for fruit-weight was also found in other *Capsicum* mapping populations.

Lee *et al.* (2008) developed CAPs marker, which are found to be associated with pendant and erect fruiting habit of *Capsicum*, suggesting these markers could be used for marker assisted breeding. Barchi *et al.* (2009) detected *fs10.1* for fruit elongation and mapped on chromosome 10. Borovsky and Paran (2011) developed Near Isogenic Lines (NILs) for *fs10.1* and mapped it in a BC_4F_2 population. Tsaballa *et al.* (2011) isolated and characterized Ovate-like genes (*CaOvate*) and observed high similarity with other *OVATE* genes of Solanaceae species especially tomato, emphasizing its role in determining fruit shape in pepper.

In *Capsicum*, diverse colors fruit such as white, yellow, orange, red and chocolate are found. The chilli pepper is also being used to extract the natural colors. Although, over 30 different pigments have been identified, there is a lot of scope in improvement of *Capsicum* for carotenoid and nutrient content (Bosland and Votava 2000). Hurtado-Hernandez and Smith (1985) reported three independent loci (*cl*,

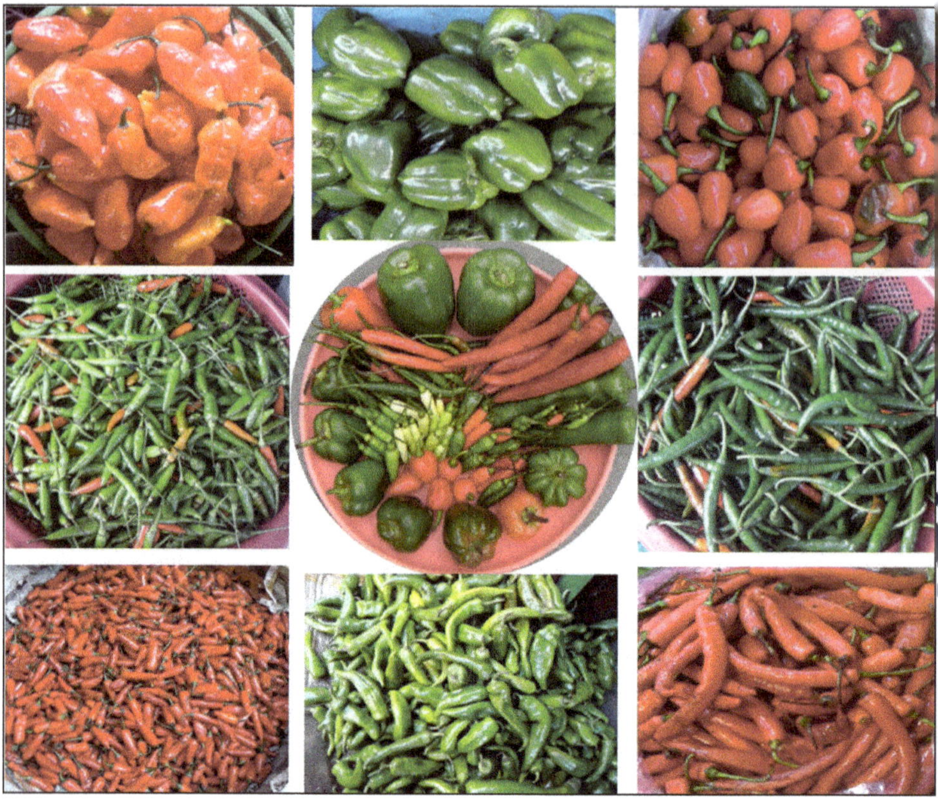

Figure 8.1: Diversity of the *Capsicum* Germplasm.

c2 and *y*) which govern the mature pepper fruit in different allelic combination. However, later with linkage analyses found that c2 and y loci correspond to genes that encode phytoene synthase (*Psy*) and capsanthin capsorubin synthase (*Ccs*), respectively (Lefebvre *et al.*, 1998, Popovsky and Paran 2000, Thorup *et al.*, 2000, Huh *et al.*, 2001). Kim *et al.* (2010) found that a splicing mutation in the phytoene synthase (*Psy*) gene resulted in orange coloration of Habanero pepper fruits, while the deletion of *Ccs* gene is reported to cause yellow and orange fruit color (Lefebvre *et al.*, 1998, Lang *et al.*, 2004).

Anthocyanin also controls pepper color and found to be governed by the incompletely dominant gene "A". Ben-Chaim *et al.* (2003) mapped "A" locus onto pepper chromosome 10 and detected two anthocyanin loci found to be associated with a major quantitative trait locus, *fs10.1*, for fruit shape. Ha *et al.* (2007) observed that with high levels of carotenoids, *Psy*, *Pds*, and *Ccs* genes were highly expressed in peppers, whereas one or two of these genes were not expressed with lower levels of total carotenoids. Rodriguez-Uribe *et al.* (2012) performed study on *Psy*, *LcyB*, *CrtZ-2*, and *Ccs* genes and their products in seven orange-colored *C. annuum* cultivars and suggested there might be a non-structural gene which controls the color development in *Capsicum* fruits. A linkage map was constructed by using

SSR, SCAR and RAPD markers where several QTLs for plant height, number of fruits per plant, ten fruits weight, fruit length, fruit width, total fruit weight and pericarp thickness were mapped in recombinant inbred line (RIL) populations of pepper (Dwivedi *et al.*, 2013).

Male Sterility

Male sterility is one of the essential characters required for chilli hybrid breeding. Male sterility reduces cost of hybrid seed production by excluding the need for manual emasculation of maternal line and eliminating impurities of the seed material originated from self-pollination. For hybrid seed breeding, identification of stable sterile lines and fertility restorer genes are important. Wang *et al.* (2004) mapped a major QTL on chromosome P6, associated with phenotypic variation for fertility restoration. In addition they also found four minor QTLs on chromosomes P5 and P2, which were linked with the same trait. Kim and Kim (2005) developed the SCAR markers which could be used for early identification of CMS genotype in *C. annuum*. Kim *et al.* (2007) concluded that a novel ORF (*orf456*) at the 3′-end of the *coxll* gene might responsible for determining the male-sterile phenotype of CMS in chilli pepper. Gulyas *et al.* (2010) reported change in *orf456* due to deletion of nucleotide base which resulted into longer transcript named, *orf507* having a possible role in microspore development.

More than 20 nuclear genes responsible for male sterility in pepper have been reported (Wang and Bosland 2006). Lee *et al.* (2008) reported that CMS in chilli pepper is restored by one major dominant nuclear gene, restorer-of-fertility (*Rf*), along with some modifier genes. They also found that these factors are influence by temperature. A co-dominant cleaved amplified polymorphic sequence marker (CAPS) named *PmsM1*-CAPS, was found to be associated with genetic male sterility (GMS) in colored pepper (paprika), and some CAPS markers were tightly linked to the *ms1* and *ms3* genes (responsible for GMS) (Lee *et al.*, 2010a,b,c). Chen *et al.* (2011) identified an anther specific gene named as *capsicum male feritile 2* (*CaMF2*) which encodes a lipid transfer protein, responsible for positive regulation of pollen germination ability in *C. annuum*. Chen *et al.* (2012) found a novel gene, *Camf1*, which expresses only in the anthers of male fertile plant and suggesting its importance in fertility of *C. annuum* L.

Bartoszewski *et al.* (2012) identified several markers linked to *ms8* locus responsible for nuclear male sterility. They used RAPD–BSA technique and found that seven markers are linked to the *ms8* locus, and four of them were converted into SCAR markers. Two COSII/CAPS markers linked to the *ms8* locus were also identied, which was located on chromosome P4. An *Rf*-linked molecular marker was employed to analyze the interaction between 6 CMS lines (A), 5 maintainers (B), and 6 restorers (C) (Ma *et al.*, 2013). They found the 6 restorers have diverse restoring abilities in individual CMS lines and concluded that the restorers can transmit the *Rf* gene or the *Rf*-linked marker to F_1 hybrids. To find out the critical genes and pathways associated with the male sterility, a CMS line 121A and it's near isogenic restorer line 121C were analyzed at transcriptome level (Liu *et al.*, 2013). Analysis of the data resulted into 53 million sequencing reads and 85,144 high quality unigenes, of which many of the differentially expressed unigenes represent a set of potential candidate genes associated with the formation or abortion of pollen.

Sequence-Based Molecular Markers and their Applications

Sequence-based molecular markers have been used in many comparative and functional genomics studies because of their preferable features like genome-wide distribution, chromosome specic location, co-dominant inheritance and reproducibility. In *Capsicum*, development of molecular markers especially the simple sequence repeats has been reported (Sanwen *et al.*, 2001, Lee *et al.*, 2004). Since the number of expressed sequence tags (ESTs) is increasing considerably in public databases with the ongoing multinational efforts of transcriptome sequencing, the EST databases provided a new source for developing SSR markers in a rapid and cost effective manner as compared from the SSRs developed form the genomic sequences. Portis *et al.* (2007) designed 348 SSRs primer pairs from 576 non-redundant EST sequences. Yi *et al.* (2006) identified a total of 1,201 SSRs which corresponds to one SSR in every 3.8 kb of the ESTs, resulting 29.2 per cent polymorphism between *C. annuum* 'TF68' and *C. chinense* 'Habanero'. A very effective conserved single-copy orthologs (COSII) markers (around a set of 2869) was developed by Wu *et al.* (2006). These markers were widely used to develop genetic maps and comparative genome analysis between many species including peppers, tomato and eggplants belonging to the Solanaceae family (Wu *et al.*, 2009a, 2009b).

The SOL Genomics Network (SGN; http://sgn.cornell.edu), was developed to perform the activities like cataloging and maintaining genetic maps and markers, assembling, analyzing, and publishing sequencing data of the Solanaceae plant species (tomato, potato, peppers and eggplant) and related families (Mueller *et al.*, 2005). Kim *et al.* (2008) developed a pepper EST database, with a total of 122,582 sequenced ESTs from 21 pepper EST libraries representing 11 different tissues, different developmental stages and conditions of stress. Tecle *et al.* (2010) developed a web interface QTL tool (solQTL), for uploading raw phenotype and genotype data to the database, which was helpful in identifying genes and alleles associated with phenotypic variation, and markers closely linked to QTLs for their utilization in breeding programmes.

Huan-huan *et al.* (2011) developed 755 SSR markers of which 127 SSR primer pairs showed polymorphism in 8 populations of *Capsicum*. Shirasawa *et al.* (2013) successfully mapped 2,245 SSRs on tomato genome. Interestingly, some of these selected SSRs which spanned the entire tomato genome showed polymorphism among the 192 *Capsicum* lines. Sugita *et al.* (2013) developed non-redundant 2- or 3-base SSR markers and obtained 1,736 genomic SSRs and 1,344 cDNA-derived SSRs.

Trnascriptome Sequencing Studies in *Capsicum* Species

Transcriptome sequencing at genome wide scale is the first step to access the gene content of a species. The transcriptome sequencing either by first-generation Sanger sequencing or by high throughput NGS approaches provide a gross idea about the gene content in a range of crop species. Initially, a *Capsicum* transcriptome database (DB, **Error! Hyperlink reference not valid.**) was developed after sequencing of *C. annuum* transcriptome from different tissues (Góngora-Castillo *et al.*, 2011). They obtained 1,324,516 raw reads from which 32,314 high quality contigs and 51,118 singletons were assembled. Functional annotation of the 75 per cent of the contigs was done resulting in 7,481 novel sequences. While using 454 GS-FLX pyrosequencing platform the transcriptome analysis of red pepper (*Capsicum annuum* L. TF68) was done by Lu *et al.* (2012). They obtained approximately 30.63 Mb of EST data with 9,818 contigs and 23,712 singletons.

Nicolai *et al.* (2012) performed transcriptome analysis using Roche 454 pyrosequencing and this consists of 23,748 contigs and 60,370 singletons. Detailed analysis identified a total of 11,849 SNPs in addition of 853 SSRs. Ashrafi *et al.* (2012) used three chilli genotypes namely Maor, Early Jalapeño and Criollo de Morelos-334 (CM334) for transcriptome sequencing. From the first assembly, they identified a total of 4,236 SNPs and 2,489 SSRs, while the second transcriptome assembly based on Illumina Genome Analyzer II resulted in 22,000 high-quality putative SNPs and 10,398 SSRs. Recently, the Pepper GeneChip array from Affymetrix in *Capsicum* for polymorphism detection and expression analysis was developed by Hill *et al.* (2013). Hybridization of genomic DNA from 40 diverse *C. annuum* lines and few lines from other cultivated species such as *C. frutescens, C. chinense* and *C. pubescens* resulted in generation of 33,401 Single Position Marker (SPP) markers within 13,323 unigenes (Hill *et al.*, 2013). Liu *et al.* (2013) constructed *De novo* transcriptome assembly in *C. frutescens* where, three candidate genes involved in the biosynthesis of capsaicinoids were identified and the sequence of these three genes namely, Dihydroxyacid dehydratase (DHAD), Thr deaminase (TD) and Prephenate aminotransferase (PAT) were predicted. They obtained 54,045 high-quality unigenes of which 4,072 SSRs were identified. Additionally, a total of 9,150 putative SNPs, which was detected between *C. frutescens* and *C. annuum*, existed in 3,349 contigs. A high throughput transcriptome profiling were done in two *Capsicum annuum* verities yielded 279,221 and 316,357 sequenced reads with a total 120.44 and 142.54 Mb of sequence data (Ahn *et al.*, 2013). Detailed sequence variant analysis identified a total of 9701 and 12,741 potential SNPs. In Table 8.4 a web databases are listed which provide bioinformatics support and analysis of *Capsicum* genetics and genomics.

Biotic Stress Tolerance

The *Capsicum* crop is affected by many factors such as fungal disease, bacterial disease, viral disease, nematodes. Several reports are available for resistance against these pathogens through many years of research.

Bacterial Spot Disease

Bacterial spot disease of pepper occurs worldwide and is major problem in tropical and subtropical regions (Jones *et al.*, 1998). The causal organism of the disease for pepper is *Xanthomonas campestris* pv. *vesicatoria* (*Xcv*). Pierre *et al.* (2000) identified AFLP markers linked to *Bs3* gene conferring resistance to *Xcv*, and mapped in a linkage map with a genetic resolution of 0.13 cM. Thereafter, a total of seven genes, 4 dominant (*Bs1* to *Bs4*) and three recessive genes (*bs5* and *bs6*, gdr) were reported (Jones *et al.*, 2002, 2004; Csillery *et al.*, 2004). Tai *et al.* (1999) detected AFLP markers associated with *Bs2* gene showing resistance against *Xcv*. Vallejos

Table 8.4: List of Web Databases Providing Bioinformatics Support for Analysis of *Capsicum* Genetics and Genomics

Database	*Institute/Affiliation*	*Country*	*Description*	*Weblonk*
Capsicum Transcriptome DB	Cinvestav Irapuato	Mexico	A collection of ESTs derived from five *C. annuum* organs (root, stem, leaf, flower and fruit) were sequenced using the Sanger method and multiple leaf transcriptomes were deeply sampled using with GS-pyrosequencing.	http://www.bioingenios.ira.cinvestav.mx:81/Joomla/
Kazusa Marker Database	Kazusa DNA Research Institute	Japan	*Capsicum annuum* EST-SSR and SNP markers	http://marker.kazusa.or.jp/Pepper/
PEPPER EST Database	Korea Research Institute of Bioscience and Biotechnology	Korea	A collection of 116,412 refined ESTs from 21 chilli pepper libraries which were constructed to represent 11 different tissues, developmental stages, or conditions of stress.	http://genepool.kribb.re.kr/pepper/
Sol Genomics Network	Boyce Thompson Institute for Plant Research	USA	A Collection SSR, RFLP, AFLP, PCR specific marker and putative genes for capsaicinoid pathway.	http://solgenomics.net/
Plant Genome Database of Japan	Kazusa DNA Research Institute	Japan	*Capsicum annuum* SSR and SNP Markers	http://pgdbj.jp/en/dna-marker-linkage-map/plant-species-list.html
SolCyc Database	Boyce Thompson Institute for Plant Research	USA	A collection genes, metabolites involved in Capsicum metabolism (Specially Capsaicinoid pathway)	http://solgenomics.net/tools/solcyc/index.pl

et al. (2010) found combine effect of the *bs5* and *bs6* genes resulted in complete resistance against P6 race.

Choi *et al.* (2007) characterized a *CaPO2* (*C. annuum* peroxidase) gene in *Arabidopsis* which provide enhanced resistance to *Xcv*. While, *CaPO2*-silenced pepper plants were highly susceptible to *Xcv* infection and showed compromised hydrogen peroxide (H_2O_2) accumulation and hypersensitive cell death in leaves. Using F_2 population derived from a cross of *C. chinense* (resistant) and *C. annuum* (susceptible). Voorrip *et al.* (2004) mapped a QTL for *Colletotrichum gloeosporioides* resistance, which is also responsible for bacterial spot disease. A *CaLOX1* gene, which encodes a 9-specic lipoxygenase, was isolated from *Xcv* infected pepper leaves (Hwang *et al.*, 2010), which over expressed in *Arabidopsis* conferred enhanced resistance to *Pseudomonas syringae* pv *tomato*, *Hyaloperonospora arabidopsidis*, and *Alternaria brassicicola*. Kim et *al.* (2012) reported that silencing of the gene *CaMLO2* in pepper can enhance resistance against *Xcv* through cell-death response, reduced bacterial growth, and accelerated reactive oxygen species burst. While its over-expression in *Arabidopsis* leads to susceptibility for *Pseudomonas syringae* pv. *Tomato* (Pst) and *Hyaloperonospora arabidopsidis*.

Phytopthora Resistance

Phytophthora capsici is arguably the most destructive pathogen to pepper (*Capsicum* sp.) which attacks all parts of the plant (Quirin *et al.*, 2005). It is assumed that, annual damage of Phytophthora blight to chilli yield in world-wide exceeds U.S. $100 million (Bosland 2008). Several resistant germplasm have been identified which confers high resistance against *Phyptopthora capsici*. These include 'AC2258' 'PI201232' and 'PI201234' from Central America, and 'CM334' from Mexico (Bosland and Lindsey 1991, Ortega *et al.*, 1992, Quirin *et al.*, 2005). Thabuis *et al.* (2004) identified 18 QTLs by using three *C. annuum* populations and transferred this resistance factors from CM-334 into a bell pepper genetic background.

Ogundiwin *et al.* (2005) detected 16 chromosomal interval containing single or clusters of resistance QTL for root rot and (or) foliar blight, suggesting a complex set of genetics involved in the resistance to *P. capsici*. Quirin *et al.* (2005) found OpD04 RAPD marker to be tightly linked to highly resistant lines, which converted into SCAR markers. Kim *et al.* (2008) developed two SSRs, one single-nucleotide amplified polymorphic marker (SNAP) and CAPS markers associated with *P. capsici* resistance. Later, Oh *et al.* (2010) found that silencing of *CaMsrB2* gene in transformed *CaMsrB2*-pepper plants leads to increased production of Reactive Oxygen Species, ultimately turns to acceleration of cell death. They found that *Pme* genes (*Pcpme* 1-9) from highly virulent *P. capsici* strain SD33 were differentially expressed in three host species in the course of *P. capsici* interaction.

Rushton *et al.* (2010) found WRKY proteins, which plays vital role in defence against biotic stresses and abiotic stresses in plants. They positively regulate resistance against bacterial disease caused by *Ralstonia solanacearum*, such that, the overexpression of *caWRKY40* in tobacco imparts resistance to *R. solanacearum* and tolerance to heat shock, while silencing leads to susceptibility to *R. solanacearum* and impaired thermo tolerance in chilli pepper (Dang *et al.*, 2013). In contrast,

Wang *et al.* (2013) observed silencing of *CaWRKY58* in pepper plants resulted in enhanced resistance to the highly virulent *R. solanacearum* strain. Wang *et al.* (2013) characterized three Polygalacturonase-inhibiting proteins (PGIPs) from peppers which plays critical role in inhibition of fungal endopolygalacturonases (PGs). Transgenic tobacco expressing *CaPGIP1* gene showed enhanced resistance to PG activity of fungi and a significant reduction in number and average size of lesions and of infection sites in the leaves.

Recently, a *P. capsici* resistance gene, *CaRGA2*, from *C. annuum*, cv. CM334 was isolated and characterized by Zhang *et al.* (2013) and expression analysis proved the involvement of *CaRGA2* gene in conferring resistance against *P. capsici*. Reeves *et al.* (2013) reported a novel disease resistance inhibitor gene (*Ipcr*), in the pepper variety NMCA10399, which inhibits resistance to *Phytophthora capsici* but not to other species of *Phytophthora*. By using F_8 RIL population Hong Truong *et al.* (2013) detected an AFLP converted SCAR marker (SA133_4) and RAPD marker (UBC553) linked to *Phytophthora* root rot resistance and mapped on chromosome 5.

Powdery Mildew

Powdery mildew is an important pathogen in pepper and caused by *Leveillula taurica*. Using doubled-haploid population from cross of H3 (resistant) and Vania (susceptible) genotype, Lefebvre *et al.* (2003) mapped powdery mildew resistance QTL. They found seven genomic regions including additive QTL and studied their epistatic interactions.

Viral Resistance

Viruses are one of the most devastating pathogen and are major constraints for capsicum yield. Several resistance genetic sources have been identified against tobacco mosaic virus, poty viruses, and cucumber mosaic viruses.

Cucumber mosaic virus (CMV) has broadest host range and large insect vector range, due to this complete control is difficult. Detection of QTLs conferring partial resistance against CMV was reported (Pochard *et al.*, 1983, Caranata *et al.*, 1997, 2002, Ben Chaim *et al.*, 2001). Kang *et al.* (2010) identified a single dominant resistance gene *Cmr1* (Cucumber mosaic resistance 1) from *C. annuum* cultivar 'Bukang' against CMV (Korean) and CMV (FNY) strains. Genetic mapping and FISH analysis showed that the *Cmr1* gene is located at the centromeric region of LG2, syntenic to the ToMV resistance locus (*Tm*-1) in tomatoes. Yao *et al.* (2013) observed an inbred line 'BJ0747-1-3-1-1' derived from a Chinese local variety confering resistance to cucumber mosaic virus (CMV) local isolate (CMVHB). They identied two stable and major QTLs that collectively explained 55 per cent of the trait variations.

Another most destructive pathogen for chilli is "Poty viruses" which includes pepper veinal mottle virus (PVMV), chilli veinal mottle virus (CVMV), potato virus Y (PVY), tobacco etch virus (TEV) and pepper mottle virus (PepMoV) (Green and Kim 1991). The *pvr2* was first characterized gene against *potyvirus* and which mapped on chromosome 4 (Murphy *et al.*, 1998; Kang *et al.*, 2005). This gene was found as a eukaryotic translation initiation factor *4E*(*eIF4E*), which codes for 228 amino acid and only two amino acids difference was observed between resistant and susceptible genotype (Ruffel *et al.*, 2002). Using doubled-haploid progeny, Carantha *et al.* (1997) detected 11 resistant QTLs for two PVY isolates and two potyvirus E. The same group developed CAPS marker tightly linked to the *Pvr4* resistance gene which showed complete resistance to the three pathotypes of PVY and PepMoV (Caranta *et al.* (1999).

Grube *et al.* (2000) detected a dominant resistant gene, *Pvr7* against the PepMoV and mapped on chromosome 10. Matsunaga *et al.* (2003) detected a RAPD marker linked to Pepper Mild Mottle Virus (PMMoV) resistant locus (*L4*) and developed a tightly linked SCAR marker "WA31-1500S' in *Capsicum* species. Rubio *et al.* (2008) developed functional markers based on SNPs at the *pvr2-eIF4E* locus that showed resistance to several potyviruses and could be useful for breeding programs. Several studies reported that double and simultaneous mutations in translation initiation factors *eIF4E* (*pvr2*) and *eIF* (iso) *4E9* (*pvr6*) are required to prevent pepper veinal mottle virus infection in pepper (Ruffel *et al.*, 2006, Hwang *et al.*, 2009, Rubio *et al.*, 2009). Arnedo-Andrés *et al.* (2002) developed SCAR markers for *Pvr4* which confers resistance against PVY in *Capsicum*. Lee *et al.* (2013) developed a new genetically dominant resistant line of chilli pepper for chilli veinal mottle virus. They identified 2 AFLP markers linked to dominant resistance which were located on chromosome 6 and through comparative mapping identified one CAPS marker closer to CAMV resistance locus.

Chilli yield is also largely affected by tobacco mosaic virus (TMV); several reports and genetic analysis indicated that resistance against TMV is regulated by several alleles of L gene (Lefebvre *et al.*, 1995, Ben-Cham *et al.*, 2001, Tomita *et al.*, 2008). Lim *et al.* (2011) found *CaWRKYb* gene, which is a positive transcription factor and plays vital role in defense-related signal transduction pathways in chilli pepper. Huh *et al.* (2012b) characterized *CaWRKYd* transcription factor and suggested its role in hypersensitive response (HR) cell death. Huh *et al.* (2012a) observed that an important transcription factor named *CaBtf3* induces transcriptional changes in defense-related genes. Hernan *et al.* (2013) reported silencing of *NPR1* genes in both *N. benthamiana* and *C. annuum* and found the plants viral symptoms increased to levels similar to those seen in wild-type plants.

Tomato spotted wilt virus (TSWV) is also a devastating virus in the chilli field. Bouitex *et al.* (1993) observed two *C. chinense* lines ('CNPH 275' and 'PI 159236') were virtually immune against one specific (TSWV-BsB) isolate but were susceptible to another isolate (TSWV-SP). Moury *et al.* (2000) reported the resistance to this virus by single dominant gene, known as *Tsw*. They detected 4 RAPD markers tightly linked to *Tsw*, of which, one RAPD marker was converted into CAPS, which further used for breeding programs. This *Tsw* gene was mapped in distal portion of chromosome 10 in *C. annuum* (Jahn *et al.* (2000). Margaria *et al.* (2007) identified, naturally occurring resistance-breaking (RB) TSWV strains and with further analysis showed that local necrotic response is not sufficient for resistance in *Capsicum* spp. carrying the *Tsw* gene. It was found that during hypersensitivity the N protein of TSWV is associated with the induction of programmed cell death (PCD) in *C. chinense* plants (Lovato *et al.* (2008).

Root- Knot Nematode (RKN) Disease

Root-knot nematodes (*Meloidogyne* species) are polyphagous pests causing severe damage to several Solanaceae crops. In *C. annuum*, many genes showing resistance to RKN is associated with several dominant genes that are thought to act independently in gene-for-gene interactions (Djian-Caporalino *et al.*, 1999, 2001). One of the first reports was characterization of nematode resistance gene N by Thies and Fery (2000, 2002). It was found that the genes *Me4*, *Mech1*, and *Mech2* were specific to certain *Meloidogyne* species or populations (Djian-Caporalino *et al.*, 2001, 2007). Further genetic analysis suggested that these nematode resistance genes are located in orthologous genomic regions in Solanaceae (Djian-Caporalino *et al.*, 2007).

Chen *et al.* (2007) characterized a nematode resistant gene *CaMi* in tomato plants, which confers enhanced resistance against the root-knot nematodes compared to untransformed susceptible plants. Fazari *et al.* (2012) developed PCR based markers associated with *Me* and *N*-genes which could be very useful for the breeding programs in pepper.

Abiotic Stress Tolerance

In field conditions, plants are exposed to different abiotic stresses such as, high temperature, cold, water deficit, salinity, heavy metals and mechanical wounding. These stresses drastically affect the plant leading to more than 50 per cent loss in crop yield. In *Capsicum*, several genes/loci have been identified for tolerance against abiotic stress and also some of them displayed response against biotic stress (principally pathogen infection).

Lee *et al.* (2003) identified SAR8.2 genes as molecular marker for pathogen infection (*Xcv*), abiotic elicitors like Ethylene, Methyl jasmonate, IAA, ABA, Salicylic acid and environmental stresses. An ERF/AP2-type transcription factor (*CaPF1*) was isolated from *Xanthomonas axonopodis* pv *glycines* 8ra infected pepper leaves by differential-display reverse transcription-PCR. (Yi *et al.*, 2004). Transgenic *Arabidopsis* plants expressing *CaPF1* displayed tolerance against freezing temperatures and enhanced resistance to *Pseudomonas syringae* pv *tomato* DC3000 (Yi *et al.*, 2004).

A *CAZFP1* gene, (Cys2/His-type zinc-nger transcription factor) was successfully isolated from an avirulent strain Bv5-4a of *Xanthomonas campestris* pv. *vesicatoria* infected pepper leaves, when transformed in *Arabidopsis* not only showed enhanced resistance against *Pseudomonas syringae* pv. *tomato*, but also the drought tolerance (Kim *et al.*, 2004). Several other repotrs indicating dual role in response to biotic and abiotic stress exist. Sohn *et al.* (2005) isolated a novel pathogen-induced RAV (Related to ABI3/VP1) transcription factor, named *CARAV1*, from *Xanthomonas campestris* pv. *vesicatoria* infected pepper leaves, when over expression in *Arabidopsis* showed tolerance to osmotic stresses by high salinity and dehydration (drought stress) along with resistance against bacterial disease. Later, it was found that CaOXR1 (*Capsicum annuum*, oxidoreductase) protein that physically interacts with the *CaRAV1* transcription factor and positively regulate *CaRAV1*-mediated plant defence during biotic and abiotic stresses (Lee *et al.*, 2010).

Hong *et al.* (2005) investigated the structural properties and expression profiles of *Ca-DREBLP1* (dehydration-responsive element binding-factor-like protein 1) gene in hot pepper, which was rapidly induced by dehydration, high salinity and, but not by cold stress. Hong *et al.* (2007) characterized the GDSL-type pepper lipase gene, named *CaGLIP1,* they proved the gene functions in disease susceptibility to *Xanthomonas campestris* pv. *vesicatoria* (*Xcv*), But when introduced in *Arabidopsis,* conferred enhanced tolerance to drought and glucose stress while differential response against oxidative stress in the form of Methyl Viologen (MV).

From the water-stressed library a gene *CaXTH3* was isolated and introduced in *Arabidopsis* which led to abnormal leaf morphology due to increased numbers of small-sized cells, resulting in disordered, highly populated mesophyll cells. In addition, the transgenic plants displayed markedly improved tolerance to severe water deficit and to lesser extent to high salinity (Cho *et al.,* 2006). Expression profile of cold stressed pepper plant was studied by Hwang *et al.* (2006), and they found up-regulation of 45 genes, simultaneously expressed in salt stress condition. They also identified an array of transcription factors such as, a bZIP protein (CaBZ1), a family of 4 ethylene-responsive element binding protein (EREBP, designated CaEREBP-C1 to C4) genes, RVA1, ring domain protein, HSF1, WRKY (CaWRKY1) protein, SAR8.2 protein precursor, late-embryogenesis abundant protein 5 (LEA5), DNAJ protein homologue and many more. A BI-1[BCL2-associated x protein (BAX) inhibitor-1] gene, named as *CaBI-1,* isolated from a heat stressed cDNA library, was found to act as anti-programmed cell death factor. Upon introducing the *CaBI-1* in tobacco displayed markedly improved tolerance to high temperature, water deficit, and high salinity compared to control plants (Isbat *et al.,* 2009).

A *sod* gene, encoding a tomato chloroplast-localized Cu/Zn SOD protein was characterized for their novel function (Chatzidimitriadou *et al.,* 2009). The *sod* gene introduced in pepper found to be tolerant to different oxidative stresses such as Methyl Viologen (MV) and drought and also to have an increased resistance to oxidative damage. Apart from this they helps in improving the regeneration efficiency of pepper explants. Zeba *et al.* (2009) isolated *Capsicum annuum* RING Zinc Finger Protein 1 (*CaRZFP1*) gene from heat stressed library and characterized in tobacco showed enhanced growth accompanied with longer vegetative growth and bigger number of leaves.

An early light-inducible protein gene (*CaELIP*) was isolated from a cDNA library of hot pepper that showed heavy metal (manganese, zinc, copper) stress-inducible expressions (Tao *et al.,* 2011). *CaELIP* also showed an endogenous circadian rhythmicity with high expression level in the morning and decreased expression level thereafter. Several genes from pepper have been identified and characterised such as *CAPIP2* (*Capsicum annuum* pathogen-induced gene), *CaPO2* (*Capsicum annuum* extracellular peroxidase 2), *CaPMEI1* (*Capsicum annuum* pectin methylesterase inhibitor protein) which confers resistance against biotic as well as abiotic stresses (Lee *et al.,* 2006, An *et al.,* 2008, Choi *et al.,* 2012). Khan *et al.* (2013) observed that *Capsicum annuum* having symbiotic relation with the fungi (*Penicillium resedanum* LK6) show less detrimental effects on osmotic stress (especially in drought) by decreasing losses in biomass as compared to non-inoculated plants.

This ultimately leads to increase in crop production in drought prone lands. Wang *et al.* (2013) found a novel peroxidise gene *CanPOD* in defence response against *Phytophtora capsici* infection. In addition, it was up-regulated after salt and drought stress treatments showing response against abiotic stress.

Comparative Mapping: Gene Discovery for Specific Traits

Comparative genetic mapping studies was performed among the plant species belonging to same family reveal similarities and differences in gene content and gene order between genera belonging to different taxa. In the Solanaceae family, mostly the comparative mapping was predicted by relating genetic maps of tomato and pepper. In one of the first report of comparative mapping, tomato RFLPs markers were used for development of linkage maps in peppers and also observed several syntenic regions between the genome of two species (Tanksley 1988, Livingstone *et al.*, 1999).

Thorup *et al.* (2004) using F_2 genetic map from cross of *C. annuum* and *C. chinense* found position of important genes for carotenoid biosynthetic pathway in pepper such as *Ccs*. Further, lycopene b-cyclase gene and lycopene cyclase locus in pepper mapped to respective corresponding homologous region in tomato. Thabuis *et al.* (2004) suggested the use of common markers which can be mapped in tomato and pepper showing chromosomal region containing disease resistance gene clusters syntenic to both the species. The genes conferring resistance to tobacco mosaic virus CMV, potyviruses and TSWV have been found to co-map in the same pepper genomic region (Lefebvre *et al.*, 1995, Caranta *et al.*, 1997a, b; Moury *et al.*, 1997). Ben Chaim *et al.* (2006) analyzed *fw*2.1 and *fw*2.2 QTL, for fruit weight, pericarp thickness and fruit shape and found synteny in both genomes. Zygier *et al.* (2005) mapped QTL for fruit weight and shape in pepper and when compared with the tomato QTL found that the pepper and tomato QTL are orthologous to each other which can be further used in marker assisted breeding program. For *P. capsici* resistance several reports are available (in Solanaceae family) stating the synteny between the major locus of pepper and potato (Leonards-Schippers *et al.*, 1994, Sandbrik *et al.*, 2000, Thabuis *et al.*, 2004). They also found that the *P. capsici* resistance locus was closely linked to R gene for nematode resistance (Lefebvre *et al.*, 2002), which shows a putative orthologous region in tomato and potato containing same R genes for resistance to nematodes (Djian-Caporalino *et al.*, 2001).

In the case of viral resistance, the common resistance loci were detected containing two potyvirus R genes; *Pvr4* and *Pvr7* and *Tsw* gene (for TSWV resistance) were mapped (Caranta *et al.*, 1999, Grube *et al.*, 2000a, Moury *et al.*, 2000, Lefebvre *et al.*, 2002, Thabuis *et al.*, 2004). It was found that this loci is an orthologous to a region of tomato chromosome 1 containing two R genes (*Cf*-1 and *Cf*-4) conferring specific resistance to *Cladosporium fulvum* (Jones *et al.*, 2002). Ruffel *et al.* (2006) performed comparative genetic mapping for *eIF4E* gene and found it is highly conserved in pepper and tomato.

Several such reports of comparative mapping with traditional breeding tools showed its importance in crop improvement. Recently available draft genome sequences of Potato and Tomato (The Potato Genome Sequencing Consortium 2011,

The Tomato genome sequencing corsortium 2012) would be beneficial for revealing orthologous genes associated with agronomically and economically important characters like fruit traits, disease resistances and other biochemical traits (Paran and Van Der Knaap 2007).

Genetic Improvement through Biotechnological Tools

Several biotechnological tools were used for the genetic improvement of Capsicum. Results of these experiments are discussed in the following section.

Tissue Culture in *Capsicum* Improvement

Tissue culture has been exploited to create genetic variability by producing haploids, somaclonal and gametoclonal variants from which crop plants can be improved. Although, being a member of Solanaceae family *Capsicum* is recalcitrant to tissue culture while, other crops such as tobacco, tomato, potato have been frequently used as a model system in tissue culture and plant genetic transformations. Gunay and Rao (1978) studied different hormonal combinations for organogenesis in *Capsicum.* Cotyledons and hypocotyls were used as explants from two *C. annuum* cultivars and a hybrid of *C. frutescens* (Bharath) and were cultured on Murashige and Skoog (Murashige and Skoog 1962) medium containing the auxins, indole-3-acetic acid (IAA), naphthaleneacetic acid (NAA), 2,4-dichlorophenoxyacetic acid (2,4-D) and the cytokinins, benzyladenine (BA), kinetin (KN), Zeatin (Zea), Zeatin (Zea), 6-benzyl 9-tetra hydropyrane adenine (SD 8339), adenine and coconut milk. Among the different factors affecting *Capsicum* regeneration, the selection of genotype for organ culture is very important. Venkataiah *et al.* (2003) reported thidiazuron (TDZ)-mediated organogenesis in ten pepper cultivars and found only *Capsicum annuum* cv.CA 960, G4 and X-235 produced maximum number of adventitious shoots. Kehie *et al.* (2012a) developed an efficient and simple protocol for *in vitro* regeneration of Naga King Chilli (*C. chinense*) from nodal segments and shoots tips with 18.16 µM Thidiazuron (TDZ) in MS medium. They found the number of shoot developed was nearly twofold more than what has been reported earlier (Sanatombi and Sharma 2008).

Several other attempts have been made on *in vitro* plant regeneration of the genus *Capsicum* through different protocols and morphogenic pathways (Reddy *et al.*, 2002, Venkataiah *et al.*, 2003, Anilkumar and Nair 2004, Peddaboina *et al.*, 2006, Khan *et al.*, 2006, Mezghani 2007). Among the choice of explants, Cotyledon was found to be the most responsive explant. Sanatombi and Sharma (2008) studied the effect of different explants in six cultivars belonging to three species of *Capsicum* (*C. annuum, C. frutescens and C. chinense*) and found leaf and cotyledons to be the most responsive explants in comparison to hypocotyls.

Other factors which influence the organogenic response are the position of the explants, plant growth regulators and growth adjuvant in culture medium, carbon source, light regime, gelling agent and temperature. Lim and Lian (2001) studied factors inûuencing protoplast isolation and culture in C. *annuum* baccatum and C. *chacoense*. They successfully isolated protoplast from cotyledon, hypocotyls and mesophyll tissues using a combination of cellulose (1 per cent), macerozyme (0.25 per cent) and 0.65 M sorbitol.

Several reports are available where *in vitro* cultured cells and tissues have been used for the production of capsaicinoids (Lindsey *et al.*, 1983, Mavituna and Park 1985, Ravishankar *et al.*, 1988, Salgado-Garciglia and Ochoa-Alejo 1990, Ochoa-Alejo and Salgardo-Garciglia 1992, Sudha and Ravishankar, 2002, Nunez-Palenius and Ochoa-Alejo 2005, Gutiérrez-Carbajal *et al.*, 2010, Kehie *et al.*, 2012b). Kothari *et al.* (2010) reviewed tissue culture and transgenic techniques used for *Capsicum* improvement.

Genetic Transformation of *Capsicum*

Genetic transformation has become an indispensable tool for improvement of crops. It has emerged as a remarkable tool for the application of modern biotechnology. Application of genetic transformation requires the development of efficient techniques for both the transfer of foreign genes into plant cells, and for regeneration of whole plants from the transformed cells (Ochoa-alejo and Ramirez-malagon 2001). Transformation method or delivery system involves the use of several technologies and requires a vector that has the capacity to shuttle isolated genetic fragments into a viable host cell (Razzaq *et al.*, 2004). *Agrobacterium tumefaciens* has been employed as the vector for genetic transformation of diverse dicotyledonous species, whereas biolistic bombardment has been a very useful technique to deliver foreign genes into plant cells of both monocotyledonous and dicotyledonous plants. In the case of chilli pepper, genetic transformation is certainly an important goal to facilitate genetic improvement against several diseases caused by phytopathogenic fungi, bacteria, and viruses, as well as for improvement against different pests and several abiotic factors. However, due to the recalcitrant nature of *Capsicum* species, advances in this area have been limited resulting in low efficiency *in vitro* plant regeneration systems (Ochoa-alejo Ramirez-malagon 2001).

The first work on chilli pepper genetic transformation was reported by Liu *et al.* (1990). They used six bell pepper cultivars (*C. annuum* L.) and one Guatemalan wild accession of *C. annuum* var. glabriusculum. Explants (hypocotyls, cotyledons and leaves) derived from in virto grown seedlings were co-cultured with individual suspensions of the wild tumorigenic strains A281 and C58 of *A. tumefaciens*, and with a disarmed strain bearing the plasmid pGV3850 containing the neomycin phosphotransferase gene (nptII) and the β-glucuronidase gene (gus) under the control of the 35S promoter from cauliflower mosaic virus. Only cotyledon and leaf tissues formed callus, leaf-like structures, and occasional shoot buds in the presence of 200 mg l^{-1} kanamycin. Sections from leaf-like structures and shoot buds showed GUS positive responses, while GUS activity was not observed in shoot buds from control explants. Wang (1991) used cotyledon, hypocotyl and leaf explants for transformation and regeneration, and transformants were able to show transient GUS activity. Lee *et al.* (1993) reported *Agrobacterium*-mediated transformation from cotyledon explants of hot pepper (*Capsicum annuum* cv. Golden Tower). Cotyledon explants were co-cultured with *Agrobacterium tumefaciens* strain LBA4404 carrying a binary vector pRok1/105 harboring the cDNA of cucumber mosaic virus I17N-satellite RNA. They obtained 4 per cent transformation frequency. Zhu *et al.* (1996) obtained transgenic sweet pepper through *Agrobacterium*-mediated transformation using *Agrobacterium* strain GV311-SE harboring cucumber mosaic cucumovirus coat protein (*cms-cp*) gene.

Kim *et al.* (1997) investigated RNA-mediated resistance to cucumber 827 mosaic virus in the progeny of transgenic plants of hot pepper that expresses RNA. Several workers have attempted to transform *Capsicum* species but with less than 0.1 per cent transformation efficiency were obtained (Jayashankar 1997). A protocol for regeneration and genetic transformation of chilli pepper (*C. annuum* L. var. Pusa jwala) was developed by Manoharan *et al.* (1998). They obtained four regenerated transgenic plants from 10 explants bearing shoot buds from a total of 200 cotyledonary explants.

Li *et al.* (2003) developed an efficient genetic transformation system using pepper cotyledons as explants through *A. tumefaciens* strain LBA 4404 with the plasmid pBI 121. High-frequency shoot regeneration and *Agrobacterium* mediated DNA transfer in red chilli has been reported by Sobhakumari and Lalithakumari (2005). Shoot tip explants were co-cultivated with *Agrobacterium* strain EHA105 carrying a T-DNA with CaMV 35S promoter and *GUS* as reporter gene. The integration of *GUS* gene in *Capsicum annuum* genome was conrmed by GUS staining, PCR and southern analysis. A new selection method for pepper transformation via callus mediated shoot transformation was developed by Lee *et al.* (2004).

Solís-Ramos *et al.* (2009) described an *Agrobacterium* mediated transformation of Habanero chilli pepper (*C. chinense*) with the gene *WUSCHEL* from *A. thaliana* under the control of an estradiol inducible promoter as a means of overcoming the somatic embryogenesis formation recalcitrant plants. This study suggests that heterologous gene *WUSCHEL* was active and involved in the somatic embryogenesis process. Transgenic pepper highly tolerant to a new CMV pathotype (CMVP1) was developed by Lee *et al.* (2009). They obtained three independent T_3 pepper lines expressing coat protein gene CMVP0-CP, highly tolerant to CMVP0 pathogen. Gururaj *et al.* (2012) reported the functional validation of putative aminotransferase gene for vanillylamine biosynthesis in heterologous system using *Agrobacterium* mediated genetic transformation studies in *C. frutescens* calli cultures.

Several researchers have attempted to transform this recalcitrant species in the last recent decade (Phillips *et al.*, 2000, Harpster *et al.*, 2002, Shin *et al.*, 2002, Lee *et al.*, 2004, Delis *et al.*, 2005, Lee *et al.*, 2009, Sharma *et al.*, 2008). A tissue culture independent *Agrobacterium* mediated *in planta* transformation has been attempted in two varieties of *C. annuum* (Kumar *et al.*, 2009).

Although some advances have been made in recent years to establish stable transformation of *Capsicum* species, the efficiency is very low when compared to other members of the Solanaceae family. Genetic transformation through *Agrobacterium tumefaciens* and other methods *viz*, particle gun bombardment, electroporation, etc. are emerging as the methods of choice for introduction of agronomically important genes for quality improvement, regulation of secondary metabolites, and for the engineering molecular farming in pharmaceutical, nutraceutical and food industry.

Conclusion

As sequencing technologies are advancing at rapid rate, and with conventional breeding knowledge, enormous information is available related to genome of *Capsicum*. Despite having several reports of QTLs/genes for different traits, only a few number of genes/QTL loci were amenable for incorporation in translational research of *Capsicum* species. For example, Mazourek *et al.* (2009) detected only *Pun1* gene which is found to be directly associated to capsaicinoid complex from over 30 QTLs. Apart from extensively studied pungency and carotenoids traits, other metabolites and bioactive compounds including whole metabolomics could be studied which will be helpful in breeding programmes for biochemical traits. The combination of high throughput NGS technologies with traditional breeding tools would be helpful for accelerating the pepper genomics research. As genome sequence of *Capsicum* is expected to become available soon, this will help to integrate the genomics assisted breeding (GAB) with the help of conventional breeding. The integration of genomic, transcriptomic, proteomic, metabolomics, translational genomics and germplasm resources with different traditional and modern molecular breeding techniques would accelerate the identification of novel genes/orthologous genes for improvement in *Capsicum*.

Acknowledgments

The authors thank to the Department of Biotechnology, Government of India, for financial assistant to Nirala Ramchiary in the form of Prestigious Ramalingaswami Fellowship.

References

Ahn YK, Tripathi S, Kim JH, Cho YI *et al.*, Transcriptome analysis of *Capsicum annuum* varieties Mandarin and Blackcluster: Assembly, annotation and molecular marker discovery. *Gene* 533: 494–499.

Aluru MR, Mazourek M, Landry LG, Curry J *et al.*, Differential expression of fatty acid synthase genes, Acl, Fat and Kas, in *Capsicum* fruit. *J. Expl. Bot.* 54: 1655–1664.2003.

Anilkumar M, Nair AS. Multiple shoot induction in *Capsicum annuum* L. cv. Early California Wonder. Plant Cell Biotech. *Mol. Biol.* 5: 95-100. 2004.

An SH, Sohn KH, Choi HW, Hwang IS *et al.*, Pepper pectin methylesterase inhibitor protein CaPMEI1 is required for antifungal activity, basal disease resistance and abiotic stress tolerance. *Planta.* 228: 61–78.2008.

Arnedo-Andres MS, Gil-Ortega R, Luis-Arteaga M, Hormaza JI. Development of RAPD and SCAR markers linked to the Pvr4 locus for resistance to PVY in pepper (*Capsicum annuum* L.). *Theo. Appl. Genet.* 105: 1067–1074. 2002.

Arumuganathan K, Earle E. Nuclear DNA content of some important plant species. *Plant Mol. Biol. Rep.* 9: 208–218. 1991.

Ashrafi H, Hill T, Stoffel K, Kozik A *et al.*, *De novo* assembly of the pepper transcriptome (*Capsicum annuum*): A benchmark for in silico discovery of SNPs, SSRs and candidate genes. *BMC Genomics*. 13: 571. 2012.

Aza-Gonza´lez C, Nunez-Palenius HG, Ochoa-Alejo N. Molecular biology of capsaicinoid biosynthesis in chili pepper (*Capsicum* spp.). *Plant Cell Rep*. 30: 695–706. 2011.

Babu BS, Pandravada SR, Prasad Rao RDVJ, Anitha K *et al.*, Global source of pepper genetic resources against arthropods, nematodes and pathogens. *Crop Prot*. 30: 389–400. 2011.

Basu SK, De AK. *Capsicum*: historical and botanical perspectives. In: De AK, editor. *Capsicum: The Genus Capsicum*. London: CRC Press. pp. 1-15. 2003.

Barchi L, Lefebvre V, Sage-Palloix AM, Lanteri S, Palloix A. QTL analysis of plant development and fruit traits in pepper and performance of selective phenotyping. *Theo. Appl. Genet*. 118: 1157–1171. 2009.

Bartoszewski G, Waszczak C, Gawronski P, Stepien I *et al.*, Mapping of the ms8 male sterility gene in sweet pepper (Capsicum annuum L.) on the chromosome P4 using PCR-based markers useful for breeding programmes. *Euphytica*. 186: 453–461. 2012.

Ben-Chaim A, Borovsky Y, Rao GU, Tanyolac B, Paran I. *fs3*.1: A major fruit shape QTL conserved in *Capsicum. Genome*. 46: 1-9. 2003.

Ben-Chaim A, Brodsky Y, Falise M, Mazourek M *et al.*, QTL analysis for capsaicinoid content in *Capsicum. Theo. Appl. Genet*. 113: 1481-1490. 2006.

Ben-Chaim A, Grube RC, Lapidot M, Jahn M, Paran I. Identification of quantitative trait loci associated with resistance to cucumber mosaic virus in *Capsicum annuum*. Theo. *Appl. Genet*. 102: 1213-1220. 2001.

Bennett DJ, Kirby GW. Constitution and biosynthesis of capsaicin. *J. Chem. Soc.* C 442–446. 1968.

Berger A, Henderson M, Nadoolman W, Duffy V *et al.*, Oral capsaicin provides temporary relief for oral mucositis pain secondary to chemotherapy/radiation therapy. *J Pain Symptom Manage*. 10: 243-248. 1996.

Blum E, Liu K, Mazourek M, Yoo EY *et al.*, Molecular mapping of the C locus for presence of pungency in *Capsicum. Genome*. 45: 702-705. 2002.

Blum E, Mazourek M, O'Connell M, Curry J *et al.*, Molecular mapping of capsaicinoid biosynthesis genes and QTL analysis for capsaicinoid content in *Capsicum. Theo. Appl. Genet*. 108: 79-86. 2003.

Boiteux LS, Nagata T, Dutra WP, Fonseca MEN. Sources of resistance to tomato spotted wilt virus (TSWV) in cultivated and wild species of *Capsicum. Euphytica*. 67(1-2) 89-94. 1993.

Borovsky Y, Paran I. Characterization of *fs10.1*, a major QTL controlling fruit elongation in *Capsicum. Theo. Appl. Genet*. 123: 657–665. 2011.

Bosland PW. *Capsicums:* Innovative uses of an ancient crop. In: Janick J, editor *Progress in new crops*. Arlington VA: Ashs Press. pp. 479–487. 1996.

Bosland, PW. Think global, breed local: Specificity and complexity of *Phytophthora capsici*. In: *19th Int. Pepper Conf. Atlantic City, NJ*. 2008.

Bosland PW, Lindsey DL. A seedling screen for *Phytophthora* root rot of pepper *Capsicum annuum*. *Plant Dis*. 75: 1048-1050. 1991.

Bosland PW, Votava EJ. *Peppers: Vegetable and spice Capsicums*. CABI Publishing New York. 2000.

Bosland PW, Walker SJ. Measuring chilli pepper heat. Guide 237, New Maxico State University, 2010. http: //aces.nmsu.edu/pubs/_h/h-237.pdf.

Caranta C, Palloix A, Gebre-Selassie K, Lefebvre V *et al.*, A complementation of two genes originating from susceptible Capsicum annuum lines confers a new and complete resistance to pepper veinal mottle virus. *Phytopathol*. 86: 739–743. 1996

Caranta C, Palloix A, Lefebvre V, Daube ze AM. QTLs for a component of partial resistance to cucumber mosaic virus in pepper: restriction of virus installation in host cells. *Theo. Appl. Genet*. 94: 431–438. 1997.

Caranta C, Thabuis A, Palloix A. Development of a CAPS marker for the *Pvr4* locus: a tool for pyramiding potyvirus resistance genes in pepper. *Genome*. 42 1111–1116. 1999.

Chatzidimitriadou K, Irini Nianiou-Obeidat I, Madesis P, Perl-Treves R, Tsaftaris A. Expression of SOD transgene in pepper confer stress tolerance and improve shoot regeneration. *Electron J. Biotech*. 12 (4). 2009. DOI: 10.2225/vol12-issue4-fulltext-10

Chaim AB, Borovsky Y, De Jong W, Paran I. Linkage of the A locus for the presence of anthocyanin and fs10.1, a major fruit-shape QTL in pepper. *Theo. Appl. Genet* 106: 8 89-94. 2003.

Chen C, Chen G, Hao Z, Cao B *et al.*, CaMF2, an anther-specic lipid transfer protein (LTP) gene, affects pollen development in *Capsicum annuum* L. *Plant Sci*. 181 439–448. 2011.

Chen CM, Hao XF, Chen GJ, Cao BH *et al.*, Characterization of a new male sterility-related gene Camf1 in *Capsicum annum* L. *Mol. Biol. Rep*. 39 (1): 737-44. 2012 doi: 10.1007/s11033-011-0793-3.

Chen RG, Li HX, Zhang LY, Zhang JH *et al.*, *CaMi*, a root-knot nematode resistance gene from hot pepper (*Capsicum annuum* L.) confers nematode resistance in tomato. *Plant Cell Rep*. 26: 895–905. 2007.

Cho SK, Kim JE, Park JA, Eom TJ, Kim WT. Constitutive expression of abiotic stress-inducible hot pepper *CaXTH3*, which encodes a xyloglucan endotransglucosylase/hydrolase homolog, improves drought and salt tolerance in transgenic *Arabidopsis* plants. FEBS Lett. 580: 3136–3144. 2006.

Choi D, Kim S, Park M, Yeom S *et al.*, The Genome Sequence of Hot Pepper (*Capsicum annuum* L.). Plant, Animal Genome Asia 2013, March, Singapore. 2013.

Choi HW, Hwang BK. The pepper extracellular peroxidase CaPO2 is required for salt, drought and oxidative stress tolerance as well as resistance to fungal pathogens. *Planta*. 235: 1369–1382. 2012.

Choi HW, Kim YJ, Lee SC, Hong JK, Hwang BK. Hydrogen peroxide generation by the pepper extracellular peroxidase *CaPO2* activates local and systemic cell death and defense response to bacterial pathogens. *Plant Physiol*. 145: 890–904. 2007.

Csillery G, Szarka E, Sardi E, Mityko J *et al*., The unity of plant defense: genetics, breeding and physiology. *Proc. 12th Eucarpia Meeting on Genetics and Breeding of Capsicum and Egg-plant*, Noordwijkerhout, the Netherlands. 147–153. 2004.

Curry J, Aluru M, Mendoza M, Nevarez J *et al*., Transcripts for possible capsaicinoid biosynthetic genes are differentially accumulated in pungent and non-pungent *Capsicum* spp. *Plant Sci*. 148: 47-57. 1999.

Dang FF, Wang YN, Yu L, Eulgem T *et al*., CaWRKY40, a WRKY protein of pepper, plays an important role in the regulation of tolerance to heat stress and resistance to *Ralstonia solanacearum* infection. *Plant Cell Environ*. 36: 757-74. 2013.

Delis M, Garbaczewska G, Niemirowicz-Szczytt K. Differentiation of adventitious buds from *Capsicum annuum* hypocotyls after co-culture with *Agrobacterium tumefaciens*. *Acta Biol. Crac*. 17: 193–198. 2005.

Díaz J, Pomar F, Bernall A, Merino F. Peroxidases and the metabolism of capsaicin in *Capsicum annuum* L. *Phytochem. Rev*. 3: 141–157. 2004.

Djian-Caporalino C, Pijarowski L, Januel A, Lefebvre V *et al*., Spectrum of resistance to root-knot nematodes and inheritance of heat stable resistance in pepper (*Capsicum annuum* L.). *Theo. Appl. Genet*. 99: 496–502. 1999.

Djian-Caporalino C, Pijarowski L, Fazari A, Samson M *et al*., High-resolution genetic mapping of the pepper (*Capsicum annuum* L.) resistance loci Me_3 and Me_4 conferring heat-stable resistance to root-knot nematodes (*Meloidogyne* spp.) *Theo. Appl. Genet*. 103: 592-600. 2001.

Djian-Caporalino C, Fazari A, Arguel MJ, Vernie T *et al*., Root-knot nematode (*Meloidogyne* spp.) Me resistance genes in pepper (*Capsicum annuum* L.) are clustered on the P9 chromosome. *Theo. Appl. Genet*. 114: 473-86. 2007.

Dwivedi N, Kumar R, Paliwal R, Kumar U *et al*., QTL mapping for important horticultural traits in pepper (*Capsicum annuum* L.). *J. Pl. Biochem. Biotech*. 2013: DOI 10.1007/s13562-013-0247-1.

Engler DE, Guri AZ, Lauritis JA, Schloemer LMP. Genetically transformed pepper plants and methods for their production. USA Patent. 5, 262, 316. 1993.

FAOSTAT. Agricultural production. 2013. http: //www.faostat.fao.org/

Fazari A, Palloix A, Wang L, Hua YM *et al*., The root-knot nematode resistance *N*-gene co-localizes in the *Me*-genes cluster on the pepper (*Capsicum annuum* L.) P9 chromosome. *Plant Breed*. 131: 665–673. 2012.

Góngora-Castillo E, Fajardo-Jaime R, Fernández-Cortes A, Garfias AEJ *et al.*, The capsicum transcriptome DB: a "hot" tool for genomic research. *Bioinformation.* 8: 043-047. 2012.

Green SK, Kim JM. Characteristics and control of viruses infecting peppers. Technical Bulletin No. 18. Asian Veg. Res. Dev. Centre, Taipei, Taiwan. 1991.

Grube RC, Blauth JR, Arnedo MA, Jahn MK. Identification of a dominant potyvirus resistance gene cluster in *Capsicum. Theo. Appl. Genet.* 101: 852-859. 2000.

Gulyas G, Shin Y, Kim H, Lee JS, Hirata Y. Altered Transcript Reveals an Orf507 Sterility-Related Gene in Chili Pepper (*Capsicum annuum* L.). *Plant Mol. Biol. Rep.* 28: 605–612. 2010.

Gunay AL, Rao PS. *In vitro* plant regeneration from hypocotyl and cotyledon explants of red pepper (*Capsicum*). *Plant Sci. Lett.* 11: 365-372. 1978.

Gururaj HB, Padma MN, Giridhar P, Ravishankar GA. Functional validation of *Capsicum frutescens* aminotransferase gene involved in vanillylamine biosynthesis using *Agrobacterium* mediated genetic transformation studies in *Nicotiana tabacum* and *Capsicum frutescens* calli cultures. *Plant Sci.* 195: 96-105. 2002. doi: 10.1016/j.plantsci.2012.06.014.

Gutiérrez-Carbajal MG, Monforte-González M, Miranda-Ham ML, Godoy-Hernández G *et al.*, Induction of capsaicinoid synthesis in *Capsicum chinense* cell cultures by salicylic acid or methyl jasmonate. *Biol. Plant.* 54: 430-434. 2010.

Harpster MH, Brummell DA, Dunsmuir P. Suppression of a ripening-related endo-1, 4-β-glucanase in transgenic pepper fruit does not prevent depolymerization of cell wall polysaccharides during ripening. *Plant Mol. Biol.* 50: 345–55. 2002.

Ha SH, Kim JB, Jong-Sug Park JS, Lee SW, Cho KJ. A comparison of the carotenoid accumulation in Capsicum varieties that show different ripening colours: deletion of the capsanthin-capsorubin synthase gene is not a prerequisite for the formation of a yellow pepper. *J. Exp. Bot.* 58: 3135–3144. 2007.

Hernan VA, Rosa U, Luisa OL, Dominique R *et al.*, A new virus-induced gene silencing vector based on Euphorbia mosaic virus-Yucatan peninsula for NPR1 silencing in Nicotiana benthamiana and *Capsicum annuum* var. *Anaheim. Biotech. Lett.* 35: 811. 2013.

Hill TA, Ashrafi H, Reyes-Chin-Wo S, Yao J *et al.*, Characterization of *Capsicum annuum* genetic diversity and population structure based on parallel polymorphism discovery with a 30K Unigene Pepper GeneChip. *PLoS ONE.* 8: e56200. 2013.

Hong JK, Choi HW, Hwang IS, Kim DS *et al.*, Function of a novel GDSL-type pepper lipase gene, *CaGLIP1*, in disease susceptibility and abiotic stress tolerance. *Planta.* 227: 539–558. 2008.

Hong JP, Kim WT. Isolation and functional characterization of the *Ca-DREBLP1* gene encoding a dehydration-responsive element binding-factor-like protein 1 in hot pepper (*Capsicum annuum* L. cv. Pukang). *Planta.* 220: 875–888. 2005.

Hong Truong HT, Kim JH, Cho MC, Chae SY, Lee HE. Identification and development of molecular markers linked to Phytophthora root rot resistance in pepper (*Capsicum annuum* L.). *Eur. J. Plant Pathol.* 135: 289–297. 2013.

Huan-huan H, Zhong-hua Z, Zheng-hai Z, Sheng-li M *et al.*, Analysis of SSRs Information in *Capsicum* spp. from EST Database. *Agr. Sci. China.* 10: 1532-1536. 2011.

Huh J, Kang B, Nahm S, Kim S *et al.*, A candidate gene approach identified phytoene synthase as the locus for mature fruit colour in red pepper (*Capsicum* spp.). *Theo. Appl. Genet.* 102: 524–530. 2001.

Huh SU, Kim KJ, Paek KH. *Capsicum annuum* basic transcription factor 3 (*CaBtf3*) regulates transcription of pathogenesis-related genes during hypersensitive response upon Tobacco mosaic virus infection. *Biochem. Biophy. Res. Comm.* 417: 910–917. 2012.

Huh SU, Choi LM, Lee GJ, Kim YJ, Paek KH. *Capsicum annuum* WRKY transcription factor d (*CaWRKYd*) regulates hypersensitive response and defense response upon Tobacco mosaic virus infection. *Plant Sci.* 197: 50-8. 2012.

Hurtado-Hernandez H, Smith P. Inheritance of mature fruit colour in *Capsicum annuum* L. *J. Heredity.* 76: 211–213. 1985.

Hwang EW, Kim KA, Park SC, Jeong MJ *et al.*, Expression profiles of hot pepper (*Capsicum annuum*) genes under cold stress conditions. *J. Biosci.* 30(5) 657-667. 2005.

Hwang IS, Hwang BK. The pepper 9-Lipoxygenase gene *CaLOX1* functions in defense and cell death responses to microbial pathogens. *Plant Physiol.* 152: 948–967. 2010.

Hwang JN, Li J, Liu WY, An SJ *et al.*, Double mutations in *eIF4E* and *eIFiso4E* confer recessive resistance to *Chilli veinal mottle virus* in pepper. *Mol. Cells.* 27: 329-336. 2009.

Isbat M, Zeba N, Kim SR, Hong CB. A BAX inhibitor-1 gene in *Capsicum annuum* is induced under various abiotic stresses and endows multi-tolerance in transgenic tobacco. *J. Pl. Physiol.* 166: 1685-1693. 2009.

Jahn M, Paran I, Hoffmann K, Radwanski ER *et al.*, Genetic mapping of the *Tsw* locus for resistance to the tospovirus tomato spotted wilt virus in *Capsicum spp.* and its relationship to the *Sw-5* gene for resistance to the same pathogen in tomato. *Mol. Pl. Microb. Interact.* 13: 673-682. 2000.

Jayashankar S, Bagga S. Phillips GC. Sweet pepper (*Capsicum annuum*) transformation using *Agrobacterium rhizogenes*. *HortSci.* 32: 454. 1997.

Jones JB, Minsavage GV, Roberts PD, Johnson RR *et al.*, A non-hypersensitive resistance in pepper to the bacterial spot pathogen is associated with two recessive genes. *Phytopathol.* 92: 273-277. 2002.

Jones JB, Lacy GH, Bouzar H, Stall RE, Schaad NW. Reclassification of the Xanthomonads associated with bacterial spot disease of tomato and pepper. *Syst. Appl. Micro.* 27: 755-762. 2004.

Jones JB, Stall RE. Diversity among xanthomonads pathogenic on pepper and tomato. *Annu. Rev. Phytopathol.* 36: 41–58. 1998.

Kang BC, Nahm SH, Huh JH, Yoo HS *et al.*, An interspecific (*Capsicum annuum* x C. *Chinense*) F2 linkage map in pepper using RFLP and AFLP markers. *Theo. Appl. Genet.* 102: 531-539. 2001.

Kang BC, Yeam I, Frantz JD, Murphy JF, Jahn MM. The *pvr1* locus in *Capsicum* encodes a translation initiation factor eIF4E that interacts with tobacco virus VPg. *Pl. Vir. J.* 42: 392–405. 2005.

Kang WH, Hoang NH, Yang HB, Kwon JK *et al.*, Molecular mapping and characterization of a single dominant gene controlling CMV resistance in peppers (*Capsicum annuum* L.). *Theo. Appl. Genet.* 120: 1587–1596. 2010.

Kehie M, Kumaria S, Tandon P. *In vitro* plantlet regeneration from nodal segments and shoot tips of *Capsicum chinense* Jacq. cv. Naga King Chili. *J. Biotech.* 2: 31–35. 2012a.

Kehie M, Kumaria S, Tandon P. Osmotic stress induced - capsaicin production in suspension cultures of *Capsicum chinense* Jacq.cv. Naga King Chili. *Acta Physiol. Plant.* 34: 2039–2044. 2012b.

Khan H, Siddique I, Anis M. Thidiazuron induced somatic embryogenesis and plant regeneration in *Capsicum annum. Biol. Plant.* 50: 789-792. 2006.

Khan AL, Waqas M, Hamayun M, Harrasi AA *et al.*, Co-synergism of endophyte *Penicillium resedanum* LK6 with salicylic acid helped *Capsicum annuum* in biomass recovery and osmotic stress mitigation. *BMC Microbiol.* 13: 51. 2013.

Kim DH, Kang JG, Kim BD. Isolation and characterization of the cytoplasmic male sterility-associated orf456 gene of chili pepper (*Capsicum annuum* L.). *Plant Mol. Biol.* 63(4): 519-32. 2007.

Kim DH, Kim BD. Development of SCAR markers for early identification of cytoplasmic male sterility genotype in chili pepper (*Capsicum annuum* L.). *Mol. Cells.* 31: 416-22. 2005.

Kim DS, Hwang BK. The pepper MLO gene, CaMLO2, is involved in the susceptibility cell-death response and bacterial and oomycete proliferation. *Plant J.* 72: 843–855. 2012.

Kim HJ, Nahm SH, Lee HR, Yoon GB *et al.*, BAC-derived markers converted from RFLP linked to *Phytophthora capsici* resistance in pepper (*Capsicum annuum* L.). *Theo. Appl. Genet.* 118: 15–27. 2008.

Kim HJ, Han JH, Kwon JK, Park M *et al.*, Fine mapping of pepper trichome locus 1 controlling trichome formation in *Capsicum annuum* L. CM334. *Theo. Appl. Genet.* 120: 1099-106. 2010.

Kim HJ, Han JH, Kim S, Lee HR *et al.*, Trichome density of main stem is tightly linked to *PepMoV* resistance in chili pepper (*Capsicum annuum* L.). *Theo. Appl. Genet.* 122: 1051–1058. 2011.

Kim M, Kim S, Kim S, Kim BD. Isolation of cDNA clones differentially accumulated in the placenta of pungent pepper by suppression subtractive hybridization. *Mol. Cells.* 11: 213-219. 2001.

Kim OR, Cho MC, Kim BD, Huh JH. A splicing mutation in the gene encoding phytoene synthase causes orange coloration in Habanero pepper fruits. *Mol. Cells.* 30: 569–574. 2010.

Kim SJ, Lee SJ, Kim BD, Paek KH. Satellite-RNA-mediated resistance to cucumber mosaic virus in transgenic plants of hot pepper (*Capsicum annuum* cv. Golden Tower). *Pl. Cell Rep.* 16: 825-830. 1997.

Kim SH, Hong JK, Lee SC, Sohn KH *et al., CAZFP1*, Cys2/His-type zinc-nger transcription factor gene functions as a pathogen-induced early-defense gene in *Capsicum annuum. Pl. Mol. Bio.* 55: 883–904. 2004.

Kosuge S, Inagaki Y, Okumura H. Pungent principles in *Capsicum. Nippon Nogei Kagaki Kaishi.* 35: 540. 1965.

Kothari SL, Joshi A, Kachhwaha S, Ochoa-Alejo N. Chilli pepper- A review on tissue culture and trangenesis. *Biotech. Adv.* 28: 35-48. 2010.

Kumar AM, Reddy KN, Sreevathsa R, Ganeshan G, Udaykumar M. Towards crop improvement in bell pepper (*Capsicum annuum* L.): transgenics (uid A: : hpt II) by a tissue culture independent *Agrobacterium* mediated *in planta* approach. *Sci. Hortic. Amsterdam.* 119: 362–70. 2009.

Kumar R, Dwivedi N, Singh RK, Kumar S, Rai VP, Singh M. A review on molecular characterization of pepper for capsaicin and oleoresin. *Int. J. Pl. Breed.* Genet. 5: 99-110. 2011.

Kyle MM, Palloix A. Proposed revision of nomenclature for potyvirus resistance genes in Capsicum. *Euphytica.* 97: 183–188. 1997.

Lang Y, Yanagawa S, Sasanuma T, Sasakuma T. Orange fruit colour in *Capsicum* due to deletion of capsanthin-capsorubin synthesis gene. *Breed. Sci.* 54: 33–39. 2004.

Lee CJ, Yoo EY, Shin J, Lee J *et al.,* Nonpungent *Capsicum* contains a deletion in the capsaicinoid synthetase gene, which allows early detection of pungency with SCAR markers. *Mol. Cells.* 19: 262–267. 2005.

Lee HR, An HJ, You YJ, Lee J *et al.,* Development of a novel codominant molecular marker for chili veinal mottle virus resistance in *Capsicum annuum* L. *Euphytica.* 193: 197–205. 2013.

Lee HR, Bae IH, Park SW, Kim HJ *et al.,* Construction of an integrated pepper map using RFLP, SSR, CAPS, AFLP, WRKY, rRAMP, and BAC end sequences. *Mol. Cells.* 22: 21-37. 2008.

Lee J, Yoon JB, Park HG. Linkage analysis between the partial restoration (pr) and the restorer-of-fertility (*Rf*) loci in pepper cytoplasmic male sterility. *Theo. Appl. Genet.* 117: 383–389. 2008.

Lee J, Han JH, An CG, Lee WP, Yoon JB. A CAPS marker linked to a genic male sterile gene in the colored sweet pepper, 'Paprika' (*Capsicum annuum* L.). *Breed Sci.* 60: 93–98. 2010a.

Lee J, Yoon JB, Han JH, Lee WP *et al.*, A codominant SCAR marker linked to the genic male sterility gene (*ms1*) in chili pepper (*Capsicum annuum*). *Pl. Breed* 129: 35–38. 2010b.

Lee J, Yoon JB, Han JH, Lee WP *et al.*, Three AFLP markers tightly linked to the genic male sterility *ms3* gene in chili pepper (*Capsicum annuum* L.) and conversion to a CAPS marker. *Euphytica.* 173: 55–61. 2010c.

Lee JM, Nahm SH, Kim YM, Kim BD. Characterization and molecular genetic mapping of microsatellite loci in pepper. *Theo. Appl. Genet.* 108: 619-627. 2004

Lee SC, Hwang BK. Identification of the pepper SAR8.2 gene as a molecular marker for pathogen infection, abiotic elicitors and environmental stresses in *Capsicum annuum. Planta.* 216: 387-396. 2003.

Lee SC, Hwang BK, Choi DS, Hwang IS. The pepper oxidoreductase CaOXR1 interacts with the transcription factor CaRAV1 and is required for salt and osmotic stress tolerance. *Pl. Mol. Biol.* 73: 409–424. 2010.

Lee SC, Kim SH, An SH, Yi SY, Hwang BK. Identication and functional expression of the pepper pathogen induced gene, *CAPIP2*, involved in disease resistance and drought and salt stress tolerance. *Pl. Mol. Biol.* 62: 151–164. 2006.

Lee SJ, Kim BD, Paek KH. *In vitro* plant regeneration and *Agrobacterium*-mediated transformation from cotyledon explants of hot pepper (*Capsicum annuum* cv Golden Tower). *Korean J. Pl. Tiss. Cult.* 20: 289-294. 1993.

Lee YH, Kim HS, Kim JY, Jung M *et al.*, A new selection method for pepper transformation: callus-mediated shoot formation. *Pl. Cell Rep.* 23: 50–8. 2004.

Lee YH, Jung M, Shin SH, Lee JH *et al.*, Transgenic peppers that are highly tolerant to a new CMV pathotype. *Pl. Cell Rep.* 28: 223–232. 2009.

Lefebvre V, Kuntz M, Camara B, Palloix A. The capsanthin-capsorubin synthase gene: a candidate gene for the *y* locus controlling the red fruit colour in pepper *Pl. Mol. Biol.* 36: 785–789. 1998.

Lefebvre V, Palloix A, Caranta C, Pochard E. Construction of an intra-specific integrated linkage map of pepper using molecular markers and doubled-haploid progenies. *Genome.* 38: 112–121. 1995.

Lefebvre V, Pflieger S, Thabuis A, Caranta C *et al.*, Towards the saturation of the pepper linkage map by alignment of three intraspecific maps including known-function genes. *Genome.* 45: 839–854. 2002.

Lefebvre V, Daubeze AM, Voort RJ, Peleman J *et al.*, QTLs for resistance to powdery mildew in pepper under natural and artificial infections. *Theo. Appl. Genet.* 107: 661-666. 2003.

Leonards-Schippers C, Gieffers W, Schafer-Pregl R, Ritter E *et al.*, Quantitative resis-tance to *Phytophthora* infestans in potato: a case study for QTL mapping in an allogamous plant species. *Genetics*. 137: 67–70. 1994.

Li D, Zhao K, Xie B, Zhang B, Luo K. Establishment of a highly efficient transformation system for pepper (Capsicum annuum L.). *Pl. Cell Rep*. 21: 785–8. 2003.

Li P, Feng B, Wang H, Tooley PW, Zhang X. Isolation of nine *Phytophthora capsici* pectin methylesterase genes which are differentially expressed in various plant species. *J. Basic Microbiol*. 51: 61-70. 2011.

Li X, Ramchiary N, Dhandapani V, Choi SR *et al.*, Quantitative trait loci mapping in *Brassica rapa* revealed the structural and functional conservation of genetic loci governing morphological and yield component traits in the A, B, and C subgenomes of Brassica species. *DNA Res*. 20: 1-16. 2013.

Lim HT, Lian YJ. Factors inuencing protoplast isolation and culture in three *Capsicum* species. *Korean J. Pl. Tiss. Cult*. 28: 141–6. 2001.

Lim JH, Park CJ, Huh SU, Choi LM *et al.*, *Capsicum annuum* WRKYb transcription factor that binds to the *CaPR*-10 promoter functions as a positive regulator in innate immunity upon TMV infection. *Biochem. Biophy. Res. Comm*. 411: 613–619. 2011.

Lindsey K, Yeoman MM, Black GM, Mavituna F. A novel method for the immobilization and culture of plant cells. *FEBS Lett*. 155: 143-149. 1983.

Liu C, Ma N, Wang PY, Fu N, Shen HL. Transcriptome sequencing and de novo analysis of a cytoplasmic male sterile line and its near-isogenic restorer line in chili pepper (*Capsicum annuum* L.). *PLoS ONE*. 8 (6): 1-12. 2013.

Liu S, Li W, Wu Y, Chen C, Lei J. *De novo* tran-scriptome assembly in chili pepper (*Capsicum frutescens*) to identify genes involved in the biosynthesis of capsaicinoids. *PLoS ONE*. 8: e48156. 2013.

Liu W, Parrott WA, Hildebrand DF, Collins GB, Williams *e.g. Agrobacterium* induced gall formation in bell pepper (*Capsicum annuum* L.) and formation of shoot-like structures expressing introduced genes. *Pl. Cell Rep*. 9: 360-364. 1990.

Livingstone KD, Lackney VK, Blauth J, Wijk VR, Jahn MK. Genome mapping in *Capsicum* and the evolution of genome structure in the *Solanaceae*. *Genetics*. 152: 1183-1202. 1999.

Lovato FA, Inoue-Nagata AK, Nagata T, de Avila AC *et al.*, The N protein of Tomato spotted wilt virus (TSWV) is associated with the induction of programmed cell death (PCD) in *Capsicum chinense* plants, a hypersensitive host to TSWV infection. *Virus Res*. 137: 245-52. 2008.

Lu FH, Cho MC, Park Y. Transcriptome profiling and molecular marker discovery in red pepper, *Capsicum annuum* L. TF68. *Mol. Biol. Rep*. 39: 3327–3335. 2012.

Ma Y, Huang W, Ji JJ, Gong ZH *et al.*, Maintaining and restoration cytoplasmic male sterility systems in pepper (*Capsicum annuum* L.). *Genet. Mol. Res*. 4: 12. 2013.

Maga JA. Capsicum. Crit. Rev. Food Sci. Nutr. 6: 177-199. 1975.

Manoharan M, Sree Vidya, CS, Lakshmi Sita G. *Agrobacterium*-mediated genetic transformation in hot chilli (*Capsicum annuum* L. var. Pusa jwala). *Pl. Sci.*131: 77-83. 1998.

Margaria P, Ciuffo M, Pacifico D, Turina M. Evidence that the nonstructural protein of Tomato spotted wilt virus is the avirulence determinant in the interaction with resistant pepper carrying the TSW gene. *Mol. Pl. Micro. Interact.* 20: 547-58. 2007.

Matsunaga H, Saito T, Hirai M, Nunome T, Yoshida T. DNA markers linked to Pepper mild mottle virus (PMMoV) resistant locus (L 4) in *Capsicum. J. Jpn. Soc. Hort. Sci.* 72: 218–220. 2003.

Mavituna F, Park JM. Growth of immobilised plant cells in reticulate polyurethane foam matrices. *Biotech. Lett.* 7: 637-640. 1987.

Mazourek M, Pujar A, Borovsky Y, Paran I *et al.*, A dynamic interface for capsaicinoid systems biology. *Pl. Physiol.* 150: 1806–1821. 2009.

Mezghani N, Jemmali A, Elloumi N, Gargouri-Bouzid R, Kintzios S. Morphohistological study on shoot bud regeneration in cotyledon cultures of pepper (*Capsicum annuum*). *Biol. Bratislava.* 2: 704–710. 2007.

Mimura Y, Inoue T, Minamiyama Y, Kubo N. An SSR-based genetic map of pepper (*Capsicum annuum* L.) serves as an anchor for the alignment of major pepper maps. *Breed. Sci.* 62: 93–98. 2012.

Minamiyama Y, Kinoshita S, Inaba K, Inoue M. Development of a cleaved amplified polymorphic sequence (CAPS) marker linked to pungency in pepper. *Pl. Breed.* 24: 288-291. 2005.

Minamiyama Y, Tsuro M, Hirai M. An SSR-based linkage map of *Capsicum annuum*. *Mol. Breed.* 18: 157–169. 2006.

Moscone EA, Baranyi M, Ebert I, Greilhuber J *et al.*, Analysis of nuclear DNA content in Capsicum (solanaceae) by flow cytometry and feulgen densitometry. *Annl. Rev. Bot.* 92: 21–29. 2003.

Moury B, Fabre F, Senoussi R. Estimation of the number of virus particles transmitted by an insect vector. *Proc. Nat. Acad. Sci. USA.* 104: 17891-17896. 2007.

Moury B, Pflieger S, Blattes A, Lefebvre V, Palloix A. A CAPS marker to assist selection of Tomato spotted wilt virus (TSWV) in pepper. *Genome.* 43: 943–951. 2000.

Mueller AL, Solow TH, Taylor N, Skwarecki B *et al.*, The SOL Genomics Network (SGN): a comparative resource for Solanaceous biology and beyond. *Pl. Physiol.* 138: 1310–1317. 2005.

Murashige T, Skoog F. A revised medium for rapid growth and bioassays with tobacco tissue cultures. *Physiol. Plant.* 15: 473-497. 1962.

Murphy JF, Blauth JR, Livingstone KD, Lackney VK, Jahn MK. Genetic mapping of the *pvr1* locus in *Capsicum* spp. And evidence that distinct potyvirus resistance loci control responses that differ at the whole plant and cellular levels. *Mol. Pl. Micro. Inter*. 11: 943-951. 1998.

Nicolai M, Pisani C, Bouchet JP, Vuylsteke M, Palloix A. Discovery of a large set of SNP and SSR genetic markers by high-throughput sequencing of pepper (*Capsicum annuum*). *Genet. Mol. Res*. 11: 2295-2300. 2012. Doi: 10.4238/2012

Nunez-Palenius HG, Ochoa-Alejo N. Effect of phenylalanine and phenylpropanoids on the accumulation of capsaicinoids and lignins in cell cultures of chili peppers (*Capsicum annum* L.). *In Vitro Dev. Biol. Plant*. 41: 801–805. 2005.

Ochoa-Alejo N, Gómez-Peralta JE. Activity of enzymes involved in capsaicin biosynthesis in callus tissue and fruits of chili pepper (*Capsicum annuum* L.). *J. Pl. Physiol*. 141: 147– 152. 1993.

Ochoa-alejo N, Ramirez-malagon R. *In vitro* chili pepper biotechnology. *In vitro* cellular and developmental biology. *Planta*. 37: 701–729. 2001.

Ochoa-Alejo N, Salgado-Garciglia R. Phenylalanine ammonia-lyase activity and capsaicin-precursor compounds in p-fluorophenylalanine-resistant and sensitive variant cells of chili pepper (*Capsicum annuum*). *Physiol. Plant*. 85: 173- 179. 1992.

Ogundiwin EA, Berke M, Massoudi TF, Black LL *et al*., Construction of 2 intraspecific linkage maps and identification of resistance QTLs for *Phytophthora capsici* root-rot and foliar-blight diseases of pepper (*Capsicum annuum* L.). *Genome*. 48: 698-711. 2005.

Oh SK, Baek KH, Seong ES, Joung YH *et al*., *CaMsrB2*, pepper methionine sulfoxide reductase *B2*, is a novel defense regulator against oxidative stress and pathogen attack. *Pl. Physiol*. 154: 245-61. 2010.

Ortega RG, Espanol CP, Zueco JC. Genetic relationships among 4 pepper genotypes resistant to *Phytophthora capsici*. *Pl. Breed*. 108: 118–25. 1992.

Paran I, Van der Knaap E. Genetic and molecular regulation of fruit and plant domestication traits in tomato and pepper. *J. Exptl. Bot*. 58: 3841–3852. 2007.

Paran I, Van der Voort JR, Lefebvre V, Jahn M *et al*., An integrated genetic linkage map of pepper (*Capsicum* spp.). *Mol. Breed*. 13: 251-261. 2004.

Peddaboina V, Christopher T, Subhash K. *In vitro* shoot multiplication and plant regeneration in four *Capsicum* species using thidiazuron. *Scientia Hort*. 2: 117-122. 2006.

Perryhttp: / /www.sciencemag.org/content/315/5814/986.short - aff-1 L, Dickau R, Zarrillo S, Holst I *et al*., Starch fossils and the domestication and dispersal of chili peppers (*Capsicum spp*. L.) in the Americas. *Science*. 315: 986–988. 2007.

Phillips GC, Valera-Montero LL, Fan Z, Jayashankar S *et al*., Chile improvement through biotechnology: *In vitro* plant regeneration and genetic transformation. New Mexico Chile Pepper Institute: Chile Conference, Las Cruces. 2000.

Pickersgill B. Chromosomes and evolution in Capsicum. In: Pochard E (ed) Capsicum 77, Comptes Rendus 2eme Congres Eucarpia Piment. Institut National de la Recherche Agronomique, Avignon-Montfavet, France. pp 27–37. 1977.

Pierre M, Noel L, Lahaye T, Ballvora A *et al.*, High-resolution genetic mapping of the pepper resis-tance locus Bs3governing recognition of the *Xanthomonas campestris* pv *vesicatora AvrBs3* protein. *Theo. Appl. Genet.* 101: 255–263. 2000.

Pochard E, Dumas de Valuix R, Florent A. Linkage between partial resistance to CMV and susceptibility to TMV in the line Perennial: analysis on androgenetic homozygous lines of *Capsicum. Eggplant News.* 2: 34–35. 1983.

Popovsky S, Paran I. Molecular analysis of the Y locus in pepper: Its relation to capsanthin-capsorubin synthase and to fruit color. *Theo. Appl. Genet.* 101: 86-89. 2000.

Portis E, Nagy I, Sasva Z, Stagelri A *et al.*, The design of *Capsicum* spp. SSR assays via analysis of *In silico* DNA sequence, and their potential utility for genetic mapping. *Pl. Sci.* 172: 640-648. 2007.

Pruthi JS. *Spices and Condiments-Chemistry, Microbiology and Technology*. New York: Academic Press Inc, USA. pp. 1-450. 1980.

Purkayastha J, Alam SI, Gogoi HK, Singh L. *Capsicum assamicum* sp. nov. Solanaceae, from Assam, northeastern India. *Ozean J. App. Sci* 5: 1. 2012.

Quirin EA, Ogundiwin EA, Prince JP, Mazourek M *et al.*, Development of sequence characterized amplified region (SCAR) primers for the detection of *Phyto.5.2*, a major QTL for resistance to *Phytophthora capsici* Leon. in pepper. *Theo. Appl. Genet.* 110: 605-612. 2005.

Razzaq, A, Zhiying M, Haibo W. Genetic transformation of wheat (*Triticum aestivum* L.): A Review. *Mol. Pl. Breed.* 2(4): 457-464. 2004.

Rao GU, Chaim AB, Borovsky E, Paran I. Mapping of yield related QTLs in pepper in an interspecific cross of *Capsicum annuum* and *C. frutescens. Theo. Appl. Genet.* 106: 1457-1466. 2003.

Ravishankar GA, Sarma KS, Venkataraman LV, Kadyan AK. Effect of nutritional stress on capsaicin production in immobilized cell cultures of *Capsicum annuum. Curr. Sci.* 57: 381-383. 1988.

Reddy OB, Giridhar P, Ravishankar GA. The effect of tricontanol on micropropagation of *Capsicum frutescens* and *Decalepis hamiltonii* W and A. *Pl. Cell Tiss. Org. Cult.* 71: 253–258. 2002.

Reeves G, Monroy-Barbosa A, Bosland PW. A novel *Capsicum* gene inhibits host-specific disease resistance to *Phytophthora capsici. Phytopathol.* 103: 472-8. 2013. Doi: 10.1094/PHYTO-09-12-0242-R

Ristaino JB. Interspecific variation among isolates of *Phytophthora capsici* from pepper and cucurbit fields in North Carolina. *Phytopathol.* 80: 1253-1259. 1990.

Rodriguez-Uribe L, Guzman I, Rajapakse W, Richins RD, O'Connell MA. Carotenoid accumulation in orange-pigmented *Capsicum annuum* fruit, regulated at multiple levels. *J. Exptl. Bot.* 63: 517–526. 2012.

Rubio M, Caranta C, Palloix A. Functional markers for selection of potyvirus resistance alleles at the pvr2-eIF4E locus in pepper using tetra-primer ARMS-PCR. *Genome.* 51: 767-71. 2008.

Rubio M, Nicolaï M, Caranta C, Palloix A. Allele mining in the pepper gene pool provided new complementation effects between *pvr2-eIF4E* and *pvr6-eIF(iso)4E* alleles for resistance to pepper veinal mottle virus. *J. Gen. Virol.* 90: 2808-14. 2009.

Ruffel S, Dussault MH, Palloix A, Moury B *et al.*, A natural recessive resistance gene against potato virus Y in pepper corresponds to the eukaryotic initiation factor 4E (eIF4E). *Plant J.* 32: 1067–1075. 2002.

Ruffel S, Gallois JL, Moury B, Robaglia C *et al.*, Simultaneous mutations in translation initiation factors *eIF4E* and *eIF*(iso)*4E* are required to prevent pepper veinal mottle virus infection of pepper. *J. Gen. Virol.* 87: 2089-98. 2006.

Rushton PJ, Somssich IE, Ringler P, Shen QJ. WRKY transcription factors. *Trends Pl. Sci.* 15: 247–258. 2010.

Salgado-Garciglia R, Ochoa-Alejo N. Increased capsaicin content in PFP resistant cells of chili pepper (*Capsicum annuum* L.). *Pl. Cell Rep.* 8: 617- 620. 1990.

Sanatombi K, Sharma GJ. *In vitro* propagation of *Capsicum chinense* Jacq. *Biol. Plant.* 52: 517-520. 2008.

Sandbrik JM, Colon LT, Wolters PJCC, Stiekema WJ. Two related genotypes of *Solanum microdontum* carry different segregating alleles for field resistance to *Phytophthora* infestans. *Mol. Breed.* 6: 215–225. 2000.

Sanwen H, Baoxi Z, Milbourne D, Cardle L, Guimei Y, Jiazhen G. Development of pepper SSR markers from sequence databases. *Euphytica.* 117: 163–167. 2001.

Seo EY, Yeom SI, Jo SH, Jeong HJ *et al.*, Ectopic expression of Capsicum-specific cell wall protein *Capsicum annuum* senescence-delaying 1 (*CaSD1*) delays senescence and induces trichome formation in *Nicotiana benthamiana. Mol. Cells.* 33: 415–422. 2013.

Sharma A, Kumar V, Giridhar P, Ravishankar GA. Induction of in vitro flowering in Capsicum frutescens under the influence of silver nitrate and cobalt chloride and pollen transformation. *Electron. J. Biotech.* 11(2): 1-7. 2008. Doi: 10.2225/vol11-issue2-fulltext-8

Shin R, Park JM, An J-M, Paek KH. Ectopic expression of Tsi1 in transgenic hot pepper plants enhances host resistance to viral, bacterial and oomycete pathogens. *Mol. Pl. Microb. Interact.* 15: 983–9. 2002.

Shirasawa K, Ishii K, Kim C, Ban T *et al.*, Development of *Capsicum* EST–SSR markers for species identification and in silico mapping onto the tomato genome sequence. *Mol. Breed.* 31: 101–110. 2013.

Sobhakumari VP, Lalithakumari D. High frequency shoot regeneration and *Agrobacterium* mediated DNA transfer in red chilli (*Capsicum annuum* L.). *Pl. Cell Biotech. Mol. Biol.* 6: 9-16. 2005.

Simonne AH, Simonne EH, Eitenmiller RR, Mills HA, Green NR. Ascorbic acid and provitamin. A contents in unusually colored bell peppers (*Capsicum annuum* L.). *J. Food Compo. Anal.* 10: 299–311. 1997.

Solís-Ramos LY, González-Estrada T, Nahuath-Dzib S, Zapata-Rodriguez LC, Castaño E. Overexpression of WUSCHEL in C. chinense causes ectopic morphogenesis. *Pl. Cell Tiss. Org. Cult.* 96: 279–87. 2009.

Stewart C, Kang BC, Liu K, Mazourek M *et al.*, The Pun1 gene for pungency in pepper encodes a putative acyltransferase. *Plant J.* 42: 675–688. 2005.

Stewart C, Mazourek M, Stellari GM, O'Connell M, Jahn M. Genetic control of pungency in *Capsicum chinense* via the *Pun1 locus*. *J. Exptl. Bot.* 58: 979–991. 2007.

Sudha G, Ravishankar GA. Influence of calcium channel modulators in capsaicin production by cell suspension cultures of *Capsicum frutescens* Mill. *Curr. Sci.* 83: 480-484. 2002.

Sugita T, Semi Y, Sawada H, Utoyama Y *et al.*, Development of simple sequence repeat markers and construction of a high-density linkage map of *Capsicum annuum*. *Mol. Breed.* 31: 909–920. 2013.

Surh YJ. Anti-tumour promoting potential of selected spice ingredients with antioxidative and anti-inammatory activities: a short review. *Food Chem. Toxicol.* 40: 1091–1097. 2002.

Tai T, Dahlbeck D, Stall RE, Peleman J, Staskawicz BJ. High-resolution genetic and physical mapping of the region containing the Bs2 resistance gene of pepper. *Theo. Appl. Genet.* 99: 1201–1206. 1999.

Tanksley SD, Bernatzky R, Lapitan NL, Prince JP. Conservation of gene repertoire but not gene order in pepper and tomato. *Proc. Natl. Acad. Sci. USA.* 85: 6419-6423. 1988.

Tao L, Zeba N, Ashrafuzzaman M, Hong CB. Heavy metal stress-inducible early light-inducible gene *CaELIP* from hot pepper (*Capsicum annuum*) shows broad expression patterns under various abiotic stresses and circadian rhythmicity. *Environ. Exptl. Bot.* 72: 297-303. 2011.

Tewksbury JJ, Reagan KM, Machnicki NJ, Carlo TA *et al.*, Evolutionary ecology of pungency in wild chilies. *Proc. Natl. Acad. Sci. USA.* 105: 11808–11811. 2008.

Tecle IY, Menda N, Buels RM, van der Knaap E, Mueller LA. solQTL: a tool for QTL analysis, visualization and linking to genomes at SGN database. *BMC Bioinform.* 11: 525. 2010.

Thabuis A, Lefebvre V, Bernard G, Daubeze AM *et al.*, Phenotypic and molecular evaluation of a recurrent selection program for a polygenic resistance to *Phytophthora capsici* in pepper. *Theo. Appl. Genet.* 109: 342–351. 2004.

The Potato Genome Sequencing Consortium. Genome sequence and analysis of the tuber crop potato. *Nature.* 2011; DOI: 10.1038/nature10158

The Tomato Genome Consortium. The tomato genome sequence provides insights into fleshy fruit evolution. *Nature.* 485, 635–641. 2012.

Thies JA, Fery RL. Characterization of resistance conferred by the N gene to Meloidogyne arenaria races 1 and 2, M. hapla, and M. javanica in two sets of isogenic lines of *Capsicum annuum. J. Amer. Soc. Hort. Sci.* 125: 71–75. 2000.

Thies JA, Fery RL. Heat stability of resistance to southern root-knot nematode in bell pepper genotypes homozygous and heterozygous for the N gene. *J. Amer. Soc. Hort. Sci.* 127(3): 371–375. 2002.

Thorup T, Tanyolac B, Livingstone K, Popovsky S *et al.*, Candidate gene analysis of organ pigmentation loci in the Solanaceae. *Proc. Nat. Acad. Sci. USA.* 97: 11192–11197. 2000.

Tomita R, Murai J, Miura Y, Ishihara H *et al.*, Fine mapping and DNA fiber FISH analysis locates the tobamovirus resistance gene L3 of *Capsicum chinense* in a 400-kb region of R-like genes cluster embedded in highly repetitive sequences. *Theo. Appl. Genet.* 117: 1107-18. 2008.

Tsaballa A, Pasentsis K, Darzentas N, Tsaftaris A. Multiple evidence for the role of an *Ovate*-like gene in determining fruit shape in pepper. *BMC Pl.* Biol. 11: 46. 2011.

USDA-ARS. Grin species records of Capsicum. Beltsville, Maryland: Natl. Germplasm Resour. *Lab.* 2011.

Vallejos CE, Jones V, Stall RE, Jones JB *et al.*, Characterization of two recessive genes controlling resistance to all races of bacterial spot in peppers. *Theo. Appl. Genet.* 121: 37–46. 2010.

Venkataiah P, Christopher T, Subhash K. Thidiauron induced high frequency adventitious shoot formation and plant regeneration in *Capsicum annum* L. *Pl. Biotech.* 5: 245–250. 2003.

Voorrips RE, Finkers R, Sanjaya Lia. QTL mapping of anthracnose (*Colletotri-chum* spp.) resistance in a cross between. *Capsicum annuum* and *C. chinense. Theo. Appl. Genet.* 109: 1275–1282. 2004.

Wang D and Bosland PW. The genes of *Capsicum. HortSci.* 41(5): 1169-1187. 2006.

Wang JE, Liu KK, Li DW, Zhang YL *et al.*, A novel peroxidase *CanPOD* gene of pepper is involved in defense responses to *Phytophtora capsici* infection as well as abiotic Stress Tolerance. *Int. J. Mol. Sci.* 14, 3158-3177. 2013.

Wang W, Yang M, Pan N, Chen ZH. Plant regeneration and transformation of sweet pepper (*Capsicum frutescens*). *Acta Bot. Sin.* 33: 780–6. 1991.

Wang LH, Zhang BX, Lefebvre V, Huang SW, Daubeze AM,Palloix A. QTL analysis of fertility restoration in cytoplasmic male sterile pepper. *Theo. Appl. Genet.*109: 1058–1063. 2004.

Wang X, Zhu X, Tooley P, Zhang X. Cloning and functional analysis of three genes encoding polygalacturonase-inhibiting proteins from *Capsicum annuum* and transgenic CaPGIP1 in tobacco in relation to increased resistance to two fungal pathogens. *Pl. Mol. Biol.* 81: 379-400. 2013.

Wu F, Mueller LA, Crouzillat D, Petiard V, Tanksley SD. Combining bioinformatics and phylogenetics to identify large sets of single-copy orthologous genes (COSII) for comparative, evolutionary and systematic studies: a test case in the euasterid plant clade. *Genetics*. 174: 1407–1420. 2006.

Wu F, Eannetta NT, Xu Y, Durrett R *et al.*, A COSII genetic map of the pepper genome provides a detailed picture of synteny with tomato and new insights into recent chromosome evolution in the genus *Capsicum*. *Theo. Appl. Genet.* 118: 1279–1293. 2009.

Wu F, Eannetta NT, Xu Y, Tanksley SD. A detailed synteny map of the eggplant genome based on conserved ortholog set II (COSII) markers. *Theo. Appl. Genet.* 2009b. Doi: 10.1007/s00122-008- 0590-9

Yao M, Li N, Wang F, Ye Z. Genetic analysis and identication of QTLs for resistance to cucumber mosaic virus in chili pepper (*Capsicum annuum* L.) *Euphytica*. 193: 135–145. 2013.

Yarnes SC, Ashrafi H, Reyes-Chin-Wo S, Hill TA, Stoffel KM, Van Deynze A. Identification of QTLs for capsaicinoids, fruit quality, and plant architecture-related traits in an interspecific *Capsicum* RIL population. *Genome*. 56(1): 61-74. 2013.

Yi G, Lee J, Lee S, Choi D, Kim BD. Exploitation of pepper EST–SSRs and an SSR-based linkage map. *Theor. Appl. Genet*. 114: 113–130. 2006.

Yi SY, Kim JH, Joung YH, Lee S *et al.*, The Pepper Transcription Factor *CaPF1* Confers Pathogen and Freezing Tolerance in *Arabidopsis*. *Pl. Physiol.* 136: 2862–2874. 2004.

Zeba N, Isbat M, Kwon NJ, Lee MO *et al.*, Heat-inducible C3HC4 type RING zinc finger protein gene from *Capsicum annuum* enhances growth of transgenic tobacco. *Planta*. 229: 861–871. 2009.

Zhang YL, Jia QL, Li DW, Wang JE *et al.*, Characteristic of the Pepper CaRGA2 Gene in Defense Responses against *Phytophthora capsici* Leonian. *Intl. J. Mol. Sci.* 14: 8985-9004. 2013.

Zhu YX, Ou-Yang WJ, Zhang YF, Chen ZL. Transgenic sweet pepper plants from *Agrobacterium* mediated transformation. *Pl. Cell Rep*. 16: 71-75. 1996.

Zygier S, Ben Chaim A, Efrati A, Kaluzky G *et al.*, QTLs mapping for fruit size and shape in chromosomes 2 and 4 in pepper and a comparison of the pepper QTL map with that of tomato. *Theo. Appl. Genet*. 111: 437–445. 2005.

2016, Biotechnological Tools for Genetic Resources Pages 275–308
Editor: Pradip Chandra Deka
Published by: Daya Publishing House, NEW DELHI

Chapter 9

Hairy Roots and their Multiple Applications

Pradip C. Deka[1]* and Pallavi Dwivedi[2]

[1]Biotechnology Department,
Sir Padampat Singhania University, Bhatewar, Udaipur – 313 601, Rajasthan
[2]Biotechnology Department,
Amity University, Somathne, Panvel, Mumbai – 410 206, Maharashtra
**E-mail: deka.pradip47@gmail.com*

ABSTRACT

Agrobacterium rhizogenes induces hairy root disease in plants. The neoplastic (cancerous) roots produced by A. rhizogenes infection, when cultured in hormone free medium, show high growth rate and genetic stability. These genetically transformed root cultures can produce levels of secondary metabolites comparable to that of intact plants. Several elicitation methods can be used to further enhance the production and accumulation of secondary metabolites. Thus hairy root culture offer promise for high production and productivity of valuable secondary metabolites in many plants. Hairy roots can also produce recombinant proteins from transgenic roots, and thereby hold immense potential for pharmaceutical industry. Hairy root cultures can also be used to elucidate the intermediates and key enzymes involved in the biosynthesis of secondary metabolites. In addition, hairy roots offer promise for phytoremediation due to their abundant neoplastic root proliferation property. Various applications of hairy root cultures and potential problems associated with them are discussed.

Keywords: *Hairy roots, In vitro culture, T-DNA, Agrobacterium rhizogenes, Bioreactor, Secondary metabolite, Phytoremediation.*

Introduction

Hairy root is a disease of higher plants caused by the bacterium *Agrobacterium rhizogenes*, a gram negative soil born bacterium. When the bacterium infects the plant, the pathogen transfers a DNA segment (T-DNA region bounded by 25 bp direct oligonucleotide repeats) from its large root-inducing (Ri) plasmid into the infected plant. The T-DNA integrates into the nuclear genome of the host plant. The T-DNA carries a set of genes that code for enzymes for the phytohormone auxin control and cytokinin biosynthesis (*iaaM, iaaH, ipt*) and also for opines (an unusual aminoacids). Expression of these new hormones induces the formation of proliferated roots. These roots emerge at the wound sites and are called hairy roots (HR) (Gaudin *et al.*, 1994).The mechanism of transfer of T-DNA from *A. rhizogenes* to the host plant is similar to the mechanism involved in *A. tumefaciens*, which causes crown gall disease in the infected plants.

The hairy roots have unique characteristics like fast hormone independent growths, lack of geotropism, lateral branching, and genetic stability. Further, hairy roots can be cultured under *in vitro* conditions indefinitely. Because of these characteristics hairy roots cultures were investigated for several decades to exploit the possibilities of their commercial use. One of the objectives was to exploit the production of high value secondary metabolites (Giri and Narasu 2006). Long term aseptic hairy root cultures have been established from more than 200 plant species, having the ability to synthesize a wide variety of secondary metabolites and to adjust their metabolic activities in response to biotic and abiotic stress (Guillon *et al.*, 2006). However, it is important to note that not every hairy root culture displays these characteristics. Further, many researchers have experienced problems with hairy root initiation and maintenance. But the overwhelming positive results have generated hope for its utilization.

In some species, regeneration of whole plants has been possible from the hairy roots. Transgenic plants have been obtained in 89 different plant taxa, representing 79 species from 55 genera and 21 families, through *A. rhizogenes* mediated transformation (Tefer 1984, Christey 2001). The transgenic plants show a characteristic phenotype, called HR syndrome, which include reduced apical dominance in both stems and roots, shortened internode, high groth rate of roots in culture, wrinkled leaves with increased width to length ratio, plagiotropic roots, with altered geotropism, altered flower morphology, late flowering, reduced fertility and reduced pollen and seed production (Spena *et al.*, 1987, Christey 1997).

Hairy Root Induction and Selection

Procedures for induction and selection of hairy roots are described in the following section.

Establishment of Hairy Root Culture System

Establishment of hairy root culture system involves several requirements. These include: the bacterial strain of *Agrobacterium rhizogenes*, an appropriate explant, a proper antibiotic to eliminate redundant bacteria after cocultivation, and a suitable culture medium. On the basis of types of opines produced, *A. rhizogenes* strains can be divided into five lines: octopine, agropine, nopaline, mannopine, and cucumopine (Zhou *et al.*, 1998). Owing to their strongest hairy root induction ability, agropine strains are the most often used strains. Explants from leaf, stem, shoot tip, stalk, petiole, cotyledon, hypocotyls, tubers, and protoplast can be used to induce hairy oots (Mugnier 1988, Han *et al.*, 1993, Drewes *et al.*, 1995, Giri *et al.*, 2001, Krolicka t *al.*, 2001, Azian *et al.*, 2002). However, selection of right type of explants and its ge are critical for the success of induction of hairy roots. Juvenile material is the preferred choice.

For induction of hairy roots, explants are separately wounded and cocultivation or inoculated with *A. rhizogenes*. After 2-3 days, the explants are transferred into olid media with antibiotics, such as cefotaxime sodium, carbencilli disodium, vancomycin, ampicilin sodium, claforan, streptomycin sulfate, or tetracycline. Antibiotics are used to kill or eliminate the redundant bacteria at a concentration anging from 100 to 500 g/ml (Spano *et al.*, 1981, Drewes *et al.*, 1995, Giri *et al.*, 2001, Krolicka *et al.*, 2001). Depending on the plant species and type of explants used, hairy roots are normally induce within a week to over a month. Hairy roots thus induced can be sub-cultured on phytohormone-free medium.

To activate the virulence genes of *A. rhizogenes* and to enhance the transfer of foreign genes into the plant genomes, acetosyringone (ranging from 10 to 150 μM) has been used (Satchel *et al.*, 1985, Gelvin 2000, Tao and Li 2006, Kumar *et al.*, 2006).

For high production of secondary metabolites, optimization of the nutrients in the culture medium and physical factors of the culture, are equally important. Factors such as carbon source and its concentration, the ionic concentration of the medium, phytohormones, light, temperature, pH of the medium and inoculums are known to influence growth and secondary metabolism (Christen *et al.*, 1992, Toivonen *et al.*, 1992, Rhodes *et al.*, 1994, Arroo *et al.*, 1995, Bhadra *et al.*, 1995, Vanhale *et al.*, 1998, Morgan *et al.*, 2000). Supplementation of auxin and elicitors often increases the levels of secondary metabolites (Dymov *et al.*, 1997, Pittaalvarez *et al.*, 1998, Rijhwani *et al.*, 1998, Singh *et al.*, 1998, Vanhala *et al.*, 1998). In view of the above findings, it is important to determine the requirements of nutrient conditions for hairy root culture of each species and each clones.

Estrada-Navarrete *et al.* (2007) developed an *A. rhizogenes*-mediated hairy root transformation protocol for *Phaseolus vulgaris*, a recalcitrant plant species. However the efficiency of hairy root transformation by this method is highly variable, and the transformation frequency never goes beyond 70 percent. By utilizing radical severed, cotyledon-bearing common bean (*P. vulgaris*) young seedlings as explants, Khandual and Reddy (2014) obtained 100 per cent transformation through *A. rhizogenes*. The same protocol was reported to be equally effective for soybean (Khandual and Reddy, 2014)

A different technique called sonication-assisted *Agrobacterium*-mediated transformation (SAAT) was developed to induce hairy roots in those plant species which are difficult to transform (Trick and Finer, 1997).

Reporter Gene

To monitor transfer of genes from *A. rhiziogenes* to the plants, a gene which expresses in the plant and can be easily identified is required. Accordingly, a gene named β-glucuronidase (*GUS*) which fulfills this requirement has been identified. This gene is transferred from *A. rhizogenes* into hairy roots, and it can be easily analyzed by histological assay. Thus this gene is called as reporter gene (Jefferson *et al.*, 1987, Hosoki *et al.*, 1994). It is the most common means of monitoring in most of the plant systems. In some cases, neomycin phosphotransferase II (NPT-II) encoding the kanamycine-resistance enzyme has been used (Han *et al.*, 1993, Qin *et al.*, 1994). However, sometimes both GUS and NPT-II were used (Christey *et al.*, 1992, Azlan *et al.*, 2002). Another gene named green fluorescent protein (GFP) was also used as reporter gene in *Catharanthus roseus* L. (Hughes *et al.*, 2002).

Infection Condition

The infection condition and the choice of the *A. rhizogenes* strain are of paramount importance for the success of transformation. The strain virulence has strong repercussions on the properties (morphology, growth rate and metabolite level) of the transformed plant tissue. The strain LBA 9402 has showed stronger infective ability, while the strain R1601 generated a faster growing clone on *Rheum palmatum*

Selection of Hairy Root Line

The site of integration of T-DNA into the host plant genome is usually uncertain. Therefore, hairy roots obtained after integration of T-DNA show different accumulation pattern of secondary metabolites. After analyzing 45 hairy root clones of *Duboisia leichhardtii* F, it was observed that there was considerable variation in growth rate, alkaloid content, and productivity among the clones (Mano *et al.* 1989). Usually sub-culturing of hairy roots is easy and they remain stable over time. However, certain amount of heterogeneity has been reported, even in hairy roots obtained from the same root tips. Therefore, it is important to follow a stringent selection process to obtained high secondary metabolite producing hairy root line (Yukimune *et al.*, 1994).

Agrobacterium rhizogenes Genes and Induction of Hairy Roots

Development of hairy roots in higher plants by *A. rhizogenes* is caused by the transfer of one or two fragments of T-DNA from a root-inducing (R_i) plasmid to the host plant genome (White *et al.*, 1985, Huffman *et al.*, 1984, Jouanin 1984). Among the 18 ORFs located in the R_i T-DNA (14), four coincide with genetic loci (*rol*A, B, C, D). These genes correspond to ORFs 10, 11, 12, and 15 of TL-DNA (14). Two other ORFs, ORF13 and ORF14 also play significant roles in the induction of roots on carrot disks and tobacco leaf segments (Capone *et al.*, 1989).

When inserted individually, *rol* genes affect plants growth and development, each with its distinctive features. Individually they do not show HR syndrome, which develops probably due to the synergistic action of these genes (Schmulling *et al.*, 1988, Lemcke and Schmulling 1998). The *rol*C gene has been most widely studied because its effects are the most advantageous for improving ornamental and horticultural traits. Effect of this gene include: reduced apical dominance, altered leaf morphology, reduced seed production, dwarfness, increase in lateral shoots, smaller flowers, advanced flowering, better rooting capacity (Schmulling *et al.*, 1988). The *rol*B show flower heterostyly, abundant adventitious rooting (Spana *et al.*, 1987, Cardarelli *et al.*, 1987). Transgenic *rol*A plants show wrinkled leaves and reduced internode length (Schmulling *et al.*, 1988, Sinkar *et al.*, 1988). The *rol*D have been shown to consist primarily in a strong acceleration and stimulation of flowering, while rolD has been shown to promote flowering.

Although formation of hairy from infected cells is regulated by *rol*A, *rol*B and *rol*C genes, the role of rolB gene in thought to be the most important (Spene *et al.*, 1987, Akoi and Syono 1999). Some possible mechanisms of action of the *rol* genes are discussed.

Mechanism of Action of *rol*A Gene

The rolA gene has been proposed to be involved in the metabolism of gibberellins in transgenic tobacco roots (Meyer *et al.*, 2000, Dehio *et al.*, 1993). This could explain the dwarfing of these plants, since a similar phenotype was observed by applying inhibitors of gibberellins synthesis (Dehio *et al.*, 1993). The rolA gene was also reported to be responsible for changes in polyamine metabolism by inhibiting their conjugation (Sun *et al.*, 1991, Martin-Tanguy 1996).

Mechanism of Action of *rol*B Gene

The rolB gene produces abundant lateral roots in plants. RolB protein was suggested to be β-glucosidase. This enzyme has the capacity to Increase the level of free indoleacetic acid (IAA) by releasing it from its inactive glucose conjugates (Estruch *et al.*, 1991). The function of RolB protein as a tyrosine phosphatase or as an auxin-binding protein has been proposed (Filippini *et al.*, 1994, 1996). However, no direct evidence has been provided between these functions and adventitious rooting. Therefore the auxin effects observed in rolB-transformed plants could be due to an altered perception of the hormone stimuli (Pistelli *et al.*, 2010).

Moriuchi *et al.* (2004) reported that *rol*B might function as a transcriptional coactivator/mediator. Although the exact role of such activity on adventitious root induction is not known, protein of *rol*B family may alter developmental plasticity in higher plants by association with plant proteins (Moriuchi *et al.*, 2004).

Increase in the anthraquinone (AQ) production in *rol*B and *rol*C-transformed plant cultures indicate that this might be involved in plants secondary metabolism (Bulgakov *et al.*, 2002b). Similarly, involvement of tyrosine phosphorylation in plant secondary metabolism was reported (Kiselev *et al.*, 2007).

The signaling pathway by which the rolB gene activates plant defense reactions does not depend on oxidative signals. In fact the stimulatory effect of the gene on stilbene production was abolished when the *rol*B-calli were cultivated in the presence of either phenylarsine oxide (PAO) and Na-orthovanadate inhibitors of Try phosphatases (Kiselev *et al.*, 2007). These results indicate that Try phosphorylation indeed is involved in the stimulatory function of the *rol*B gene. Try phosphorylation has been identified to be involved in critical functions in plants, regulating activity of MAP kinase, transcription factors and reactive oxygen species (ROS) signaling (Laloi *et al.*, 2004).

Mechanism of Action of the *rol*C Gene

The gene *rol*C affects the plant size and architecture. These include apical dominance, decreased height, internode length, male fertility, an increased number of flowers, changes in leaf size, colour and shape (Smith *et al.*, 2006). They produce essentially similar phenotypes in all the analyzed plant species. The reduction in height has been observed at different degrees of dwarfness among independent transformants carrying the same *rol*C gene construct (Kiyokawa *et al.*, 1996). These differences are dependent on several factors like, site of integration, copy number, mutation, somaclonal variation and changes in expression level (Kiyokawa *et al.*, 1996, Giovannini *et al.*, 1997).

The effect of *rol*C gene on plant morphology may be due to cytokinin-beta-glucoside activity that increases cytokinin levels (Estruch *et al.*, 1991, Casanova *et al.*, 2003). Moreover, significant increase of some carbohydrate isoforms in *rol*C transformed cells of ginseng has been reported. Increase in the level of activity of β-and α-D-galactosidase and 1,3-β-D-glucanase were detected in *rol*C transformed cells compared to control cells (Bulgakov *et al.*, 2002).

Stimulatory effect of *rol*C gene on secondary metabolism was demonstrated in tropane alkaloids, pyridine alkaloids, indole alkaloids, ginsennosides, and anthraquinone phytoalexins (Bonhomme *et al.*, 2000, Bulgakov *et al.*, 1998, Bulgakov *et al.*, 2002b, Bulgakov *et al.*, 2003). Usually *rol*C gene-mediated signal did not interfere with general plant defense pathways. An inhibitory effect of *rol*C gene has been reported on rabdosiin and rosmarinic acid production in *Eritrichium scriccum* and *Lithospermum crythrorhizon* hairy roots (Bulgakov *et al.*, 2005). The inhibitory action may be due to interference of *rol*C gene product with different regulatory backgrounds existing in plants. One of the possible targets of *rol*C gene could be protein phosphatases enzyme.

Mechanism of Action of *rol*D Gene

The *rol*D gene stimulates the reproductive phase transition in plants. RolD protein has been suggested to exert its effect on increased flowering through changes in the concentration of plant hormones in transformed plants (Mauro *et al.*, 1996). In transgenic tobacco, the *rol*D gene induces earliness in the flowering process and increase in the number of flowers speculated to be due to accumulation of proline or depletion of ornithine (Mauro *et al.*, 1996). High proline concentration in tomato flowers led to believe that proline-mediated role of *rol*D in flowering (Trovato *et al.*, 2001). An increase in the amount of proline could affect the biosynthesis of hydroxyproline rich glycoproteins (HRGPs, extensions and arabinogalactan proteins). These proteins are structural constituents of the plant cell wall and are thought to play a key role in the regulation of cell division, cell wall assembly and cell extension (Varner and Lin, 1989).

Mechanism of Action of ORF13

The sequence of ORF13 is highly conserved in the agropine, mannopine, cucumopine and mikinopine- type R_i plasmids (Aoki *et al.*, 1994, Fruendt *et al.*, 1998). Although it was thought to be involved in hormone signaling pathways, most subsequent studies excluded hormone-relate biochemical function for ORF13 (Lemcke and Schmulling 1998). ORF13 expression leads to the formation of spikes (protrusion between minor veins) on leaves and petals of tobacco (Meyer *et al.*, 2000). Increased cell division in the vegetative shoot apical meristems and accelerated formation of leaf primordial were observed in plants expressing ORF13 (Stieger *et al.*, 2004). It has been proposed that ORF13 confers meristematic competence to cells infected by *A. rhizogenes* by inducing the expression of KNOX genes and promotes the transition of infected cells from the G_1 to the S phase by binding to RB (retinoblastoma) (Stieger *et al.*, 2004).

Elicitation

Application of biotic or abiotic stress on plant tissues in cultures has been shown to have an effect on the secondary metabolite accumulation. The process of elicitation involves treatment of the cultures with a physical and a chemical agent that will cause phytoalexin production leading to defense mechanisms in the plant cells. The eliciting agents are classified into two categories: abiotic elicitors (physical, mineral and chemical factors), and biotic elicitors (factors of plant or pathogen origin) (Yoshikawa 1978). In nature secondary metabolites are generally produced as a defense mechanism against pathogenic and insect attack. Therefore, elicitors are used to enhance the production of secondary metabolites while the plant tissues are grown in culture. Elicitor is mainly used when the hairy roots cultures have reached its stationary phase, usually around 2-3 weeks after inoculation. Some examples of application of elicitors for increased production of secondary metabolites are shown in Table 9.1.

Application of Hairy Roots

Hairy roots have been identified to have several applications. Some of the important applications of hairy roots are described (Figure 9.1).

Functional Analysis of Genes

Lotus japonicas were transformed by infection with *A. rhizogenes* containing gene constructs for the expression of hairpin RNAs (hpRNAs) having sequences complimentary to the GUS coding region (Kumagai *et al.*, 2003). In the transformed lines the GUS activity decreased by more than 60 percent. This result suggested that transient RNA silencing by hairy root transformation provides a powerful tool for loss-of-function analysis of genes that are expressed in roots. In another study, Hughes *et al.* (2002) transformed hairy roots of *Catharanthus roseus* with a GFP gene controlled by glucocorticoid-inducing promoter. The inducible promoter showed a tightly controlled, reversible, and dose-dependent response to the glucocorticoid dexamethasone in the hairy roots. Several experiments have demonstrated that when different promoters are fused with *GUS* gene, and transferred to hairy roots show different expression patterns. For example, when expression of *GUS* gene fused with alcohol dehydrogenase (Adh) promoter introduced into hairy roots of soybean and tested in different conditions (cold temperature, wounding anoxia and absicsic acid treatment), it showed differential expression (Preiszner *et al.*, 2001). Similarly, Carron *et al.* (1994) introduced an antisense dihydroflavonol reductase

Table 9.1: Elicitors (Biotic and abiotic) Used on Hairy Root Cultures for Enhanced Production of Metabolites

Plant Species	*Metabolites (Medicinal properties)*	*Medicinal Properties*	*Elicitor (Type)*	*Fold Increase in Metabolite Content*	*References*
Ammi majus	Coumarine, furocoumarine		Benzo (1,2,3) – thiadiazole-7-carbothionic acid S–methyl easter (abiotic)	1.3	Staniszewska *et al.*, 2003
Aracheis hypogaea	Resveratrol and trans-resveratrol	Antioxidant and athero-sclerosis prevention	Sodium acetate, 10.2 mM (abiotic)	60.0	Medina-Bolivar *et al.*, 2007
Artemisia annua	Artemisinin	Anti-malarial	Oligosaccharides from Colletotricum gloeosporoides (fungus), 0.4 mg/l (biotic)	1.5	Wang *et al.*, 2006
			Polysaccharide fraction of the yeast, 2 mg/l (biotic)	3.0	Putalin *et al.*, 2007
			Chitosan, 150 mg/l (biotic)	6.0	–do-
Azadirachta indica	Azdirachtin	Pesticide	Salicylic acid, 100 mM (biotic)	6.0	Satvide *et al.*, 2007
Beta vulgaris	Peroxidase		$CaCl_2$ (5 mM)	1.2	Rudrappa *et al.*, 2005
			Jasmonic acid, 100 mM (biotic)	9.0	–do-
Centella asiatica	Asiaticoside	Anti-inflammato-ry	MeJA, 0.1 µM (biotic)	*de novo* accumulation	Kim *et al.*, 2007
Hyoscyamus niger	Polyamines, tropane alkaloids	Mydriatic, parasympatho-lytic, antiparkinsonian	MeJA, 50 µM (biotic)	2.0	Zhang *et al.*, 2007
Oxalis tuberosa	Harmaline, harmine		Phytosphtora cinnamon (biotic)	1.3	Bais *et al.*, 2003
Pasax ginseng	Total saponin	Tonic, stimulant, adaptogenic	$NiSO_{4,}$ 20µM (abiotic)	1.2	Jeong *et al.*, 2006
			Selenium 0.5 mM (abiotic)	1.3	–do-
			NaCl 1 per cent (abiotic)	1.2	–do-

Contd...

Table 9.1–*Contd...*

Plant Species	*Metabolites (Medicinal properties)*	*Medicinal Properties*	*Elicitor (Type)*	*Fold Increase in Metabolite Content*	*References*
			Oligosaccharides from *Paris polyphylla* (plant), 30 mg/l (biotic)	1.5	Wang *et al.*, 2006
			Methyl jasmonate (abiotic)	3.8	Kim *et al.*, 2009
Pharbitis nil	Umbelliferone, scopoletin, skimmin		$CuSO_4$ (abiotic), MeJA (biotic)		Yaoya *et al.*, 2004
Portulaca oleracea	Dopamine	Anti-parkinsonian (100 Mmol)	Methyl jasmonate	4.3	Moghadam *et al.*, 2013
Salvia miltiorrhiza	Tanshinone	Antioxidant and anti-inflammatory	Sorbital, 50g/l(abiotic)	4.5	Shi *et al.*, 2007
			Yeast elicitor (biotic), Ag (abiotic)	1.2	Staniszewska *et al.*, 2003, Yan *et al.*, 2005, Ge *et al.*, 2005
			Yeast extract + Ag + Methyl jasmonate (biotic)	2.2	Cheng *et al.*, 2013
Silybum marianum	Silymarin		Ag, 2 mM (abiotic)	2.0	Khilili *et al.*, 2010
Scopolia parviflora	Scopolamine		*Pseudomonas aeruginosa, Basillus ceeus, Staphylococcus aureus* (biotic)	1.5	Jung *et al.*, 2003
Solanum tuberosum	Sesquiterpene (rishitin, lubimin, phytuberin, phytuberol), lypoxygenase		*Rhizoctonia bataticola,* MeJa (biotic), B cyclodextrin (abiotic)	2.0	Komaraiah *et al.*, 2003

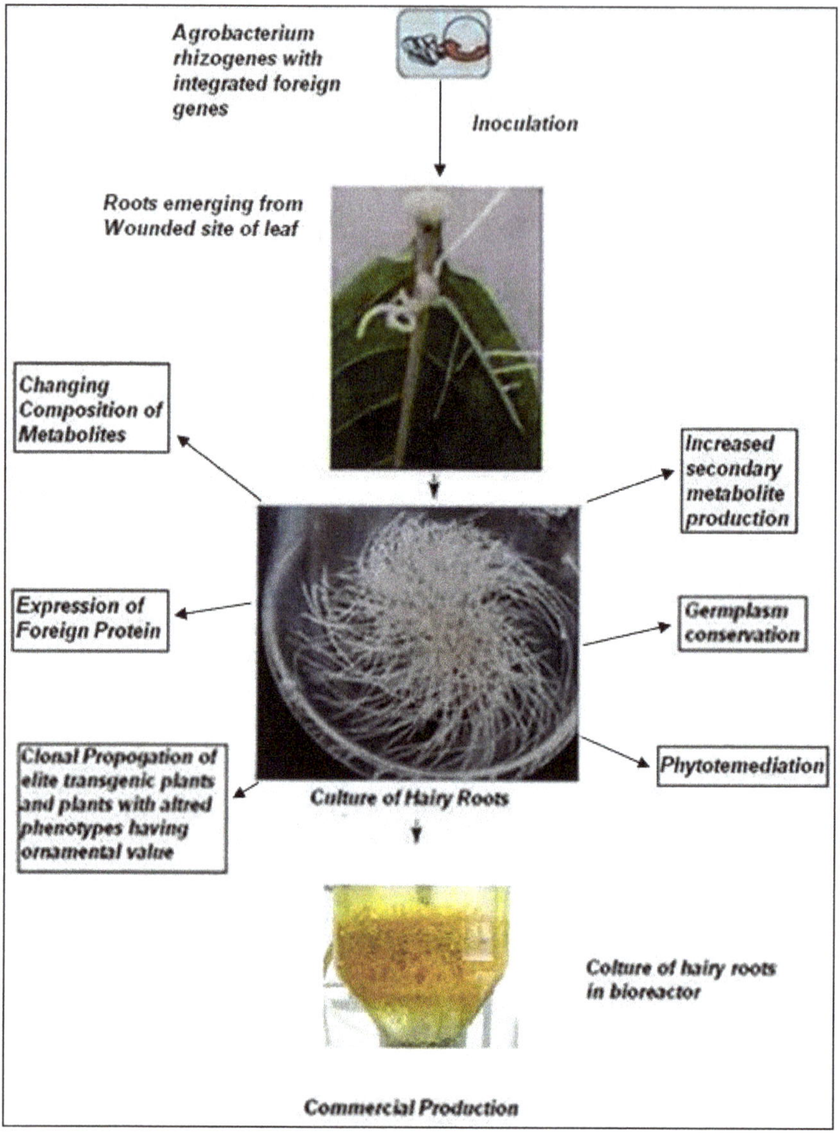

Agrobacterium rhizogenes with integrated foreign genes
Inoculation
Roots emerging from Wounded site of leaf
Changing Composition of Metabolites
Increased secondary metabolite production
Expression of Foreign Protein
Germplasm conservation
Clonal Propogation of elite transgenic plants and plants with altred phenotypes having ornamental value
Phytotemediation
Culture of Hairy Roots
Colture of hairy roots in bioreactor
Commercial Production

Figure 9.1: Biotechnological Prospects for Hairy Root Research.

Agrobacterium rhizogenes **transfers the T-DNA segment from its large plasmid (Ri) into the plant genome after leaf infection. A few days later, roots emerge from the inoculation site of the leaf. Hairy roots develop in agitated liquid culture. To become an acceptable biotechnological process, hairy root cultures must be scaled-up in a bioreactor in order (a) to produce valuable metabolites from medicinal plants, (b) to increase the production of secondary metabolites by chemical means, (c) to introduce foreign genes into plant genomes to produce recombinant proteins or to overexpress proteins that are otherwise limiting to metabolic pathways, (d) to uptake heavy metals from phytoremediation systems, and (e) to conserve germplasm through artificial seeds, (f) clonal propagation of elite transgenic plants, and (g) clonal propagation of plants with altered phenotypes having ornamental value.**

(DFR) gene into the hairy roots of *Lotus corniculatus* and effectively downgraded tannin biosynthesis.

Expression of Foreign Proteins

Possibility of production of industrial and therapeutic protein in plants has been studied intensely for its commercial value. Diaz *et al.* (1995a) reported introduction and expression of pea lectin gene in white clover (*Trifolium repens*) hairy roots. Sharp and Doran (2001b) reported that expression of murine-lgG1 in the hairy roots of tobacco and increase in the production of the antibody by increasing the dissolved oxygen tension to 150 per cent air saturation. Menzel *et al.* (2003) introduced three genes (responsible for poly 3-hydroxybutyrate, PHB, synthesis) from the bacteria *Ralstonia eutropha* into hairy roots of sugar beet. Twenty transgenic hairy root clones produced up to 55 mg high molecular PHB per gram of dry weight.

In vitriculture, antiviral traits are important economic factors. Plants transformed with virus protein often show resistance to virus infection. Transformation of grapevine hairy roots with coat protein of grapevine chrome mosaic nepovirus was reported (Torregrosa *et al.*, 1997). However, they could not regenerate the whole plants from the hairy roots. The fact that coat protein genes can be expressed in the hairy roots, indicate that this approach could be viable for the development of virus resistant plants in future.

Production of Secondary Metabolites

Hairy roots have several advantages for the production of secondary metabolites. These include: highly productive under hormone-free cultural conditions, fast growth, low doubling time, ease of maintenance, ability to synthesize a range of chemical compounds, and stability in culture. These roots can also synthesize more than one metabolite and therefore, prove economical for commercial production processes. Many medicinal plants have been transformed successfully by *A. rhizogenes* and hairy roots induced show a relatively high productivity of secondary metabolites. Sevon (2002) has summarized the most important alkaloids produced by hairy roots of various plants. A list of important secondary metabolites produced in hairy root cultures of different plant species is presented in Table 9.2.

Sometimes, the efficiency of secondary metabolite production by hairy roots is not found to be of desirable level for commercial production. In such cases, new approaches have been made for improving the production of secondary metabolites. Such approaches are designed to increase the level of enzymes involved in the metabolism and which consequently result in the accumulation of the target product.

Based on the type of gene to transfer, two different transformation methods are used. The first method utilizes the foreign genes that encodes enzyme activities not normally present in a plant. This may cause the modification or diversion of plant metabolic pathways. Two direct repeats of a bacterial lysine decarboxylase gene expressed in the hairy roots on tobacco markedly increased cadaverine and anabasine (Fecker *et al.*, 1993). Similarly, production of anthraquinone and alizarin in hairy roots of *Rubia peregrine* was enhanced by the introduction of isochorismata

Table 9.2: Plant Species Transformed by *A. rhizogenes* for the Production of Secondary Metabolites

Plant Species	*Secondary Metabolites*	*Medicinal* Property	References
Arachis hypigaea	Resveratrol	Anti-inflamatory, anti-oxidant, anti-cancerous	Kim et al., 2008
Arbus precatorium	Glycyrrhizin	Diuretic, tonic, alexitric, anti-fertility	Dixit and Vaidy 2010
Artemisia annua	Artemisinin	Anti-malarial	Weathers et al., 2005
Atropa belladonna	Tropane alkaloids (hyoscamine, atropine, hyoscine)	Anti-parkinsonian	Richter et al., 2005
Beta vulgaris	Betalains	Aphrodisiac, laxative	Pavlov et al., 2002a, b
	Peroxidase		Rudrappa et al., 2005
Camptotheca acuminate	Camptothecin	Anti-cancer, anti-viral	Lorence et al., 2004
Catharanthus roseus	Indole alkaloid (vinblastive, vincristine)	Anti-cancerous	Ayora-Talavera et al., 2002
Datura innoxia	Tropane alkaloids (scopolamine, hyoscyamine)	Nacrotic, anti-cholinergic, anti-spasmodic	Dechaux and Boitelconti 2005
Datura metal	–do–	–do–	Mayaro et al., 2003
Datura stromonium	–do–	–do–	Pavlo et al., 2009
Fagopyrum esculentum	Rutin	Anti-oxidant, anti-carcinogenic, anti-thromobotic	Kim et al., 2010
Ginko biloba	Ginkgolides	Aging disorders	Ayadi and Tremouillaux-Guiller 2003
Glycyrrhiza palliflora	Flavonoids	Anti-Gastric ulcer, anti-inflammatory, anti-tumor	Li et al., 2002
Glycyrrhiza uralensis	–do–	–do–	Zhang et al., 2009
Gmelina arborea	Verbascoside	Aging disorder, anti-inflammatory, wound healing	Dhakulkar et al., 2005
Gynostemma pentaphyllum	Gypenoside	Detergent	Chang et al., 2005
Panax ginseng	Phytosterols,ginsennosides	Tonic, stimulant, adaptogenic	Kim et al., 2014
Salvia broussonetii	Diterpens	Antioxidant, anti-inflammatory	Frage et al., 2005
S. cinnabarina	p-sitosterol, ursolic acid		Savona et al., 2003
S. inolucrata	Apigenin, total flavonoids		Li et *al.*, 2006

Contd.

Table 9.2–*Contd...*

Plant Species	*Secondary Metabolites*	*Medicinal Property*	*References*
S. miltiorrhiza	Cryptotanshinone, tanshinone -I, IIA and IIB, lithospermic acid B,diterpenoid,tanshinones	Antioxidant, anti- inflammatory	Chen *et al.*, 2001, Zhing *et al.*, 2004, Yan *et al.*, 2005, Ge *et al.*, 2005
S. sclarea	Ortonaphtoquinone diterpens		De Felice *et al.*, 2004
S. wagneriana	Rosmarinic acid		Pistelli *et al.*, 2010
Solanum khasianum	Solasodin	Barth control	Jacob and Malpathak 2004

synthase (Lodhi *et al.*, 1996). The hairy roots of *Atropa belladonna* transformed with the rabbit P450 2E1 gene led to increased production of the metabolites (Banerjee *et al.*, 2002). Ayora-Talavera *et al.* (2002) reported increased production of ajmalicine and cantharanthine or serpentine and campesterol by the hairy roots of *Catharanthus roseus* harboring hamstar 3-hydroxy 3-methylglutaryl coenzyme A (CoA) reductase (HMGR) cDNA without the membrane-binding domain.

The second method enhances the overexpression of enzymes that are already present in a plant. When tobacco putrescine N-methyltransferase (PMT) gene was transformed into *Datura metel* and *Hyoscyamus muticus,* the enzyme catalyzed the first committed step in the tropane alkaloid pathway, stimulated the growth of transgenic roots and enhanced accumulation of tropane alkaloid. To overcome the deficiency of oxygen in the hairy root culture, two genes namely Adh and pyruvate decarboxylase, were transferred into the hairy roots of *Arabidopsis thaliana*. The transformed hairy roots lines could maintain similar growth rate under conditions of low oxygen to the rate achieved with full aeration (Shiao *et al.,* 2002). Thus the problem of oxygen deficiency in hairy root culture caused by poor mixing and mass transfer could be solved.

Production of Compounds not Found in Untransformed Roots

Sometime, hairy roots produce new compounds which are not found in the untransformed roots. Such compounds having industrial or pharmaceutical value can be exploited further for commercial production. Nishikawa *et al.* (1997) reported that transformed hairy roots of *Scutellaria baicalensis* accumulated glucoside conjugates of flavonoids instead of glucose conjugates accumulated in untransformed roots.

Changing Composition of Metabolites

Composition of several metabolites has been reported to have changed in the hairy roots culture lines. For example, expression of an *Antirrhinum* dihydroflavavonol reductase gene resulted in changes in condensed tannin structure and accumulation in hairy root culture of *L. conrniculatus* (Bavage *et al.,* 1997). In another study, selected hairy roots culture lines indicated alteration of monomerlevels during growth and development without changes in composition.

As a Tool for Phytoremediation

Phytoremediation takes advantage of the ability of plants and associated micro-organisms to remove, contain, or render harmless inorganic as well as organic contaminants (Cunningham *et al.,* 1996). Phytoremediation studies carried out with whole plants provide useful information related to the removal capabilities of the plant species under study and also about the phytotoxic effects of the contaminant. In vitro cultures of roots are of particular interest for studying the interaction of contaminants with the plant system. Isolated organ culture permit the characterization of the uptake capability of the roots while avoiding the interference of translocation to other plant tissues. The drawback of root cultures is their low growth rate, which can impair experimental procedures. However, the in vitro culture of transformed roots (hairy roots) can overcome this drawback. Flocco and Giulietti (2007) reported development of a protocol for application of hairy root culture of *A. lapathifolia* for studying the removal of organic compounds like phenol, a model organic contaminant. A. lapathifolia roots contain high levels of peroxidases enzyme that are known to be involved in the detoxification of plenols and other aromatic compounds. The cultures were exposed to different concentrations of the contaminant and the remaining amounts of it, and some physiological parameters were monitored at different time intervals. The experimental procedure permitted the estimation of the capability of the plant species to remove the contaminant and also the main variables that may affect the remediation process. Such information is essential for assessing the feasibility of a remediation process prior to its field application. Thus hairy root culture constitutes a valuable tool for phytoremediation research.

For Germplasm Conservation

Artificial seed are considered to be good material for ex-situ conservation of germplasm. Hairy roots can be used for the production of artificial seeds. This provides an effective tool for ex-vitro conservation of germplasm. Hairy roots in the form of artificial seeds are reliable delivery system for clonal propagation of elite plants with genetical uniformity, high yield and low production cost. Artificial seed were produced from hairy roots of horseradish (Nakashimada *et al.*, 1995) and Ajuge reptans (Uozumi 2004). While cryopreserved root-tips derived from the hairy roots of *Panex gensing* (Yoshimatsn *et al.*, 1996) and shoot tips of HRs regenerants of horseradish were regenerated (Phunchindawan *et al.*, 1997).

Hairy root induced from rare medicinal plants can be used for regeneration of whole plants, making them an alternative and complimentary ex-site biodiversity conservation method. For germplasm conservation, development of long term preservation technique for hairy root cultures is essential. Hairy root cultures have been stored at ambient, low and –zero temperatures with success. Stable alkaloid production was observed in transgenic *Catharanthus roseus* hairy roots after five-year maintenance in liquid cultures (Peebles *et al.*, 2009).

Regeneration of whole Plants

Regeneration of transgenic plants depends mostly on the *in vitro* cultural conditions for each species. But genotype and juvenility of the explants are equally important. Transformed roots can be regenerated into somatic embryos following the addition of the appropriate phytohormone. Han *et al.* (1993) reported regeneration of shoots from the hairy roots of *Robinia pseudoacacia* following the addition of 10 µmol/l α-NAA (naphthalene acetic acid) and 5 µmol/l 6-BAP (benzyl aminopurine). Cho and Wildholm (2002) reported induction of somatic embryos from the hairy roots of *Astragalus sinicus* when the medium was supplemented with 2,4-dichlorophenoxy acetic acid (7.5 to 10.0 mg/l).

Transformed roots are able to regenerate genetically stable plants as transgenics or clones. This property of rapid growth and high plantlet regeneration frequency allow clonal propagation of elite plants. in addition, the altered phenotype of hairy root regenerants (hairy root syndrome) is useful in plant breeding programme with plants of ornamental interest (Giri and Narasu, 2000).

Medicinal Plants Transformed by *A. rhizogenes*

Agrobacterium rhizogenes has been successfully used to transform medicina plants and for production of secondary metabolites. Some important medicina plants having potential for secondary metabolite production through hairy roo transformation are discussed.

Basil (*Ocimum basilicum*)

Ocimum basilicum (sweet basil) plants are valued for their pharmaceutica properties. Among the different secondary metabolites found in *Ocimum* species rosemarinic acid (RA), having antioxidant property, is one of the most abundant Suspension hairy root cultures of sweet basil obtained from the leaves accumulate RA up to 10 mg/g dry weight, a value up to 11 times higher than in callus culture or in the leaves of the donor plant (Bais *et al.*, 2002).

To maximize the production of secondary metabolites, HR cultures of *O. basilicum* were exposed to salicylic acid, jasmonic acid, chitosan and fungal cell wall elicitors. Among the different elicitors tested, application of fungal cell wal elicitor from *Phytophthora cinnamoni* has increased the production of RA to 2.67 fold compared to untreated control (Bais *et al.*, 2002).

Echinacea (*Echinacea* spp.)

The genus *Echinacea* has nine species and is widely grown and used for the immunostimulant property. Several caffeic acid derivatives (CADs) such as cichoric acid, caftaric acid, chlorogenic acid and caffeic acid have been identified in *Echinacea* species. They are believed to have immunostimulatory activity (Hu and Kitts 2000 Bergeron *et al.*, 2002).

The method of transformed HR cultures of *E. purpurea* was established by infecting different types of explants with three strains of *A. rhizogenes* (Wang *et al.*, 2006). Higher concentrations of polysaccharides were detected in transformed HR than in nontransformed roots. Accumulation of secondary metabolites could be increased by change and/or addition of nutritional ingredients, hormones or precursors (Wang *et al.*, 2006). Liu *et al.* (2006) reported production of significant amounts of CADs (especially cichoric acid and caftaric acid) by the HR of *E. purpurea*.

Abbasi *et al.* (2007) has demonstrated a definite positive effect of light on root growth, cell viability and PAL (phenylalanine ammonia lysate) activity in relation to the biosynthesis of CADs in *E. purpurea*. The photoregulation of CADs biosynthesis in *E. purpurea* HR may offer additional advantages of quantitative and qualitative improvements of these medicinally important metabolites.

Ginseng (*Panax ginseng*)

Panax ginseng is of Chinese origin and is well known for its use in oriental medicine. Crude ginseng root extracts have tonic, stimulatory and adoptogenic properties, mainly due to the presence of numerous saponins and sapogenins (Tang and Eisenbrand 1992).

Successful induction and establishment of *P. ginseng* rhizomes HR after *A. rhizogenes* infection has been reported (Inomata *et al.*, 1993, Vazquez-Flota *et al.*, 1994). These transformed roots exhibited a more rapid growth and higher levels of ginsenosides than the normal cultured roots obtained by hormonal control. Jeong *et al.* (2004) demonstrated that the growth of *P. ginseng* HR is strongly influenced by the inoculums size and its age.

Pavlov *et al.* (2002a, b) reported that the *P. ginseng* root lines produced the highest levels of ginsenosides at the third day of culture, when they were culture in the presence of methyl jasmonate and when the cultures were in the advanced progressive deceleration growth phase. To improve the productivity of useful metabolites, several elicitors were used in *P. ginseng* HR cultures. These include: salicylic acid (SA), acetylsalicylic acid (ASA), yeast elicitor and bacterial elicitor. In general, elicitor treatments were found to inhibit the growth of the HR, but enhance ginseng saponin biosynthesis (Jeong *et al.*, 2005). Also, addition of 20 µM $NiSO_4$ increased ginseng saponine content and productivity (Jeong and Park 2006). It was also reported that sodium chloride added into the media increased the amount of synthesized ginseng saponins. These results suggest that application of elicitors can reduce the processing time for the generation of ginseng saponin in HR culture.

Oligosaccharides [for example, heptasaccharide (HS), octasaccharide (OS) etc.] from plant and microbial sources represent a class of the most widely recognized elicitors, acting as inducers of plant defense responses and playing regulatory roles in plant growth and development (John *et al.*, 1997, Vorwerk *et al.*, 2004). Therefore, these compounds were tested as elicitors in HR of *P. ginseng* to see their effect in the induction of secondary metabolites. Separate addition of HS and OS to HR cultures of *P. ginseng* increased the root biomass dry weight by more than 70 per cent and the total saponin content of roots by more than 1-fold (Zhou *et al.*, 2007). These results suggest that HS and OS may have activities like plant growth regulators in plant cell cultures.

Mint (*Mentha* spp.)

The genus *Mentha* includes more than 25 species, and is widely cultivated for their essential oil. This valuable product is mainly composed of monoterpens and is largely used in the food, cosmetics and pharmaceutical industries. The quality of oil depends on the composition of the monoterpene, and therefore emphasis has been made to develop strains producing better quality oil.

Regeneration of HR and shoots from *M. piperita* after infection with *A. rhizogenes* was first reported by Inoue *et al.* (2003). The regenerated plants showed HR syndrome. Hairy roots was also induced in *M. pulegium* (clone line MPH-4), a species containing high levels of endogenous phenolics, by *A. rhizogenes* infection. The inoculated explants exhibited higher levels of total phenolic components and guaiacol peroxidase activity. Enhancement of phenolics production was more apparent when explants were treated with polymeric dye R-478. Polymeric dyes are widely used in textile industry and are known environmental pollutants. Polymeric dyes have a structure analogous to common polycyclic aromatic hydrocarbons (PAHs). Plants that show an inherent tolerance to these dyes are currently being investigated for use in phytoremediation. The response of *M. pulegium* line MPH-4 to *A. rhizogens* and polydye R-478 has created interest to study the possible use of this clone in phytoremediation (Strycharz and Shetty 2002).

Saga (*Salvia officinalis*)

The genus *Salvia* includes more than 900 species. Some of them are known for their medicinal potential and are commercially used. Only few are cultured *in vitro.* Kintzios (1999) demonstrated the possibility to manipulate the *in vitro* production of rosmarinic acid (RA) in cell cultures of *S. officinalis* and *S. fruticosa*. Chen *et al.* (1999) reported production of RA and lithospermic acid B from transformed cells of *S. miltiorrhiza*. In 2003, Savona identified a new sccoisopimarane diterpenoid in *S. cinnabarina,* while Bisio (2004) described other new terpenoids in *S. wagneriana* having interesting biological activity.

Several HR lines were obtained from *S. wagneriana, S. cinnabarina, S. jamensis* through single transformation event. Several elicitors were used to enhance the production of secondary metabolites from these HR lines grown in liquid medium. Screening of the secondary metabolites produced by *S. wagneriana* does not reflect any of the secondary metabolites produced by the matured plants. However, it showed presence of diterpenes, ursolic acid, p-sitosterol, caffeic acid and other flavonoids different from the available reference material (Pistelli *et al.*, 2012).

Potential Problems

Hairy roots have been recognized as a potential tool for various applications. However, there exist certain potential problems which need to be solved. Some of these problems are presented in the following section.

Different Regulation of Secondary Metabolism in Related Species

Normally related plant species share the same pathways for the production of secondary metabolites, and their regulation may differ according to different pattern. For example, the tropane alkaloid was increased in the hairy roots of two related species, *D. metel* and *H. muticus* (Moyano *et al.*, 2003). But different patterns of accumulation were observed in the two species mentioned above. Both hyoscyamine and scopolamine were accumulated in the hairy roots of *D. metel,* whereas only hyoscyamine levels increased in *H. muticus*. This indicates that the same pathway in two related species is regulated differently. Mitra *et al.* (2002) reported expression of 4- Hydroxycinnamoly-CoA hydratase (HCHL) in the hairy roots of *Datura stromonium,* although it was not expressed in the normal mature plants.

Depending on the genotype of the recipient HR, expression of the transferred gene may differ. Carron *et al.* (1994) reported that antisense DFR downregulated tannin biosynthesis in two genotypes (S33 and S50) of *L corniculatus,* bur accumulated high levels of tannins in the third genotype (S41).

Overexpression of Key Enzymes Does not Always Improve Secondary Metabolism

In the biosynthesis of shikonin, two key enzymes encoding chorismate pyruvate-lysate and HMGR, are assumed to be involved. Genes controlling this two enzymes were transferred to the hairy roots of *Lithospermum erthrorhizon*. However, accumulation of sikonin remained unchanged, even with high expression of both the enzymes (Koehle *et al.*, 2002).

Reduction of Chromosome Numbers during Sub-Culture

The number of chromosome may be reduced in certain HR cultures and thereby affect production of the secondary metabolites. For example, after four months of culture the chromosome number of *Onobrychis viciaefolia* was found to have reduced from 85 to 23.5 percent, and after eight months to only 4.1 percent cells had normal chromosome number (Xu *et al.*, 1996).

Co-suppression of Endogenous and Foreign Genes

Transfer of more copies of the gene(s) does not result in greater expression of the task enzyme and a corresponding increase in the product(s). For example, *Catharanthus roseus* hairy roots having hamster HMGR cDNA expressed a different alkaloid production pattern. One of the clone (236) having more copies of the gene HMGR, had the lowest HMGR activity but increased levels of ajmalicine and catharanthine. Another clone (19), with low copy number of HMGR, expressed more HMGR and produced more campesterol and serpentine, but had a low level of ajmalicine and showed no accumulation of catharanthine.

Loss of Expression of Foreign Gene after Long Period Culture

Hairy roots of *Cinchona officinalis* transformed with tryptophan decarboxylase (TDC) and strictosidine synthase (STR) produced high amounts of tryptamine and strictosidine at the beginning of the culture. However, they completely lost their capacity to accumulate alkaloids, after one year in culture, without any change in the growth and morphology (Geerlings *et al.*, 1999).

Alternation in the Morphology of the Regenerated Plants

Plants regenerated from hairy roots often have altered morphological characters. The changes include an extremely abundant and plagiotropic root system, wrinkled leaves, reduced internoe length and leaf size, reduced apical dominance, and an increased ability of leaf explants to differentiate roots in phytohormone-free medium (Tepfer 1984, Taylor *et al.*, 1985, Cardarelli *et al.*, 1987, Spano *et al.*, 1988, Hamamoto *et al.*, 1990). Apparently these changes have originated from either the insertion of foreign DNA or somaclonal variations, rather than from the expression of T-DNA genes in the transformants (Han *et al.*, 1993). Further, compared to untransformed plants, the transgenic plants show higher mortality.

Difficulties in Scaling-Up

The present established culture systems are based on flask or small-scale bioresctors. Many attempts have been made to develop economical bioreactors containing airlift, bubble column, mist, dual, and wave reactors (Du *et al.*, 2003, Lin *et al.*, 2003, Palazon *et al.*, 2003, Souret *et al.*, 2003, Kintzios *et al.*, 2004, Suresh *et al.*, 2004). Except few, most of the existing culture systems could not resolve the cost benefit ratio, making them impractical for commercial use. To overcome this issue, future research should focus on the establishment of effective and economical scale-up culture system. While designing the bioreactor following points should be considered: it should permit the growth of interconnected tissues unevenly distributed throughout the vessel, rheological characteristics of heterogeneous system, oxygen consumption and excretion of products to the medium. Once such breakthrough is achieved, commercial application of hairy roots shall be a reality. Few examples on modifications made in the major types of bioreactors for increased production of biomass and secondary metabolite from hairy roots are discussed.

Stirred Tank Bioreactor

In stirred tank bioreactors, the aeration and medium currency is regulated by morter-derived impeller or turbine blades. Usually the temperature, pH, amount of dissolved oxygen, and nutrient concentration can be better controlled within this reactor. In general, the impellers used in this reactor produce a high-shear stress compared to other type (Hilton and Rhodes 1990, Kim and Yoo 1993). For hairy root culture, the impeller must be operated with restricted power input and speed to minimize the shear stress. Improvement in the impeller performance by modifying internal reactor geometry has been reported (Kondo *et al.*, 1989, Uuzumi *et al.*, 1993, Doran 1999). In *Catharanthus trichophyllus*, hairy roots cultured in stirred bioreactors showed similar alkaloid composition as found in normal roots (Doran 1999). Success in hairy root culture of *Swertia chirata* and Panax ginseng in stirred-tank reactor was successful only when a stainless-steel mesh fitted inside the culture vessel (Keil *et al.*, 2000, Jeong *et al.*, 2003).

Airlift Bioreactor

In airlift bioreactors, aeration and liquid currency are driven by externally supplied air. Therefore this type of reactor is useful for culturing plant cells and organs, which are sensitive to shear stress. However, this reactor is not suitable for high-density culture because of insufficient mixing process inside the reactor. Kintzios *et al.* (2004) reported 200 times increase in puerarin accumulation from *Pueraria phaseoloides* hairy root culture grown in 2.5 L airlift reactor compared to 250 ml shake flask culture. In *Asteagalas membranaceas*, hairy roots cultured in 30 L airlift reactor accumulated more astragaleside, compared to when cultured in 10 L bioreactor (Du *et al.*, 2003). In *Panax gensing*, growth of hairy roots was reported to have increased several times when cultured in stirred bioreactor compared to flask cultivation (Jeong *et al.*, 2002, 2003). Growth and production of hyescyamine and scopolamine in the culture of hairy roots of Datura metel was enhanced by the treatment of permeabilizing agent Tween 20 in an airlift bioreactor with root anchorage (Cusido *et al.*, 1999).

Bubble Column Bioreactor

The bubble column reactor creates less shear stress compared to other stirred type reactor, and thus useful for hairy root culture. In this case, the bubbling rate needs to be gradually increased with the growth of hairy roots. However, at a high tissue density level, the bubble column has been observed to reduce growth performance (Kwok *et al.*, 1995). Tescione *et al.* (1997) reported that in bubble column hairy root culture of *Solanum tuberosum*, stagnation and channeling of gas through the bed of growing roots exists, however, the gas-liquid interface was not the dominant resistance factor to oxygen mass transfer and oxygen uptake of growing tips increase with the oxygen tension of the medium. Inclusion of polyurethane foam in the vessel of air-sparged bioreactor reduces the entrapping of gas by hairy roots, which in-turn improves biomass and alkaloid production in *Duboisia leichhardtii* hairy root culture (Muranaka *et al.*, 1993). In *Artemisia annua* hairy root culture, the bubble column reactor was reported to be superior to mist reactor for biomass concentration, whereas mist reactors produce significantly more artemisinin (Kim *et al.*, 2002, Souret *et al.*, 2003). High density culture of red beet hairy roots was obtained by a radial flow reactor, which consists of a cylindrical vessel with a radial flow of medium (Kino-Oka *et al.*, 1999).

Liquid-Dispersed Bioreactor

Bioreactors used for hairy root culture can be classified as either liquid-phase or gas-phase. The liquid-dispersed bioreactors provide sufficient oxygen supply to roots and low sheer stress environment compared to reactors in which the roots remained submersed in a liquid medium (McKetuey *et al.*, 1993). In liquid-dispersed bioreactors, roots are exposed to ambient air or gas mixture, and the nutrient liquid, which is dispersed as spray or mist onto the top of the root bed (Williams *et al.*, 2000, Kim *et al.*, 2002). The sprayed liquid and mist are drained from the bottom of the bioreactor to a reservoir and is re-circulated. The degree of distribution of liquid varies according to the mechanism of liquid delivery at the top of the reactor chamber. Various types of liquid-dispersed bioreactors are developed for the hairy root culture. These include: nutrient mist (Dilovio *et al.*, 1992, Whitney 1992, Buer *et al.*, 1996, Wilson 1997), droplet (Kim *et al.*, 2002, Wilson 1997), trickle-bed or tricking film (Whitney 1992, Taya *et al.*, 1998), and drip tube (Holmes 1997). In all these bioreactors, certain types of support like glass beads, rasching rings, steel wire scaffolding, polyurethane foam, horizontal mesh trays, and cylindrical stainless steel mesh, to the roots are provided (Taya *et al.*, 1989, Whitney 1992, Wilson 1997, Holmes 1997, Kim *et al.*, 2002). Bais *et al.* (2002) reported production of twice as much aesculin in acoustic mist bioreactor grown hairy root cultures of *Cicborium intybus* compared to roots grown in bubble column and nutrient sprinkle reactors (Bais *et al.*, 2002). *Artemisia annua* hairy roots grown in nutrient mist reactors produce nearly three times as much artemisinin as roots grown in bubble column reactor (Kim *et al.*, 2001). Apparently a higher level of artemisinin was produced due to a response to the increased osmotic strength of the medium within the mist reactor, as the medium becomes concentrated due to water evaporation (Kim *et al.*, 2001). However, in general, the mist reactor accumulates lower biomass than does the bubble column reactor due to insufficient nutrient availability (Kim *et al.*, 2002).

Balloon Type Bubble Bioreactor

Son *et al.* (1999) designed a balloon-type bubble reactor (BTBB) which was found to be superior to the bubble column bioreactor and stirred tank bioreactor for biomass growth of hairy root culture of *Taxas caspidota* (Son *et al.*, 2000), *Beta valgaris* (Shin *et al.*, 2002), *Panax ginseng* (Yu *et al.*, 2000), and adventitious roots of *Panex ginseng* (Yu *et al.*, 2002). The fresh weight of ginseng hairy-like adventitious root culture in 20 L BTBB was three-times higher than that of the stirred tank reactor (Son *et al.*, 1999). In a 20 L bioreactor, the maximum biomass production of 2.2 kg fresh weight was obtained after 42 days of inoculation of 240 gm adventitious root cultures of ginseng (Choi *et al.*, 2000). Growth of biomass in mountain ginseng cell line, maintained by the CBN Biotech Co., Korea, increased 30 fold after 42 days of culture. Pilot scale 500 and 1000 L stainless steel bioreactors was designed according to BTBB type for commercial production of saponin from hairy root culture of ginseng by the CBN Biotech Co., Korea. In the 1000 L reactor, the saponine content increased by six times (33.6 mg/g) (Choi *et al.*, 2008).

Conclusion

Plants are rich source of different bioactive molecules having pharmaceutical and industrial application. Medicinal plants are mostly growing wild. Habitat loss and indiscriminate collection has let to severe loss of genetic diversity of important medicinal plants. Thus the use of tissue culture technology under controlled environment can overcome some of these problems. Further genetic engineering techniques can be applied on tissue culture grown plants to enhance the production of bioactive compounds for commercial production.

Significant progress has been made in the use of tissue culture and genetic transformation to modify pathways for the biosynthesis of target metabolites. Hairy roots are unique in their genetic and biosynthetic stability and their fast growth offers an additional advantage to use as a continuous source for the production of valuable secondary metabolites. The oncogenic effect of Agrobacterium *rhizogenes* has been recently clarified. The RolA protein was suggested to act as a transcription factor and is implicated in the metabolism of gibberellins. The *rolC* stimulatory effect on secondary metabolism was demonstrated by investigations with different groups of secondary metabolites, such as tropane alkaloids, pyridine alkaloids, indole alkaloids, and ginsenosides. The rolB protein is a β-glucosidase which has a crucial effect on the formation of both lateral and adventitious roots while recently the *rolB* gene, introduced in *Vitis amurensis* cells induced calli able to increase resveratrol production. *RolD* protein stimulates the reproductive phase transition in plants and it is more related to flowering process.

Evidences accumulated so far on molecular mechanism of hairy root development suggest that certain strains of *A. rhizogenes* with selected pool of *Rol* genes when used for transformation results into more driven results in order to optimize metabolite production.

The number of plant species successfully transformed by *A. rhizoenes* for the establishment of hairy roots is more than 190 from 41 families (Kuzovkina and

Schneider 2006). Hairy root cultures offer many advantages, particularly for the production of wide range of metabolites continuously at high rate (Grzegorczyc *et al.*, 2006). Large scale culture feasibility and long term stability make this biotechnological approach not only a reliable source of secondary metabolites, but also an effective tool to study the biosynthetic pathways of complex plant products (Rubins 1998, Peebles *et al.*, 2007). However scaling-up hairy roots to industrial levels poses a great challenge.

References

Abbasi BH, Tian CL, Murch SJ, *et al.*, Light-enriched caffeic acid derivatives biosynthesis in hairy root cultures of *Echinacca purpurea*. *Plant Cell Rep.* 8: 1367-1372. 2007.

Aoki S, Kawaoka A, Sekine M, *et al.*, Sequence of the cellular T-DNA in the untransformed genome of *Nicotiana glauca* that is homologous to ORFs 13 and 14 of the R_i plasmid and analysis of its expression in genetic tumors of *N. glauca* x *N. langsdorffii*. *Mol Gen. Genet.* 243: 706-710. 1994.

Aoki S, Syono K. Synergistic function of rolB, rolC, ORF13, and ORF14 of TL-DNA of A. rhizogenes in hairy root induction in Nicotiana tabacum. *Plant Cell Physiol.* 40: 252-256. 1999.

Arroo RRJ, Develi A, Meijers H, Van-de-Westerio E, Kemp AK, Croes AF. Effect of exogenous auxin on root morphology and secondary metabolism in *Tagetes patula* hairy root cultures. *Physiol. Plant.* 93: 233-240. 1995.

Ayora-Talavera T, Chappell J, Lozoya-Gloria E, Loyola-Vargas VM. Overexpression in *Catharanthus roseus* hairy roots of a truncated hamster 3-hydroxy -3-methylglutaryl-CoA reductase gene. *Appl. Biochem. Biotechnol.* 97: 135-145. 2002.

Azian GJ, Marziah M, Radzali M, Johari R. Establishment of *Physalis minima* hairy roots culture for the production of physalins. *Plant Cell Tiss. Org. Cult.* 69: 271-278. 2002.

Bais HP, Surest B, Raghavarao GA. Performance of hairy root culture of *Cichorium intybus* in bioreactors of different contigurations. *In vitro Cell Dev. Biol. Plant.* 38: 538-580. 2002.

Bais HP, Walker TS, Schweizer HPB, *et al.*, Root specific elicitation and antimicrobial activity of rosmarinic acid in hairy root cultures of *Ocimum basilicum. Plant Physiol. Biochem.* 40: 983-995. 2002.

Banerjee S, Shang TQ, Wilson AM *et al.*, Expression of functional mammalian P450 in hairy root cultures. *Biotechol. Bioeng.* 77: 462-466. 2002.

Bavage AD, Davis IG, Robbins MP, Morris P. Expression of an Antirrhinum dihydroflavonol reductase gene results in changes in condensed tannin structure and accumulation in root cultures of *Lotus corniculatus*. *Plant Mol. Genet.* 35: 443-458. 1997.

Bensaddel L, Villarreal ML, Fliniaux MA. Induction and growth of hairy roots for the production of medicinal compounds. *J. Integ. Biosci.* 3: 2-9. 2008.

Bergeron C, Gafner S, Batcha LL *et al.*, Stabilization of caffeic acid derivatives in *Echinacea purpurea* glycin extract. *J. Agric. Food Chem.* 50: 3967-3970. 2002.

Bhadra R, Shanks JV. Statistical design of the effect of inoculum conditions on growth of hairy root cultures of *Catharanthus roseus*. *Biotechnol. Tech.* 9: 681-686. 1995.

Bisio A, De-Tommasi N, Romussi G. Diterpenoids from *S. wagneriana*. *Planta Medica.* 70: 452-457. 2004.

Bonhomme V, Matta DL, Fliniaux MA. Effect of the rolC gene on hairy roots: induction developmentand tropane alkaloid production by *Atropa belladonna*. *J. Nat. Prod.* 63: 1249-1252. 2000.

Buer CS, Correl KJ, Smith TC *et al.*, Development of a nontoxic acoustic window nutrient-mist bioreactor and relevant growth data. *In vitro Cell Dev. Biol. Plant.* 32: 299-304. 1996.

Bulgakov VP, Khodakovskaya NV, Labetskaya NV *et al.*, The impact of plant rolC oncogene on ginsenoside production by ginseng hairy root cultures. *Phytochem.* 49: 1929-1934. 1998.

Bulgakov VP, Kusaykin M, Tchernoded GK *et al.*, Carbohydrate activities of the rolC gene transformed and nontransformed ginseng cultures. *Fitoterapia.* 73: 638-643. 2002.

Bulgakov VP, Tchernoded GK, Mischenko NP *et al.*, Effect of salicylic acid, methyl jasmonate, ethephon and cantharidin on anthraquinone production by *Rubia cordifolia* callus cultures transformed with the rolB and rolC genes. *J. Biotech.* 97: 213-221. 2002b.

Bulgakov VP, Tchernoded GK, Mischenko NP *et al.*, Effect of Ca^{+2} channel blockers and protein kinase/phosphatase inhibitors on growth and anthraquinone production in *Rubia cordifolia* callus cultures transformed by the rolB and rolC genes. *Planta.* 217: 349-355. 2003.

Bulgakov VP, Veselova MV, Tchernoded GK, *et al.*, Inhibitory effect of the *A. rhizogenes* rolC gene on rabdosiin and RA production in *Eritrichium sericeum* and *Lithospermum erythrorhizon* transformed cell culture. *Planta.* 221: 471-478. 2005.

Capone I, Spano L, Cardarelli M, *et al.*, Upstream noncoding region which confers polar expression to R_i plasmid root inducing gene rolB. *Plant Mol. Biol.* 13: 43-52. 1989.

Cardarelli M, Mariotti D, Pomponi M. Agrobacterium rhizogenes T-DNA genes capable of inducing hairy root phenotype. *Mol. Gen. Genet.* 209: 475-480. 1987.

Carron TR, Robbins MP, Morris P. Genetic modification of condensed tannin biosynthesis in *Lotus corniculatus*. 1. Heterologous antisense dihydroflavonol reductase down-regulates tannin accumulation in hairy root cultures. *Theo. Appl. Genet.* 87: 1006-1015. 1994.

Casanova E, Zuker A, Trillas MI *et al.*, The rolC gene in carnation exhibits cytokinin and auxin like activities. *Sci. Hort.* 97: 321-331. 2003.

Chen H, Chen F, Zhang YL *et al.*, Production of lithospermic acid B and rosmarinic acid in hairy root cultures of *S. miltiorrhiza*. *J. Ind. Microb. Biotech.* 22: 133-138. 1999.

Chio YE, Kim TS, Pake KY. Types and designs of bioreactors for hairy root culture. In: Dutta Gupta (Ed.), *Plant tissue culture engineering*. Springer, Amsterdam, pp. 161-172. 2008.

Cho HJ, Wildholm JM. Improved shoot regeneration protocol for hairy roots of the legume *Astragalus sinicus*. *Plant Cell Tiss. Org. Cult.* 69: 259-269. 2002.

Choi SM, Son SH, Yum SR, *et al.*, Pilot scale culture of adventitious roots of ginseng in a bioreactor system. *Plant Cell Tiss. Org. Cult.* 62: 187-193. 2000.

Christen P, Aoki T, Shimomura K. Characteristics of growth and tropane alkaloid production in Hyoscyamus albus hairy roots transformed with *A rhizogenes*. *Plant Cell Rep.* 11: 597-600. 1992.

Christey MC, Sinclair BK. Regeneration of transgenic kale (*Brassica oleracea*), rape (*B. napus*) and turnip (*B. campestris*) via *A rhizogenes* mediated transformation. *Plant Sci.* 87: 161-169. 1992.

Christey MC. Transgenic crop plants using *Agrobacterium rhizogenes* mediated transformation. In: *Hairy root: culture and applications* (Doran PM ed.). Academic Publisher, Amsterdam. pp. 99-111. 1997.

Christey MC. Use of Ri-mediated transformation for production of transgenic plants. *In vitro Cell Dev. Biol. Plant.* 37: 687-700. 2001.

Cunningham SD, Anderson TA, Schwab AP, Hsu FC. Phytoremediation of soils contaminated with organic pollutants. *Adv. Agron.* 56: 55-114. 1996.

Cusido RN, Palazon J, Pinal MT. *Datura metel*: in vitro production of tropane alkaloids. *Planta Med.* 65: 144-148. 1999.

Davioud E, Kan C, Hanon J, *et al.*, Production of Indole alkaloids by in vitro root culture of *C. trichophyllus*. *Phytochem.* 28: 2675-2680. 1998.

Dechaux C, Biotel-Conti M. A strategy for over accumulation of scopolamine in *Datura innoxia* hairy root culture. *Acta Biologica. Coriensia Ser. Botanica.* 47: 101-107. 2005.

Dehio C, Grossmann K, Schell J *et al.*, Phenotype and hormonal status of transgenic tobacco plants overexpressing the rolA gene of *A. rhizogenes* T-DNA. *Plant Mol. Biol.* 23: 1199-1210. 1993.

Dhakulkar S, Gopinath TR, Bhargava S, Bapat VA. Induction of hairy root in *Gmelina arborea* and production of verbascoside in hairy roots. *Plant Sci.* 169: 812-818. 2005.

Diaz CL, Longman TJJ, Stam HC, Kijne JW. Sugar-bindinh activity of pea lectin expressed in white clover hairy roots. *Plant Physiol.* 109: 1167-1177. 1995.

Dilovio AA, Cheetam RD, Weathers PJ. Growth of transformed roots in a nutrient mist bioreactor: reactor performance and evaluation. *Appl. Micrbiol. Biotechnol.* 37: 457-462. 1992.

Dixit AK, Vidya S. *Agrobacterium rhizigenes* induced hairy root development and its effect on production of glycyrrhizin in *Abrus precatorius. Int. J. Curr. Res.* 6: 33-38. 2010.

Doran PM. Design of mixing system for plant cell suspensions in stirred reactors. *Biotechnol. Prog.* 15: 319-335. 1999.

Drewes FE, Staden JV. Initiation of and solasodine production in hairy root culture of *Solanum mauritianum. Plant Growth Regul.* 17: 27-31. 1995.

Du M, Wu XJ, Ding J *et al.*, Astrogaloside IV and polysaccharide production by hairy roots of *Astragdus membranaceus. Biotechnol. Lett.* 25: 1853-1856. 2003.

Dymov SI, Vitavskaya OS, Demetskaya AV, Kostenyuk IA. The effect of methyl jasmaonate on the biomas increase and intracellular biosynthesis of indole alkaloids in the transgenic culture of *Catharanthus roseus. Cytol. Genet.* 31: 14-17. 1997.

Estrada-Navarrete G, Alvarado-Affantranger X, Olivares JE *et al.*, Fast, efficient and reproducible genetic transformation of *Phaseolus* spp. by *A. rhizogenes. Nature protocols.* 2: 1819-1824. 2007.

Estruch JJ, Schell J, Spena A. The protein encoded by rolB plant oncogene hydrolysis indole glucosidases. *EMBO J.* 10: 3125-3128. 1991.

Fecker LF, Ruegenhagen C, Berlin J. Increased production of cadaverine and anabasine in hairy root cultures of *Nicotiana tabaccum* expressing a bacterial lysine decarboxylase gene. *Plant Mol. Biol.* 23: 11-21. 1993.

Filippini F, Rossi V, Martin O *et al.*, A plant oncogene as a phosphatase. *Nature.* 379: 499-500. 1996.

Fillppini F, Lo Schiavo F, Terzi M *et al.*, The plant oncogene rolB alters binding of auxin to plant cell membrane. *Plant Cell Physiol.* 35: 767-771. 1994.

Flocco CG, Giulietti AM. In vitro hairy root cultures as a tool for phytoremediation research. *Methods Biotechnol.* 23: 161-173. 2007.

Fruendt C, Meyer AD, Ichikawa T, *et al.*, A tobacco homologue of the R_i plasmid ORF13 gene causes cell proliferation in carrot root disc. *Mol. Gen. Genet.* 259: 559-568. 1998.

Fu CX, Zhao DX, Xue XT *et al.*, Transformation of Saussureo involucrate by *A. rhizogenes*: hairy root induction and syringing production. *Proc. Biochem.* 40: 3789-3794. 2005.

Gaudin V, Vrain T, Jouanin L. Bacterial genes modifying hormonal balances in plants. *Plant Physiol. Biochem.* 32: 11-29. 1994.

Gelvin SB. *Agrobacterium* and plant genes involved in T-DNA transfer and integration. *An. Rev.Plant Phys. Plant. Mol.* Biol. 51: 223-256. 2000.

Giovannini A, Secchioni N, Rabaglio M *et al.*, Characterization of ornamental Datura plants transformed by *A. rhozogenes*. *In Vitro Cell. Dev. Biol. Plant*. 33: 101-106. 1997.

Giri A, Narasu ML. Transgenic HRs: recent trends and applications. *Biotech Adv.* 18: 1-22. 2000.

Giri A, Ravindra ST, Dhingra V, Narasu ML. Influence of different strains of *A. rhizogenes* on induction of hairy roots and artemisinin production in *Artemisia annua*. *Curr. Sci.* 81: 378-382. 2001.

Guillon S, Tremnouillaux-Guiller J, Patil PK *et al.*, Hairy root research: recent scenario and exciting prospects. *Curr Opin. Plant. Biol.* 9: 341-346. 2006.

Han KH, Keathley DE, Davis JM, Gordon MP. Regeneration of a transgenic woody legume (*Robinia pseudoacacia*) and morphological alternations induced by *A. rhizogenes*- mediated transformation. *Plant Sci.* 88: 149-157. 1993.

Hilton MG, Rhodes MJ. Growth and hyccyamine production of hairy root culture of *Datura stramonium* in a modified stirred tank reactor. Appl. Microbial. Biotechnol. 33: 132-138. 1990.

Holmes P, Li SL, Green KD, *et al.*, Drip-tube technology for continuous culture of hairy roots with integrated alkaloid extraction. In: Doran (Ed.) *Hairy roots: culture and applications*. Horwood Academic, Amsterdam, 1997. pp. 201-208.

Hosoki T, Kigo T. Transformation of Brussels sprouts (*Brassica loeracea*) by *A rhizogenes*-harbouring a reporter, β-glucuronidase gene. *J. Jpn. Sco. Hort. Sci.* 63: 589-592. 1994.

Hu C, Kitts DD. Studies on the antioxidant activity of *Echinacea* root extract. *J. Agric. Food Chem.* 48: 1466-1472. 2000.

Hu ZB, Du M. Hairy root and its application in plant genetic engineering. *J. Integra. Plant Biol.* 48: 121-127. 2006.

Huffman GA, White FF, Gordon MP, *et al.*, Hairy root inducing plasmid: physical map and homology to tumor-inducing plasmids. *J. Bacteriol.* 157: 269-276. 1984.

Hughes EH, Hong SB, Shanks JV, San KY, Gibon SI. Characterization of an inducible promoter system in *Catharanthus roseus* hairy roots. *Biotechnol. Prog.* 18: 1183-1186. 2002.

Jacob A, Malpathak N. Green hairy root cultures of *Solanum khasianum* Clarke- a new route to in vitro solasodine production. *Curr. Sci.* 87: 1442-1447. 2004.

Jefferson RA, Kavanagh TA, Bevan MW. GUS fusion b-glucurronidase as sensitive and versatile gene fusion marker in higher plants. *EMBO J.* 6: 3901-3907. 1987.

Jeone GT, Park DH, Hwang B *et al.*, Studies on mass production of transformed *Panex ginseng* hairy roots in bioteactors. *Appl. Biochem. Biotechnol.* 98: 115-1127. 2002.

Jeong GT, Purk DH, Hwang B, Woo JC. Comparison of growth characteristics of *Panex ginseng* hairy roots in various bioreactors. *Appl. Biochem. Biotechnol.* 107: 493-503. 2003.

Jouanin L. Restriction map of an agropine-type R_i plasmid and its homologies with T_i plasmid. *Plasmids*. 12: 91-102. 1984.

Kevers C, Jacques PH, Thonart PH, Gaspar TH. In vitro root culture of *Panas ginseng* and *P. quinquefolium*. *Plant Growth Regul*. 27: 173-178. 1999.

Khandual S, Reddy PM. Rapid, efficient and high performance protocol for *A. rhizogenes*-mediated hairy root transformation of the common bean *Phaseolus vulgaris*. *Adv. Biosci. Biotech*. 5: 333-339. 2014.

Kiel M, Hartle B, Guillaume S, Psiorz M. Production of amarogentin in root cultures of *Swertia chirata*. *Planta Med*. 66: 452-457. 2000.

Kim Y, Wyslouzil BE, Weathers PJ. A comparative study of mist and bubble column reactors in the in vitro production of artemisinin. *Plant Cell Rep*. 20: 451-455. 2001

Kim YH, Yoo YS. Development of a bioreactor for high density culture of hairy roots. *Biotechnol. Letts*. 7: 859-862. 1993.

Kim YJ, Weathers PJ, Wyslouzil BE. Growth of *Artemisia annua* hairy roots in liquid and gas-phase reactor. *Biotechnol. Bioeng*. 80: 454-464. 2002.

Kim YK, Kim YB, Romijuddin Md, Lee S, Kim SU, Park SU. Enhanced triterpene accumulation in Panax ginseng hairy roots overexpressing mevalonate-5-pyrophosphate decarboxylase and farnesyl pyrophosphate synthase. *ACS Synth. Biol*. 2014. doi: 10.1021/sb400194g.

Kino-Cka M, Hitaka Y, Taya M, Tone S. High density culture of red beet hairy roots by considering medium flow condition in a bioreactor. *Chem. Eng. Sci* 54: 3179-3186. 1999.

Kintzios S, Makri O, Pistola E *et al*., Seale-up production of *Pueraria phaseoloides* in air-lift bioreactor. *Biotechnol. Letts*. 26: 1057-1059. 2004.

Kintzios S, Nikolaou A, Skoula M. Somatic embryogenesis and rosmarinic acid accumulation in *S. officinalis* and *S. fruticosa* callus cultures. *Plant Cell Rep*. 18: 462-466. 1999.

Kiselev KV, Dubrovina AS, Veselova MV *et al*., The rolB gene indiced overproduction of resveratrol in *Vitis amurensis* transformed cells. *J. Botech*. 123: 681-692. 2007.

Kiyokawa S, Kikuchi Y, Kamada H *et al*., Genetic transformation of *Begonia tuberhybrida* by R_i rol gene. *Plant Cell. Rep*. 15: 606-609. 1996.

Komaraiah P, Reddy GV, Reddy PS *et al*., Enhanced production of antimicrobial sesquiterpenes and lipoxygenenase metabolites in elicitor-treated hairy root cultures of *Solanum tuberosum*. *Biotechnol. Lett*. 25: 593-597. 2003.

Kondo O, Honda H, Taya M, Kabayashi T. Comparison of growth of carrot hairy root in various bioreactors. *Appl. Microbiol. Biotechnol*. 32: 291-294. 1989.

Krolicka A, Staniszewska I, Bielawaki K, Malinski E, Szafranek J, Lojkowaska E. Establishment of hairy root cultures of Ammi majus. *Plant Sci*. 160. 259-264. 2001.

Kumar V, A Sharma A, Prasad BCN, Gururaj HB, Ravishankar GA. *A. rhizogenes* mediated genetic transformation resulting in hairy root formation in enhance by untrasonication and acetosyringone treatment. *Electron J. Biotechn.* 9: 349-357. 2006.

Kwok KH, Doran PM. Kinetic and stoichiometric analysis of hairy roots in a segmented bubble column reactor. *Biotechnol. Prog.* 11: 429-435. 1995.

Laloi C, Apel K, Danon A. Reactive oxygen signaling: the latest news. *Curr. Opin. Biol.* 7: 323-328. 2004

Lemcke K, Schmulling T. Gain of function assays identify normal genes from A. rhizogenes TL-DNA that alter plant morphogenesis or hormone sensitivity. *Plant J.* 15: 423-433. 1998.

Liu CZ, Abbasi BH, Gao B *et al.*, Caffeic acid derivatives production by hairy root cultures of *Echinacca purpurea*. *J. Agric. Food Chem.* 54: 8456-8460. 2006.

Lodhi AH, Bongaerts RJM, Verpoorte R, Coomber SA, Charlwood BV. Expression of bacterial isochorismate synthesis in transgenic root cultures of Rubia peregrine. *Plant Cell Rep.* 15: 54-57. 1996.

Makashimeda Y, Uozemi N, Koboyashi T. Production of plantlets for use as artificial seeds from horseradish hairy roots fragmented in a blender. *J. Ferm. Bioengg.* 79: 458-464. 1995.

Mano Y, Ohkawa H, Yamada Y. Production of tropane alkaloid by hairy root cultures of *Duboisia leichhardii* transformed by *A. rhizogenes*. *Plant Sci.* 59: 191-201. 1989.

Martin-Tanguy J, Sun LY. Attenuation of the phenotype caused by the root-inducing, left-hand, transferred DNA and its rolA gene. *Plant Physiol.* 111: 259-267. 1996.

Mauto ML, Trovato M, De Paolis A *et al.*, The plant oncogenic rolD stimulates flowering in transgenic tobacco plants. *Dev. Biol.* 180: 693-700. 1996.

Mayer A, Tempe J, Costantino P. Hairy roots: a molecular overview. Functional analysis of *A. rhizogenes* T-DNA genes. In: Stacey and Keen (Ed.): *Plant microbe interactions*. APS Press. St. Paul. pp. 93-139. 2000.

McKeluey SH, Gehrig JH, Holler KA, Curtis WR. Growth of plant root cultures in liquid-gas-dispersed reactor environment. *Biotechnol. Prog.* 9: 317-322. 1993.

Menzel G, Haroloff HJ, Jung C. Expresion of bacterial poly (3-hydroxybutyrate) synthesis genes in hairy roots of sugar beet (*Beta vulgaris*). *Appl. Mocrobiol. Biotechnol.* 60: 571-576. 2003.

Moghadam YA, Piri K, Bahramnejad B, Habib P. Methyl jasomonate and salicylic acid effects on the dopamine production in hairy cultures of *Portulaca oleracea* (Purslan). *Bull. Environ. Pharmacol Life Sci.* 2: 89-94. 2013.

Morgan JA, Barney CS, Penn AH, Shanks JV. Effect of buffered media upon growth and alkaloid production of *Catharanthus roseus* hairy roots. *Aool. Microbiol. Biotechnol.* 53: 262-265. 2000.

Moriuchi H, Okamoto C, Nishihama R *et al.*, Nuclear localization and interaction of rolB with plant 14-3-3 proteins correlates with induction of adventitious roots by the oncogenic rolB. *Plant J.* 38: 260-275. 2004.

Moyano E, Jouhikainen K, Tammela P *et al.*, Effect of pmt gene overproduction on tropane alkaloid production in transformed root cultures of *Datura metel* and *Hyoscyamus muticus*. *J. Expt. Bot.* 54: 203-211. 2003.

Mugnier J. Establishment of new axenic hairy root lines by inoculation with *Agrobacterium rhizogenes*. *Plant Cell Rep.* 7: 9-12. 1988.

Muranaka T, Kazuoka T, Ohkawa H, Yamada Y. Characteristics of scopolamic-releasing hairy root clones of *Duboisia leichhardtii*. *Biosci. Biotech. Bioche.* 57: 1398-1413. 1993.

Nishikawa K, Ishimuru K. Flovonoids in rot cultures of Scutellaris baicalensis. *J. Plant Physiol.* 151: 63-636. 1997.

Nuutila AM, Lindqvist AS, Kauooinen V. Growth of hairy root culture of strawberry in different types of bioreactors. *Biotechnol. Techn.* 11: 363-366. 1994.

Park SU, Facchini PJ. *Agrobacterium rhizogenes*-mediated transformation of opium poppy (*Papaver sominiferum*) and California poppy (*Eschseholzia californica*) root culture. *J. Expt. Biol.* 51: 1005-1016. 2000.

Pavlov A, Baker J, Weber J, Bley T. Hyoscyamine biosynthesis in *Datura stromonium* hairy root in vitro system with different ploidy levels. *App. Biochem. Biotech.* 157: 210-225. 2005.

Pavlov A, Georgier V, Kovatcheva P. Relationship between type and age of inoculum and betalains biosynthesis by *B. vulgaris* hairy root culture. *Biotech. Lett.* 25: 307-309. 2002a.

Pavlov A, Kovatcheve P, Georgiev V *et al.*, Biosynthesis and radical scaverging activity of betalanins during cultivation of red beet (*Beta vulgaris*) hairy root cultures. *Zeitschrift fur Naturforschung*. 57: 640-544. 2002b.

Peebles CA, Sander GW, Li M *et al.*, Five year maintenance of the inducible expression of anthranilacte synthesis in *C. roseus* hairy roots. *Biotech. Bioengg.* 102: 1521-1525. 2009.

Phunchindawan M, Hivata K, Sakai A, Miyamoto K. Cryopreservation of encapsulated shoot primodial induced in horseradish (*Armoracia resticana*) hairy root cultures. *Plant Cell Rep.* 16: 469-473. 1997.

Pistelli L, Giovannini A, Ruffoni B, Bertoli A, Pistelli L. Hairy root cultures for secondary metabolites production. In: Giardi, Rea, Berra (Ed.), Bio-farms for nattraceuticals: functional food and safety control by biosensors. *Springer Sci.* 2010. pp.167-184.

Pittaaalvarez SI, Giulietti AM. Noval biotechnological approaches to obtain asopolamine and hyoscyamine: the influence of biotic elicitors and stress agents on cultures of transformed roots of *Brugmansia candida*. *Phytother. Res.* 12: 18-20. 1998.

Preiszner J, Van-Toai TT, Huynh L, Bolla RI, Yen HH. Structure and activity of a soybean Adh promoter in transgenic hairy roots. *Plant Cell Rep.* 20: 763-769. 2001.

Qin MB, Li GZ, Yun Y, Ye HE, Li GF. Induction of hairy roots from *Artemisia annua* with *A. rhizogenes* and its culture *in vitro*. *Acta Bot. Sin*. 36: 165-170. 1994.

Rhodes MJC, Parr AJ, Giulietti A, Aird ELH. Influence of exogenous hormones on the growth and secondary metabolite formation in transformed root cultures. *Plant Cell Tiss. Org. Cult*. 38: 143-151. 1994.

Richav D, Rothe G, Fabina AK *et al.*, Over-production of tropinone reductases alter alkaloid composition of *Atropa belladonna* root culture. *J. Exptl. Bot*. 56: 645-652. 2005.

Rijhwani S, Shanks JV. Effect of elicitor dosage and exposure time on biosynthesis of indole alkaloids by *Catharanthus roseus* hairy root cultures. *Biotechnol. Prog*. 14: 442-445. 1998.

Savona M, Mascarello C, Bisio A *et al.*, *S. cinnabarina* Martens et Galeotti: optimization of the extraction of a new compound, tissue culture and hairy root transformation. *Agric. Medit*. 133: 28-35. 2003.

Schmulling T, Schell J, Spena A. A single gene from *A. rhizogenes* influence plant development. *EMBO J*. 7: 2621-2629. 1998.

Sevon N, Oksman C, Kirsi M. *Agrobacterium rhizogenes*-mediated transformation: root cultures as a source of alkaloids. *Planta Med*. 68: 859-868. 2002.

Sharp JM, Doran PM. Strategies for enhancing monoclonal antibody accumulation in plant cell and organ cultures. *Biotechnol. Prog*. 17: 979-992. 2001.

Shiao TL, Ellis MH, Dolferus R, Dennis ES, Doran PM. Overexpression of alcohol dehydrogenase or pyruvate decarboxylase improves growth of hairy roots at reduced oxygen concentrations. *Biotechnol. Bioengg*. 77: 455-461. 2003.

Shin KS, Murthy HM, Ko JY, Pack KY. Growth and betacyanin production by hairy roots of *Beta vulgaris* in airlift bioreactor. *Biotechnol. Letts*. 24: 2067-2069. 2002.

Singh G, Gavrieli J, Oakley JS, Curtis WR. Interaction of methyl jasmonate, wounding and gungal elicitation during sesquiterpene induction in *Hyoscyamus mutucus* in root cultures. *Plant Cell Rep*. 17: 391-395. 1998.

Sinkar VP, Pythoud F, White FF *et al.*, RolA locusof the R_i plasmid directs developmental abnormalities in transgenic tobacco plants. *Genet. Dev*. 2: 688-697. 1988.

Sivanesan I, Jeong BR. Induction and establishment of adventitious and hairy root cultures of *Plumbego zeylanica*. *African J. Biotech*. 27: 29-43. 2009.

Slightom JL, Durand-Tardif M, Jouanin L, *et al.*, Nucleotide sequence analysis of TL-DNA of *A. rhizogenes* agropine type plasmid. *J. Biol. Chem*. 261: 108-121. 1986.

Smith AG, John KE, Gardner N. Dwarfing ornamentally crops with the rolC gene. In: Texixeira de Silva (Ed.), *Floriculture, Ornamental and Plant Biotechnology*. 2006. pp. 54-59.

Son SH, Choi SM, Lee YH *et al.*, Large scale growth and taxane production in cell cultures of *Taxus cuspidate* using a noval bioreactor. *Plant Cell Rep*. 19: 628-633. 2000.

Son SH, Choi SM, Soo JH *et al.*, Induction and culture of mountain ginseng adventitious roots and AFLP analysis for identifying mountain ginseng. *Biotechnol. Biopros. Eng*. 4: 119-123. 1999.

Souret FF, Kim Y, Wyslouzil BE *et al.*, Scale-up of *Artemisia annua* hairy root cultures produce complex pattern of terpenoid gene expression. *Biotechnol. Bioeng*. 83: 653-667. 2003.

Spana A, Schmulling T, Konez C *et al.*, Independent and synergistic activity of rolA, B and C loci in stimulating abnormal growth in plants. *EMBO J*. 6: 3891-3899. 1987.

Spano L, Mariotti D, Cardarelli M, Branco C, Constantino P. Morphogenesis and auxin sensitivity of transgenic tobacco with different compliments of Ri T-DNA. *Plant Physiol*. 87: 479-483. 1981.

Spena A, Schmulling T, Koncz C *et al.*, Independent and synergistic activity of rolA, B and C loci in stimulating abnormal growth in plants. *EMBO J*. 6: 3891-3899. 1987.

Stachel SE, Messens E, Van-Montagu M, Zambryski P. Identification of the signal molecules producedby wonded plant cells which activate the T-DNA transfer process in *A tumefaciens*. *Nature*. 318: 624-629. 1985.

Stieger PA, Meyer Ad, Kathmann P *et al.*, The ORF13 T-DNA gene of *A. rhizogenes* confers meristematic competence to differentiated cells. *Plant Physiol*. 135: 1798-1808. 2004.

Strycharz S, Shetty K. Peroxidase activity and phenolic content in elite clonal lines of Mentha pulegium in response to polymeric dye R-478 and *A. rhizogenes*. *Process Biochem*. 37: 805-812. 2002.

Sun LY, Monneuse MO, Martin-Tanguy J *et al.*, Changes in flowering and the accumulation of polyamines and hydroxycinnamic acid-polyamine conjugate in tobacco plants transformed by the rolA locus from the R_i TL-DNA of *A. rhizogenes*. *Plant Sci*. 80: 145-156. 1991.

Sung LS, Huang SY. Lateral root bridging as a strategy to enhance L-DOPA production in *Stizolobium hassjoo* hairy root cultures by using a mesh hindcave mist tricking bioreactor. *Biotech. Bioeng*. 94: 441-447. 2006.

Tao J, Li L. Genetic transformation of *Torenia fournier* mediated by *A rhizogenes*. *South Aff. J. Bot*. 72: 211-216. 2006.

Taya M, Yoyama, Kondo O, Kobayeshi T. Growth characteristics of plant hairy roots and their culture in bioreactors. *J. Chem. Eng. Japan*. 22: 84-89. 1989.

Tepfer D. Transformation of several species of higher plants by *Agrobacterium rhizogenes*: sexual transmission of the transformed genotype and phenotype. *Cell*. 37: 959-967. 1984.

Tescine ID, Ramakrishnan D, Curtis WR. The role of liquid mixing and gas-phase dispersion in a submersed sperged root culture. *Enzyme Micro. Technol*. 20: 207-213. 1997.

Toivonen L, Laakso S, Rosenqvst H. The effect of temperature on hairy root cultures of *Catharanthus ruseus*: growth, indole alkaloid accumulation and membrane lipid composition. *Plant Cell Rep*. 11: 395-39. 1992.

Torregrosa L, Bouquet A. *Agrobacterium rhizogenes* and *A. tumefaciens* co-transformation to obtain grapevine hairy roots producing the coat protein of grapevine chrome mosaic nepovirus. *Plant Cell Tiss. Org. Cult*. 49: 53-62. 1997.

Trick HN, Finner JJ. Sonication-associated *Agrobacterium*-mediated transformation. *Transgenic Res*. 6: 329-336. 1997.

Trovato M, Maras B, Linhares F *et al*., The plant oncogenic rolD encodes a functional ornithine cyclodeaminase. *PNAS*. 698: 13449-13453. 2001.

Uozuni N. Large-scale production of hairy roots. *Adv. Biochem. Engg./Biotech*. 91: 75-103. 2004.

Uzumi N, Kohketsu K, Kobayashi T. Growth and kinetic parameters of *Aguga* hairy roots in feed-batch culture on monosccharide medium. *J. Chem. Tech. Biotech*. 57: 155-161. 1993.

Vanhale L, Eeva M, Lapinjoki S, Hiltunen R, Oksman-Caldentey KM. Effect of growth regulators on transformed root cultures of *Hyoscyamus muticus*. *J. Plant Physol*.153. 204-209. 1998

Varner JE, Lin LS. Plant cell wall architecture. *Cell*. 56: 231-239. 1989.

Wang B, Zhang G, Zhu L *et al*., Genetic transformation of *Echinacca purpurea* with *A. rhizogenes* and bioactive ingredient analysis transformed cultures. *Colloids and Surfaces B: Biointerfaces*. 53: 101-104. 2006.

Weathers TE, Bunk G, McCoy MC. 2005. The effect of phytohormones on growth and artemisinin production in *Artemisia annua* hairyroots. *In vitro Cell. Dev. Biol. Plant*. 41: 47-53.

White FF, Taylor BH, Huffmman GA *et al*., Molecular and genetic analysis of the transferred DNA regions of the root-inducing plasmid of *A. rhizogenes*. *J. Bacteriol*. 164: 33-44. 1985.

Whitney PJ. Noval bioreactor for the growth of roots transformed by *A. rhizogenes*. *Enzyme Microb. Technol*. 14: 13-17. 1992.

Williams GR, Doran PM. Hairy root culture in a liquid-dispersed bioreactor: characterization of spatial heterogeneity. *Biotech. Prog*. 16: 391-401. 2000.

Wilson PDG. The pilot-scale cultivation of transformed roots. In: Doran PM (Ed.). *Hairy roots: culture and application*. Harweod Academia, Amsterdam. pp. 179-190. 1997.

Wink M, Alfermann AW, Franke R *et al*., Sustainable bioproduction of phyto-chemicals by plant *in vitro* cultures: anticancerous agents. *Plant Genet. Resour*. 3: 90-100. 2005.

Yang YK. Exogenous auxins and phytamines enhance growth and vosmarinic acid production in hairy root cultures of *Nepeta cataria*. *Plant Omica*. 3: 190-193. 2010.

Yoshikawa M. Diverse modes of action of biotic and abiotic phytoalexin elicitors. *Nature*. 275. 546-547. 1978.

Yoshikawa T, Furaya T. Saponin production by cultures of *Panax ginseng* transformed with *A. rhizigenes*. *Plant Cell Rep*. 6: 449-453. 1987.

Yoshimatsu K, Yamaguchi H, Shimorura K. Traits of *Panex ginseng* hairy roots after cold storage and cryopreservation. *Plant Cell Rep*. 15: 555-560. 1996.

Yu KW, Gao WY, Son SH, Pack KY. Improvement of ginsenoside production by jasmonic acid and some other elicitors in hairy root culture of *Panax ginseng*. *In vitro Cell Dev. Biol. Plant*. 36: 424-428. 2000.

Yu KY, Gao W, Hahn EJ, Pack KY. Jasmonic acid improves ginsenoside accumulation in adventitious root culture of *Panax ginseng*. *Biochem. Engg. J*. 11: 211-215. 2002.

Yukimune Y, Hara Y, Yamada Y. Tropane alkaloid production in root cultures of Duboisia myoporoides obtained by repeated selection. Biosci. *Biotech. Biochem*. 58: 1443-1446. 1994.

Zhaug HC, Liu JM, Lu HY, Gao SL. Enhanced flavonoid production in hairy root cultures of *Glycyrrhiza uralensis* by combining overexpression of chalcone isomerase gene with the elicitation treatment. *Plant Cell Rep*. 28: 1205-1213. 2009.

Zhou L, Wang J and Yang C. Progress on plant hairy root culture and its chemistry. Introduction and culture of plant hairy roots. *Nat. Products Res. Dev*. 10: 87-95. 1998.

2016, Biotechnological Tools for Genetic Resources Pages 309–345
Editor: Pradip Chandra Deka
Published by: Daya Publishing House, NEW DELHI

Chapter 10

Application of High Throughput Molecular Techniques for Breeding of Farm Animals against Major Diseases

Albin M. Ahmed[1]*, Anindya Mukhopadhya[1,2] and Bojlul Bahar[1,2]

[1]School of Veterinary Medicine,
[2]School of Agriculture and Food Science,
University College Dublin, Belfield, Dublin 4, Ireland
**E-mail: albin.mostaque@gmail.com*

ABSTRACT

Farm animals play an important role in the agricultural and rural economy worldwide. Diseases affecting farm animals negatively impact animal health and productivity of the farm. Frequent uses of drugs to control diseases often lead to the development of resistant strains of the infectious agent and contamination in the food and ecosystem and hence breeding of farm animals resistant to the diseases and pets are necessary. There are convincing evidences on the existence of genetic resistance in different farm animal species which can be explored for breeding of resistant animals for a number of economically important diseases. Traditionally, identification of resistant/susceptible animal is based on conspicuous phenotypes. However, there is only limited number of robust phenotypic markers available which can be effectively explored for identification of resistant/susceptible animals against a wide range of diseases. Therefore, molecular markers are being increasingly explored for this purpose. Molecular techniques enable understanding and establishment of a biochemical basis of disease resistance/susceptibility in animals which have the potential to identify resistant/susceptible animals for complex disease traits. This review focuses on few economically important diseases of farm animals in India, where high-throughput molecular techniques can be potentially explored.

Keywords: *Farm animal, Animal breeding, Disease resistance, Molecular markers, Molecular techniques.*

Introduction

Farm animals play an important role in the rural economy of the developing countries throughout the world. They contribute through the production of meat, milk, eggs, wool and skin. The livestock industries contribute about $1.4 trillion annually to the global economy and employ about 1.3 billion people across the world (Thornton, 2010). The livestock products share 33 per cent of the total protein consumed by human and 17 per cent of the total calories consumed (Rosegrant *et al.*, 2009). The role of farm animals in many developing countries goes beyond food production as they are used for draught power, producing manure and a mean for rural transport. In developing countries including India, large ruminants generate manure that contributes about 50 per cent of the total nitrogen supply in agriculture (Smith 2012). Many of the farm animal species play an important link in nutrient recycling as they return the nutrients back to the soil in the form of manure, which is later used by the plant. They also transport nutrients in the form of food from the pasture and grasslands and release in the croplands in the form of manure.

Livestock production contributes more than one-fourth of the share of agricultural in the total gross domestic product of India and it provides employments to more than 20 million people (Singh and Meena, 2012). Compared to other agricultural products, contribution of the livestock industry in Indian economy has substantially increased over the last few years and this trend is likely to continue in the near future (Singh and Meena 2012). India has the largest combined population of farm animals in the world. The major farm animal populations in India (as in 2007) are as follows: cattle 199 million, buffalo 105 million, goat 141 million, sheep 72 million, pig 11 million and poultry 649 million (Kumar *et al.*, 2012). Among the major farm products, the total milk production in India was about 127.3 million tones in 2012 (Kumar *et al.*, 2012). Despite such a huge production, India is yet to attain self-sufficiency in milk on a per capita basis. Even with the current productivity level of milk in the country, India needs another 14-15 year to be self-sufficient in milk production (Kumar *et al.*, 2012). The animal husbandry sector in India is yet considered as a traditional, primitive and unexplored (Singh and Meena, 2012).

Breeding Farm Animals for Resistance against Diseases and Pests

The health of farm animals directly influences the productivity and the farm income (Jovanovic *et al.*, 2009). Until now, the breeding of farm animals mainly focused to improve productivity traits such as milk, meat and eggs while little or no attention was paid on identification, selection and breeding of farm animals for the environmental adaptability and resistance to pests and parasites. Highly adaptable genotypes are often associated with low productivity (Taneja 1999, Duclos and Hiemstra, 2010). Therefore, constant selection pressure for high productivity resulted in loosing of the elite resistant genotypes with greater environmental adaptability.

A common practice of managing the incidences of infection in farm animals is through applications of drugs. However, excessive use of chemicals for treating of farm animals are frequently associated with adverse side effects within the host, development of highly drug resistant disease causing organisms and the adverse impact of veterinary drug residues in human health, the environment and ecosystem (Bartley *et al.*, 2004, Gibson and Bishop 2005, Papadopoulos 2008). Vaccination protocols in domesticated animals are a highly effective strategy for animal health management however; currently there is a lack of effective vaccination for many of the viral strains affecting major farm animals. Frequent vaccination is also associated with the development of new and more virulent viral strains (Jovanovic *et al.*, 2009). Considering the facts that excessive uses of synthetic drugs have negative impact on the human health, environment and ecosystem and vaccination for a wide range of diseases affecting farm animals is lacking, there is a need of identification, selection and breeding of farm animals for resistant traits (Gibson and Bishop, 2005).

For successful breeding of farm animals for resistance to diseases and pests, accurate identification of animals with resistance/susceptible characteristics is really a challenging task. While the resistance refers to the ability of the host to resists infection with no impact in its health and productivity, the tolerance refers to a limited adverse effect in the host due to infection. About 40 major infectious diseases have been identified those are of great concern for health and productivity of farm animals worldwide (Jovanovic *et al.*, 2009). Animal's response to the infectious agents may vary at the levels of species, breed and individual (Jovanovic *et al.*, 2009). Hence, disease resistance is a relative term; some animal may be resistant to one disease while susceptible to others. It is now widely recognized that the disease incidence even varies within or between breeds of farm animals, which further necessitate proper identification and selection of resistant animals for breeding purposes. Resistant breeding program was successfully employed in farm animals in many developed nations including Australia, where breeding sheep for resistance to gastrointestinal nematode infection, a major parasite of sheep was highly successful (Karlsson and Greeff, 2006, 2012).

The mechanism underlying genetic resistance/susceptibility of farm animals against diseases and pests is poorly understood. For genetic selection of animals, a long-term goal is to identify and characterize the quantitative trait loci (QTL), single genes or closely linked loci, which controls the underlying resistance to a particular disease. The resistance/susceptibility in farm animals is a polygenic trait and a multi-factorial nature underlying resistance/susceptibility traits make it difficult to identify and select resistant animals for breeding purposes (Hiendleder *et al.*, 2005). However, with the advancement of genomic technologies, it is likely that the underlying mechanisms of resistance/susceptibility in a wide range of farm animal species will be understood and advance strategies for the identification and selection of resistant animals for breeding purposes will be developed. The genome sequence of the farm animals including cattle, buffalo, sheep, pig and chicken are being enriched and publicly available. Successful applications of genomic technologies are already reported for most of the economically important farm animals (Huang and Khatib 2010, Cox *et al.*, 2012, McCabe *et al.*, 2012, O'Loughlin *et al.*, 2012).

Molecular Techniques in Animal Breeding

Traditionally, identification and selection of farm animals are performed on the basis of various phenotypic traits. In this approach, the underlying biochemical and cellular mechanisms behind the phenotypic trait are mostly unknown. Due to the lack of large number of phenotypic markers, which can be effectively used for predicting the performance and health of animals, application of this approach for a wide range of diseases and pests is often not practical. However, with the advancement of genomic technologies, many of these interesting phenotypic traits are being dissected to the level of DNA of the individual animal and the underlying cellular and biochemical processes are being known. Classical examples are the identification of quantitative trait loci (QTL) associated with complex phenotypes such as milk yield (Mateescu and Thonney 2010) and meat quality (Gutiérrez-Gil *et al.*, 2008) in farm animals. Finding of robust genetic, biochemical and phenotypic markers to enable identification and selection of farm animals for production and adaptability traits are still remain a big challenge.

For the identification and characterization of disease resistance phenotype in farm animals, a number of genomic techniques hold great potential. These techniques can be broadly classified as a) structural genomic techniques and b) functional genomic techniques. This review mostly addresses the aspect of characterization of disease resistance phenotype in farm animals using functional genomic approach that includes analyzing the gene expression of one or few candidate genes or a global gene expression profiling.

Gene Expression Analysis of One or Few Candidate Genes

Molecular technique used for analysis of one or few genes is described in the following section.

Quantitative Real Time PCR (Polymerase Chain Reaction)

The quantitative real time PCR (qPCR) is a molecular technique generally used to amplify and quantify a target DNA molecule. This method can be used for detection of the expression level of a particular gene. The quantification may be either absolute or relative (Livak and Schmittgen 2001). The qPCR is based on the principle of conventional PCR however; the abundance of the transcript is detected during the progression of the reaction on a real time basis (Figure 10.1). Detection of the transcript abundance is done with non-specific fluorescent dye such as SYBR Green or using sequence specific DNA probes labeled with fluorescent reporter such as TaqMan. The non-specific fluorescent dye generally binds to any double stranded DNA and emits fluorescence, which is being monitored on a real time basis during progression of the PCR. An increase in the abundance of double stranded DNA due to PCR amplification results in a proportionate increase of fluorescence intensity, which is measured at the end of each PCR cycle.

In the qPCR technique based on the use of sequence specific DNA fluorescent reporter probes utilizes gene specific primers and sequence specific probe which bind to the DNA template that contains the complimentary nucleotide sequence (Heid *et al.*, 1996). As the PCR cycle progresses, the amplicon of the target DNA increases in number and greater number of reporter dyes released in free from and the fluorescent is recorded on a continuous basis. The major advantages of

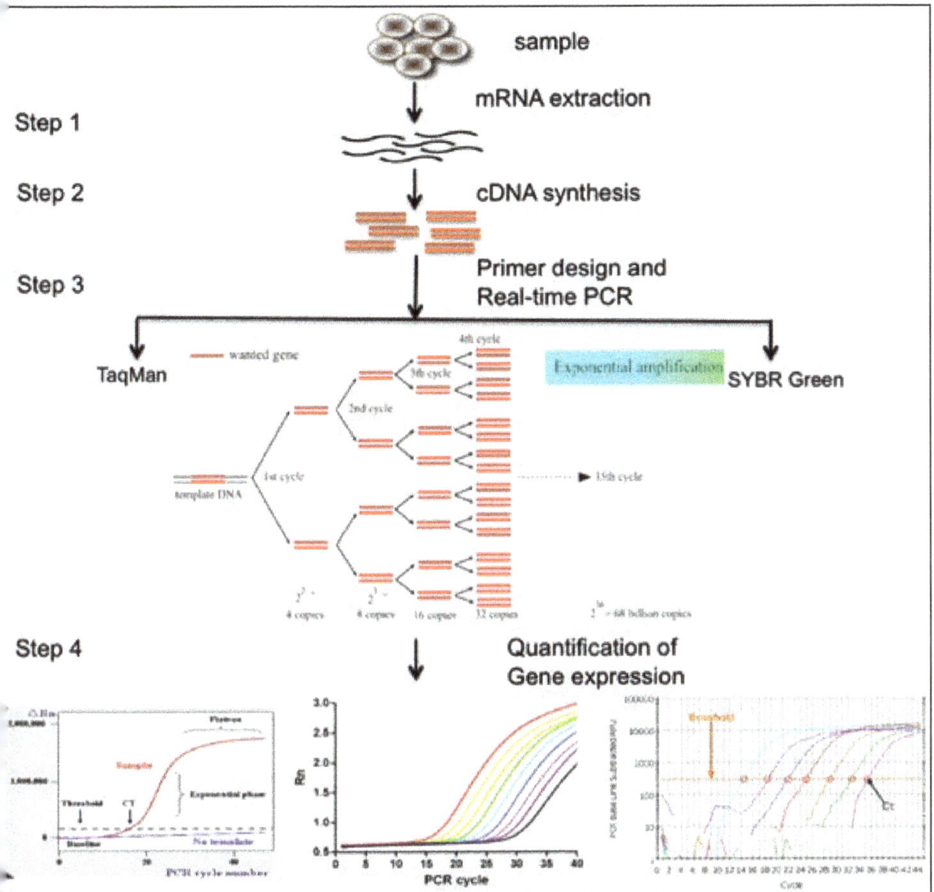

Figure 10.1: Outline of different Steps of a Quantitative Real-Time Reverse Transcriptase Polymerase Chain Reaction (qPCR) Experiment.

the qPCR technique include: i) generation of quantitative gene expression data with an accurate dynamic range of 7 to 8 log orders of magnitude (Morrison *et al.*, 1998), ii) post-amplification manipulation does not require (Wong and Medrano 2005), iii) highly sensitive and can detect up to a single transcript copy, and iv) relatively less quantity of RNA is required for the experiment. The disadvantages of qPCR technique include: i) requirement of expensive equipments and reagents, ii) relatively low throughput and iii) requirement of prior sequence data for primer design.

Gene Expression Analysis of Large Number of Genes

For large-scale analysis of gene expression, the available molecular techniques can be classified into two broad groups: a) those based on hybridization of nucleic acid and b) those based on sequencing of nucleic acid. Hybridization based techniques such as microarrays generally involve use of fluorescent labeled DNA which hybridized with the target DNA through complementary base pairing.

Hybridization based approaches are generally high throughput and relatively inexpensive, however they require prior knowledge of the genome sequence and there are greater chances of unspecific hybridization resulting in background noise (Okoniewski and Miller 2006).

Microarrays

Microarrays are based on nucleic acid hybridization principle where arrays comprised of a collection of DNA probes that are spotted on a solid support ideally in a glass or silicon platform and are used to detect the presence of gene transcripts (Gresham *et al.*, 2008). The DNA probes attached in the solid surface can be chemically synthesized or pre-made. Microarrays constitute a number of spots where each spot contains large number of specific DNA probes for hybridization with the test DNA. The probes are typically short sections of gene those can hybridize with mRNA/cDNA through complementary base pairing. Any un-hybridized gene transcripts are washed out and those successfully hybridized with the probe are detected through fluorescent color development. Various steps of a microarray experiment (Figure 10.2) involve harvesting of tissue samples, isolation of total RNA/mRNA, synthesis of single strand cDNA, tagging of cDNA with fluorescent

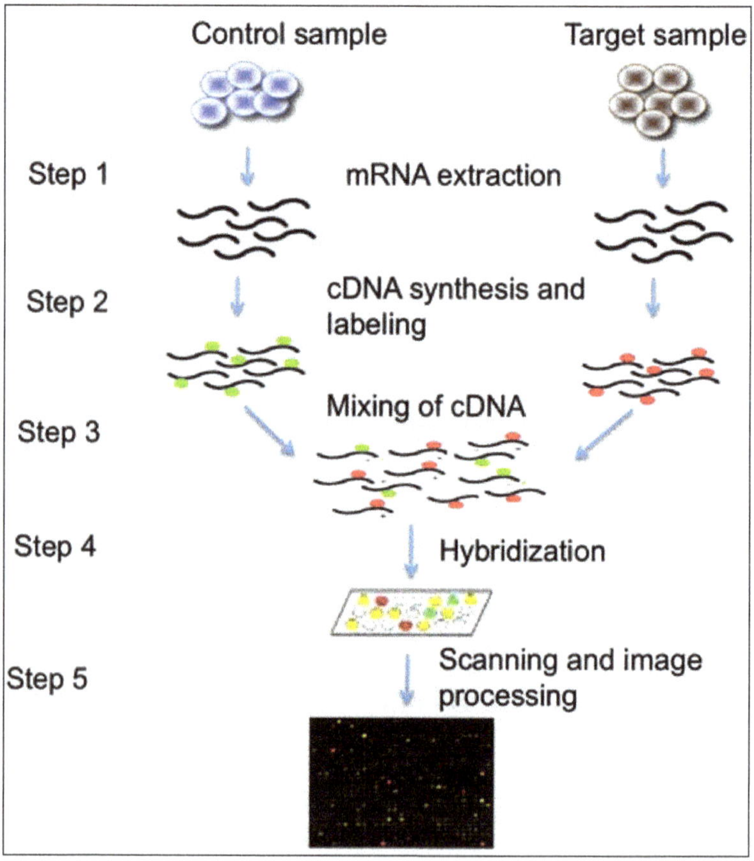

Figure 10.2: Outline of different Steps of a Microarray Experiment.

labels, hybridization, scanning and bioinformatics. Microarrays are considered as a powerful tool for gene expression analysis since about 10^5-10^6 probes may be present in a microarray making it a high-throughput gene expression analytical technique. The main advantages of microarray technology are: i) high-throughput nature enable screening of gene expression for thousands of genes in a single experiment, ii) relatively easy, fast and cost effective method, iii) availability of cross species platforms. Some of the disadvantages include: i) inherent difficulty in monitoring the probe hybridization efficiency and avoidance of cross hybridization, ii) prior sequence data is needed, iii) background noise affect the real gene expression, and the abundance of gene transcript many not always indicate the expression of protein.

Techniques based on sequencing of nucleic acid mostly rely on Sanger sequencing of cDNA or expressed sequence tags (ESTs), which are generally low throughput and are non-quantitative as summarized in Table 10.1. To overcome these disadvantages, tag based gene expression profiling methods were developed which included a) serial analysis of gene expression (SAGE), b) cap analysis of gene expression (CAGE) and c) massively parallel signature sequencing (MPSS). These tag-based sequencing approaches are high throughput and can provide precise, 'digital' gene expression levels. However, most are based on expensive Sanger sequencing technology, and a significant portion of the short tags cannot be uniquely mapped to the reference genome. Moreover, only a portion of the transcript is analysed and many transcript variants are generally indistinguishable from each other. These disadvantages limit the use of traditional sequencing technology in annotating the structure of transcriptome.

RNA Sequencing

RNA sequencing is a novel high-throughput technique based on sequencing of the nucleic acids, which enable mapping of the entire transcript profile and can quantify the abundance of different transcripts. The transcriptome, which represents the sum total of the gene transcripts present in a cell/tissue/organ, reveals the functional element of the genome of the individual. This is often highly relevant for understanding of the resistance/susceptibility mechanism underlying a particular disease. The idea behind performing transcriptomic profiling is to a) catalogue different species of the gene transcripts (mRNA, non-coding RNAs and small RNAs), b) to know the structure and composition of the gene transcripts, c) to know the post-translational modifications such as splicing pattern and d) to evaluate the changing pattern in gene expression in terms of the transcript copies and types (Wang *et al.*, 2009).

RNA sequencing (RNA-seq) enables mapping and quantitative estimation of different transcripts. It enables deep sequencing of the transcripts (Wang *et al.*, 2009). It involves the sequencing of cDNA obtained from mRNA, using any next generation sequencing (NGS) platform followed by mapping of the sequence reads to a reference genome (Nagalakshmi *et al.*, 2008). It is a powerful approach, which produces data on transcriptome sequences, enabling annotation of the genome while also providing gene expression data (Nagalakshmi *et al.*, 2010). High quality of total RNA is used for RNA-seq library preparation. Briefly, mRNA is purified from the

Table 10.1: Comparison of different Types of Advanced Molecular Techniques of Gene Expression Analysis

Characteristics	*Expression Arrays*	*Tiling Arrays*	*cDNA or EST Sequencing*	*RNA-seq*
Principle	Hybridization	Hybridization	Sanger sequencing	Next generation sequencing
Resolution	NA	Up to 100 bp	Single base	Single base
Throughput	High	High	Low	High
Reliance on genomic sequence	Yes	Yes	No	In some cases
Sensitivity (Signal: Noise)	Moderate	Low	High	High
Discovery of novel transcript	No	Yes	Yes	Yes
Dynamic range to quantify gene expression level	Up to few hundred folds	Up to few hundred folds	NA	> 8000 fold
Ability to distinguish different isoforms	Limited	Limited	Yes	Yes
Ability to distinguish SNPs, mutations, allelic expression	Limited	Limited	Yes	Yes
Quantity RNA required	High	High	High	Low
Cost for mapping transcriptomes of large genome	High	High	High	Relatively low
Downstream bioinformatic requirement	Low	High	Low	Very high
Species dependent	Yes	Yes	No	No
Ability to generate information of more than one species at a time	No	No	No	Yes

total RNA followed by fragmentation of mRNA. First and second strands of cDNA are synthesized from the fragmented mRNA using random primers followed by ligation of specific adapters in one or both ends of the double stranded cDNA. This adapter ligated cDNA is further amplified using PCR and subjected to sequencing in a high throughput manner. Different steps of RNA-seq experiment are outlined in Figure 10.3. Sequencing typically results in generation of millions of fragment reads with individual fragment length of about 30-400 bp. There are a number of high throughput sequencing technologies available which include Illumina IG, Applied Biosystems SOLiD and Roche 454 Life Science.

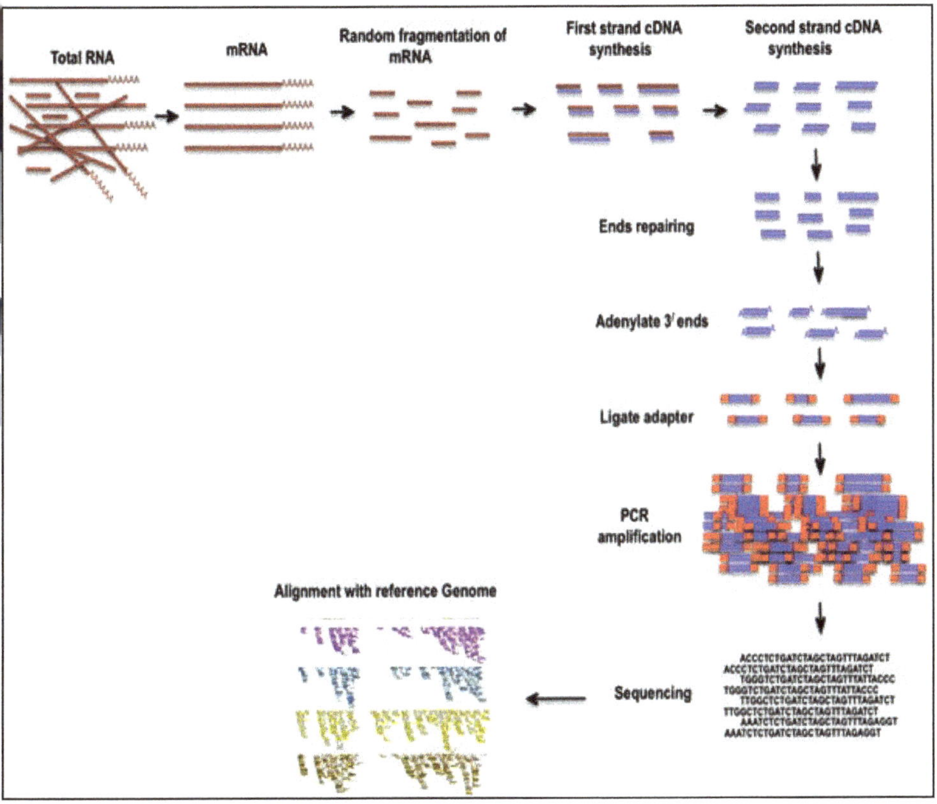

Figure 10.3: Outline of different Steps of an RNA Sequencing (RNA-seq) Experiment.

An important step of the RNA-seq methodology includes the analysis of the short length sequence read and their identification. This is often performed through alignment of the sequence read with a reference genome, which typically contains the well-annotated genome sequences. Following proper identification of the gene transcripts and quantitative evaluation of their abundance, the profile of the whole transcriptome containing the structural and functional constituent of the transcripts are obtained. This information is further analyzed to have a comprehensive understanding on the difference in the transcriptome profile of individual animals with resistance/susceptibility profile.

Application of Molecular Techniques in Breeding for Resistance in Farm Animals

Various molecular techniques used for breeding for resistance in farm animals are described in the following sections.

Cattle

Among the livestock species, cattle are economically most important farm animals worldwide as they produce major share of milk, meat, hide and manure. Cow's milk has the major contribution to the dairy industry and accounts for more than two-third of the total value of the output of livestock industry (Kumar *et al.*, 2012). In developing countries like India, cattle are also used for ploughing of farmland and transportation of goods. India has the highest number of cattle in the world (Khan and Iqubal 2010) with about 13 per cent of the global cattle population (Singh and Meena, 2012). However, compared to the developed and many other developing countries, the productivity of Indian cattle is just marginal (Birthal and Parthasarathy 2002). India produces largest quantity of milk with an annual contribution of more than Rs 2500 million (Singh and Meena, 2012), however, milk yield per animal is less than half of the world's average (Birthal and Parthasarathy 2002).

Prevalence of tropical and subtropical climates across the Indian subcontinent makes the incidences of diseases quite common in cattle. Few major diseases affecting cattle production caused by a range of infectious agents are listed in Table 10.2. *Bos taurus* and *Bos indicus* are the two main species of cattle and there are about 800 breeds of these two species recognized worldwide. Of these breeds, there are a number of cattle breeds reported to have genetic resistance to the major diseases. For instance, some breeds of *B. indicus* (Sahiwal, Brahman) and interspecies crosses between *B. indicus* and *B. taurus* cattle were more resistance to parasite infestation such as tick than breeds of *B. taurus* and the crosses within different breeds of *B. taurus*. Existence of genetic variability that imparts genetic resistance to a number of major diseases of cattle within the breeds/species is extensively reported in the literatures (Freeman *et al.*, 2005, Mulder *et al.*, 2011).

Genetic variability for disease resistance present within and between the cattle breeds can be explored for identification, selection and breeding of disease resistant animals (Bishop *et al.*, 2002, Nicholas 2005). With the availability of bovine genome sequence, a number of genomic techniques including sequencing and hybridization were applied to understand the disease resistance mechanism in cattle (Zhang *et al.*, 2012). Large scale screening of mutation in the genome through the use of SNP chips enabled identification of genetic markers for resistance/susceptibility to diseases. In last few years, numerous genome wide association studies (GWAS) were conducted to establish the association of disease phenotype with the SNP markers associated with the resistance to numerous diseases in cattle including mastitis (Sahana *et al.*, 2013), caratoconjuctivitis, a bacterial disease caused by *Moraxellabovis* (Kizilkaya *et al.*, 2013) and bovine tuberculosis (Finlay *et al.*, 2012) and paratuberculosis (Minozzi *et al.*, 2012). SNP markers hold great potential for identification and selection of cattle breed and their utilization for breeding of cattle against a variety of disease

Table 10.2: Major Diseases and Parasites of Cattle and Underlying Mechanism of Genetic Resistance

Infectious Agent	*Disease*	*Genetic Variation*	*References*
Virus	Foot-and-mouth disease	BoLA-DRB3 gene polymorphism is related to resistance and susceptibility	Lei *et al.*, 2012
	Rinderpest	*Bos indicus* (zebu) are more resistance than *Bos taurus*	Freeman *et al.*, 2005
	Bovine leukemia	BoLA-DRB3 alleles are associated with resistance and susceptibility	Miyasaka *et al.*, 2011
Bacteria	Paratuberculosis (Johnes)	PGLYRP1 polymorphism is associated with resistance to Johnes disease	Pant *et al.*, 2011
	Mastitis	Marker assisted breeding for mastitis resistance	Mulder *et al.*, 2011
	Tuberculosis	*Bos indicus* (zebu) are more resistance than *Bos taurus*	Vordermeier *et al.*, 2012b
	Brucellosis	Existence of natural resistance and susceptibility. Nramp1 gene associated with natural resistance	Paixao *et al.*, 2012
	Salmonellosis	Friesian calves are more resistant than Jersey	Wray and Sojka 1978
	Dermatophilosis	BoLA DRB3 gene is associated with resistance in Brahman Zebu cattle	Maillard *et al.*, 2006
Protozoa	Trypanosomosis	N'darma cattle are more resistant than Zebu cattle	Roberts and Gray 1973
	Theileria (*Theileria annulata*)	Sahiwals (*Bos indicus*) are more resistant than Holstein–Friesian (*Bos taurus*)	Jensen *et al.*, 2008
	Theileria (*T. sergenti*)	Japanese Black are more resistant than Holstein.	Terada *et al.*, 1997
	Babesia	*Bos indicus* are more resistant than *Bos taurus* and their cross	Bock *et al.*, 2008
Nematodes	Helminthosis	N'dama are tolerant than Boran cattle	Hanotte *et al.*, 2003
Ticks	Ticks	*Bos indicus* are resistant than the cross breed (*Bos indicus* x *Bos taurus*)	Wambura *et al.*, 1998

and pest (Jolly 2002). However, most disease resistant traits are more complex than originally thought as those are controlled by large numbers of genes and are often characterized by complex biochemical and cellular events, it is also necessary to understand the underlying molecular events of resistance/susceptibility in the host.

Among the major diseases of cattle throughout the world, mastitis of dairy cows causes an extensive economic loss. Mastitis is a chronic inflammatory condition of the mammary gland (Kaneene and Scott 1990). It causes serious losses in productivity and in extreme cases death of the animal and hence considered as a disease with major economic significance in the dairy farming. Due to the multi-factorial nature underlying the susceptibility of mastitis in dairy cows which is influenced by the type of genetic/breed, environmental and farm management practices, it still remains a major challenge to effectively control mastitis. Of the hundreds of different pathogens of broad phylogenic spectrum which can cause mastitis in dairy cows two major pathogen species are *Escherichia coli* and *Staphylococcus spp*. The clinical symptoms range from the alteration in milk composition to the presence of excessive somatic cells in the mammary gland secretion (Heringstad *et al.*, 2000). Antibiotics are frequently used to reduce the incidence of mastitis; however antibiotics are sometime less effective and their extensive use is associated with the danger of emergence of antibiotic resistant bacterial strains (Myllys *et al.*, 1998).

Genomic techniques including microarray based gene expression profiling (Table 10.3) were previously explored to understand the genes involve in the immune signaling in mastitis of resistant/susceptible breeds of dairy (Sugimoto *et al.*, 2006, Zheng *et al.*, 2006, Rinaldi *et al.*, 2010). Specific gene expression profile of somatic cells present in milk and presence of some inflammatory cytokines and acute phase proteins in the milk were reported to indicate the susceptibility of the host and hence can be explored for diagnosis of early onset of mastitis. If the disease is detected at an early stage of development, a complete cure may be possible following appropriate therapeutic and management practices. Incidences of mastitis was found to be associated with an elevated level of pro-inflammatory cytokines including interleukin (IL)-1β, IL-8, IL-12, interferon gamma (IFN)-γ and tumor necrosis factor (TNF)-α in milk. There are a number of microarray platform (Table 10.3) specifically designed to study the gene expression profile associated with mastitis in dairy cows (Rinaldi *et al.*, 2010).

Table 10.3: Bovine Microarray Platforms Specifically Designed for Screening of Gene Expression in Mastitis and Deposited in the Gene Expression Omnibus (GEO) Database

Platform	*Transcript*	*Technology*	*Description*
GPL8776	13,257	Oligo (spotted)	UIUC Bos taurus 13.2K 70-mer oligoarray
GPL2112	24,128	Oligo (in situ)	Affymetrix Bovine Genome Array
GPL3301	46,490	Oligo (in situ)	USDA Bovine 60mer 344K array
GPL6497	20,736	cDNA (spotted)	AgResearch Bos taurus clone array

Some dairy breeds such as Montbeliarde, Abondance, Simmental, Brown Swiss have lower incidence of clinical mastitis relative to other dairy breeds such as Holstein and Holstein-Friesian crosses (Rupp and Boichard 2003, Govignon-Gion *et al.*, 2012). In India, the local breeds (*Bos indicus*) exhibited very less mastitis compared to the Holstein and Jersey breeds (Joshi and Gokhale 2006). Identification of resistant animals to mastitis based on genetic marker alone is not highly effective. A number of candidate genes including diglyceride acyltransferase (*DGAT1*) (Grisart *et al.*, 2002), ATP-binding cassette sub-family G member 2 (*ABCG2*) (Cohen-Zinder *et al.*, 2005), lactoferrin (*LTF*) and lysozyme (*LYZ*) (Seyfert *et al.*, 1996) were found to have association with resistance to mastitis. There are more than 70 mastitis related quantitative trait loci (QTL) identified (Ogorevc *et al.*, 2009). Recently, transcriptome profiling using the RNA-seq technology was performed in somatic cells isolated from bovine milk at various stages of lactation and revealed differences in the global gene expression profile (Wickramasinghe *et al.*, 2012). This profiling technology holds great promise to understand the complex biochemical signaling mechanism involve in resistance/susceptibility to mastitis (Rinaldi *et al.*, 2010).

Among the various parasite infestation in cattle, ticks are a serious problem that can adversely affect the health of the animals and reduce the productivity of the herd quite substantially (Jonsson 2006). Tick infestation results in reduction in live weight gain and anemia. Globally, economic damage caused by ticks and tick-borne diseases annually is about $18 billion (De Castro, 1997). The dominant species of tick in the tropical and subtropical countries is *Rhipicephalus microplus*. Acaricides are mainly used to control tick infestation in cattle farms. The emergence of acaricide resistant tick strains and increasing cost of acaricides necessitated breeding of resistant animals. The genetic variation in tick resistance within and between breeds was previously reported (Latif 1984, Farooq *et al.*, 2010). In general, the zebu cattle (*Bos indicus; e.g.* Brahman and Nelore, Cholistani breeds) have greater resistance to ticks compared to the European cattle (*Bos taurus;* Holstein and Angus) or African cattle (*e.g.* Tuli) (Mwangi *et al.*, 1998, Wambura *et al.*, 1998, da Silva *et al.*, 2007). The heritability of host resistance to cattle tick infestation is estimated to be 39-49 per cent in British breed animals (Wharton *et al.*, 1970), while in the cross breed of Africander and Brahman was as high as 82 per cent (Seifert 1971). Application of microarray to profile the immune response of *Bos taurus* and *Bos indicus* cattle to ticks through experimental infestation with *R. microplus* was reported (Piper *et al.*, 2009). Recently, RNA-seq was applied to profile the transcriptome of leukocyte from taurine (Holstein and Jersey) and indicine (Cholistai) cattle (Huang *et al.*, 2012). Transcriptome profile of Holstein and Jersey cattle revealed only small differences while a major difference between the taurine and the indicine cattle was quite evident. Such transcriptome profile particularly those relevant to the immune pathways might be linked to a greater resistance to diseases including tick in Cholistani cattle. These breed specific transcriptome profile might be useful in identification and further characterization of resistance/susceptibility of different breeds to infestation by *R. microplus*.

Buffalo

The domestic water buffalo (*Bubalus bubalis*) is a large bovine species contributing significantly to the agricultural output in India and Southeast Asia (Vijh *et al.*, 2008). Based on morphological, behavioral, geographical criteria and number of chromosomes, water buffaloes are categorized into two groups: river buffalo and swamp buffalo (Sangwan 2012). River buffaloes are large in size and prefer to stay in clear water while the swamp buffaloes are stocky animals (Vignesh *et al.*, 2012). The global buffalo population is estimated to be about 180 million of which approx. 97 per cent belongs to Asia and about 56 per cent to India alone (Sangwan 2012).

Buffalo contributes about 5 per cent of the total milk production of the world. In India, buffalo contributes about 60 per cent of the total milk production, even though the buffalo population is only one-third of total cattle population (www.ikisan.com). Buffalo contributes substantially to Indian economy by producing 60.9 million metric tons of milk, over 1.6 million tons of meat and using approximately 8 million buffalos as draught power (Sangwan 2012). The buffalo milk is preferred over cow because of higher protein and fat percentage and high profitability due to low cost of production relative to dairy (Vijh *et al.*, 2008). Compared to cattle, water buffaloes are more resistant to diseases and parasites, and have higher adaptability to extreme environments, that make them suitable for tropical region. Because of its body structure and resilience, the water buffalo is often considered as better work animal than cattle.

More than a dozen buffalo breeds have been characterized worldwide. In India, the important buffalo breeds include: Murrah, Nili-Ravi, Surti, Jaffarabadi, Bhadawari, Mehsana, Nagpuri Toda, Pandharpuri and Godavari (Sangwan 2012). These breeds differ in resistance and susceptibility to various diseases (Mingala *et al.*, 2009, Vignesh *et al.*, 2012). Few potential genetic mechanisms underlying the resistance/susceptibility of buffalo to various diseases are highlighted in Table 10.4. In general, the African buffaloes (*Syncerus caffer*) are highly tolerant to many infectious diseases than Asian buffaloes.

Table 10.4: Major Diseases and Parasites of Buffalo with Underlying Mechanism of Genetic Resistance

Infectious Agent	*Disease*	*Genetic Variation*	*References*
Bacteria	Brucella abortus	Nramp1 are associated with resistance	Capparelli *et al.*, 2007, Borriello *et al.*, 2006
	Mastitis	Polymorphism in *TLR4* is associated with resistance	Gulhane and Sangwan 2012
	Anaplasma	Toda breed is more resistant than Murrah	Vignesh *et al.*, 2012
Protozoa	Theileria	Toda breed is more resistant than Murrah	Vignesh *et al.*, 2012
Nematodes	Helminthosis	African buffalo (*Syncerus caffer*) varies in resistance character	Ezenwa *et al.*, 2010
Ticks	Ticks	Swamp buffalo are more resistant	Mingala *et al.*, 2009

Although in many aspects buffaloes are more advantageous than the cattle, relatively less scientific investigation is reported on this species. Substantial progress has been made towards the whole genome sequencing of buffalo, however a well annotated buffalo genome is yet to be publicly available. An annotated genome sequence will facilitate application of high throughput molecular methods for better understanding of the disease resistance. Recent studies have highlighted the potential of high-throughput method for identification of transcripts and SNPs in buffaloes (Jakhesara *et al.*, 2012, Rajput *et al.*, 2012). However, these technologies are yet to be explored for identification of disease resistance in buffalo. The management of health and infectious diseases of buffaloes and cattle are different, although buffaloes are currently being managed only like those of cattle. For a successful adaptation of a cattle-based strategy for the health management of buffaloes, it is necessary to comprehend their immune system and clearly understand the various facets involved in disease resistance/susceptibility. The studies identifying the physiological processes involved in health and disease of buffaloes will not only contribute to the improvement in the management of buffalo herds, but will also provide an insight into the underlying mechanisms resulting in the differences in disease resistance (Thanislass *et al.*, 2009).

Among the major disease of buffaloes, brucellosis is caused by a facultative intracellular pathogen *Brucella abortus*. Brucellosis causes serious economic losses and the eradication process is limited due to latent infection, prolonged incubation of the pathogen, incomplete protection provided by vaccines and difficulties in distinguishing serologically between vaccinated and naturally infected animals (Borriello *et al.*, 2006). To overcome brucellosis infection in water buffalo, a genetic selection approach has been identified through selection of the disease-resistant genotypes for breeding. The *Nramp1* gene, a member of a large family of genes coding for metal ion-transporting proteins, has been identified as a candidate for selective breeding program to tackle brucellosis infection (Capparelli *et al.*, 2007).

Similar to cattle, mastitis is also an important and persistent problem in buffalo population causing economic losses due to drop in milk production and cost of treatment and culling processes (Dhakal and Thapa, 2002). Buffaloes are relatively less susceptible to mastitis when compared with cow and somatic cell counts were much lower in the milk of mastitis infested buffaloes (Moroni *et al.*, 2006, Kavitha *et al.*, 2009). While the genetic polymorphism in *TLR4* was reported to be associated with mastitis in buffalo (Gulhane and Sangwan 2012), a number of studies have also reported potential candidate genes including MHCII-DRB3, β-defensin, lectoferrin, neutrophilschemokine receptors, interleukins, TLR to effect the genetic resistance/susceptibility to mastitis in buffaloes (Petrovski *et al.*, 2006, Kumar *et al.*, 2011). To our knowledge, no study was performed yet to characterize the disease resistance/susceptibility in buffaloes utilizing high throughput molecular techniques, although there is a recent report of high throughput sequencing technology for identification of SNPs in African buffaloes (Le Roex *et al.*, 2012).

Sheep and Goat

Farming of small ruminants such as sheep and goats are mostly distributed across the tropical, subtropical, temperate and arid and semi arid regions of the world. High prolificacy, adaptability and versatile nature of sheep and goats make them critically important resource for societies of various geographical regions. Sheep farming is quite wide spread in most developed countries within the EU,

America, Canada, Australia and New Zealand, while goat farming is more common in the developing nations including India (Glimp, 1995). Since the domestication of sheep about 8000-11000 years ago (Tapio *et al.*, 2006), different breeds were selected based on environmental adaptability, productivity (wool, meat and milk) and to a lesser extent the resistance to various infectious diseases (Meadows *et al.*, 2005). Presently, there are about 1400 breeds of sheep and about 500 breeds of goat available worldwide (Mirkena 2010). Sheep and goats are both members of *Caprinae* subfamily of *Bovidae*.

Sheep and goats are infected by a number of infectious agents (Table 10.5) which causes a substantial economic damage to the farmers. Major diseases of sheep include scrapie, footrot, mastitis and gastrointestinal nematode infections. Many of these diseases result in lamb loss, reduction in weight gain, lameness, reduction in wool production and additional cost on medicines for disease management. Goats are relatively more resistant diseases such as footrot (Hunt *et al.*, 2008). Relatively greater number of scientific literature is available describing the diseases of sheep compared to goats (Bishop and Morris, 2007).

Table 10.5: Major Diseases of Sheep and Goat and Existence of Genetic Resistance

Ilnfectious Agent	*Disease*	*Existence of Genetic Resistance*	*References*
Bacteria	Footrot	Goats are more resistant than sheep. Romney sheep breed are more resistant than Merino breed	Emery *et al.*, 2008
	Mastitis	Somatic cell counts in milk can be used for selection of resistant animals	Bishop and Morris 2007
	Paratuberculosis	Rajasthani crossbreed goats are more resistant than Barbari and Jamunapari breed. Nramp and MHC alleles are associated with resistance	Reddacliff *et al.*, 2008, Singh *et al.*, 2009
	Dermatophilosis	Selection of resistant sheep within Merino breeds.	Raadsma *et al.*, 1994
	Cowdriosis) (heart water	Creole goat breed are resistant	Matheron *et al.*, 1987
Nematodes	Helminthosis	Texel, Red Masai, Barbados Blackbelly, Santa Ines, Garole sheep are more resistant.	Nimbkar *et al.*, 2003, Sayers *et al.*, 2008
Plathyhelminth	Liver fluke	Indonesian Thin Tail sheep breed are more resistant	Roberts *et al.*, 1997

Footrot is a chronic, necrotic disease that causes lameness, sensitivity with hoof trimming, bleeding and pungent odor in sheep and goat. It causes a poor weight gain and reduction in the productivity. Footrot causes significant economic losses worldwide in both sheep and goat production (Nieuwhof and Bishop 2005). It is caused by two bacterial species; *Dichelobacter nodosus* and *Fusobacteri anecrophorum* (Bennett and Hickford 2011). Presence of highly humid environment, wet weather and moist soil conditions favor spread of the disease. Existences of heritable genetic variation against footrot in different breeds of sheep were previously reported

Nieuwhof *et al.*, 2008). In a previous report Merino breed of sheep was highly susceptible while Romney was somewhat tolerant to footrot (Emery *et al.*, 2008). Variation in the MHC class II genes were reported to influence the resistance/susceptibility of sheep to footrot (Bishop and Morris, 2007). To our knowledge, there are no reports on application of high throughput molecular technique for investigation of the mechanism of footrot tolerance in sheep.

Gastrointestinal nematode (GIN) infection in sheep is a considerable health and economic concern worldwide. GIN infection causes inefficient feed utilization of the host, which subsequently leads to protein deficiency, anemia, reduced appetite, poor weight gain, diarrhea and mortality (Sargison, 2012). The treatment of gastrointestinal nematode infection in ruminants with anthelmintics alone costs more than $3 billion per year globally (Jackson *et al.*, 2009). In temperate climates the species accounting for the majority of GIN infections in sheep belong to the genus *Teladorsagia (or Ostertagia), Trichostrongylus, Nematodirus* and *Haemonchus* (Sargison 2012). Two dominant abomasal nematode species; *Teladorsagia circumcincta* and *Haemonchus contortus* impact most negatively on sheep production (Good *et al.*, 2006, Patten *et al.*, 2011).

Treatment with anthelmintics is the conventional method of controlling GIN infection in sheep (Cooper *et al.*, 2012). However, this approach is facing uncertainty due to emergence of anthelmintic resistant nematode species (Papadopoulos *et al.*, 2012) and consumers concern for chemical residue free animals product. Alternative methods of minimizing GIN infections include: grazing management, nutritional boost through protein supplementation, use of parasitic microfungi against the nematode, vaccines and selection of resistant animals (Sayers and Sweeney 2005). Selection of resistant animals is thought to be a potential alternative for reducing GIN infection (Eady *et al.*, 2003). Existence of breeds with superior resistance to GIN infection (Table 10.6) holds great potential for genetic selection and breeding for animals, which are both optimal for resistance and production/quality traits.

In India, the Garole sheep breed was reported to be more resistant to GIN infection compared to other breeds (Nimbkar *et al.*, 2003). The genetic variation for resistance to GIN infection among goat breeds is limited and usually the indigenous breeds are more resistant compared to the imported breeds. In Australia, establishment of relatively more resistant Marino sheep flock to GIN infection by Rylington Merinos resistant breeding programme showed success in selective breeding (Karlsson and Greeff 2006, 2012). Similar approach was adopted in New Zealand for establishing resistant and resilient Romney sheep flocks (Bisset *et al.*, 2001, Morris 2009). The physiological markers such as fecal egg counts, worm burden, nematode specific antigens IgA, IgE and molecular markers for genes encoding interferon gamma gene (*IFNG*) and the MHC DR β-chain gene (*MHCII-DRB1*) are proposed for the identification of resistant animals. As disease resistance is a complex trait, it is necessary to identify and characterize other relevant genetic markers involved in resistance/susceptibility to GIN infection.

The application of high-throughput molecular techniques in sheep is limited. A recent study adopted tag based approach to characterize the transcriptome of resistant and susceptible sheep from Scottish Blackface breed in response to

Table 10.6: Sheep/Goat Breeds that Exhibited Resistance to Nematode Infections

Sheep/Goat Breed	*Region*	*Comparison Breed*	*Nematode Species*	*References*
Texel	Western Europe	Suffolk	*T. circumcincta*	Sayers *et al.*, 2008, Good *et al.*, 2006
Florida Native	USA	Suffolk or Rambouillet	*H. contortus*	Bradley *et al.*, 1973
Red Maasai	Africa	Romney Marsh, Dooper, Blackheaded Somali	*H. contortus* and *mixed*	Mugambi *et al.*, 1997
Red Maasai	South Africa	Sabi	*H. contortus*	Matika *et al.*, 2003
Gulf Coast Native sheep	USA	Other breeds of USA	*H. contortus*	Amarante *et al.*, 1999
Dorper	USA	Katahdin and Suffolk	Mixed	Burke and Miller 2004
Black Belly	France	INRA 401	*H. contortus* and *T. colubriformis*	Gruner *et al.*, 2003
Jamunapari	India	Barbari	Mixed	Chauhan *et al.*, 2003
Santa Ines	Brazil	Suffolk and Ile de France	*H. contortus*	Amarante *et al.*, 2005
Garole	India	Deccani and Bannur	Mixed gastrointestinal nematodes, *H. contortus*	Nimbkar *et al.*, 2003

experimental infection with *T. circumcincta* (Pemberton *et al.*, 2011). This study identified a large number of differentially expressed genes associated with inflammation and cell activation in the susceptible animals when compared with the resistant animals. This study further concluded that the susceptibilty of the animals are associated with dysfuction of T cell differentiation and regulations.Other studies attempted profiling of the whole transcriptome of resistant and susceptible animals to GIN infection for identification of differentially expressed genes (Diez-Tascon *et al.*, 2005, Keane *et al.*, 2007).

Pig

Pig is an economically important farm animal which is also used as an important model for biomedical research for certain human diseases due to their genetic and physiological similarity to humans (Prather 2013). Infectious diseases in pig are mainly caused by bacteria and viruses (Table 10.7) which can negatively impact in the pig production worldwide. Gram-negative bacteria such as *Escherichia coli, Salmonella* causing diarrhoea and pneumonia are very common in pig. These infections often result in decreased weight gain and occasional death of the animal (Fairbrother *et al.*, 2005). Among the viruses, African swine fever virus and foot-and mouth disease virus can adversely affect pig production. Medication and vaccination are although practiced to control bacterial and viral infection, emergence of resistant bacterial/ viral strains are common in pig farms. Presence of genetic component responsible for resistance/susceptibility in pig was previously reported (Table 10.7). However, genetic selection of disease resistance animals has not been widely practiced in pig farms due to various reasons: Firstly, selection of animals was biased towards production traits such as meat production, while the disease traits were almost ignored. Secondly, selection of resistant animal is hardly effective since disease resistance is a polygenic trait. Thirdly, due to lack of well-characterized genetic markers and underlying mechanism of disease resistance is mostly unknown.

Table 10.7: Major Diseases of Pig and Existence of Genetic Resistance

IInfectious Agent	*Disease*	*Existence of Genetic Resistance*	*References*
Virus	African swine fever	Individual animals varies on their survival	Jovanovic *et al.*, 2009
	Porcine reproductive and respiratory syndrome	Chinese Dapulian breed are more resistant than Duroc X Landrace X Yorkshire crossbreed	Jiang *et al.*, 2013
	Atrophic rhinitis	Genetic variation in resistance and susceptibility	Reiner *et al.*, 2002
Bacteria	Diarrhoea	A number of genes differentially expressed between resistant and susceptible animals	Bao *et al.*, 2012
	Post-weaning diarrhoea	Polymorphisms in *FUT1* gene is associated with resistance	Luo *et al.*, 2010

Availability of porcine genome sequence will provide great opportunities to identify and characterize the genes associated with resistance to major diseases in pig as well as identification of novel marker of resistance/susceptibility which can be effectively used in breeding programs. A number of studies have suggested that resistance to infection by certain pathogen is heritable in pig (Lundeheim 1979, Henryon *et al.,* 2001). Moreover, occurrence of enteric, respiratory and chronic pleuritis diseases significantly varies among different pig breeds including Landrace, Yorkshire, Hamshire and Duroc (Lundeheim 1988). This finding suggested that selection of resistant pigs could be effective in controlling various diseases. However, the observed variation in disease resistance may be influenced by some other factors such as genetic background, environmental factors etc. Therefore, understanding of the genetic basis of resistance to infectious diseases and identification of genetic markers that can be used for breeding purpose are important. There are many ways to identify the molecular markers of disease resistance, but integration of sequencing, association of whole genome, functional genomics and immunology is necessary to understand the molecular mechanism of disease resistance.

Pig has been extensively used as a medical model for studies relating to renal transplantation (Giraud *et al.,* 2011), cardiovascular-related diseases (Zaragoza *et al.,* 2011), atherosclerosis and Cystic Fibrosis (Stoltz *et al.,* 2013). The porcine model has also been helpful in exploring the advances in induced pluripotent stem cell (iPSCs) technologies and therefore the pig is considered as an attractive model for the research on regenerative medicine and stem cell research (Ezashi *et al.,* 2012). Due to the close resemblance of the internal anatomy and physiology of pigs with humans, the porcine model has been used for evaluation of food bioactives and their effect on the digestive system as well as systemic effects (Meurens *et al.,* 2012). A number of well-characterized mucosal inflammatory diseases of humans such as inflammatory bowel disease (IBD), celiac disease and food allergy share a similar etiology to weaning piglets, since in both organisms, there is a loss of tolerance to commensal bacteria and antigens (Bailey *et al.,* 2006). The weaning period in pigs is characterised by undesirable morphological, physiological, microbiological and immunological changes in the gastrointestinal environment, which increase the susceptibility to intestinal dysfunction and enteric infections resulting in poor growth performance (Pluske *et al.,* 1997, Kim *et al.,* 2012). The post-weaning period is also associated with an increase in proliferation of strains of enterotoxigenic *E. coli* (*ETEC*) and decrease in proliferation of *Lactobacilli* numbers in ileum and colon in weaned piglets, evaluated by a non-culture based 16s rRNA qPCR technology (Heo *et al.,* 2013). Interestingly, recent studies have identified the above-mentioned disruption associated with humans suffering from mucosal inflammatory diseases of gut.

There are growing evidences to suggest that early nutrition and environmental stress has a long term effect on the architecture and functionality of the gastro-intestinal tract (Lalles 2012). Studies based on nutrition and epigenetics have suggested a link between early nutrition and later chronic diseases, particularly metabolic syndromes like insulin resistance, type-2 diabetes, obesity, hypertension and cardiovascular disease (Canani *et al.,* 2011). There are enough evidences present now to demonstrate that maternal and early postnatal nutritional deficiencies or excesses do have a permanent effect on genes implicated in energy homeostasis and epigenetic modifications that involve modulation of gene expression and finally affect offspring phenotype. Additionally, the influence of stress early in life is another important factor to be considered as it is now well established that it leads to long lasting alterations in both intestinal and colonic mucosal functions (Lalles 2012).

Candidate gene approach identifies the major genes that play roles in disease resistance and focused on SNPs of those genes in resistant and susceptible animals. But the disease traits being polygenic it is likely that many genes are actively involved in the disease resistance process. Hence, it is necessary to apply high throughput methods to identify the whole set of genes that contributes to disease resistance. The completion of swine genome sequencing and development of high throughput methods such as microarray, RNA-seq, ChIP-seq, SNP chip facilitates identification of key genes and SNPs associated with disease resistance. Microarray and RNA-seq data can be used to map expressed quantitative trait loci (eQTL) associated with disease resistance.

In pig, the susceptibility against the bacteria *Escherichia coli* is a good example of disease resistance. Pathogenic *E. coli* strain can cause diarrhoea in young piglets, which can cause high morbidity and mortality up to 50 per cent. Although vaccination of sows against *E. coli* infection is possible it may not be a cost effective way of control. Moreover, rapid use of drugs in food-producing animals is also a matter of public concern. This necessitated demand for alternative control strategies such as breeding of resistant pigs. Evidence of genetic control factor for resistance to *E. coli* infection in pig has been reported earlier (Gibbons *et al.*, 1977). A single allele responsible for adhesion factor receptors determines the binding of various *E. coli* strains (Gibbons *et al.*, 1977). Pigs lacking these receptors have been reported to be resistant (Gibbons *et al.*, 1977). Further characterization of resistance to *E. coli* infection in pig using high-throughput molecular method will help in more accurate identification of resistant animals for breeding.

Another economically important disease in pig is porcine reproductive and respiratory syndrome (PRRS). PRRS in pig is caused due to PRRS viral infection and probably the most costly disease in pig industries of Europe and North America. Piglets infected with PRRS virus, develop diarrhea and become highly susceptible to respiratory infections. Breed differences have been reported to PRRS infection in pig (Vincent *et al.*, 2006, 2005, Ait-Ali *et al.*, 2007, Petry *et al.*, 2007), which may be used for selection of resistant animals/breeds for breeding purpose. Applications of high-throughput molecular methods are suggested for functional characterization of PRRS disease in pig. Another important disease in pigs in the classical swine fever (CSF), caused by classical swine fever virus (CSFV), and the symptoms include pyrexia, respiratory and gastrointestinal inflammation, haemorrhages and ataxia with moderate to high mortality depending on the strain and age of pigs (Depner *et al.*, 2006). Thus, the full-genome sequencing has the potential to facilitate the research into virulence markers and genetic modification of CSFV for DIVA (Differentiating Infected from Vaccinated Animals) vaccine development as well as provide measures to control future CSF outbreaks (Leifer *et al.*, 2010).

The rapid evolution of the genomic technologies provides a tremendous opportunity for quantitative trait loci and expression quantitative trait loci (eQTL) discovery and development of applications beneficial for the pig industry (Fan *et al.*, 2011). While accessibility to the molecular data for applying genomics to pig breeding is no longer unachievable, the major hurdle is to overcome the development of analysis methods and tools for translating these methods into practical applications for genetic improvements. Another limiting factor is the cost of implementing these technologies within the pig breeding industry, which is still not well estimated. Although technological innovations are being implemented by breeding companies, other approaches will be needed to make these advances available in an economically feasible way. The discovery of causative variants through eQTL analysis is also considered to be a great boon to the pig industry (Cleveland *et al.*, 2012). Inclusion of causative variants into analyses provides the advantage of increasing selection accuracy and these studies are expected to reveal genomic markers controlling genetic variation in economically important pig phenotypes by enhancing our knowledge of the underlying trait (Ernst *et al.*, 2013).

Poultry

Production of domestic birds such as chicken, ducks, turkeys and geese for meat and/or eggs are included in poultry farming. Poultry is one of the most important and fastest growing components of global meat production and egg production. Globally, >50 billion chickens are reared annually as a source of meat and egg. In India, about 70 per cent of the poultry products are produced by organized poultry farming sector. In the last decade, consumers demand for broiler in India has risen steadily to 2.65 million metric tons in 2010 from 1.25 million metric tons in 2001. Similarly, the total egg production was increased to 61.5 billions in 2010-2011 from 36.6 billion in 2000-2001 (www.worldpoultry.net).

There are about 150 different diseases and pests of poultry are reported in the database (www.thepoultrysite.com) of which few major groups of diseases and pests of chicken, the major poultry species are presented in Table 10.8. In chickens, Newcastle disease also known and Ranikhet disease in India is one of the major poultry disease which causes substantial economic loss. Newcastle disease is caused by avian paramyxovirus also known as Newcastle disease virus (NDV) which was first reported in 1926 in poultry from Java, Indonesia and Newcastle-upon-Tyne. The NDV is made up of single stranded RNA genome of approximately 15 kb that encodes six genes (Chambers *et al.*, 1986). The NDV can affect a number of bird species including chicken and ducks and causes large-scale mortality due to fatal failure of the respiratory and neuronal systems. The NDV is highly contagious and infection spreads through inhalation in the air or ingestion with the food (Seal *et al.*, 2000).

Presence of genetic variation which imparts tolerance/resistance to NDV in different breeds of chicken was reported in the literature (Cole and Hutt 1961, Hassan *et al.*, 2004). An Iranian study with experimental infection of different breeds of chickens with virulent strain of NDV demonstrated that one breed (Mandarah) had higher resistance with just 20 per cent mortality while other breeds; Sina (85 per cent), Dandrawi (100 per cent) and Gimmizah (100 per cent) had high degree of susceptibility to Newcastle disease (Hassan *et al.*, 2004). In order to understand the role of NDV infection on transcriptional processes within cells, avian cells were subjected to experimental infection with NDV and the gene transcripts were analyzed using a cDNA microarray (Munir *et al.*, 2005). This study revealed that transcriptional silencing of a number of cytoskeletal proteins and genes involve in the cellular apoptotic process might contribute to the susceptibility of the host to NDV infection (Munir *et al.*, 2005). The host responses to experimental infection of the chickens were also analyzed by using transcriptional profiling using microarray technique (Rue *et al.*, 2011). In the spleens, an early response of the NDV infection was evident with an increase in the transcriptional activation of genes involved in the innate antiviral and pro-inflammatory pathways. These included numerous genes of type 1 and type II interferons, cytokines (IL1B and IL6) and chemokines and inducible nitric oxide synthase (Rue *et al.*, 2011).

Table 10.8: Major Diseases of Poultry and Existence of Genetic Resistance

Infectious Agent	*Disease*	*Existence of Genetic Resistance*	*References*
Virus	Newcastle disease	Breed differences in resistance	Hassan *et al.*, 2004
	Marek's disease	An allele of MHC locus is used for selection of resistant birds	Briles *et al.*, 1977, Longenecker *et al.*, 1977
	Avian leukosis	B alleles of MHC locus plays a major role to resistance	Bacon 1987
	Infectious brusal disease	Breed differences in resistance	Hassan *et al.*, 2004
	Rous sarcoma	Selection of resistant bird is possible	Gyles and Brown 1971
Bacteria	Compylobac-teriosis	Differences in resistance in four inbred lines	Boyd *et al.*, 2005
	Salmonellosis	Genetic variation in resistance	Barrow *et al.*, 2004, Bumstead and Millard 1992
Protozoa	Coccidiosis	Genetic variation in resistance	Pinard-Van Der Laan *et al.*, 1998
Nematodes	Ascaridia galli	Breed differences in resistance	Schou *et al.*, 2003

Another important disease of poultry with major economic significance is the Marek's disease (MD) is caused by Marek's disease virus in chicken and turkey. MD is characterised by immuno-suppression and development of tumors in a range of organs of the infected birds. The mortality within the infected flock can be 100 per cent, which can result in serious economic damage to the poultry industry (Davies *et al.*, 2009). Currently, there is no treatment available for prevention or complete cure of MD. Vaccinations at early stage (about 1-day old chicks) are recommended. However, due to a rapid emergence of virulent strains of the virus, the vaccination often remains ineffective and hence alternative control strategies are sought. Presence of genetic variants to impart tolerance to MD in chicken was reported (Cole 1968). It have been reported that chickens heterozygous or homozygous for the B21 allele of MHC locus are somewhat tolerant to MD (Briles *et al.*, 1977, Longenecker *et al.*, 1977). However, the genetic potential of MD resistance in poultry is yet to be explored completely.

Coccidiosis in chickens caused by protozoan infection is another economically important disease in poultry farming. The economic loss for coccidiosis is due to negative effects on weight gain and feed conversion efficiency of the birds. Usually coccidiosis is controlled by in-feed medication, however due to restriction in the use of anti-coccidial drugs and occurrences of drug resistance, alternative strategies are needed. There are about seven species of protozoan parasites *Eimeria* can infect chickens and coccidiosis. In out bred chicken populations, genetic variation for tolerance to *Eimeria* infection was reported (Pinard-Van Der Laan *et al.*, 1998, however, in inbred lines also the existence of genetic variation against different coccidiosis causing virulent strains of protozoa were also reported (Bumstead and Millard 1992). To our knowledge, only very limited number of high-throughput molecular techniques were applied to understand the genomic mechanism of resistance/susceptibility of coccidiosis in different breeds of chickens which can help identification, selection and breeding of resistant chickens.

Conclusion

Genetic variability present in the different species and breeds of farm animals can be explored for breeding of resistant animals for a number of economically important diseases. Studies have demonstrated that breeding of resistant/tolerant farm animals can provide a cost effective and environment friendly solution of controlling the diseases. However, identification of genetically resistant animal is challenging due to lack of robust markers. Identification of novel molecular markers associated with disease resistance has potential to aid resistant breeding in farm animals. However, the resistance/susceptibility to infectious agents is a complex phenotype controlled by a large number of genes with small individual affect highly influenced by environment. Hence, identification of whole set of genes and SNPs, biochemical signaling pathways associated with disease resistance are necessary. High throughput molecular techniques are being increasingly applied to dissect the underlying molecular mechanisms of resistance/susceptibility to various diseases in major farm animal species. In the near future, extensive application of these technologies particularly those enable profiling of whole transcripts and proteins and metabolites will help in pinpoint the exact mechanism of disease resistance, which will tremendously help in identification, selection and breeding of farm animals for numerous infectious agents.

References

Ait-Ali T, Wilson AD, Westcott DG, Clapperton M *et al.*, Innate immune responses to replication of porcine reproductive and respiratory syndrome virus in isolated Swine alveolar macrophages. *Viral Immunol.* 20: 105-118. 2007.

Amarante A, Bricarello P, Huntley J, Mazzolin L, Gomes J. Relationship of abomasal histology and parasite-specific immunoglobulin A with the resistance to *Haemonchus contortus* infection in three breeds of sheep. *Vety. Parasitol.* 128: 99-107. 2005.

Amarante A, Craig T, Ramsey W, El-Sayed N *et al.*, Comparison of naturally acquired parasite burdens among Florida Native, Rambouillet and crossbreed ewes. *Vety. Parasitol.* 85: 61-69. 2009.

Bacon LD. Influence of the major histocompatability complex on disease resistance and productivity. *Poultry Sci.* 66: 802-811. 1987.

Bailey M, Haverson K. The postnatal development of the mucosal immune system and mucosal tolerance in domestic animals. *Vety. Res.* 37: 443-453. 2006.

Bao W, Ye L, Pan Z, Zhu J *et al.*, Microarray analysis of differential gene expression in sensitive and resistant pig to Escherichia coli F18. *Animl. Genet.* 43: 525-534. 2012.

Barrow P, Bumstead N, Marston K, Lovell M, Wigley P. Faecal shedding and intestinal colonization of Salmonella enterica in in-bred chickens: the effect of host-genetic background. *Epidemiol. Infec.* 132: 117-126. 2004.

Bartley D, Jackson F, Jackson E, Sargison N. Characterisation of two triple resistant field isolates of Teladorsagia from Scottish lowland sheep farms. *Vety. Parasitol.* 123: 189-199. 2004.

Bennett GN, Hickford JG. Ovine footrot: new approaches to an old disease. *Vety. Microbiol.* 148: 1-7. 2011.

Birthal P, Parthasarathy RP. Economic contributions of the livestock subsector in India. *In: Technology option for sustainable livestock production in India.* ICRISAT-Patancheru, Hyderabad. pp. 12-19. 2002.

Bishop S, Chesnais J, Stear M. Breeding for disease resistance: issues and opportunities. *Proceedings of the 7th World Congress on Genetics Applied to Livestock Production*, Montpellier, Institut National de la Recherche Agronomique (INRA), France pp 1-8. 2002.

Bishop SC, Morris CA. Genetics of disease resitance in sheep and goats. *Small Ruminant Res.* 70: 48-59. 2007.

Bisset S, Morris C, McEwan J, Vlassoff A. Breeding sheep in New Zealand that are less reliant on anthelmintics to maintain health and productivity. *New Zealand Vety. J.* 49: 236-246. 2001.

Bock R, Vos AJ, Kingston T, McLellan D. Effect of breed of cattle on innate resistance to infection with *Babesia bovis, B bigemina* and *Anaplasma marginale. Australian Vety. J.* 75: 337-340. 2008.

Borriello G, Capparelli R, Bianco M, Fenizia D *et al.*, Genetic resistance to Brucella abortus in the water buffalo (*Bubalus bubalis*). *Infect. Immunl.* 74: 2115-2120. 2006.

Boyd Y, Herbert EG, Marston KL, Jones MA, Barrow PA. Host genes affect intestinal colonisation of newly hatched chickens by *Campylobacter jejuni. Immunogenet.* 57: 248-253. 2005.

Bradley R, Radhakrishnan C, Patil-Kulkarni C, Loggins P. Responses in Florida Native and Rambouillet lambs exposed to one and two oral doses of *Haemonchus contortus. Amer. J. Vety. Res.* 34: 729-735. 1973.

Briles W, Stone HA, Cole R. Marek's disease: effects of B histocompatibility alloalleles in resistant and susceptible chicken lines. *Science*. 195: 193-195. 1977.

Bumstead N, Millard B. Variation in susceptibility of inbred lines of chickens to seven species of Eimeria. *Parasitol*. 104: 407-413. 1992.

Burke J, Miller J. Relative resistance to gastrointestinal nematode parasites in Dorper, Katahdin, and St. Croix lambs under conditions encountered in the south-eastern region of the United States. *Small Ruminant. Res*. 54: 43-51. 2004.

Canani RB, Di-Costanzo M, Leone L, Bedogni G *et al.*, Epigenetic mechanisms elicited by nutrition in early life. *Nutril. Res. Rev*. 18: 1-8. 2011.

Capparelli R, Alfano F, Amoroso MG, Borriello G *et al.*, Protective effect of the Nramp1 BB genotype against *Brucella abortus* in the water buffalo (*Bubalus bubalis*). *Infect. Immunity* 75: 988-996. 2007.

Chambers P, Millar NS, Bingham RW, Emmerson PT. Molecular cloning of complementary DNA to Newcastle disease virus and nucleotide sequence analysis of the junction between the genes encoding the haemagglutinin-neuraminidase and the large protein. *J. Gen. Virol*. 67: 475–486. 1986.

Chauhan K, Rout P, Singh P, Mandal A *et al.*, Susceptibility to natural gastro-intestinal nematode infection in different physiological stages in Jamunapari and Barbari goats in the semi-arid tropics. *Small Ruminant. Res*. 50: 219-223. 2003.

Cleveland MA, Hickey JM, Forni S. A common dataset for genomic analysis of livestock populations. *G3: Genes Genomes Genet*. 2: 429-435. 2012.

Cohen-Zinder M, Seroussi E, Larkin DM, Loor JJ *et al.*, Identification of a missense mutation in the bovine ABCG2 gene with a major effect on the QTL on chromosome 6 affecting milk yield and composition in Holstein cattle. *Genome Res*. 15: 936-944. 2005.

Cole RK. Studies on genetic resistance to Marek's disease. *Avian Diseases*. 12: 9-28. 1968.

Cole RK, Hutt FB. Genetic differences in resistance to Newcastle disease. *Avian Diseases*. 5: 205-214. 1961.

Cooper K, Whelan M, Kennedy D, Trigueros G *et al.*, Anthelmintic drug residues in beef: UPLC-MS/MS method validation, European retail beef survey, and associated exposure and risk assessments. *Food Addit. Contamit. Part A*. 29: 746-760. 2012.

Cox LA, Glenn JP, Spradling KD, Nijland MJ *et al.*, A genome resource to address mechanisms of developmental programming: determination of the fetal sheep heart transcriptome. *J. Physiol*. 590: 2873-2884. 2012.

Da Silva AM, De Alencar MM, De Almeida RLC, De Sena OMC *et al.*, Artificial infestation of Boophilus microplus in beef cattle heifers of four genetic groups. *Genet. Mol. Biol*. 30: 1150-1155. 2007.

Davies G, Genini S, Bishop S, Giuffra E. An assessment of opportunities to dissect host genetic variation in resistance to infectious diseases in livestock. *Animal.* 3: 415-436. 2009.

De Castro JJ. Sustainable tick and tickborne disease control in livestock improvement in developing countries. *Vety. Parasitol.* 71: 77-97. 1997.

Depner K, Strebelow G, Staubach C, Kramer M *et al.,* Case report: the significance of genotyping for the epidemiological tracing of classical swine fever (CSF). *Deutsche Tierarztliche Wochenschrift.* 113: 159-162. 2006.

Dhakal I, Thapa B. Economic impact of clinical mastitis in the buffaloes in Nepal. *Buffalo J.* 18: 225-234. 2002.

Diez-Tascon C, Keane OM, Wilson T, Zadissa A *et al.,* Microarray analysis of selection lines from outbred populations to identify genes involved with nematode parasite resistance in sheep. *Physiol. Genomics.* 21: 59-69. 2005.

Duclos D, Hiemstra SJ. State of local cattle breeds in Europe. *In: Local cattle breeds in Europe* (Hiemstra SJ, de Haas Y, Maki-Tanila A and Gandini G Eds.) Wageningen Academic Publishers, Wageningen. pp. 42-57. 2010.

Eady S, Woolaston R, Barger I. Comparison of genetic and nongenetic strategies for control of gastrointestinal nematodes of sheep. *Livestock Prod. Sci.* 81: 11-23. 2003.

Emery D, Stewart D, Clark B. The comparative susceptibility of five breeds of sheep to foot-rot. *Australian Vety. J.* 61: 85-88. 2008.

Ernst CW, Steibel JP. Molecular advances in QTL discovery and application in pig breeding. *Trends Genet.* 29: 215-224. 2013.

Ezashi T, Telugu B, Roberts R. Induced pluripotent stem cells from pigs and other ungulate species: an alternative to embryonic stem cells? *Reprodt. Domestic Anim.* 47: 92-97. 2012.

Ezenwa VO, Etienne RS, Luikart G, Beja-Pereira A, Jolles AE. Hidden consequences of living in a wormy world: nematode-induced immune suppression facilitates tuberculosis invasion in African buffalo. *Amer. Naturalist.* 176: 613-624. 2010.

Fairbrother JM, Nadeau â, Gyles CL. *Escherichia coli* in postweaning diarrhea in pigs: an update on bacterial types, pathogenesis, and prevention strategies. *Anim. Health Res. Rev.* 6: 17-39. 2005.

Fan B, Gorbach D, Rothschild M. The pig genome project has plenty to squeal about. *Cytogenet. Genome Res.* 134: 9-18. 2011.

Farooq U, Samad HA, Sher F, Asim M, Khan MA. Cholistan and Cholistani breed of cattle. *Pakistan Vety. J.* 30: 126-130. 2010.

Finlay EK, Berry DP, Wickham B, Gormley EP, Bradley DG. A genome wide association scan of bovine tuberculosis susceptibility in Holstein-Friesian dairy cattle. *PLoS One.* 7: e30545. 2012.

Freeman A, Bradley D, Nagda S, Gibson J, Hanotte O. Combination of multiple microsatellite data sets to investigate genetic diversity and admixture of domestic cattle. *Anim. Genet.* 37: 1-9. 2005.

Gibbons R, Sellwood R, Burrows M, Hunter P. Inheritance of resistance to neonatal *E. coli* diarrhoea in the pig: examination of the genetic system. *Theo. Appl. Genet.* 51: 65-70. 1997.

Gibson J, Bishop S. Use of molecular markers to enhance resistance of livestock to disease: a global approach. *Rev Sci Et Tech-Off Intl Des Epizooties* 24: 343-353. 2005.

Giraud S, Favreau F, Chatauret N, Thuillier R *et al.*, Contribution of large pig for renal ischemia-reperfusion and transplantation studies: the preclinical model. *J. Biomed. Biotech.* 201: 5321–5327. 2011. doi: 10.1155/2011/532127

Glimp HA. Meat goat production and marketing. *J. Anim. Sci.* 73: 291-295. 1995.

Good B, Hanrahan J, Crowley B, Mulcahy G. Texel sheep are more resistant to natural nematode challenge than Suffolk sheep based on faecal egg count and nematode burden. *Vety. Parasitol.* 136: 317-327. 2006.

Govignon-Gion A, Dassonneville R, Baloche G, Ducrocq V. Genetic evaluation of mastitis in dairy cattle in France. *Interbull. Bull.* 46: 121-126. 2012.

Gresham D, Dunham MJ, Botstein D. Comparing whole genomes using DNA microarrays. *Nature Rev.* 9: 291-302. 2008.

Grisart B, Coppieters W, Farnir F, Karim L *et al.*, Positional candidate cloning of a QTL in dairy cattle: identification of a missense mutation in the bovine DGAT1 gene with major effect on milk yield and composition. *Genome Res.* 12: 222-231. 2002.

Gruner L, Aumont G, Getachew T, Brunel J *et al.*, Experimental infection of Black Belly and INRA 401 straight and crossbred sheep with trichostrongyle nematode parasites. *Vety. Parasitol.* 116: 239-249. 2003.

Gulhane A, Sangwan M. Polymorphism in TLR4 gene and its association with mastitis in Murrah buffaloes. *Ind. J. Biotech.* 11: 330-332. 2012.

Gutiérrez-Gil B, Wiener P, Nute GR, Burton D *et al.*, Detection of quantitative trait loci for meat quality traits in cattle. *Anim. Genet.* 39: 51-61. 2008.

Gyles N, Brown C. Selection in chickens for retrogression of tumors caused by Rous sarcoma virus. *Poultry Sci.* 50: 901-905. 1971.

Hanotte O, Ronin Y, Agaba M, Nilsson P *et al.*, Mapping of quantitative trait loci controlling trypanotolerance in a cross of tolerant west African N'Dama and susceptible east African Boran cattle. *Proc. Natl. Acad. Sci. USA.* 100: 7443-7448. 2003.

Hassan MK, Afify MA, Aly MM. Genetic resistance of Egyptian chickens to infectious bursal disease and Newcastle disease. *Tropl. Anim. Health Prod.* 36: 1-9. 2004.

Heid CA, Stevens J, Livak KJ, Williams PM. Real time quantitative PCR. *Genome Res.* 6: 986-994. 1996.

Henryon M, Berg P, Jensen J, Andersen S. Genetic variation for resistance to clinical and subclinical diseases exists in growing pigs. *J. Anim. Sci.* 73: 375-388. 2001.

Heo JM, Opapeju FO, Pluske JR, Kim JC *et al.*, Gastrointestinal health and function in weaned pigs: a review of feeding strategies to control post-weaning diarrhoea without using in-feed antimicrobial compounds. J. *Anim. Physiol. Anim. Nutri.* 97: 207-237. 2013.

Heringstad Br, Klemetsdal G, Ruane J. Selection for mastitis resistance in dairy cattle: a review with focus on the situation in the Nordic countries. *Livestock Prod. Sci* 64: 95-106. 2000.

Hiendleder S, Bauersachs S, Boulesteix A, Blum H *et al.*, Functional genomics: tools for improving farm animal health and welfare. *Rev Sci Et Techn-Off Intl Des Epizooties*. 24: 355-377. 2005.

Huang W, Khatib H. Comparison of transcriptomic landscapes of bovine embryos using RNA-Seq. *BMC Genomics*. 11: 711. 2010.

Huang W, Nadeem A, Zhang B, Babar M *et al.*, Characterization and comparison of the leukocyte transcriptomes of three cattle breeds. *Plos One*. 7: e302444. 2012. doi: 10.1371/journal.pone.0030244

Hunt PW, McEwan JC, Miller JE. Future perspectives for the implementationm of genetic markers for parasite resistance in sheep. *Trop. Biomed.* 25: 18-33. 2008.

Jackson F, Bartley D, Bartley Y, Kenyon F. Worm control in sheep in the future. *Small Ruminant Res.* 86: 40-45. 2009.

Jakhesara SJ, Ahir VB, Padiya KB, Koringa PG *et al.*, Tissue-specific temporal exome capture revealed muscle-specific genes and SNPs in Indian buffalo (*Bubalus bubalis*). *Genomics, Proteomics Bioinformatics* 10: 107-113. 2012.

Jensen K, Paxton E, Waddington D, Talbot R *et al.*, Differences in the transcriptional responses induced by Theileria annulata infection in bovine monocytes derived from resistant and susceptible cattle breeds. *Intl. J. Parasitol.* 38: 313-325. 2008.

Jiang C, Xing F, Xing J, Jiang Y, Zhou E. Different expression patterns of PRRSV mediator genes in the lung tissues of PRRSV resistant and susceptible pigs. *Devel. Comp. Immunol.* 39: 127-131. 2013.

Jolly R. Mannosidosis in cattle and its control. *New Zealand Vety. J.* 50: 90-90. 2002.

Jonsson N. The productivity effects of cattle tick (*Boophilus microplus*) infestation on cattle, with particular reference to *Bos indicus* cattle and their crosses. *Vety. Parasitol.* 137: 1-10. 2006.

Joshi S, Gokhale S. Status of mastitis as an emerging disease in improved and periurban dairy farms in India. *Annl. New York Acad. Sci.* 1081: 74-83. 2006.

Jovanovic S, Savic M, Zivkovic D. Genetic variation in disease resistance among farm animals. *Biotech. Anim. Hus.* 25: 339-347. 2009.

Kaneene JB, Scott H. The national animal health monitoring system in Michigan III. cost estimates of selected dairy cattle diseases. *Prevent. Vety. Med.* 8: 127 140. 1990.

Karlsson L, Greeff J. Selection response in fecal worm egg counts in the Rylington Merino parasite resistant flock. *Anim. Prod. Sci.* 46: 809-811. 2006.

Karlsson L, Greeff J. Genetic aspects of sheep parasitic diseases. *Vety. Parasitol.* 189 104-112. 2012.

Kavitha KL, Rajesh K, Suresh K, Satheesh K, Syama Sundar N. Buffalo mastitis-risk factors. *Buffalo Bull.* 28: 134-137. 2009.

Keane OM, Dodds KG, Crawford AM, McEwan JC. Transcriptional profiling of *Ovis aries* identifies Ovar-DQA1 allele frequency differences between nematode resistant and susceptible selection lines. *Physiol. Genomics.* 30: 253-261. 2007.

Khan N, Iqubal MA. Livestock revolution and its impacts on the sustainability of marginal and small farmers in India: a case study. *J. Geography* 5: 95-108. 2010.

Kim J, Hansen CF, Mullan B, Pluske J. Nutrition and pathology of weaner pigs Nutritional strategies to support barrier function in the gastrointestinal tract *Anim. Feed Sci. Tech.* 173: 3-16. 2012.

Kizilkaya K, Tait RG, Garrick DJ, Fernando RL, Reecy JM. Genome-wide association study of infectious bovine keratoconjunctivitis in Angus cattle. *BMC Genomics* 14: 23. 2013. doi: 10.1186/1471-2156-14-23

Kumar R, Yadav B, Singh R. Antibiotic resistance and pathogenicity factors in Staphylococcus aureus isolated from mastitic Sahiwal cattle. *J. Biosci.* 36: 175-188. 2011.

Kumar A, Joshi PK, Jongeneel RJ. Structural changes in the Indian dairy section. In *Asian livestock: challenges, opportunities and the response* (Ahuja V Ed.), *Proc Intl Policy Forum,* Intl. Livestock Res. Inst. FAO, pp. 51-71. 2012.

Kumar A, Joshi PK and Jongeneel RJ (2012). Structural changes in the Indian dairy section. In: *Asian livestock: challenges, opportunities and the response* (Ahuja V Ed.), *Proc Intl Policy Forum,* Intl. Livestock Res. Inst. FAO, pp. 51-71. 2012.

Lalles JP. Long term effects of pre- and early postnatal nutrition and environment on the gut. *J. Anim. Sci.* 90: 421-429. 2012.

Latif A. Resistance to natural tick infestations in different breeds of cattle in the Sudan. *Intl. J. Trop. Insect Sci.* 5: 95-97. 1984.

Le Roex N, Noyes H, Brass A, Bradley DG *et al.,* Novel SNP discovery in African Buffalo, *Syncerus caffer,* using high-throughput sequencing. *PLoS ONE.* 7: e48792. 2012. doi: 10.1371/journal.pone.0048792

Lei W, Liang Q, Jing L, Wang C *et al.,* BoLA-DRB3 gene polymorphism and FMD resistance or susceptibility in Wanbei cattle. *Mol. Biol. Rep.* 39: 9203-9209. 2012.

Leifer I, Hoffmann B, Höper D, Rasmussen TB *et al.,* Molecular epidemiology of current classical swine fever virus isolates of wild boar in Germany. *J. Gen. Virol.* 91: 2687-2697. 2010.

Livak KJ, Schmittgen TD. Analysis of relative gene expression data using real time quantitative PCR and the 2-AACT method. *Methods*. 25: 402-408. 2001.

Longenecker B, Pazderka F, Gavora J, Spencer J *et al.*, Role of the major histocompatibility complex in resistance to Marek's disease: restriction of the growth of JMV-MD tumor cells in genetically resistant birds. *Avian Immunol. Adv. Exptl. Med. Biol.* 88: 287-298. 1997.

Lundeheim N. Genetic analysis of respiratory diseases in pigs. *Acta Agril. Scandinavica*. 29: 209-215. 1997.

Lundeheim N. Health disorders and growth performance at a Swedish pig progeny testing station. *Acta Agril. Scandinavica*. 38: 77-88. 1988.

Luo Y, Qiu X, Li H, Zhang Q. Association between the polymorphism in FUT1 gene and the resistance to PWD and ED in three pig breeds. *Asian-Australasian J. Anim. Sci*. 23: 1268-1275. 2010.

Maillard J, Martinez D, Bensaid A. An amino acid sequence coded by the exon 2 of the BoLA DRB3 gene associated with a BoLA class I specificity constitutes a likely genetic marker of resistance to dermatophilosis in Brahman zebu cattle of martinique (FWI). *Annl. New York Acad. Sci.* 791: 185-197. 2006.

Mateescu RG, Thonney ML. Genetic mapping of quantitative trait loci for milk production in sheep. *Anim. Genet*. 41: 460-466. 2010.

Matheron G, Barre N, Camus E, Gogue J. Genetic resistance of Guadeloupe native goats to heartwater. *Onderstepoort J. Vety. Res*. 54: 337-340. 1987.

Matika O, Nyoni S, Van Wyk J, Erasmus G, Baker R. Resistance of Sabi and Dorper ewes to gastro-intestinal nematode infections in an African semi-arid environment. *Small Ruminant. Res*. 47: 95-102. 2003.

McCabe MS, Waters SM, Morris DG, Kenny DA *et al.*, RNA-seq analysis of differential gene expression in liver from lactating dairy cows divergent in negative energy balance. *BMC Genomics*. 13: 193. 2012.

Meadows J, Li K, Kantanen J, Tapio M *et al.*, Mitochondrial sequence reveals high levels of gene flow between breeds of domestic sheep from Asia and Europe. *J. Heredity*. 96: 494-501. 2005.

Meurens F, Summerfield A, Nauwynck H, Saif L and Gerdts V. The pig: a model for human infectious diseases. *Trends Microbiol*. 20: 50-57. 2012.

Mingala CN, Konnai S, Cruz LC, Onuma M, Ohashi K. Comparative moleculo-immunological analysis of swamp-and riverine-type water buffaloes responses. *Cytokine*. 46: 273-282. 2009.

Minozzi G, Williams JL, Stella A, Strozzi F *et al.*, Meta-analysis of two genome-wide association studies of bovine paratuberculosis. *PLoS ONE*. 7: e32578. 2012.

Mirkena T, Duguma G, Haile A, Tibbo M *et al.*, Genetics of adaptation in domestic farm animals: a review. *Livestock Sci*.132: 1-12. 2012.

Miyasaka T, Takeshima S, Matsumoto Y, Kobayashi N *et al.*, The diversity of bovine MHC class II DRB3 and DQA1 alleles in different herds of Japanese Black and Holstein cattle in Japan. *Gene*. 472: 42-49. 2011.

Moroni P, Sgoifo Rossi C, Pisoni G, Bronzo V *et al.*, Relationships between somatic cell count and intramammary infection in buffaloes. *J. Dairy Sci.* 89: 998-1003. 2006.

Morris C. Review of genetic parameters for disease resistance in sheep in New Zealand and Australia. *Proc. Aust. Assoc. Anim. Breed. Genet*. 18: 263-271. 2009.

Morrison TB, Weis JJ, Wittwer CT. Quantification of low-copy transcripts by continuous SYBR Green I monitoring during amplification. *Biotechniques*. 24: 954-962. 1998.

Mortazavi A, Williams BA, McCue K, Schaeffer L, Wold B. Mapping and quantifying mammalian transcriptomes by RNA-Seq. *Nature Methods*. 5: 621-628. 2008.

Mugambi J, Bain R, Wanyangu S, Ihiga M *et al.*, Resistance of four sheep breeds to natural and subsequent artificial *Haemonchus contortus* infection. *Vety. Parasitol.* 69: 265-273. 1997.

Mulder H, Lidauer M, Vilkki J, Stranden I, Veerkamp R. Marker-assisted breeding value estimation for mastitis resistance in Finnish Ayrshire cattle. *J. Dairy Sci.* 94: 4164-4173. 2011.

Munir S, Sharma JM, Kapur V. Transcriptional response of avian cells to infection with Newcastle disease virus. *Virus Res. 107*: 103-108. 2005.

Mwangi E, Stevenson P, Ndung'u J, Stear M *et al.*, Studies on host resistance to tick infestations among trypanotolerant *Bos indicus* cattle breeds in east Africa. *Annl. New York Acad Sci*. 849: 195-208. 1998.

Myllys V, Asplund K, Brofeldt E, Hirvela-Koski V *et al.*, Bovine mastitis in Finland in 1988 and 1995—changes in prevalence and antimicrobial resistance. *Acta Vetera Scandinavica*. 39: 119-126. 1998.

Nagalakshmi U, Wang Z, Waern K, Shou C *et al.*, The transcriptional landscape of the yeast whole genome defined by RNA sequencing. *Science*. 320: 1344-1349. 2008.

Nagalakshmi U, Waern K, Snyder M. RNA-seq: a method for comprehensive transcriptome analysis. *Curr. Protl. Mol. Biol*. 89: 4.11.1-4.11.13. 2010.

Nicholas FW. Animal breeding and disease. *Phil. Trans. Roy. Soc. B. Biol. Sci.* 360: 1529-1536. 2005.

Nieuwhof G, Bishop S. Costs of the major endemic diseases of sheep in Great Britain and the potential benefits of reduction in disease impact. *Anim. Sci*. 81: 23-29. 2005.

Nieuwhof G, Conington J, Bunger L, Haresign W, Bishop SC. Genetic and phenotypic aspects of foot lesion scores in sheep of different breeds and ages. *Animal*. 2: 1289-1296. 2008.

Nimbkar C, Ghalsasi P, Swan A, Walkden-Brown S, Kahn L. Evaluation of growth rates and resistance to nematodes of Deccani and Bannur lambs and their crosses with Garole. *Anim. Sci.* 76: 503-516. 2003.

Ogorevc J, Kunej T, Razpet A, Dovc P. Database of cattle candidate genes and genetic markers for milk production and mastitis. *Anim. Genet.* 40: 832-851. 2009.

Okoniewski MJ, Miller CJ. Hybridization interactions between probesets in short oligo microarrays lead to spurious correlations. *BMC Bioinformatics.* 7: 276. 2006. doi: 10.1186/1471-2105-7-276

O'Loughlin A, Lynn DJ, McGee M, Doyle S *et al.*, Transcriptomic analysis of the stress response to weaning at housing in bovine leukocytes using RNA-seq technology. *BMC Genomics.* 13: 250. 2012.

Paixao T, Martinez R, Santos R. Polymorphisms of the coding region of Slc11a1 (Nramp1) gene associated to natural resistance against bovine brucellosis. *Arquivo Brasileiro de Medicina Veterinaria e Zootecnia.* 64: 1081-1084. 2012.

Pant S, Verschoor C, Schenkel F, You Q *et al.*, Bovine PGLYRP1 polymorphisms and their association with resistance to Mycobacterium avium ssp. paratuberculosis. *Anim. Genet.* 42: 354-360. 2011.

Papadopoulos E. Anthelmintic resistance in sheep nematodes. *Small Ruminant Res.* 76: 99-103. 2008.

Papadopoulos E, Gallidis E, Ptochos S. Anthelmintic resistance in sheep in Europe: a selected review. *Vety. Parasitol.* 189: 85-88. 2012.

Patten T, Good B, Hanrahan JP, Mulcahy G, de Waal T. Gastrointestinal nematode control practices on lowland sheep farms in Ireland with reference to selection for anthelmintic resistance. *Irish Vety. J.* 64: 4. 2011. doi: 10.1186/2046-0481-64-4

Pemberton J, Beraldi D, Craig B, Hopkins J. Digital gene expression analysis of gastrointestinal helminth resistance in Scottish blackface lambs. *Mol. Ecol.* 20: 910-919. 2011.

Petrovski K, Trajcev M and Buneski G. A review of the factors affecting the costs of bovine mastitis: review article. *J. South African Vety. Assoc.* 77: 52-60. 2006.

Petry D, Lunney J, Boyd P, Kuhar D *et al.*, Differential immunity in pigs with high and low responses to porcine reproductive and respiratory syndrome virus infection. *J. Anim. Sci.* 85: 2075-2092. 2007.

Pinard-Van DLM, Monvoisin J, Pery P, Hamet N, Thomas M. Comparison of outbred lines of chickens for resistance to experimental infection with coccidiosis (*Eimeria tenella*). *Poultry Sci.* 77: 185-191. 1998.

Piper EK, Jonsson NN, Gondro C, Lew-Tabor AE *et al.*, Immunological profiles of *Bos taurus* and *Bos indicus* cattle infested with the cattle tick, Rhipicephalus (Boophilus) microplus. *Clinical Vaccine Immunol.* 16: 1074-1086. 2009.

Pluske JR, Hampson DJ, Williams IH. Factors influencing the structure and function of the small intestine in the weaned pig: a review. *Livestock Prod. Sci.* 51: 215-236. 1997.

Prather RS. Pig genomics for biomedicine. *Nature Biotech.* 31: 122-124. 2013.

Raadsma H, Egerton J, Wood D, Kristo C, Nicholas F. Disease resistance in Merino sheep. III. Genetic variation in resistance to footrot following challenge and subsequent vaccination with an homologous rDNA pilus vaccine under both induced and natural conditions. *J. Anim. Breed Genet.* 111: 367-390. 1994.

Rajput S, Kumar P, Roy B, Verma A *et al.,* Identification of some unknown transcripts from SSH cDNA library of buffalo follicular oocytes. *Animal.* 1: 1-10. 2012.

Reddacliff L, Beh K, McGregor H, Whittington R. A preliminary study of possible genetic influences on the susceptibility of sheep to Johne's disease. *Australian Vety. J.* 83: 435-441. 2008.

Reiner G, Melchinger E, Kramarova M, Pfaff E *et al.,* Detection of quantitative trait loci for resistance/susceptibility to pseudorabies virus in swine. *J. Gen. Virol.* 83: 167-172. 2002.

Rinaldi M, Li RW, Capuco AV. Mastitis associated transcriptomic disruptions in cattle. Vety. *Immunol. Immunopathol.* 138: 267-279. 2010.

Roberts C, Gray. Studies on trypanosome-resistant cattle. II. The effect of trypanosomiasis on N'Dama, Muturu and Zebu cattle. *Tropl. Anim. Health Prod.* 5: 220-233. 1973.

Roberts J, Estuningsih E, Widjayanti S, Wiedosari E *et al.,* Resistance of Indonesian thin tail sheep against Fasciola gigantica and F. hepatica. *Vety. Parasitol.* 68: 69-78. 1997.

Rosegrant M, Fernandez M, Sinha A, Alder J *et al.,* Looking into the future for agriculture and AKST (Agricultural Knowledge Science and Technology). In: *Assessment of Agricultural Knowledge, Science and Technology for Development* (Mclntyre BD *et al.,* Ed.) Island Press, Washington. 2009.

Rue CA, Susta L, Cornax I, Brown CC *et al.,* Virulent Newcastle disease virus elicits a strong innate immune response in chickens. *J. Gen. Virol.* 92: 931-939. 2011.

Rupp R, Boichard D. Genetics of resistance to mastitis in dairy cattle. *Vety. Res.* 34: 671-688. 2003.

Sahana G, Guldbrandtsen B, Thomsen B, Lund MS. Confirmation and fine-mapping of clinical mastitis and somatic cell score QTL in Nordic Holstein cattle. *Anim. Genet.* 44: 620-626. 2013. doi: 10.1111/age.12053

Sangwan M. Analysis of genetic diversity of Indian buffalo breeds by DNA markers. *J. Buffalo Sci.* 1: 91-101. 2012.

Sargison ND. Pharmaceutical treatments of gastrointestinal nematode infections of sheep-Future of anthelmintic drugs. *Vety. Parasitol.* 189: 79-84. 2012.

Sayers G, Sweeney T. Gastrointestinal nematode infection in sheep- a review of the alternatives to anthelmintics in parasite control. *Anim. Health Res. Rev.* 6: 159-171. 2005.

Sayers G, Good B, Hanrahan J, O'donovan J *et al.*, Breed differences in mucosal and systemic antibody response to nematode infection in sheep: an important role for IgE? *Parasitol.* 135: 71-80. 2008.

Schou T, Permin A, Roepstorff A, Sorensen P, Kjaer J. Comparative genetic resistance to Ascaridia galli infections of 4 different commercial layer-lines. *British Poultry Sci.* 44: 182-185. 2003.

Seal BS, King DJ, Sellers HS. The avian response to Newcastle disease virus. *Dev. Comp. Immunol.* 24: 257-268. 2000.

Seifert G. Variations between and within breeds of cattle in resistance to field infestations of the cattle tick (Boophilus microplus). *Crop Pasture Sci.* 22: 159-168. 1971.

Seyfert HM, Henke M, Interthal H, Klussmann U *et al.*, Defining candidate genes for mastitis resistance in cattle: the role of lactoferrin and lysozyme. *J. Anim. Breed. Genet.* 113: 269–276. 1996.

Singh KM, Meena MS. Livestock value chains: prospects, challenges and policy implications. In: *Status of agricultural development in eastern India* (Bhatt BP, Sikka AK, Mukharjee J, Islam A and Dey A Eds), ICAR, pp. 493-508. 2012.

Singh P, Singh S, Singh A, Sohal J. Variability in susceptibility of different Indian goat breeds with respect to natural and experimental infection of Mycobacterium avium subspecies paratuberculosis. *Ind. J. Small Ruminants.* 15: 35-43. 2009.

Smith J. Health at the livestock-policy interface. In: *Asian livestock: challenges, opportunities and the response* (Ahuja V Ed.). *Proc. Intl. Policy Forum,* Intl. Livestock Res. Inst. FAO. pp. 23-28. 2012.

Stoltz DA, Rokhlina T, Ernst SE, Pezzulo AA *et al.*, Intestinal CFTR expression alleviates meconium ileus in cystic fibrosis pigs. *J. Clinical Investn.* 123: 2685-2693. 2013.

Sugimoto M, Fujikawa A, Womack JE, Sugimoto Y. Evidence that bovine forebrain embryonic zinc finger-like gene influences immune response associated with mastitis resistance. *Proc. Natl. Acad. Sci.USA.* 103: 6454-6459. 2006.

Taneja VK. Dairy breeds and selection. In: *Smallholder dairying in the tropics.* (Falvey L and Chantalakhana C Eds.), Intl. Livestock Res. Inst. Nairobi. Kenya. 1999.

Tapio M, Marzanov N, Ozerov M, Cinkulov M *et al.*, Sheep mitochondrial DNA variation in European, Caucasian, and central Asian areas. *Mol. Biol. Evol.* 23: 1776-1783. 2006.

Terada Y, Kariya Y, Terui S, Shioya S *et al.*, Comparison of resistance to theileria sergenti infection between Holstein and Japanese black cattle under grazing conditions. *Japan Agril. Res. Qutly.* 31: 219-224. 1997.

Thanislass J, Yuvaraj G, Reddy KS. Characterization of TLR4 signaling in water buffalo (*Bubalus bubalis*). *Vety. Res. Comm.* 33: 97-102. 2009.

Thornoton PK. Livestock production: recent trends, future prospects. *Philo. Trans. Roy. Soc. B. Biol. Sci.* 365: 2853-2867. 2010.

Vignesh A, Raj GD, Dhanasekaran S, Tirumurugaan K, Raja A. Comparative *in vitro* toll-like receptor ligand induced cytokine profiles of Toda and Murrah buffaloes- identification of tumour necrosis factor alpha promoter polymorphism. *Vety Immunol. Immunopathol.* 150: 189-197. 2008.

Vijh R, Tantia M, Mishra B, Kumar STB. Genetic relationship and diversity analysis of Indian water buffalo (*Bubalus bubalis*). *J. Anim. Sci.* 86: 1495-1502. 2008.

Vincent A, Thacker B, Halbur P, Rothschild M, Thacker E. *In vitro* susceptibility of macrophages to porcine reproductive and respiratory syndrome virus varies between genetically diverse lines of pigs. *Viral Immunol.* 18: 506-512. 2005.

Vincent A, Thacker B, Halbur P, Rothschild M, Thacker E. An investigation of susceptibility to porcine reproductive and respiratory syndrome virus between two genetically diverse commercial lines of pigs. *J. Anim. Sci.* 84: 49-57. 2006.

Vordermeier M, Ameni G, Glass EJ. Cytokine responses of Holstein and Sahiwal zebu derived monocytes after mycobacterial infection. *Trop. Anim. Health Prod* 44: 651-655. 2011.

Vordermeier M, Ameni G, Berg S, Bishop R *et al.*, The influence of cattle breed on susceptibility to bovine tuberculosis in Ethiopia. *Comp. Immunol. Microbiol. Inf Diseases.* 35: 227–232. 2012.

Wambura P, Gwakisa P, Silayo R, Rugaimukamu E. Breed-associated resistance to tick infestation in *Bos indicus* and their crosses with *Bos taurus*. *Vety. Parasitol* 77: 63-70. 1998.

Wang Z, Gerstein M, Snyder M. RNA-seq: a revolutionary tool for transcriptomics *Natl. Rev. Genet.* 10: 57-63. 2009.

Westermann AJ, Gorski SA, Vogel J. Dual RNA-seq of pathogen and host. *Natl. Rev Microbiol.* 10: 618-630. 2012.

Wharton R, Utech K, Turner H. Resistance to the cattle tick, *Boophilus microplus* in a herd of Australian Illawarra shorthorn cattle: its assessment and heritability *Crop Pastu. Sci.* 21: 163-181. 1970.

Wickramasinghe S, Rincon G, Islas-Trejo A, Medrano JF. Transcriptional profiling of bovine milk using RNA sequencing. *BMC Genomics.* 13: 45. 2012.

Wilhelm BT, Landry JR. RNA-seq quantitive measurement of expression through massively parallel RNA-sequencing. *Methods.* 48: 249-257. 2009.

Wong ML, Medrano JF. Real-time PCR for mRNA quantitation. *Biotechniques.* 39 1-11. 2005.

Wray C, Sojka W. Experimental Salmonella typhimurium infection in calves. *Res. Vety. Sci.* 25: 139-143. 1978.

Zaragoza C, Gomez-Guerrero C, Martin-Ventura JL, Blanco-Colio L *et al.*, Animal models of cardiovascular diseases. *J. Biomed. Biotech.* 2011: 1-13. 2011.

Zhang H, Wang Z, Wang S, Li H. Progress of genome wide association study in domestic animals. *J. Anim. Sci. Biotech.* 3: 26. 2012. doi: 10.1186/2049-1891-3-26

Zheng J, Watson AD, Kerr DE. Genome-wide expression analysis of lipopolysaccharide-induced mastitis in a mouse model. *Infec. Immunl.* 74: 1907-1915. 2006.

2016, Biotechnological Tools for Genetic Resources *Pages* **347–372**
Editor: **Pradip Chandra Deka**
Published by: **Daya Publishing House, NEW DELHI**

Chapter 11

Microbial Fuel Cells for Bioenergy Production through Wastewater Treatment

Archana Gajbhiye

Department of Biotechnology,
Sir Padampat Singhania University, Bhatewar,
Udaipur – 313 601, Rajasthan
E-mail: archana.yg@gmail.com

ABSTRACT

The conversion of biomass into electricity through the metabolic activity of microorganisms is possible through the bioreactor known as microbial fuel cell (MFC). It can be an effective operational technology for sustainable generation of bioenergy from wastewater treatment. The principle of electricity generation in MFC is the transfer of electrons generated during the microbial metabolic activity through anode to cathode. The mechanism of electron donation to anode by microorganisms is dependent upon either electrochemical activity of bacteria or the mediators for translocation of electrons from microbes to anode. Since the efficiency and performance depends on the composition of the wastewater, the designs of the MFCs vary. For designing an efficient MFC it is important to have information on various parameters, and thus knowledge and understanding of both biology and engineering is essential. Recent advances made in designing of efficient MFCs has regenerated interest on its practical applications. Various parameters involved in research on MFCs such as: microbial population, designs of MFCs, factors affecting the efficiency of the MFCs and recent developments and applications of MFC are discussed in this article.

Keywords: *Microbial fuel cell, MFC, Bioreactor, Bioenergy, Renewable energy, Wastewater treatment.*

Introduction

Microbial fuel cells (MFC) are bio-electrochemical reactors wherein bacteria oxidize various organic and inorganic compounds in the anode chamber and generate protons and electrons, which are transported to the cathode to reduce oxygen to water. It is a process where bacterial oxidation of organic matter and nutrients is coupled to the generation of electric energy. It is a new technology for direct production of electricity from organic waste. This technology can be a promising alternative for renewable energy from wastewater treatment based upon its advantages. There is a direct generation of electricity without any additional conversion step, it can be operated at a range of temperature and are efficient at low substrate concentration levels, in terms of both electricity generation and organic removal, it can improve biodegradation of organics and it can be diversified with new functions such as hydrogen production, desalination, and heavy metal removal. The technology requires more research to overcome the limitations such as efficiency improvement for wastewater treatment and cost reduction. Till date various models have been proposed for efficient energy production with a lot of potential for their commercial utilization. In the past decade, researchers have made significant progress towards understanding fundamental issues of microbiology, electrochemistry and reactor architecture in MFCs (Arends and Verstraete, 2012). A review of the development in microbial fuel cell and its commercial utilization is presented in this paper.

Working Principle of MFC

A typical microbial fuel cell (Figure 11.1) consists of anodic and cathodic chambers partitioned by a proton exchange membrane (Wilkinson, 2000, Gil *et al.*, 2003). The bacterial metabolism is involved in the energy generation, where chemical energy is converted into electrical energy in MFCs. In the anodic chamber the microbes oxidize the added substrates and generate electrons, protons and carbon dioxide as an oxidation product. In cellular metabolism the natural electron acceptor is oxygen or inorganic compounds like sulphate, nitrate etc. This electron acceptor is replaced by MFC anode, which helps in transfer of electrons to cathode through a resistor. The protons enter the cathodic chamber through the proton exchange membrane or the salt bridge, where it combines with electrons and oxygen to form water. This whole process of generation of electrons and its flow through electrodes leads to generation of electricity and an off gas CO_2.

The representative electrode reactions (Equation 1 and 2) using acetate as a substrate are given as follows:

Anodic reaction: $CH_3COO^- + 2H_2O \longrightarrow 2CO_2 + 7H^+ + 8e^-$ (1)

Cathodic reaction: $O_2 + 4e^- + 4H^+ \longrightarrow 2H_2O$ (2)

Electric current generation is made possible by keeping microbes separated from oxygen or any other end terminal acceptor other than the anode and this requires an anaerobic anodic chamber. Under closed circuit condition, the available power of MFC (P_{cell}) depends on the cell voltage (V_{cell}) and cell current (I_{cell}) as in equation 3. The voltage depends upon the resistance according to the Ohm's law (equation

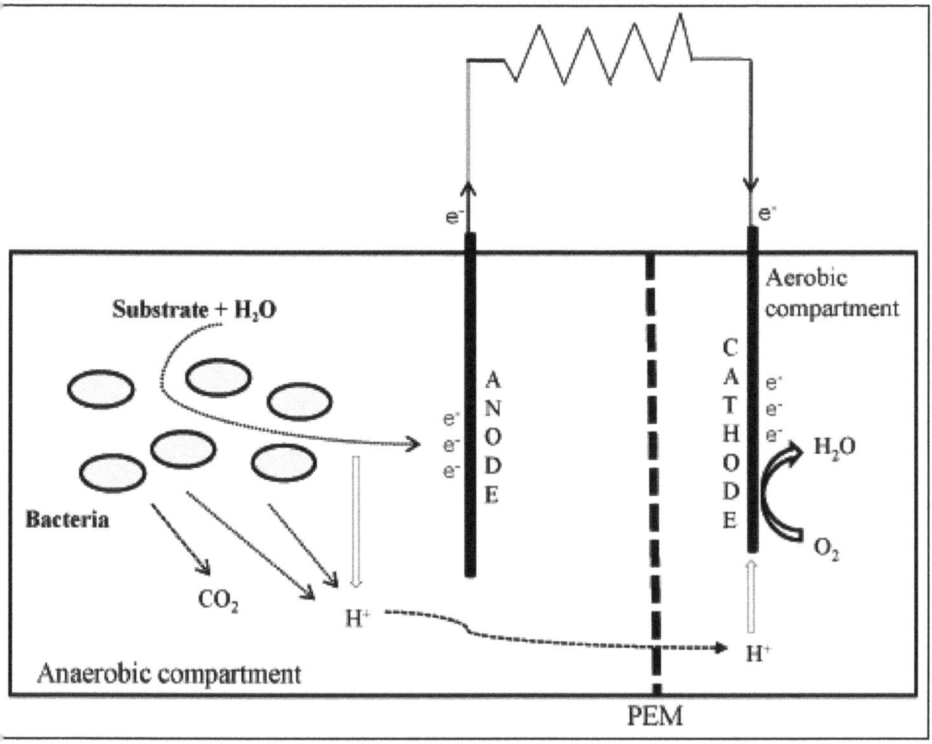

Figure 11.1: Representative Design of a Typical Microbial Fuel Cell. The anodic and cathodic chambers partitioned by a proton exchange membrane.

4). The ideal cell voltage is the difference in the potentials of the oxidant and fuel compounds ($E_{ox} - E_{red}$), however irreversible losses (overpotential, η) are incurred as a result of kinetic limitations (equation 5) (Katz *et al.*, 2003).

$$P_{cell} = V_{cell} \times I_{cell} \quad (3)$$

$$V_{cell} = I_{cell} \times R \quad (4)$$

$$V_{cell} = (E_{ox} - E_{red}) - \eta \quad (5)$$

The mechanism of transport of electrons from membrane bound proteins to the anode is a major area, which need to be understood. It has been proposed that the microbes transfer their electrons to anode as it is the necessity of every living cell to dispose the electrons liberated during oxidative substrate degradation (Schroder, 2007). Two major principles are proposed for electron transport from bacterial cell to the anode *viz.* mediated and mediator less electron transport.

Mediated MFCs

For the generation of electrode potential there is an absolute requirement of transfer of electrons to the anode from the bacteria. Most microbes are electrochemically inactive due to the cell membrane embedded proteins involved in electron transport. Therefore an electron transport mechanism from microbe to anode is required, which can be established via different mechanisms *viz.* through electron mediators or redox shuttles (Rabaey *et al.*, 2004, Rabaey *et al.*, 2005a). The electron mediators preferentially gets reduced during the metabolic oxidation of the organic compounds, and the reduced form of the mediator is then re-oxidized at the working electrode (anode), which is maintained at a sufficiently high electric potential (Figure 11.2). Chemical mediators, such as neutral red (NR) or anthraquinone-2,6-disulfonate (AQDS), can be added to the system to allow electricity production by bacteria, which otherwise cannot use the electrode (Park and Zeikus, 1999; Bond *et al.*, 2002).

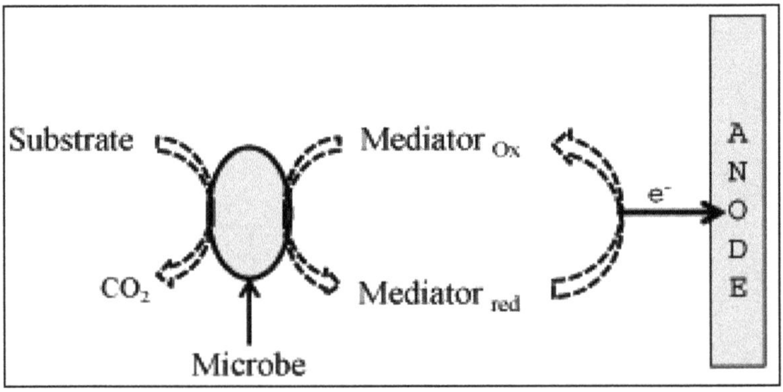

Figure 11.2: Mechanism of Electron Transfer to Anode in Mediated MFC. The mechanism of electron transport is the mediators or redox shuttles. The electron mediators accept electron from microbial cell, get reduced and then re-oxidized at electrode by transferring the electron to anode.

Hydrogenase enzyme could be directly involved in electron transfer towards electrodes in combination with a mobile redox shuttle (McKinlay and Zeikus, 2004). Many fermentative microorganisms identified in MFCs, like *Clostridium butyricum* and *Enterococcus faecium* possess hydrogenase enzyme (Park *et al.*, 2001, Rabaey *et al.*, 2004). Hydrogenases have a role in reducing neutral red (dye) at the bacterial surface.

Mediator Less MFCs

If no exogenous mediators are added to the system, the MFC is classified as a "mediator-less" MFC even though the mechanism of electron transfer may not be known (Logan, 2004). The principle of electron transfer to anode in mediator-less MFCs is the electrochemically active (ECA) bacteria. There may be two possible mechanisms of electron transfer: direct membrane associated electron transfer (Bond and Lovely, 2003), or by electrically conductive bacterial appendages known as nanowires (Reguera *et al.*, 2005, Gorby *et al.*, 2006) produced by the bacteria (Figure 11.3). The electrochemical activity in bacteria was proposed due to the presence of ECA compounds on the cell surface such as cytochromes (Kim *et al.*, 1999a). Multiheme *c*-type chromosomes are thought to play a major role in ETS and outer membrane cytochromes are believed to be the contact point to externally located Fe(III) and Mn(IV)-bearing minerals. The genome analysis of *S. oneidensis* strain MR-1 suggested the presence of 42 possible cytochrome *c* genes (Heidelberg *et al.*, 2002, Meyer *et al.*, 2004) whereas in *Geobacter sulfurreducens* presence of more than 100 genes was reported (Methe *et al.*, 2003, Moon *et al.*, 2004). These c type cytochromes are located on the outer membrane in both the organisms. This supports the quite apparent role of cytochrome *c* in extracellular electron exchange.

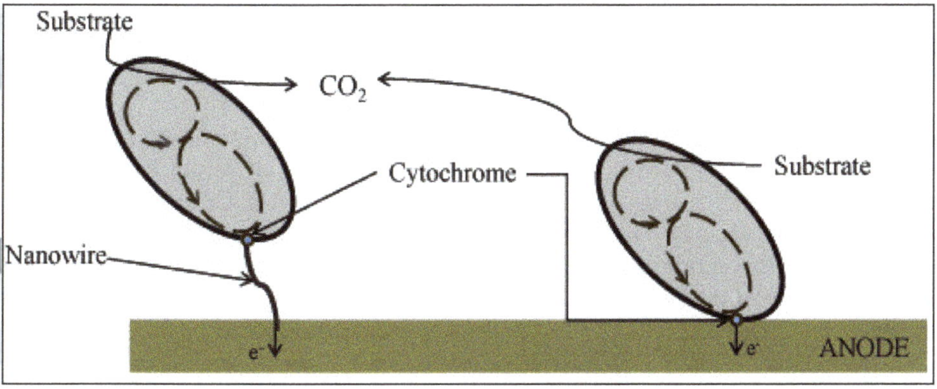

Figure 11.3: Mechanism of Electron Transfer in Mediator-less MFC. The electrons transfer is direct from microbial cell to anode which can be a direct membrane associated electron transfer or through electrically conductive bacterial appendages known as nanowires produced by the bacteria.

Microbial Communities in MFCs

Microorganisms are the most important component in MFCs. Metabolic activities is the part of all cellular organisms, microorganisms has no exceptions. In all metabolic activities the electrons generated are finally transported to oxygen in the case of aerobic organisms and to inorganic compounds in the case of anaerobic organisms. Many microorganisms possess the property of transferring the electrons generated from the metabolic processes to the anode. This property has been reported in microbial communities inhabiting the soil, wastewater, activated sludge, fresh water sediments, and marine sediments (Niessen *et al.*, 2006; Zhang *et al.*, 2006).

Several bacterial species are known to produce electrical current in microbial fuel cells. Important among them are *Shewanella putrefaciens* using lactate, pyruvate and formate as electron donor (Kim *et al.*, 1999b; Park and Kim, 2001), *Clostridium butyricum* and *Clostridium beijerinckii* by using glucose, starch, lactate and molasses (Park *et al.*, 2001; Niessen *et al.*, 2004a), *Geobacter sulfurreducens* by using acetate and hydrogen (Caccavo *et al.*, 1994; Yang *et al.*, 2010), *Rhodoferax ferrireducens* by using glucose (Chaudhuri and Lovley, 2003), *Geobacter metallireducens* by using acetate (Min *et al.*, 2005a) and *Rhodopseudomonas palustris* by using acetate, lactate, valerate, fumarate, ethanol, glycerol and yeast extract (Xing *et al.*, 2008). *Alcaligenes faecalis, Enterococcus gallinarum* and *Pseudomonas aeruginosa* are known to generate electricity by producing their own mediators, using glucose as an electron donor (Rabaey *et al.*, 2004). To date, *Enterobacter cloacae* is the only pure culture that is known to generate electricity directly from more complex electron donors, such as cellulose (Rezaei *et al.*, 2009).

Microbial flora of MFC found to vary with the design of the cell as well as the mechanism of the microorganisms by which it donates the electron to the anode. Usually the respiratory or the electron transport chain (ETC) is present in the plasma membrane through which the oxidative transfer of electron takes place and is donated to the anode. Bacteria known to use this pathway are *Geobacter metallireducens* (Vandevivere and Verstraete, 2001), *Aeromonas hydrophila* (Pham *et al.*, 2003) and *Rhodoferax ferrireducens* (Chaudhuri and Lovley, 2003).

In MFCs used in wastewater treatment, the major bacterial population contributing the electricity generation was found to be of phyla *Proteobacteria, Firmicutes*, and *Bacteroidetes* (Ishii *et al.*, 2012, Park *et al.*, 2014). Of the *Proteobacteria*, members of the class *Deltaproteobacteria* were found to be important for electricity generation in the anode biofilm. The *Geobacter* biofilms (Srikanth *et al.*, 2007) and Bacteroidetes biofilm (Ishii *et al.*, 2012) were also suggested to be important function in MFC.

The genera *Geobacter* and *Desulfobulbus* have been found in Plant MFCs (De Schamphelaire *et al.*, 2010). In the PMFC, electrons, protons and carbon dioxide are produced by oxidation of organic compounds lost by plant roots in the anode. The electrons that are transferred to the anode electrode are consumed in the cathode compartment by typically reduction of oxygen to water (Strik *et al.*, 2011).

MFC Designs

Two categories of designs of microbial fuel cells are available, research type and application type. Several different models have been constructed, indicating their utility and efficiencies. So far the designs developed purely for research goals are difficult to implement at commercial scale. The construction and analysis of MFCs requires knowledge of different scientific and engineering fields, ranging from microbiology and electrochemistry to materials and environmental engineering. Consideration of the parameters such as mode of operation, efficiency and cost involvement is important for designing of MFC's for its application in commercial scale.

The standard model of MFC consists of an anodic chamber and a cathodic chamber separated by a proton exchange membrane (Figures 11.1 and 11.4). The anodic chamber is the centre of metabolism and electron generation containing the waste organic material mixed with the microbial system and cathode chamber is the oxidation centre that contains an oxidizing agent such as dissolved oxygen.

Based upon the structure, till date four major designs of MFCs are proposed *viz.* two chambered, single chambered, upflow mode and stacked microbial fuel cell.

Two Chambered MFC System

Two chambered MFCs are comparatively inexpensive and thus most widely used. The traditional H shaped design consists of an anodic and a cathodic chamber connected via proton exchange membrane (PEM) or a salt bridge (Figure 11.4). This

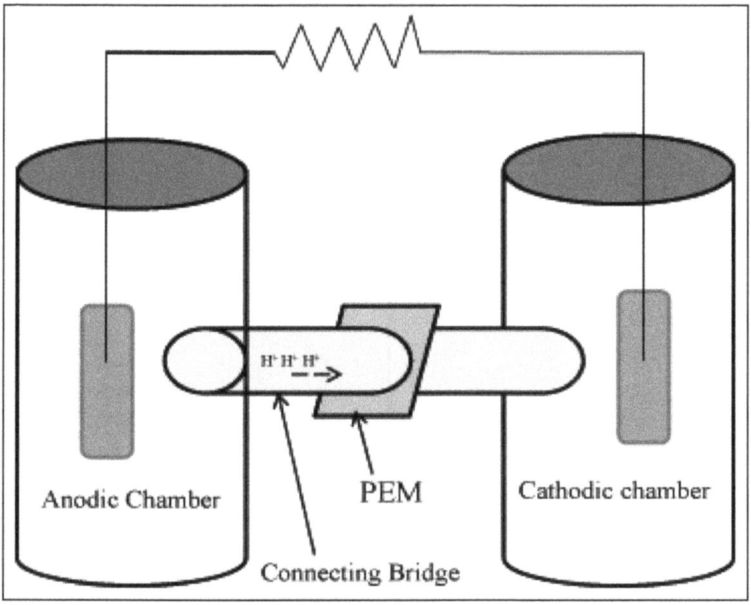

Figure 11.4: Schematic Design of Two Chambered MFC. The traditional H shaped design consisting of an anodic and a cathodic chamber connected via proton exchange membrane (PEM) or a salt bridge.

type of MFC system is suitable for lab operations and can be operated both as batch and continuous manner. The electrons generated during the metabolism are driven to the anode while the protons get transported selectively through the PEM to the cathodic chamber. The selective use of PEM blocks the passage of oxygen from the cathodic chamber to anodic chamber. This lab scale design is easy for construction and operation, but difficult for large scale operations. A flat plate MFC (FPMFC) was designed by Min and Logan (2004) using a combined electrode/PEM system. The reactor consisted of a single channel formed between two nonconductive plates that were separated into two halves by the electrode/PEM assembly. Each electrode was placed on opposite sides of the PEM, with the anode facing the chamber containing the liquid phase and the cathode facing a chamber containing only air. A miniature microbial fuel cell (mini-MFC) model with high output power per device with a cross-section of 2.0 cm^2 and volume of 1.2 cm^3 was demonstrated by Ringeisen *et al.* (2006).

Single Chambered MFC System

Single chamber MFCs are more practical and less expensive than the conventional two-compartment system. The one compartment fuel cell designed by Park and Zeikus (2003) was composed of a rubber bunged bottle with a center-inserted anode and a window-mounted air cathode containing an internal, proton-permeable porcelain layer. In this model the protons are transferred from the anolyte solution to the porous air-cathode (Figure 11.5). A single chamber microbial fuel cell (SCMFC) containing eight graphite electrodes (anodes) and a single air cathode with a continuous flow system was designed by Liu *et al.* (2004).

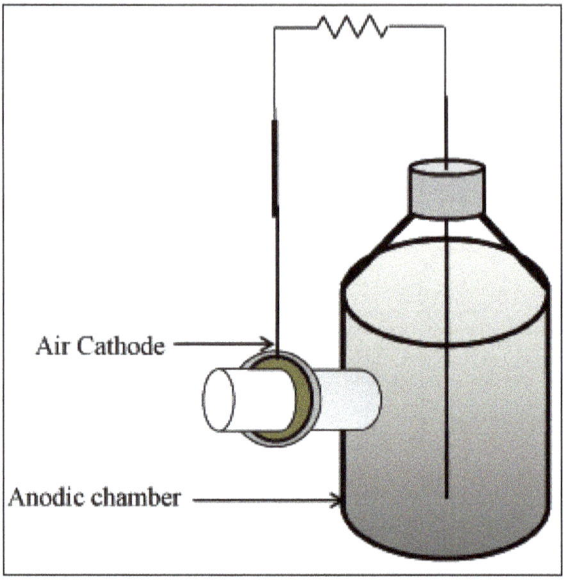

Figure 11.5: Schematic Representation of Single Chambered MFC. A rubber bunged bottle is used with an anode fixed in the centre of the bottle. The bottle design consists of a window-mounted air cathode containing an internal, proton-permeable porcelain layer.

The possibility of designing a MFC for power generation containing carbon electrodes in the presence and absence of a polymeric proton exchange membrane using bacteria present in domestic wastewater as the biocatalyst, was studied by Liu and Logan (2004). According to the design, the anode is placed inside a plastic cylindrical chamber and a cathode is placed outside. The anode was made of carbon paper without wet proofing and the cathode was either a carbon electrode/PEM assembly fabricated by bonding the PEM directly onto a flexible carbon-cloth electrode, or a standalone rigid carbon paper without PEM (Liu and Logan, 2004, Liu *et al.*, 2005a, Cheng *et al.*, 2006). A tubular, single-chambered, continuous microbial fuel cell (MFC) that generates high power outputs using a granular graphite matrix as the anode and a ferricyanide solution as the cathode was designed by Rabaey *et al.* (2005b).

Upflow Mode MFC System

A membrane-less, upflow microbial fuel cell was developed by Jang *et al.* (2004). This model consisted of cylinder-shaped reactor made of polyacrylic plastic with the disc shaped graphite felt anode and cathode placed at the bottom and top, respectively (Figure 11.6). The layers of glass wool and glass bead were sandwiched in between the electrodes. The feed stream is supplied from the bottom of the anode and the effluent comes out through the cathode. This system works in continues

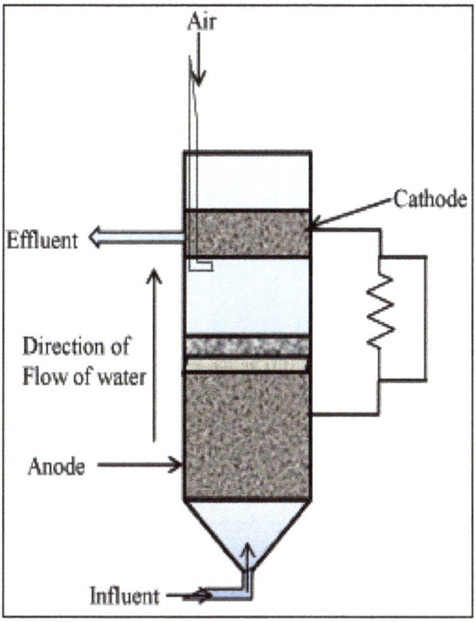

Figure 11.6: Model Representation for Upflow Mode MFC. This model consists of a cylinder shaped reactor with an anode and cathode discs placed at the bottom and top of the reactor.

node. Another model of an upflow microbial fuel cell system with a U-shaped cathode inside the anode chamber was developed by He *et al.* (2005). In this model both the anodic and the cathodic chambers were filled with the activated carbon granules passing the catholyte through the cathode chamber.

Stacked Microbial Fuel Cell

The MFC stack consisting of six individual MFC units (Figure 11.7) was developed by Aelterman *et al.* (2006). They were constructed of 12 identical Perspex frames. Each MFC unit consisted of anode and cathode, separated by an Ultrex cation exchange membrane. The anode and cathode electrodes consisted of graphite granules to collect the electrons (type 00514, diameter between 1.5 and 5 mm, Le Carbone, Belgium) and a graphite rod (5 mm diameter, Morgan, Belgium) to connect to the external circuit. All six of these MFCs were placed parallel to each other, separated by five rubber sheets, with anode and cathode at alternate positions.

Studies on stacked MFCs for increasing power generation, scaling up of the process and parameters involved in overall voltage output etc. have been carried out by various researchers (Oh and Logan, 2007; Li *et al.*, 2008; Dekker *et al.*, 2009; Ledezma *et al.*, 2013). To design more convenient stacked microbial fuel cells (MFCs), a baffled single-chambered MFC with two groups of electrodes sharing only one anode chamber was designed by Li *et al.* (2008).

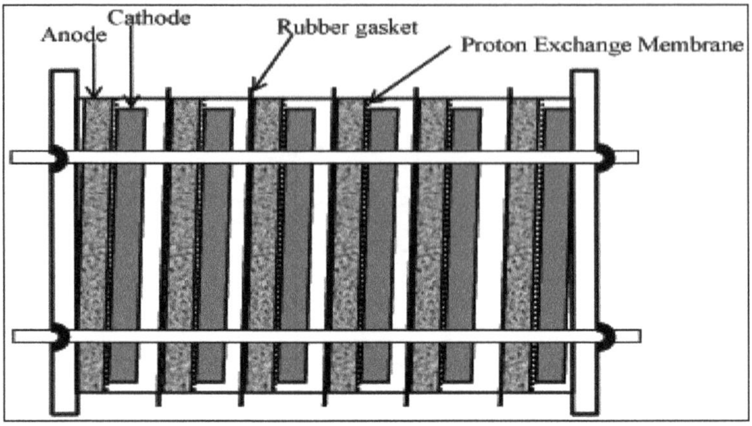

Figure 11.7: Model Representation for Stacked MFC.
This representative model shows the stack of six individual MFC units. Each MFC unit consisting of anode and cathode, separated by cation exchange membrane.

Components Associated with Performance

The major concern in the development of MFC's is the generation of energy *i.e.* power output in a reasonable utilizable amount. Different components of MFCs are responsible for the performance of MFC. The parameters like MFC design, electrode material, the metabolic properties of microorganisms, particularly the paths and mechanisms of biochemical energy conversion and the redox potential (Schroder, 2007) contribute significantly in the performance of MFC. The power generation of an MFC is also affected by many factors including the operating conditions like microbe type, fuel biomass type and concentration, ionic strength, pH, temperature and reactor configuration (Liu *et al.*, 2005b).

Ideal and Actual Performance of MFC

The ideal performance of MFC depends on the electrochemical reactions that occur between the organic substrate at low potential such as glucose and the final electron acceptor with a high potential such as oxygen (Rabaey and Verstraete 2005). The electrode reactions for various types of MFCs and their corresponding redox potentials of those substrates involved in electrode reactions (Madigan *et al.*, 2000, Hernandez and Newman, 2001, Straub *et al.*, 2001, Rabaey and Verstraete, 2005) are presented in Table 11.1. The ideal potentials of MFCs can be calculated by the Nernst equation that relates the standard reduction potential ($E°$) to the reduction potential (E) at any concentration of oxidized and reduced species in the cell (equation 6). For these reactions it ranges from several hundred mV to over 1000mV. Since the biochemical rate and mechanism of electron generation and its further transfer to the anode varies among the microbes and also under different growth conditions, there is always a possibility of variation in the voltage generation. The actual cell potential is always lower than its equilibrium potential because of irreversible losses. The equation 7 reflects various irreversible losses in actual MFC, where $\eta_{act,c}$ and $\eta_{act,a}$ are activation polarization losses on the cathode and anode respectively (Appleyby

Table 11.1: The Electrode Reactions for Various Types of MFCs and the Corresponding Redox Potentials

Oxidation/Reduction Pairs	*E° (mV)*
H^+/H_2	–420
$NAD^+/NADH$	–320
S^0/HS^-	–270
SO_4^{2-}/H_2S	–220
$Pyruvate^{2-}/Lactate^{2-}$	–185
2,6-AQDS/2,6-AHQDS	–184
$FAD/FADH_2$	–180
Menaquinione ox/red	–75
Pyocyanin ox/red	–34
Humic substances ox/red (Straub *et al.*, 2001)	–200 to +300
Methylene blue ox/red	+11
$Fumarate^{2-}/Succinate^{2-}$	+31
Thionine ox/red	+64
Cytochrome b(Fe^{3+})/Cytochrome b(Fe^{2+})	+75
Fe(III) EDTA/Fe(II) EDTA	+96
Ubiquinone ox/red	+113
Cytochrome c(Fe^{3+})/Cytochrome c(Fe^{2+})	+254
O_2/H_2O_2	+275
Fe(III) citrate/Fe(II) citrate	+372
Fe(III) NTA/Fe(II) NTA	+385
NO_3^-/NO_2^-	+421
$Fe(CN)_6^{3-}/Fe(CN)_6^{4-}$	+430
NO_2^-/NH_4^+	+440
O_2/H_2O	+820

Abbreviations: 2,6-AQDS: Anthraquinone 2,6 disulphonate; 2,6-AHQDS: Anthrahydroquinone 2,6 disulphonate; FAD: Ferredoxine adenosine dinucleotide; EDTA: Ethylene diamine tetraacetic acid.

and Foulkes, 1989). $\eta_{conc,c}$ and $\eta_{conc,a}$ are concentration polarization in cathodic and anodic chambers, respectively. Ohmic losses η_{ohm} occur because of resistance to the flow of ions in the electrolyte and resistance to flow of electrons through the electrode. Since both the electrolyte and the electrodes obey Ohm's law, it can be expressed as iR_i, in which i is the current flowing through the MFC, and R_i is the total cell internal resistance of the MFC.

$$E = E^o + \frac{RT}{nF} \ln \frac{[\text{Electron acceptor}]}{[\text{Electron donor}]} \tag{6}$$

$$V_{cell} = E_{cathode} - |\eta_{act,c} + \eta_{conc,c}| - E_{anode} - |\eta_{act,a} + \eta_{conc,a}| - iR_i \tag{7}$$

Electrode Material

For better performance of MFCs selection of the electrode material plays an important role since different anode materials result in different activation polarization losses. The anodic material and its structure can directly affect bacteria attachment, electron transfer and substrate oxidation. The choice of anodic materials depends on their conductivity, biocompatibility and chemical stability in the reactor solution. Various materials such as non-corrosive stainless steel mesh, compact graphite plates, rods, granules, fibrous materials, glassy carbon, platinum and platinum black have been used as anodes due to their stability in microbial mixture, high conductivity and high specific surface area (Tanisho *et al.*, 1989). The carbon electrodes are highly versatile and are available as compact graphite plates, rods, or granules, as fibrous material (felt, cloth, paper, fibers, foam), and as glassy carbon. The simplest materials for anode electrodes are graphite plates or rods as they are inexpensive, easy to handle, and have a defined surface area (Logan *et al.*, 2006). Platinum and platinum black electrodes are superior to graphite, graphite felt and carbon-cloth electrodes for both anode and cathode constructions, but are comparatively expensive (Ringeinsen *et al.*, 2007). One drawback of using Pt or Pt black electrodes is that their activities are reduced by the formation of a PtO layer at the electrode surface at positive potentials (Dam and Bruijn, 2007).

A breakthrough is needed in creating inexpensive electrodes that resist fouling (Du *et al.*, 2007). In an attempt to improve the MFC performance in order to increase the current density output, the electrode modifications were investigated by several research groups. Use of modified graphite along with immobilized neutral red has increased the current density of an *E. coli* MFC from 1.41µA/cm^2 to 3.1µA/cm^2 (Park *et al.*, 2000). An increase of 100-folds in current output by using NR-woven graphite and Mn (IV) graphite anode compared to the woven graphite anode alone has also been reported (Park and Zeikus, 2002, 2003). NR and Mn(IV) served as mediators in their MFC reactors. Schroder *et al.* (2003) investigated the function of a polyaniline overlay on a Pt black anode. Their current density increased from 0.84 mA^{-1} cm^{-2} with Pt black anode to 1.45 mA^{-1} cm^{-2} with a polyaniline coated Pt black anode. The fluorinated polyanilines poly (2-fluoroaniline) and poly (2,3,5,6-tetrafluoroaniline) are reported to be comparatively superior than polyaniline as electrode modifiers due to their protection effect from becoming poisoned by metabolic by-products (Niessen *et al.*, 2004b, 2006). These conductive polymers form a redox active biocompatible layer that serves as dissolved mediators due to their structural similarities to conventional redox mediators (Schroder *et al.*, 2003). A maximum power density of 42mW/m^2 has been reported when used carbon nanotubes (CNT), with the addition of polyaniline (PANI) as an anode electrode in an *E. coli* microbial fuel cell (Qiao *et al.*, 2007).

Other oxygen cathodes made of materials as iron(II) phthalocyanine (FePc) and cobalt tetramethoxyphenylporphyrin (CoTMPP) can also be used as they are inexpensive and are efficient alternatives for use in MFCs because they demonstrate similar performances as Pt oxygen electrodes (Zhao *et al.*, 2005, 2006). In the electrode of the cathode reaction, the power density of the MFC was 379mW/m^2 by adding a platinum cathode and 369mW/m^2 by adding a CoTMPP cathode (Cheng *et al.*, 2006).

The performance of microbial fuel cells can be increased by electrode material modification. Lowy *et al.* (2006) demonstrated the performance of a seafloor microbial fuel cell increased to a power density of 95mW/m^2 when used an AQDS modified graphite electrode with coated manganese ions (Mn^{2+}) and nickel ions (Ni^{2+}). Another modified electrode made of carbon nanotube/polyaniline carbon paper (CNT/PANI carbon paper) executed a larger power density with about 1574mW/m^2 at the condition of voltage being 1.18V and current as 12.8mA (Wang *et al.*, 2013). In addition to the electrode material modification, the contact area of the electrode also affects the performance of the MFC (Logan *et al.*, 2007, Oh and Logan, 2006). Using a carbon brush in an air-cathode MFC for a reaction volume of carbon brush of 9.6×103m^2/m^3 a maximum power density of 2.4×10^3mW/m^2 was produced (Logan *et al.*, 2007).

pH Buffer and Electrolyte

Microbial fuel cells (MFCs) traditionally operate at pH values between 6 and 8. During the operation of the MFCs, the pH may change in the anodic and cathodic chambers, affecting the power output. The possible reasons being the differences in the rate of production and consumption of protons at the anode and cathode respectively. If the reaction rate of proton, electron and oxygen at the cathode equals the production of protons at the anode, theoretically no pH shift should be observed. Whereas, the protons generated at anode need to be transported to cathode through PEM. At the initial stages of MFC operation, the rate of proton transport through the membrane is slower than its production rate in the anode and its consumption rate in the cathode chambers, which results in the pH difference (Gil *et al.*, 2003). However, the pH difference increases the driving force of the proton diffusion from the anode to the cathode chamber and finally a dynamic equilibrium forms. Out of the total pool of protons generated during the biodegradation of the organic substrate some gets transported to the cathodic chamber and are able to react with dissolved oxygen while some remain in the anodic chamber. Gil *et al.* (2003) detected a pH difference of 4.1 (9.5 at cathode and 5.4 in anode) after 5-hour operations with an initial pH of 7 without buffering. With the addition of a phosphate buffer (pH 7.0), pH shifts at the cathode and anode were both less than 0.5 unit and the current output was increased about 1 to 2 folds. The possible reason of increase in current might be the addition of buffer which may compensate the slow proton transport rate and improved the proton availability for the cathodic reaction. Jang *et al.* (2004) supplied an HCl solution to the cathode and found that the current output increased by about one fold. This again suggested that the proton availability to the cathode is a limiting factor in electricity generation. Increasing ionic strength by adding NaCl to MFCs also improves the power output (Jang *et al.*, 2004, Liu *et al.*, 2005b), possibly due to the fact that NaCl enhanced the conductivity of both the anolyte and the catholyte. Tolerance to pH change upto pH 10.0 has been shown in the air cathode design (He *et al.*, 2008). The possible reason of this tolerance may be attributed to the neutralization by the bacterial metabolism which constantly produces weak acids. A current output of more than 14 A/m^2 may be obtained by decreasing the pH of the cathodic compartment to pH 1.0 in an air cathode design (Erable *et al.*, 2009).

Oxygen is the most desirable terminal electron acceptor in MFCs not only for its high standard reduction potential, but also because of practical considerations for environmental deployment (Wang, 2005). Regardless of the catalyst, the electrochemical effects of acidity on oxygen reduction reaction (ORR) will indirectly affect the working potential range (Spendelow and Wieckowski, 2007) of the MFC. According to the Nernst equation, the potential of ORR should shift +59mV for each pH unit in the acidic direction (*i.e.* the driving force for the fuel cell reaction increases with decreasing pH). Decreasing the overall operational pH of a MFC from neutral pH would be a fundamental parameter that could be changed to generate significant increases in current output from MFCs.

Membrane

Cation exchange membranes (CEM) are used as separators in two chambered MFCs comprising an anodic and cathodic compartments. The selection of the membrane is based on its permeability to chemicals such as oxygen, ferricyanide, other ions, or organic matter used as the substrate (Logan *et al.*, 2006). The most commonly used CEM is Nafion™ (Dupont Co., USA). The only limitation to Nafion membrane is its sensitivity to (bio) fouling by ammonium. Alternatively Ultrex CMI-7000 (Membranes International Incorp., Glen Rock, NJ) membranes are also well suited for MFC applications and are considerably more cost-effective than Nafion™ (Rabaey *et al.*, 2004). The market for ion exchange membranes is constantly growing, and more systematic studies are necessary to evaluate the effect of the membrane on performance and long-term stability (Rozendal *et al.*, 2006).

The MFC as a Wastewater Treatment Process

The selection of wastewater treatment is closely related to the standards and/or expectations set for the effluent quality. These processes are designed to achieve improvements in the quality of the wastewater, which is done at three major levels, primary (mechanical), secondary (biological) and tertiary treatment. The secondary treatment process is dependent upon either aerobic or anaerobic biological activities in the bioreactors. From economic point of view it is an energy intensive and expensive process. This call for the investigation and exploration of cost effective technologies that can be accomplished through several strategies including: i) implementing energy efficient equipment and practices, ii) recovering energy during treatment processes, and iii) optimizing treatment methods to minimize overall disposal costs of wastewater effluents and biosolids (sludge). This strategy can be very well adapted through the concept of MFCs by extending the conventional wastewater treatment processes to generation of biofuel. In an aerobic process, microorganisms degrade organic contaminants and utilize all the energy generated in the metabolism for growth and maintenance. This leads to increase in biomass and a large amount of sludge that needs to be disposed of, which is an expensive process. With this respect MFCs has several advantages. In comparison to the aerobic wastewater treatment only a small part of the energy is required by the microorganisms in MFCs for their growth. It generates less excess sludge (almost 50-90 per cent) in a more stable condition than the aerobic treatment process (Holzman, 2005). Moreover the amount of power generated by MFCs in the wastewater treatment process can potentially supplement half of the electricity needed in a conventional treatment process.

The success of specific MFC applications in wastewater treatment depends on the concentration and biodegradability of the organic matter in the influent wastewater and thereby the purity level of the effluent which should meet the standards of the appropriate authorities (Logan *et al.*, 2006). It is for this reason that MFCs should be optimized not only for power generation, but also for the rate of fuel oxidation with the fuel concentration to treat wastewater and efficiency in terms of effluent quality. MFCs have been studied as an alternative energy process using wastewater as a fuel (Kim *et al.*, 2004; Liu *et al.*, 2004; Min and Logan 2004; Min *et al.*, 2005a; Oh and Logan, 2005; Yokoyama *et al.*, 2006; You *et al.*, 2006). It is worth mentioning that an oligotrophic MFC can be operated with a fuel concentration (as BOD value) as low as 5 mg/l (Moon *et al.*, 2005; Phung *et al.*, 2004). As a method of wastewater treatment, it is important to evaluate the overall performance of MFCs in terms of biochemical oxygen demand (BOD), or chemical oxygen demand (COD), or total organic carbon (TOC) removal. COD removal is a common measure of wastewater treatment efficiency, and Coulombic efficiency is a measure of MFC efficiency which is calculated from the COD removal (Logan *et al.*, 2006). The COD removal efficiency can be calculated as the ratio between the removed and influent COD. This parameter measures how much of available fuel has been converted in the MFC, either into electrical current (via Coulombic efficiency) or biomass (via growth yield). MFCs are highly efficient as a biological treatment system at low to moderate loading rates, which can achieve high COD removal, depending on the substrate (Liu and Logan, 2004). The comparative MFC efficiencies with different parameters as MFC design and the substrate used are given in Table 11.2. In some cases removal of COD was found to be up to 80 per cent (Liu *et al.*, 2004) and a Coulombic efficiency as high as 80 per cent (Kim *et al.*, 2005). In addition to easily assimilable organic contaminants, some xenobiotics were also reported to be metabolizable under microbial fuel cell conditions (Jang *et al.*, 2006).

Composition of the wastewater is very important for designing the treatment method. The chemical as well as biological composition of wastewater varies according to the source. Municipal wastewater, sanitary wastes, brewery and food manufacturing wastewater, food processing wastewater, swine wastewater and corn stover are all great biomass sources for MFCs because they are rich in different organic matters that can also serve as fuel to MFCs (Suzuki *et al.*, 1978, Liu *et al.*, 2004, Oh and Logan, 2005, Min *et al.*, 2005b, Zuo *et al.*, 2006). The removal of carbon along with nitrogen and sulfur is essential for wastewater treatment process for which different microbes may be utilized. Carbon compounds are utilized as the nutrients and there by removal of carbon is possible. Denitrification and sulfur removal is also reported through the application of MFC (Rabaey *et al.*, 2006, Clauwaert *et al.*, 2007; Vilar-Sanz *et al.*, 2013). MFCs with specific type of microbes having the ability to remove sulfides as required in wastewater treatment have been reported (Rabaey *et al.*, 2006). Breweries are ideal for the implementation of microbial fuel cells, as their wastewater composition remain always the same. These constant conditions allow bacteria to adapt and become more efficient. Currently, Fosters, an Australian beer

Table 11.2: Efficiency of Wastewater Treatment and Power Output in different Designs of Microbial Fuel Cell

MFC Design	*Substrate*	*Power Output*					*References*
		BOD Removal (per cent)	*COD Removal (per cent)*	*Coulombic Efficiency (per cent)*	*Power Density (mW/m^2)*	*Current (mA/m^2)*	
Single chamber microbial fuel cell (SCMFC)	Acetate, lactate, and glucose	–	80	<12	26	–	Liu *et al.*, 2004
Single chamber microbial fuel cell (SCMFC)	Domestic wastewater	90–95	–	19.1–32	538–766	–	Cheng *et al.*, 2006
Single-chamber MFC without air cathode	Glucose	–	–	11	19	–	Nimje *et al.*, 2012
Single-chamber MFC	Sewage sludge	–	–	–	788	1750	Park and Zeikus, 2003
Single-chamber microbial	Acetate	–	–	3-7	506	2200	Liu *et al.*, 2005a
fuel cell	Butyrate	–	–	2-5	305	770	
Tubular, single-chambered, continuous microbial fuel cell (MFC)	Acetate	–	–	75 ± 5	$90x10^3$ mW/m^3	–	Rabaey *et al.*, 2005b
	Glucose	–	–	59 ± 4	$66\ x10^3$ mW/m^3	–	
	Digester effluent	–	–	–	$59\ x10^3$ mW/m^3	–	
	Domestic wastewater	–	–	–	$48\ x10^3$ mW/m^3	–	
Baffled single-chambered MFC	Artificial glucose wastewater	–	Upto 88	5	133	–	Li *et al.*, 2008
One-chambered MFC	Pre-fermented wastewater	–	–	–	371±10	53.5± 1.4 mA/l	Oh and Logan, 2005
Two-chambered MFC	Cereal wastewater	–	95	–	81±7	25±2 mA/l	Oh and Logan, 2005

Contd...

Table 11.2–*Contd...*

MFC Design	*Substrate*	*Power Output*					*References*
		BOD Removal (per cent)	*COD Removal (per cent)*	*Coulombic Efficiency (per cent)*	*Power Density (mW/m²)*	*Current (mA/m²)*	
Two-chambered MFC	Domestic wastewater. Primary clarifier effluent and anaerobic digester sludge	–	–	80	30–40	–	Kim *et al.*, 2005
Two chambered	Glucose	–	–	7	1.7	–	Jia *et al.*, 2008
Dual-chambered membrane MFC	Yamuna river samples, sucrose	–	–	71–77	220.66	–	Devasahayam and Masih, 2012
Two-chamber system	Glucose (with PEM)	–	–	40–55	262±10	–	Liu and Logan, 2004
	Glucose (without PEM)	–	–	9–12	494±21	–	
	Wastewater (with PEM)	–	–	28	28±3	–	
	Wastewater (without PEM)	–	–	20	146±8	–	
Mediator-less and membrane-less microbial fuel cell (ML-MFC)	Synthetic wastewater and actual sewage	87	88	–	10.9	–	Ghangrekar and Shinde, 2007
Membrane-less Microbial fuel cell	Modified artificial wastewater containing glucose and glutamate	–	90	–	1.3	6–9	Jang *et al.*, 2004
Upflow microbial fuel cell (UMFC)	Artificial wastewater	–	90	0.7–8.1	170	–	He *et al.*, 2005
Closed circuit design	Primary clarifier effluent	–	98	26.5±2.1	640±10	–	Shehab *et al.*, 2013
Hybrid, air-biocathode microbial fuel cell-membrane bioreactor (MFC-MBR)	Pre-filtered domestic wastewater	–	97	–	380	–	Malaeb *et al.*, 2013
Flat plate MFC (FPMFC)	Domestic wastewater	–	42	–	72±1	–	Min and Logan, 2004
Stacked Microbial Fuel Cells	Sterile synthetic Influent containing 0.75–1.00 g/L sodium acetate	–	–	71.6 ± 0.4	258×10^3 mW/m³	–	Aelterman *et al.*, 2006
MFC stack of four cells	–	–	–	–	144×10^3 mW/m³	–	Dekker *et al.*, 2009

company, has begun testing out an MFC to clean its wastewater while generating electricity and clean water (Coates and Wrighten, 2010). Sewage wastewater can also be converted via microbial fuel cells to decompose the waste organic material contained within it. It has been demonstrated that MFCs can reduce (upto 80 per cent) the amount of organic material present in sewage wastewater (Liu *et al.*, 2004).

MFCs have also been used for desalination, which is otherwise a high energy requiring process (Mohankrishna *et al.*, 2010, Luo *et al.*, 2012, Kim and Logan, 2011, Chen *et al.*, 2012a). Capacitive deionization (CDI) technology based MFC have been investigated for desalination of salty water (Yuan *et al.*, 2012, Feng *et al.*, 2013). CDI is an electrochemically controlled method for deionization by the adsorption of ions in the electrical double layer region at an electrode-solution interface that requires a low external power supply. Hence, MFC-CDI has been suggested as the energy saving technology to remove low level dissolved ions from aqueous solutions for the water and wastewater treatment processes (Feng *et al.*, 2013). A hybrid device called microbial electrolysis desalination cell (MEDC), which is a combination of the microbial electrolysis cell and the microbial desalination cell, has been developed to desalinate salty water (Mehanna *et al.*, 2010, Luo *et al.*, 2011, Chen *et al.*, 2012a, b, Zhu and Logan, 2014). However, several factors such as; sharp pH decrease and Cl(-) accumulation in the anode chamber, limit the MEDC development. A hybrid, air-biocathode microbial fuel cell-membrane bioreactor (MFC-MBR) system was suggested for simultaneous wastewater treatment and ultrafiltration to produce water for direct reclamation with removals of 97 per cent of the soluble chemical oxygen demand, 97 per cent NH_3-N, and 91 per cent of total bacteria (Malaeb *et al.*, 2013).

Conclusion

Wastewater composition varies according to its sources. Therefore, for the efficient operation and utilization of microbial fuel cells for wastewater treatment a proper understanding of all of its components including the composition of wastewater is very essential. MFCs are more suitable for low to medium strength wastewater and the treatment time is longer. Hence for the treatment of high strength wastewater the conventional anaerobic digestion treatment process may be adapted for faster processing. Compared to the conventional treatment process the sludge formation would also be reduced. Nitrogen removal and desalination is also performed by MFCs. To achieve the maximum output for BOD or COD removal along with power density appropriate MFC design may be adopted based on the wastewater composition. An extensive research has been done on various aspects of MFCs during past decade, yet its commercialization is still under development. Newer electrochemically active bacterial population may be explored for increasing the efficiency of wastewater treatment and to reduce the time of treatment process. Wastewater treatment process is energy requiring process, whereas MFCs would generate energy, which is helpful in cost reduction of the overall wastewater treatment.

References

Aelterman P, Rabaey K. The Pham H, Boon N, Verstraete W. Continuous Electricity Generation at High Voltages and Currents Using Stacked Microbial Fuel Cells. *Environ. Sci. Technol.* 40: 3388-3394. 2006.

Appleby AJ, Foulkes FR. *Fuel cell handbook.* New York: Van Nostrand Reinhold. 1989.

Arends JBA, Verstraete W. 100 years of microbial electricity production: three concepts for the future. *Microbial Biotech.* 5(3): 333-346. 2012.

Bond DR, Lovley DR. Electricity production by *Geobacter sulfurreducens* attached to electrodes. *Appl. Environ. Microbiol,* 69: 1548-1555. 2003.

Bond DR, Holmes DE, Tender LM, Lovley DR. Electrode-reducing microorganisms that harvest energy from marine sediments. *Science.* 295: 483-485. 2002.

Caccavo F Jr, Lonergan DJ, Lovley DR, Davis M, Stolz JF, McInerney MJ. *Geobacter sulfurreducens* sp. nov., a hydrogen- and acetate-oxidizing dissimilatory metal-reducing microorganism. *Appl. Environ. Microbiol.* 60(10): 3752-3759. 1994.

Chaudhuri SK, Lovley DR. Electricity generation by direct oxidation of glucose in mediatorless microbial fuel cells. *Nat. Biotech.* 21: 1229-1232. 2003.

Chen S, Liu G, Zhang R, Qin B, Luo Y, Hou Y. Improved performance of the microbial electrolysis desalination and chemical-production cell using the stack structure. *Bioresour. Technol.* 116: 507-511. 2012a.

Chen S, Liu G, Zhang R, Qin B, Luo Y. Development of the microbial electrolysis desalination and chemical-production cell for desalination as well as acid and alkali productions. *Environ. Sci. Technol.* 46(4): 2467-72. 2012b.

Cheng S, Liu H, Logan BE. Increased performance of single-chamber microbial fuel cells through an improved cathode structure. *Electrochem. Comm.* 8: 489-494. 2006.

Clauwaert P, Rabaey K, Aelterman P, DeSchamphelaire L, Pham TH, Boeckx P, Boon N, Verstraete W. Biological denitrification in microbial fuel cells. *Environ. Sci. Technol.* 41: 3354-3360. 2007.

Coates JD, Wrighton K. Microbial Fuel Cells: Plug-in and Power-on Microbiology. *Microbe Magazine,* 2010.

Dam VAT, de Bruijn FA. The stability of PEMFC electrodes-Platinum dissolution vs. potential and temperature investigated by quartz crystal microbalance. *J. Electrochem. Soc.* 154: B494-B499. 2007

De Schamphelaire L, Cabezas A, Marzorati M, Friedrich MW, Boon N, *et al.,* Microbial community analysis of anodes from sediment microbial fuel cells powered by rhizodeposits of living rice plants. *Appl. Environ. Microbial.* 76: 2002–2008. 2010.

Dekker A, Heijne AT, Saakes M, Hamelers HVM, Buisman CJN. Analysis and improvement of a scaled-up and stacked microbial fuel cell. *Environ. Sci. Technol.* 43: 9038–9042. 2009.

Devasahayam M, Masih SA. Microbial fuel cells demonstrate high coulombic efficiency applicable for water remediation. *Ind. J. Exptl. Biol.* 50(6): 430-438. 2012.

Du Z, Li H, Gu T. A state of the art review on microbial fuel cells: a promising technology for wastewater treatment and bioenergy. *Biotechnol. Adv.* 25: 464–482. 2007.

Erable B, Etcheverry L, Bergel A. Increased power generation from a two chamber microbial fuel cell with a low-pH air cathode compartment. *Electrochem. Comm.* 11: 619-622. 2009.

Feng C, Hou CH, Chen S, Yu CP. A microbial fuel cell driven capacitive deionization technology for removal of low level dissolved ions. *Chemosphere.* 91: 623–628. 2013.

Ghangrekar MM, Shinde VB. Performance of membrane-less microbial fuel cell treating wastewater and effect of electrode distance and area on electricity production. *Bioresour. Technol.* 98(15): 2879-2885. 2007.

Gil GC, Chang IS, Kim BH, Kim M, *et al.*, Operational parameters affecting the performance of a mediatorless microbial fuel cell. *Biosens. Bioelectron.* 18: 327–334. 2003.

Gorby YA, Yanina S, McLean JS, Rosso KM *et al.*, Electrically conductive bacterial nanowires produced by *Shewanella oneidensis* strain MR-1 and other microorganisms. *PNAS USA.* 103(30): 11358-11363. 2006.

He Z, Huang Y, Manohar AK, Mansfeld F. Effect of electrolyte pH on the rate of the anodic and cathodic reactions in an air–cathode microbial fuel cell. *Bioelectrochem.* 74(1): 78–82. 2008.

He Z, Minteer SD, Angenent LT. Electricity generation from artificial wastewater using an upflow microbial fuel cell. *Environ. Sci. Technol.* 39: 5262–5267. 2005.

Heidelberg JF, Paulsen IT, Nelson KE, Gaidos EJ, *et al.*, Genome sequence of the dissimilatory metal ion-reducing bacterium *Shewanella oneidensis*. *Nat. Biotech.* 20: 1118–1123. 2002.

Hernandez ME, Newman DK. Extracellular electron transfer. *Cell Mol. Life Sci.* 58(11): 1562-1571. 2001.

Holzman DC. Microbe power. *Environ. Health Persp.* 113: A754-A757. 2005.

Ishii S, Suzuki S, Norden-Krichmar TM, Nealson KH, Sekiguchi Y, Gorby YA, Bretschger O. Functionally stable and phylogenetically diverse microbial enrichments from microbial fuel cells during wastewater treatment. *PLoS ONE,* 7(2): e30495. 2012.

Jang JK, Chang IS, Moon H, Kang KH, Kim BH. Nitrilotriacetic acid degradation under microbial fuel cell environment. *Biotechnol. Bioengg.* 95: 772-774. 2006.

Jang JK, Pham TH, Chang IS, Kang KH, *et al.*, Construction and operation of a novel mediator-and membraneless microbial fuel cell. *Process Biochem,* 39: 1007-1012. 2004.

Jia, YH, Tran HT, Kim DH, Oh SJ, Park DH, Zhang RH, Ahn DH. Simultaneous organics removal and bio-electrochemical denitrification in microbial fuel cells. *Bioprocess Biosyst. Engg*. 31: 315-321. 2008.

Katz E, Shipway AN, Willner I. Biochemical fuel cells. In: *Handbook of Fuel Cells – Fundamentals, Technology and Applications* (Vielstich W, Gasteiger HA, Lamm A Eds.), John Wiley and Sons Ltd., New York. p. 1. 2003.

Kim BH, Ikeda T, Park HS, Kim HJ, Hyun MS, Kano K, Takagi K, Tatsumi H. Electrochemical activity of an Fe(III)-reducing bacterium, *Shewanella putrefaciens* IR-1, in the presence of alternative electron acceptors. *Biotechnol. Tech.* 13(7): 475-478. 1999b.

Kim BH, Kim HJ, Hyun MS, Park DH. Direct electrode reaction of Fe (III)-reducing bacterium, *Shewanella putrifaciens*. *J. Microbiol Biotech*. 9: 127-31. 1999a.

Kim BH, Park HS, Kim HJ, Kim GT, Chang IS, Lee J, *et al.*, Enrichment of microbial community generating electricity using a fuel-cell type electrochemical cell. *Appl. Microbiol Biotech*. 63: 672–81. 2004.

Kim JR, Min B, Logan BE. Evaluation of procedures to acclimate a microbial fuel cell for electricity production. *Appl. Microbiol Biotech*. 68: 23-30. 2005.

Kim Y, Logan BE. Series assembly of microbial desalination cells containing stacked electrodialysis cells for partial or complete seawater desalination. *Environ. Sci. Technol*. 45(13): 5840-5845. 2011.

Ledezma P, Greenman J, Ieropoulos I. MFC-cascade stacks maximise COD reduction and avoid voltage reversal under adverse conditions. *Bioresour. Technol*. 134: 158-165. 2013.

Li Z, Yao L, Kong L, Liu Hong. Electricity generation using a baffled microbial fuel cell convenient for stacking. *Bioresour. Tech*. 99(6): 1650-1655. 2008.

Liu H, Logan BE. Electricity generation using an air-cathode single chamber microbial fuel cell in the presence and absence of a proton exchange membrane. *Environ. Sci. Technol*. 38: 4040-4046. 2004.

Liu H, Cheng S, Logan BE. Power generation in fed-batch microbial fuel cells as a function of ionic strength, temperature, and reactor configuration. *Environ. Sci. Technol*. 39(14): 5488-5493. 2005b

Liu H, Cheng S, Logan BE. Production of electricity from acetate or butyrate using a single-chamber microbial fuel cell. *Environ. Sci. Technol*. 39: 658–62. 2005a

Liu H, Ramnarayanan R, Logan BE. Production of electricity during wastewater treatment using a single chamber microbial fuel cell. *Environ. Sci. Technol*. 28: 2281-2285. 2004.

Logan BE, Cheng S, Watson V, Estadt G. Graphite fiber brush anodes for increased power production in air-cathode microbial fuel cells. *Environ. Sci. Technol*. 41: 3341-3346. 2007.

Logan BE, Hamelers B, Rozendal R, Schroder U, Keller J, Verstraete W, Rabaey K. Microbial fuel cells: methodology and technology. *Environ. Sci. Technol.* 40: 5181-5192. 2006.

Logan BE. Extracting hydrogen and electricity from renewable resources. *Environ Sci. Technol.* 38: 160a-167a. 2004.

Lowy DA, Tender LM, Zeikus JG, Park DH, Lovley DR. Harvesting energy from the marine sediment-water interface II – Kinetic activity of anode materials. *Biosens. Bioelectron.* 21: 2058-2063. 2006.

Luo H, Jenkins PE, Ren Z. Concurrent desalination and hydrogen generation using microbial electrolysis and desalination cells. *Environ. Sci. Technol.* 45: 340–344. 2011.

Luo H, Xu P, Ren Z. Long-term performance and characterization of microbial desalination cells in treating domestic wastewater. *Bioresour. Technol.* 120. 187–193. 2012.

Madigan MT, Martinko JM, Parker J. *Brock biology of microorganisms*. Upper Saddle River: Prentice Hall, 2000.

Malaeb L, Katuri KP, Logan BE, Maab H, Nunes SP, Saikaly PE. A hybrid microbial fuel cell membrane bioreactor with a conductive ultrafiltration membrane biocathode for wastewater treatment. *Environ. Sci. Technol.* 47: 11821–11828. 2013.

McKinley JB, Zeikus JG. Extracellular iron reduction is mediated in part by neutral red and hydrogenase in *Escherichia coli*. *Appl. Environ. Microbiol.* 70(6): 3467-3474. 2004.

Mehanna M, Saito T, Jingling Y, Hickner MA, Cao X, Huang X, Logan BE. Using microbial desalination cells to reduce water salinity prior to reverse osmosis. *Energy Environ. Sci.* 3(8): 1114–1120. 2010.

Methe BA, Nelson KE, Eisen JA, Paulsen IT, Nelson W, Heidelberg JF, Wu D, Wu M, Ward N, Beanan MJ *et al.*, The genome of Geobacter sulfurreducens: insights into metal reduction in subsurface environments. *Science*. 302: 1967-1969. 2003

Meyer TE, Tsapin AI, Vandenberghe I, de Smet L, Frishman D, Nealson KH, Cusanovich MA, van Beeumen JJ. Identifiaction of 42 possible cytochrome c genes in the *Shewanella oneidensis* genome and characterization of six soluble cytochromes. *OMICS*. 8: 57-77. 2004.

Min B, Logan BE. Continuous electricity generation from domestic wastewater and organic substrates in a flat plate microbial fuel cell. *Environ. Sci. Technol* 38: 5809-5814. 2004.

Min B, Cheng S, Logan BE. Electricity generation using membrane and salt bridge microbial fuel cells. *Water Res.* 39: 1675-1686. 2005a.

Min B, Kim JR, Oh SE, Regan JM, Logan BE. Electricity generation from swine wastewater using microbial fuel cells. *Water Res.* 39: 4961-4968. 2005b.

Mohanakrishna G, Venkata Mohan S, Sarma PN. Bio-electrochemical treatment of distillery wastewater in microbial fuel cell facilitating decolorization and desalination along with power generation. *J. Hazard Mater.* 177: 487-494. 2010.

Moon H, Chang IS, Jang JK, Kim KS, Lee J, Lovitt RW, Kim BH. On-line monitoring of low biochemical oxygen demand through continuous operation of a mediator-less microbial fuel cell. *J. Microbiol. Biotech.* 15: 192-196. 2005.

Moon H, Chang IS, Kang KH, Jang JK, Kim BH. Improving the dynamic response of a mediator-less microbial fuel cell as a biochemical oxygen demand (BOD) sensor. *Biotech. Lett.* 26: 1717-1721. 2004.

Niessen J, Harnisch F, Rosenbaum M, Schroder U, Scholz F. Heat treated soil as convenient and versatile source of bacterial communities for microbial electricity generation. *Electrochem. Comm.* 8: 869-873. 2006.

Niessen J, Schroder U, Scholz F. Exploiting complex carbohydrates for microbial electricity generation – a bacterial fuel cell operating on starch. *Electrochem. Comm.* 6(9): 955-958. 2004a.

Niessen J, Schroder U, Rosenbaum M, Scholz F. Fluorinated polyanilines as superior materials for electrocatalytic anodes in bacterial fuel cells. *Electrochem. Comm.* 6: 571-575. 2004b.

Nimje VR, Chen CY, Chen HR, Chen CC, Huang YM, Tseng MJ, Cheng KC, Chang YF. Comparative bioelectricity production from various wastewaters in microbial fuel cells using mixed cultures and a pure strain of *Shewanella oneidensis*. *Bioresour. Technol.*104: 315-323. 2012.

Oh SE, Logan BE. Hydrogen and electricity production from a food processing wastewater using fermentation and microbial fuel cell technologies. *Water Res.* 39: 4673-4682. 2005.

Oh SE, Logan BE. Proton exchange membrane and electrode surface areas as factors that affect power generation in microbial fuel cells. *Appl. Microbiol. Biotech.* 70: 162-169. 2006.

Oh SE, Logan BE. Voltage reversal during microbial fuel cell stack operation. *J. Power Sources.* 167: 11-17. 2007.

Park DH, Kim BH. Growth properties of the iron-reducing bacteria, *Shewanella putrefaciens* IR-1 and MR-1 coupling to reduction of Fe(III) to Fe(II). *J. Microbiol.* 39: 273-278. 2001.

Park DH, Zeikus JG. Impact of electrode composition on electricity generation in a single-compartment fuel cell using *Shewanella putrefaciens*. *Appl. Microbiol. Biotech.* 59: 58–61. 2002.

Park DH, Zeikus JG. Improved fuel cell and electrode designs for producing electricity from microbial degradation. *Biotech. Bioengg.* 81: 348-355. 2003.

Park DH, Zeikus JG. Utilization of electrically reduced neutral red by *Actinobacillus succinogenes*: physiological function of neutral red in membrane-driven fumarate reduction and energy conservation. *J. Bacteriol.* 181: 2403-2410. 1999.

Park DH, Kim SK, Shin IH, Jeong YJ. Electricity production in biofuel cell using modified graphite electrode with Neutral Red. *Biotech. Lett.* 22: 1301-1304. 2000.

Park HS, Kim BH, Kim HS, Kim HJ, Kim GT, Kim M, *et al.*, A novel electrochemically active and Fe(III)-reducing bacterium phylogenetically related to *Clostridium butyricum* isolated from a microbial fuel cell. *Anaerobe,* 7: 297-306. 2001.

Park TJ, Ding W, Cheng S, Brar MS, Ma APY, Tun HM, Leung FC. Microbial community in microbial fuel cell (MFC) medium and effluent enriched with purple photosynthetic bacterium (Rhodopseudomonas sp.) *AMB Express.* 4: 22. 2014.

Pham CA, Jung SJ, Phung NT, Lee J, Chang IS, Kim BH, *et al.*, A novel electrochemically active and Fe(III)-reducing bacterium phylogenetically related to *Aeromonas hydrophila,* isolated from a microbial fuel cell. *FEMS Microbiol. Lett.* 223: 129–34. 2003.

Phung NT, Lee J, Kang KH, Chang IS, Gadd GM, Kim BH. Analysis of microbial diversity in oligotrophic microbial fuel cells using 16SrDNAsequences. *FEMS Microbiol. Lett.* 233: 77-82. 2004.

Qiao Y, Li CM, Bao SJ, Bao QL. Carbon nanotube/polyaniline composite as anode material for microbial fuel cells. *J. Power Sources.* 170: 79-84. 2007.

Rabaey K, Verstraete W. Microbial fuel cells: novel biotechnology for energy generation. *Trends Biotech.* 23: 291-298. 2005.

Rabaey K, Boon N, Hofte M, Verstraete W. Microbial phenazine production enhances electron transfer in biofuel cells. *Environ. Sci. Technol.* 39(9): 3401-3408. 2005a.

Rabaey K, Boon N, Siciliano, SD, Verhaege M, Verstraete W. Biofuel cells select for microbial consortia that self-mediate electron transfer. *Appl. Environ. Microbiol.* 70: 5373–5382. 2004.

Rabaey K, Clauwaert P, Aelterman P, Verstraete W. Tubular microbial fuel cells for efficient electricity generation. *Environ. Sci. Technol.* 39(20): 8077-8082. 2005b.

Rabaey K, Van De Sompel K, Maignien L, Boon N, Aelterman P, Clauwaert P, *et al.*, Microbial fuel cells for sulfide removal. *Environ. Sci. Technol.* 40: 5218-5224. 2006.

Reguera G, McCarthy KD, Mehta T, Nicoll JS, Tuominen MT, Lovley DR. Extracellular electron transfer via microbial nanowires. *Nature.* 435: 1098-1101. 2005.

Rezaei F, Xing D, Wagner R, Regan JM, Richard TL, Logan BE. Simultaneous cellulose degradation and electricity production by *Enterobacter cloacae* in a microbial fuel cell. *Appl. Environ. Microbiol.* 75(11): 3673-3678. 2009.

Ringeisen BR, Henderson E, Wu PK, Pietron J, Ray R, Little B, *et al.*, High power density from a miniature microbial fuel cell using *Shewanella oneidensis* DSP10. *Environ. Sci. Technol.* 40: 2629-2634. 2006.

Ringeisen BR, Ray R, Little B. A miniature microbial fuel cell operating with an aerobic anode chamber. *J. Power Sources.* 165: 591-597. 2007.

Rozendal RA, Hamelers HVM, Buisman CJN. Effects of membrane cation transport on pH and microbial fuel cell performance. *Environ. Sci. Technol.* 40: 5206-5211. 2006.

Schroder U, Nieben J, Scholz F. A generation of microbial fuel cells with current outputs boosted by more than one order of magnitude. *Angew. Chem. Intl. Ed.* 42: 2880-2883. 2003.

Schroder U. Anodic electron transfer mechanisms in microbial fuel cells and their energy efficiency. *Phys. Chem.* 9: 2619-2629. 2007.

Shehab N, Li D, Amy GL, Logan BE, Saikaly PE. Characterization of bacterial and archaeal communities in air-cathode microbial fuel cells, open circuit and sealed-off reactors. *Appl. Microbiol. Biotech.* 97(22): 9885-9895. 2013.

Spendelow JS, Wieckowski A. Electrocatalysis of oxygen reduction and small alcohol oxidation in alkaline media. *Phys. Chem.* 9: 2654-2675. 2007.

Srikanth S, Marsili E, Flickinger MC, Bond DR. Electrochemical characterization of *Geobacter sulfurreducens* cells immobilized on graphite paper electrodes. *Biotech. Bioengg.* 99(5): 1065–1073. 2007.

Straub KL, Benz M, Schink B. Iron metabolism in anoxic environments at near neutral pH. *FEMS Microbiol. Ecol.* 34(3): 181-186. 2001.

Strik DPBTB, Timmers RA, Helder M, Steinbusch KJJ, Hamelers HVM, Buisman CJN. Microbial solar cells: applying photosynthetic and electrochemically active organisms. *Trends Biotech.* 29(1): 41-49. 2011.

Suzuki S, Karube I, Matsunaga T. Application of a biochemical fuel cell to wastewater. *Biotech. Bioengg. Symp.* 8: 501-511. 1978.

Tanisho S, Kamiya N, Wakao N. Hydrogen evolution of *Enterobacter aerogens* depending on culture pH: mechanism of hydrogen evolution from NADH by means of membrane bound hydrogenase. *Biochem. Biophys. Acta.* 973: 1-6. 1989.

Vandevivere P, Verstraete W. Environmental applications. In: *Basic Biotechnology* (Ratledge C., Kristiansen B. Eds), Cambridge University Press. p. 531-557. 2001.

Vilar-Sanz A, Puig S, Garcia-Lledo A, Trias R, Balaguer MD, Colprim J, Baneras L. Denitrifying bacterial communities affect current production and nitrous oxide accumulation in a microbial fuel cell. *PLoS One.* 8: e63460. 2013.

Wang B. Recent development of non-platinum catalysts for oxygen reduction reaction. *J. Power Sources.* 152: 1-15. 2005.

Wang CT, Huang RY, Lee YC, Zhang CD. Electrode material of carbon nanotube/polyaniline carbon paper applied in microbial fuel cells. *J. Clean Energy Technol.* 1: 206-210. 2013.

Wilkinson S. Gastrobots: benefits and challenges of microbial fuel cells in food powered robot applications. *Auton. Robot.* 9: 99-111. 2000.

Xing D, Ren N, Rittmann BE. Genetic diversity of hydrogen-producing bacteria in an acidophilic Ethanol-H_2-Coproducing system, analyzed using the [Fe]-Hydrogenase gene. *Appl. Environ. Microbiol.* 74: 1232-1239. 2008.

Yang TH, Coppi MV, Lovley DR, Sun J. Metabolic response of *Geobacter sulfurreducens* towards electron donor/acceptor variation. *Microbial Cell Factories*. 9: 90. 2010.

Yokoyama H, Ohmori H, Ishida H, Waki M, Tanaka Y. Treatment of cow-waste slurry by a microbial fuel cell and the properties of the treated slurry as liquid manure. *Animal Sci. J.* 77: 634-638. 2006.

You SJ, Zhao QL, Jiang JQ, Zhang JN, Zhao SQ. Sustainable approach for leachate treatment: electricity generation in microbial fuel cell. *J. Environ Sci. Health, Part A: Environ Sci. Engg. Toxic Hazard Substance Control*, 41: 2721-2734. 2006.

Yuan L, Yang X, Liang P, Wang L, Huang ZH, Wei J, Huang X. Capacitive deionization coupled with microbial fuel cells to desalinate low concentration salt water. *Bioresour. Technol.* 110: 735-738. 2012.

Zhang E, Xu W, Diao G, Shuang C. Electricity generation from acetate and glucose by sedimentary bacterium attached to electrode in microbial-anode fuel cells. *J. Power Sources*. 161: 820-825. 2006.

Zhao F, Harnisch F, Schroder U, Scholz F, Bogdanoff P, Herrmann I. Application of pyrolysed iron(II) phthalocyanine and CoTMPP based oxygen reduction catalysts as cathode materials in microbial fuel cells. *Electrochem. Comm.* 7: 1405-1410. 2005.

Zhao F, Harnisch F, Schroder U, Scholz F, Bogdanoff P, Herrmann I. Challenges and constraints of using oxygen cathodes in microbial fuel cells. *Environ. Sci. Technol.* 40(17): 5193-5199. 2006.

Zhu X, Logan BE. Microbial electrolysis desalination and chemical-production cell for CO_2 sequestration. *Bioresour. Technol.* 159: 24-29. 2014.

Zuo Y, Maness PC, Logan BE. Electricity production from steam exploded corn stover biomass. *Energy Fuel*. 20: 1716-1721. 2006.

2016, Biotechnological Tools for Genetic Resources *Pages* 373–405
Editor: Pradip Chandra Deka
Published by: Daya Publishing House, NEW DELHI

Chapter 12

Female Genital Tuberculosis and its Relationship with Infertility

Venkanna Bhanothu* and Jane P. Theophilus

Department of Zoology, Osmania University, Hyderabad – 500 007, Telengana
**E-mail: banothu.venkanna@gmail.com*

ABSTRACT

Female Genital Tuberculosis (FGTB) which is commonly implicated as a cause of infertility is a symptom-less, rare disease with non-specific, mild clinical pictures and low index of clinical suspicion. Genital tuberculosis (GTB) represents an uncommon form of extra pulmonary tuberculosis (TB) and remains a major health problem in developing countries. There are no reliable confirmatory investigative procedures to ascertain the cause of infertility. Demonstration of the etiologic agent by Hematoxylin and Eosin (H and E) staining or Ziehl-Neelsen's (Z-N) staining for acid fast bacilli (AFB), smear microscopy and culture of sputum and other body fluid specimens were often not possible. Inefficacy of costly tests and negligence has resulted in the disease often not being diagnosed. Early detection of the disease and development of inexpensive methods are of current importance. The review attempts to summarize the information available on examinations and procedures necessary for the early, cost effective and sensitive diagnosis of infection and disease. Molecular biology techniques continue to evolve rapidly, and many laboratories have been reluctant to introduce these new methods due to concerns that the technology would become outda ted. In consequence, the vast majority of clinical bacteriology laboratories do not currently use any molecular diagnostics, although such technology is becoming more widespread in specialized regional laboratories, as well as in national reference laboratories. Presently, molecular biology offers a wide repertoire of techniques and permutations. Recently, important advances have been achieved in these fields that have led to substantial improvements in the accuracy and the timing of the diagnosis of FGTB. The review brings out the importance of multigene/multi PCR and allow for a better identification of latently infected individuals who are at risk of developing active tuberculosis, they also offer the possibility for a rapid diagnosis of active tuberculosis in infertile patients. Compared to Z–N staining and culturing on L-J media, multi-gene/multi primer PCR improved the detection rate of suspected FGTB where the estimated cost and time of diagnosis are marginal. FGTB can be diagnosed if multi-gene PCR is considered in the evaluation of infertile patients in areas where tuberculosis is endemic. Site specific sampling, irrespective of sample type and amplification of the 19-kDa antigen gene in combination with TRC4 element as a successful multi-gene PCR for the diagnosis of FGTB and differentiation of mycobacteria infection among endo-ovarian tissue biopsies and PAFs taken from infertile women are suggested.

Keywords: *Female genital tuberculosis, Diagnosis of FGT, Multi-gene/multi-primer PCR Infertility, Vaccination.*

Introduction

Tuberculosis (TB) is an ancient communicable disease which is still one of the biggest killers among infectious diseases, despite the worldwide use of a live attenuated vaccine and several antibiotics. TB can also affect female reproductive health and is a diagnostic challenge. It was in the middle of 18th Century that tuberculous gynaecological manifestations received attention when Morgagni (the famous morbid anatomist) described the signs of genital tuberculosis (GTB) in women. In 1744, the first case of genital TB was reported (Morgagni, 1744), following a postmortem examination of a 20-year-old woman who died of TB, whose uterus and fallopian tubes were found to be filled with caseous material. In 1847, Kiwish first described a case of tuberculosis of uterus. The manifestations of tuberculosis in gynaecology were published as a monograph by Hagar in 1886 (Broune and Willium, 1962). The clinical interest of gynaecologists was aroused after the accidental finding of tuberculous lesions, by Sutherland in 1943 (Broune and Willium, 1962), in specimens of endometrium, obtained during routine investigations for sterility and menstrual disorders. Since the beginning of the 20th century, the incidence of TB in general and GTB in particular has been steadily declining in developed countries but remains a major health problem in many developing countries, where, GTB is responsible for a significant proportion of females presenting primary and secondary infertility. In addition to infertility TB also gives rise to a number of sequalaes including chronic pelvic pain, menstrual disturbances, postmenopausal bleeding (Neonakis *et al.*, 2011), pelvic adhesions, pelvic masses, amenorrhea, irregular vaginal discharge, an adnexal lump and fever (Namavar *et al.*, 2001, Tripathy and Tripathy 2002, Gatongi *et al.*, 2005; Ali and Abdallah, 2012). However none of these are specific for GTB (Singh *et al.*, 2008, Sharma *et al.*, 2009). Therefore, GTB is called "the great pretender" because it resembles the presentation of advanced ovarian carcinoma (Botha and van der Merwe, 2008) and it lead to various complications like abortions, low conception rates, increase incidences of ectopic pregnancy and miscarriages. It generates worrying effects, causing irreversible damage to the fallopian tube with potential consequences of causing infertility and making it untreatable both by medical and surgical methods (Varma, 1991).

Female genital tuberculosis (FGTB) a chronic disease, often has a low-grade symptomatology with very few specific complaints. The worldwide incidence of infertility in GTB varies from 10-87 per cent (Namavar *et al.*, 2001, Tripathy and Tripathy 2002), being highly endemic in India (Gupta *et al.*, 2007), with an incidence of 58 per cent (Dam *et al.*, 2006) and majority of the patients in the reproductive age group (15–45 years) (Parikh *et al.*, 1997). The disease is responsible for 5 per cent of all female pelvic infections and occurs in 15-20 per cent cases of extra pulmonary tuberculosis (EPTB) (Saraswat *et al.*, 2010). In 80-90 per cent cases, it affects women with menstrual irregularities accounting for about 27 per cent of manifestations of FGTB (Chakrabarti *et al.*, 1998). The pathogenicity and mechanism of host response to FGTB is very controversial and still unclear. The bacilli reach the genital tract by three principal routes. The initial invasion occurs with a few bacilli which slowly colonize and multiply locally without causing many symptoms. Primary infection of the genitalia may rarely occur from direct inoculation during sexual intercourse (Gatongi *et al.*, 2005) with an infected partner suffering from tuberculous lesions of the genitalia (Angus *et al.*, 2001). Once the genital tract is colonized, granulomata containing viable tubercle bacilli form within various pelvic organs. Granulomas are compact, organized aggregates of immune cells consisting of blood-derived infected and uninfected macrophages, foamy macrophages, epithelioid cells (uniquely differentiated macrophages), and multinucleated giant cells (Langerhans cells) surrounded by a ring of lymphocytes. The tuberculosis lesions are highly dynamic and shaped by both, immune response elements and the pathogen (Figure 12.1). This co-evolutionary perspective emphasizes the mutual shaping of the tissue microenvironment, which, at the same time, allows propagation and transmission of *Mycobacterium tuberculosis*, yet restricts tissue damage to safeguard survival of the host. After the development of tubercular hypersensitivity, these generally become clinically silent for 1–10 years or even longer before infection in this location is reactivated or becomes clinically manifested, if symptoms occur at all (Simon *et al.*, 1977). It is known that tuberculous foci may exist in the body and remain undetected for a long time. It usually remains silent and physical signs are usually not present, hence the disease remains largely undiagnosed or specific investigations are not undertaken to rule out the problem.

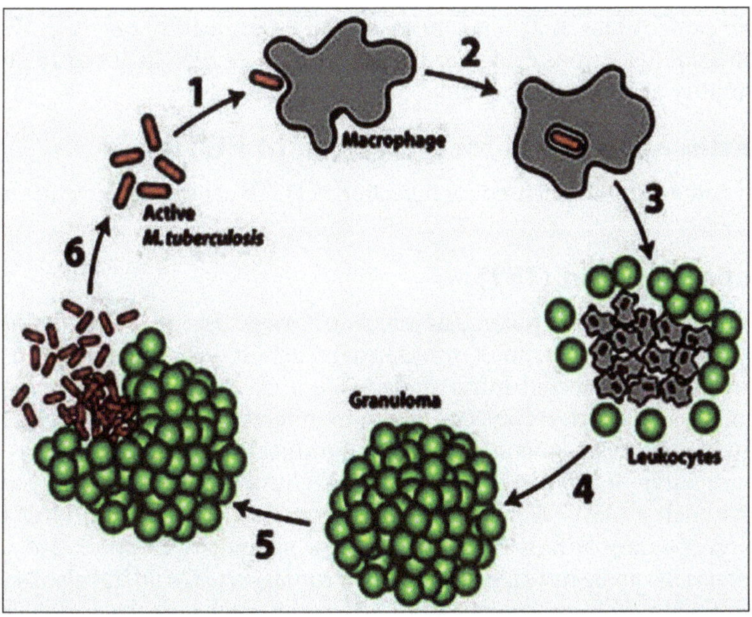

Figure 12.1: Recycling and Re-activation of Tuberculosis Infection.

Once an active disease is established, irreversible tubal and endometrial damage can occur. However, during the pre-clinical stage, an insidious, low-grade inflammation is quite likely to alter the function of fallopian tubes, uterus and of the endometrium which leads to subtle damage and functional loss of the uterus and the tubes. The signs, symptoms and altered immune responses of FGTB patients mimic those of immuno-suppressed individuals, so diagnostic awareness may prevent unnecessary treatment and morbidity (Eastwood *et al.*, 2001). Literature on female genital tuberculosis (FGTB) is presented in Table 12.1

FGTB and Infertility

FGTB is major cause of infertility and is multifaceted condition with a myriad of causes, diagnosis and treatment. The incidence of female infertility is rising and varies from 10 to 20 per cent (Romero Ramos *et al.*, 2008). If the occurrence of mycobacterial infection coincides with puberty, primary infertility is caused while if infection occurs later in life, secondary infertility is seen. In earlier studies, infertility was reported in 44 per cent of patients with genital tuberculosis, pelvic pain in 25 per cent, leucorrhoea in about 5 per cent of cases, and abnormal vaginal bleeding in 18 per cent cases and post-menopausal bleeding in 2 per cent of patients presenting with genital tuberculosis. Rare symptoms included an abdominal mass or unexplained ascites. Most cases of confirmed genital tuberculosis had perfectly normal clinical examination (43 per cent) and about a quarter of cases presented with an adnexal mass (23.6 per cent). Tripathy and Tripathy, (1998) observed primary and secondary infertility in 58 per cent cases, pelvic pain in 18 per cent and leucorrhoea in 26 per cent of the cases. The predominant menstrual symptom noted was secondary amenorrhea in 43 per cent cases followed by menorrhagia in 17 per cent cases and oligomenorrhea in 11 per cent cases. The most significant signs were pelvic mass in 21 per cent cases and an unhealthy cervix in 17 per cent cases. Tuberculous lesions elsewhere in the body were seen in about 18 per cent of cases (Tripathy and Tripathy, 1998).

Conventional Methods for Detection of FGTB

Conventional methods used for detection of FGTB are described in the following section.

Tuberculin Skin Test (TST)

The diagnosis of latent tubercular infection is made using the Tuberculin reaction test, also known as the Mantoux intradermal reaction. When the purified proteins derivative (PPD) is injected intracutaneously, a classic delayed hypersensitivity reaction occurs in infected subjects, which manifests in vivo as a dermal infiltrate and subsequent measurement of the size of induration. The intradermal reaction may be indicative of a positive PPD reaction. Unfortunately, the TST has several limitations such as low sensitivity, antigenic cross-reactivity resulting from the distribution of many antigens in BCG and low specificity (Siddiqi *et al.*, 2003). A positive reaction can be indicative not only of contact with MTB but also of previous vaccination with BCG or contact with environmental mycobacteria. Therefore, one cannot differentiate active from latent TB, BCG vaccination or infection

Table 12.1: Literature on Female Genital Tuberculosis (FGTB)

Research Data Bases/ Phrase Used for Collecting the Literature	*"Female Genital Tuberculosis"*	*"Molecular Immunology of Female Genital Tuberculosis"*	*"Evaluation of Molecular and Immunological Profile of FGTB"*	*"Molecular Profile of FGTB"*	*"immunological Profile of FGTB"*	*"Use of Genetic Material in the Detection of FGTB"*
PubMed: biomedical literature citations and abstracts	2436	4	nil	nil	nil	nil
PubMed Central: free, full text journal articles	2648	213	43	78	64	4
Books: online books	27	2	1	2	1	4271
dbGaP: genotype and phenotype	7	1	1	1	1	100
Clone: integrated data for clone resources	585358	585358	585358	585358	585358	nil
Epigenomics: Epigenetic maps and data sets	323	5	nil	nil	nil	nil
OMIA: online Mendelian Inheritance in Animals	1	nil	nil	nil	nil	133
dbVar: Genomic structural variation	1	1	nil	nil	nil	1
NLM Catalog: catalog of books, journals, and audiovisuals in the NLM collections	66	nil	nil	nil	nil	142
MeSH: detailed information about NLM's controlled vocabulary	1	nil	nil	nil	nil	nil
Google search	501000	53600	73800	844000	857000	1310

with environmental mycobacteria. False positive results may also be caused by repeated tests as a consequence of the boosting effect of continuous sensitization with PPD. TST may be negative in patients with active tuberculosis if the patient has overwhelming clinical disease, or is severely immune compromised or has co-incidental viral infection or is malnourished (Sudre *et al.*, 1996). These limitations of the TST have led to the development of alternative assays.

Interferon Gamma Release Assays

IGRAs measure a person's immune reactivity to *M. tuberculosis*. White blood cells from most persons infected with *M. tuberculosis* release IFN-γ. An individual is considered positive for *M. tuberculosis* infection if the IFN-γ response to TB antigens is above the test cut-off (after subtracting the background IFN-γ response in the negative control). It is used to diagnose latent TB infections (LTBI). Availability of IGRAs is limited by the need for a fresh blood sample and the potential for delays due to long distances from laboratories that offer these tests. TST and IGRAs do not measure the same components of the immunological response and are not interchangeable. Assessment of the accuracy of these tests is limited by lack of a standard for confirming LTBI. The level of concordance is adversely affected by prior BCG vaccination, immune reactivity to nontuberculous mycobacteria, and a prior positive TST (Mazurek *et al.*, 2001). Although there have been studies confirming the increased future risk of active TB in individuals with positive TST, the same was not true for those with a positive IGRA result. In some cases increase in IFN-γ response might be attributed to new infection or boosting following a TST and a decrease in IFN-γ response may be attributed to antimycobacterial treatment. Thus there is currently no accepted, validated biomarker in serology that can detect EPTB or PTB. Therefore, the Indian government banned serological antibody tests in 2012, and Standards for TB Care in India (STCI) and International Standards for TB Care (ISTC) discourage the use of IGRAs for the diagnosis of active TB (ISTC 2014, STCI 2014).

Chest X-Ray and Lung X-Ray

More than 75 per cent of the patients with active, culture-proven genital tuberculosis have a normal chest X-ray and lung X-ray. It is important not to use a chest X-ray and lung plain X-ray as exclusion for the diagnosis of genital tuberculosis (Saracoglu *et al.*, 1992).

Hysterosalpingograms

HSG continues to be an important diagnostic procedure to evaluate infertility in women and is the most helpful procedure in the diagnosis of genital tuberculosis in patients being investigated for infertility. Chavan *et al.* (2004) observed genital TB in 7.5 per cent of the HSGs performed for infertility. The most common features observed in HSGs are isthmo ampullary tubal occlusion (81 per cent), terminal hydrosalpinx (16 per cent), synechiae and intrauterine adhesions (16 per cent) and venous and lymphatic intravasation of dye (27 per cent) (Puri and Bansal, 2009).

Hysterolaparoscopy

A complete examination of a woman's internal pelvic structures can provide important information regarding infertility and common gynaecologic disorders. Laparoscopy and hysteroscopy are two procedures that provide a direct view of the pelvic organs (Tinelli *et al.*, 2008). Diagnostic laparoscopy is recommended to view the outside of the uterus, fallopian tubes, ovaries, and internal pelvic area. Both diagnostic and operative laparoscopy and hysteroscopy are an integral aspect of management of infertility in women.

Histopathological Studies

Haematoxylin and Eosin staining are used for histopathological studies for the reason that it works well with a variety of fixatives and displays a broad range of nuclear, cytoplasmic and extracellular matrix features. Essentially, it recognizes various tissue types and the morphologic changes. Haematoxylin (H) has a deep blue-purple colour and stains nucleic acids by a complex. Eosin (E) is a pink fluorescent red dye that stains proteins non-specifically. It is most commonly used stain for highlighting cytoplasmic materials in samples. In a typical tissue, nuclei are stained blue, and the cytoplasm, collagen, muscle fibers and extracellular matrix stains in varying degrees of pink. If abundant polyribosomes are present, the cytoplasm will have a distinct blue cast. The Golgi zone can be tentatively identified by the absence of staining in a region next to the nucleus. Thus, the stain discloses abundant structural information, with specific functional implications. Diagnosis of FGTB from tissue samples is usually made by histopathological examination (HPE) that depends on the presence of typical tuberculous granulomatous inflammation, lesion, caseous necrosis, caseating granulomas surrounded by giant epithelioid cells with or without Langerhans's giant cells, malignant lymphocytic infiltrations, plasma cells and giant polymorphonuclear cells. It is an easy, quick and cheap method that provides characteristic features of *M. tuberculosis*. However many non- tuberculous lesions can also produce granulomas, mimicking tuberculosis. Particularly, environmental mycobacteria infections such as *M. avium-intercellulare*, may be encountered, where the lesion is more diffuse, poorly formed and the lesion consists of histiocytic cells with abundant pale cytoplasm packed with organisms (multibacillary histiocytosis) (Shafer and Edlin, 1996). Sampled sites may not represent the infected area and the infected site can be simply missed due to sparse number and paucibacillary nature of mycobacteria (Thangappah *et al.*, 2011). A high false negative rate is seen due to either technical failure, inability to obtain adequate sample or wrong time of collection of the sample in relation to the disease stage (Gatongi *et al.*, 2005).This test therefore is only suggestive and not confirmatory unless acid fast bacilli are demonstrated in the lesion (Walter, 1977).

Ziehl-Neelsen's Staining Method

It is a special bacteriological stain used to identify acid-fast organisms, mainly Mycobacteria. These bacteria cannot be stained by simple stains or even by Gram staining. But can be stained by drastic measures, and once stained cannot be readily decolourized by weak mineral acids. The cell wall of Mycobacterium species, typically contain mycolic acids, which are ß-hydroxy carboxylic acids with chain

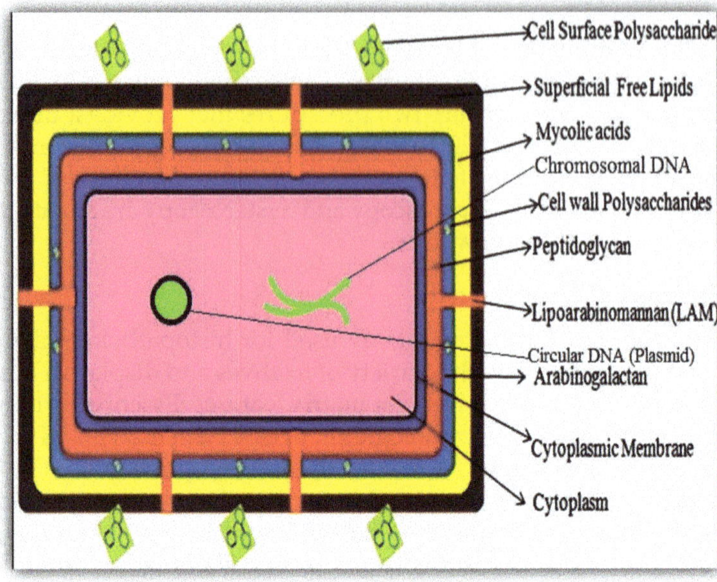

Figure 12.2: Structure of *M. tuberculosis.*

lengths of up to 90 carbon atoms. The mycolic acid and other cell wall lipids act as a barrier for the entry of dye and this coat is called lipoid capsule (Figure 12.2). This coat presents a barrier to dye entry as well as microscopic examination of AFB which requires the presence of at least 10000 organisms' ml^{-1} in the tissue or fluid specimens to get a positive result (Cheng *et al.*, 2004). With the Z-N staining, *M. tuberculosis* stains bright red/pink on pale blue background, while the tissue cells and other organisms are stained blue. Although the Z-N stain is rapid, inexpensive, easy to perform, it has high predictive value (more than 90 per cent) high specificity (98 per cent), but lacks sensitivity (Leung *et al.*, 2010) and the sample prerequisites 5000-10000 organisms ml^{-1} (Cheng *et al.*, 2004). It cannot differentiate between live versus dead bacteria and only 50 per cent of AFB positive cases were identified as total culture positive.

Selected Cultivation on Löwenstein-Jensen (L-J) Media

L-J media is a common, conventional, selective, enriched and differential media used for the isolation and cultivation of mycobacteria (Collee *et al.*, 1996). It was originally formulated by Lowenstein, containing Congo red and malachite green dyes (Lowenstein, 1931). Jensen in 1932 modified Lowenstein's medium by altering the citrate and phosphate contents, eliminating the Congo red dye and increased the malachite green concentration. It is either egg-based or agar-based solid media containing whole eggs or egg yolk or agar, potato flour, salts and glycerol solidified by inspissation. L-asparagine and potato flour are sources of nitrogen and vitamins in L-J medium. Monopotassium phosphate and magnesium sulphate enhances the growth of organism and act as buffers. Glycerol and the egg suspension provide fatty acids and protein required for the metabolism of mycobacteria. The coagulation of the egg albumin during sterilization provides a solid support for inoculation. Sodium citrate and malachite green are selective agents that prevent the growth of most contaminants and allow early growth of mycobacteria. Culture is capable of detecting as few 10^1-10^2 organisms/ml of specimen, surpassing the sensitivity of smear microscopy (Bates, 1979). Detection of positive culture on L-J medium depends lying on various factors: 1) Number of organisms in the specimen, heavy stain positive specimens may turn positive as early as 48 hours, but if bacterial load is low, then it takes longer to grow the bacilli. 2) Treatment status of the patient; if the patient is already on treatment, and then the bacilli are debilitated and may require a longer time to grow. Other factors like size of inoculums, temperature, salt concentration and pH of the medium, and CO_2 supply play a major role on the growth of the bacteria. Standard precautions and Institutional guidelines are available (Kent and Kubica, 1985; CLSI/NCCLS 2001).

Molecular Methods for Detection of FGTB

With the purpose of obtaining faster results and earlier diagnosis of tuberculosis, several molecular detection methods were used. MTB-specific nucleic acid amplification tests (NAATs) are the most frequently used molecular tests for laboratory diagnosis of tuberculosis. A range of polymerase chain reaction (PCR) techniques have been mechanized for the detection of specific nucleic acid sequences of MTB and other mycobacteria (CDCP, 1996). Targeting diverse gene stretches of *M. tuberculosis* and other mycobacteria (Verma *et al.*, 1995, Bhanu *et al.*, 2005, Thangappah *et al.*, 2011), different genes like MPB64 protein (Bhanu *et al.*, 2005), repetitive sequences (Reddi *et al.*, 1993), GC repeats (Verma *et al.*, 1995), devR (Singh *et al.*, 1999), 38-kDa protein (Kadival *et al.*, 1996), TRC4 element (Thangappah *et al.*, 2011, Sujatha *et al.*, 2001), 32-KDa protein/MPT59 α (alpha)–antigen gene (Kidane *et al.*, 2002), 19-kDa antigen gene (Mustafa *et al.*, 1995, Fletcher *et al.*, 2003), IS1081 element (Ahmed *et al.*, 1998) and 65-kDa heat shock protein-encoding gene (Brisson-Noel *et al.*, 1991) have been targeted. The most commonly used target for identification of members of the *M. tuberculosis* complex is the insertion sequence IS6110 element present in 4 to 20 copies of more than 95 per cent of MTB strains (Eisenach *et al.*, 1990, Chakravorty *et al.*, 2005). The presence of multiple copies of this element in the majority of *M. tuberculosis* strains undoubtedly enhances the sensitivity of PCR. However, the discovery of occasional *M. tuberculosis* strains from India lacking IS6110 element implies that relying only on IS6110 element based PCR is not advisable (Van Soolingen *et al.*, 1993). These tests have been repeatedly found to be reproducible, highly sensitive and specific (Soini *et al.*, 1996). With the use of amplification systems, nucleic acid sequences unique to *M. tuberculosis* can be detected directly in clinical specimens, offering better accuracy than AFB smear and greater speed than culture method (Eisenach *et al.*, 1991), and confirmative than histopathology.

Multi-Gene/Multi-Primer PCR

The genus *Mycobacterium* contains more than 90 species, as listed in J. P. Euze´by's List of bacterial names with standing in nomenclature (http://www.bacterio.cict.fr/m/mycobacterium.html), including organisms that cause serious human and animal diseases. Identication of genes encoding the virulence determinants, highly available targets in genome and highly expressing factors are currently important biomarkers for the detection of FGTB. The use of one gene within the genus *Mycobacterium* does not allow specific discrimination of the bacteria. Multi-gene/multi-primer PCR system, which involves the use of four sets of primers, each annealing to different bacterial genomic fragments, allowed discrimination between *M. tuberculosis*, *M. bovis*, and other nontuberculous mycobacteria (Del Portillo *et al.*, 1996, Mustafa *et al.*, 1999). This multi-genic approach fulfils the recent recommendations of the ad hoc committee for the re-evaluation of the definition of the bacterial species (Stackebrandt *et al.*, 2002). The approaches illustrated in this study identify *M. tuberculosis* genes that are or are potentially involved in virulence, ethiopathogenesis and diagnosis of FGTB. Biological, molecular and immunological studies have resulted in identification of more than 33 different useful proteins, some of which are specific to MTB or MTB complex (Cole *et al.*, 1998).

19-kDa protein (Rv3763, lpqH)

The 19-kDa protein is an immunodominant antigen that is recognized by T cells in sera from TB patients. It is one of the mycobacterial lipoproteins called as MTB 19-kDa lipoprotein or 19-kDa antigen (Cole *et al.*, 1998, Stenger and Modlin, 2002). It is the part of a large family of molecules sharing a common structural motif consisting of a triacyl head group attached to an amino-terminal cysteine (Young and Garbe 1991). Ashbridge *et al.* (1989) have identified and determined the sequences of the gene encoding for 19-kDa antigen and the open reading frame (ORF) region. It has been extensively studied in terms of its ability to trigger responses in innate immune cells and immune responses against cellular and humoral arms of the adaptive immunity (Neyrolles *et al.*, 2001) and cell-mediated immunity in humans (Surcel *et al.*, 1994). Experimental studies on staining of macrophages revealed that the 19-kDa protein is secreted by live *M. tuberculosis* residing within the phagolysosomal compartment and intracellular mycobacteria as well (Neyrolles *et al.*, 2001). 19-kDa lipoprotein treated macrophages showed slight increase in the phagocytosis of *M. tuberculosis*, indicating intact cellular function. When *M. tuberculosis* enters macrophages and other phagocytic cells, this surface-exposed glycolipoprotein is thought to cause host signalling events as it interacts with TLR2 (Thoma-Uszynski *et al.*, 2001). It activates macrophages via TLR2 during the acute phase of infections, resulting in a signalling cascade that results in the production of pro-inammatory cytokines, nitric oxide synthase and co-stimulatory molecule (Medzhitov *et al.*, 1997; Brightbill *et al.*, 1999). Intracellular persistence of MTB and shedding of MTB 19-kDa lipoprotein provide effective means for chronic stimulation of TLR2 and consequent inhibition of MHC-II expression, and MHC-II antigen processing (Noss *et al.*, 2001), also suggesting that macrophage responses to *M. tuberculosis* infection are down regulated. It induces TLR2 dependent production of interleukin-12 p40 (IL-12p40) when added to a macrophage cell line (Brightbill *et al.*, 1999). However, there are confusing and contradictory reports regarding host responses to this protein. It was originally noted that *M. tuberculosis* strain-I2646 did not produce the 19-kDa protein, and subsequent DNA sequence analyses demonstrated that the I2646 lpqH gene was disrupted. Increased virulence was observed when the gene for the 19-kDa lipoprotein was transformed into a strain of *M. tuberculosis* naturally defective in 19-kDa lipoprotein expression (Fifis *et al.*, 1991). Hence, 19-kDa antigen gene is selected as one molecular target in the detection of FGTB (Mustafa *et al.*, 1995, Fletcher *et al.*, 2003).

TRC4 Element

It is a conserved repetitive element, repeats at least four times in the genome of *M. tuberculosis* complex (Young and Garbe, 1991). This fragment is situated in open reading frame (Rv0697) of the *M. tuberculosis* genome (Cole *et al.*, 1998). The size of TRC4 fragment in *M. tuberculosis* genome is about 2.1 kb. The G+C content of TRC4 element is 63 per cent which was determined from the global G+C ratio of *M. tuberculosis* genome (Cole *et al.*, 1998). A small portion of the TRC4 sequence ranging from 48-76 base pairs (bp) showed 68 per cent - 80 per cent homology to others sequences. Restriction fragment length polymorphism studies have shown that it is not highly polymorphic rather shows conservative fingerprint pattern (Sujatha *et al.*, 1997). TRC4 fragment present in all the strains and specific for *M. tuberculosis* complex, was sequenced and patented by the Tuberculosis Research Centre (TRC-ICMR), Chennai, India, as an ideal target for PCR assays to identify *M. tuberculosis*; especially in strains carrying no copies of IS6110 element in extra pulmonary patients (Das *et al.*, 1995; Sujatha *et al.*, 2001). There were no significant homologies to any known insertion or transposon sequences.

MPB64 Gene

It encodes a highly specific protein secreted by MTB complex, which includes *M. tuberculosis*, *M. bovis* and *M. africanum* (Harboe *et al.*, 1986; Chaudhary *et al.*, 2010) and other mycobacterial species. *Mycobacterium tuberculosis* protein 64 (MPB64/ MPT64) encoded by the Rv1980c gene contains 228 amino acids and has a molecular mass of about 24,000 daltons (Da) (Yamaguchi *et al.*, 1989, Wang *et al.*, 2007). The size of MPB64 protein is about 24 to 26-kDa (Harboe *et al.*, 1986, Nagai *et al.*, 1991) and is highly immunogenic antigen (Yamaguchi *et al.*, 1989) found in the unheated culture fluid of only strains of the *M. tuberculosis* complex (Harboe *et al.*, 1986) and is used as potential diagnostic marker for TB (Nakamura *et al.*, 1998). Except for the MTB complex, bioinformatics analysis showed no epitopes similar to MPB64 protein, indicating its uniqueness. It is suggested (Minden *et al.*, 1986) that some polymeric epitopes as well as the mature MPB64 protein would be considered as good candidates for serodiagnosis of TB. The MPB64 gene is well characterized and a widely studied antigen (Oettinger and Andersen, 1994; Nakamura *et al.*, 1998). MPB64 protein is one of the main filtrate proteins secreted by MTB complex at an early stage during active growth of MTB strains (Oettinger and Andersen, 1994). It was also proved that MPB64 antigen is found only in viable and actively dividing cells of *M. tuberculosis* (Wang *et al.*, 2007). Viability and activity of MPB64 antigen has been confirmed by cloning and sequencing of MPB64 gene of H37Rv culture filtrate (Gennaro, 2000). MPB64 antigen is restricted to MTB complex and found as TB specific candidate (Ruiling *et al.*, 2009). The MPB64 antigen assay can specifically detect MPB64 antigen secreted by the tuberculosis-causing bacteria and suggests the presence of an organism belong to the MTB complex. MPB64 gene is selected in this study as one of the target for diagnosis of FGTB due to its high sensitivity and importance in the detection of *Mycobacterium tuberculosis* complex (Sharma *et al.*, 2011, Ghosh and Mondal 2012).

32-kDa Protein/MPT59 α (alpha)–Antigen Gene

Mycobacteria have three mycolyl-transferase enzymes, encoded by three genes, fbpA, fbpB, and fbpC, that transfer long-chain mycolic acids to trehalose derivatives, and the proteins can also bind the cell matrix protein fibronectin (Belisle *et al.*, 1997). The Fbp proteins are also found in the culture filtrate and are also known as the antigen 85A, 85B, and 85C complex or the 30- to 32-kDa proteins. 32-kDa protein is one among the mycolyl transferase complex codified by three homologous but distinct structural genes (Ag85A (Rv3804c), Ag85B (Rv1886c) and Ag85C), displaying genetic diversity in species of slow and fast growing mycobacteria (Wiker *et al.*, 1990, Kitaura *et al.*, 1993). Matsuo *et al.* (1988) did the identification of the gene encoding the 32-kDa protein of *M. tuberculosis*, which presented 77.5 per cent homology at the DNA level within the coding region with the 85A antigen gene. In the *M. tuberculosis* antigen 85 complex, the gene for antigen 85A encodes a 294 amino acid mature protein, which shows 79 per cent homology with the deduced 285-aminoacid sequence of antigen 85B (Borremans *et al.*, 1989). Ag85 complex is produced in large amounts (20 to 30 per cent [wt/wt]) of all secreted proteins by *M. tuberculosis* either extracellularly in culture or intracellularly in human mononuclear phagocytes (Lee and Horwitz 1995). Ag85 complex is involved in the final stage of mycobacterial cell wall assembly (Belisle *et al.*, 1997). Wiker *et al.* (1990) analysed NH_2-terminal amino acid sequences which revealed distinct differences among the A, B, and C components of the BCG antigen 85 complex. The 32-kDa protein was identified as antigen 85A (Rv3804c) in the Closs reference system for BCG antigens (Closs *et al.*, 1980). One of the secreted antigens from *M. tuberculosis* is MPT59. It is also known as alpha (α) antigen or antigen 85B (Ohmen *et al.*, 1994). Matsuo *et al.* (1988) recently cloned the gene encoding the α-antigen, a major protein secreted by BCG (sub strain Tokyo) and highly homologous to MPB-59 antigen in its N-terminal amino acid sequence. The fibronectin binding activity exhibited by all three components suggests that they involved in pathogenicity of disease (Abou-Zeid *et al.*, 1988). The 85 antigen complex is present in all mycobacteria, and there is considerable evidence that the complex contains both genus and species-specific epitopes (Matsuo *et al.*, 1988, Kitaura *et al.*, 1993, Matsuo *et al.*, 1990). It is abundantly secreted into the culture supernatant of a variety of mycobacterial species (Borremans *et al.*, 1989). The observation that these proteins are immunodominant, has led to the creation of a new live vaccine that was made by introducing the *M. tuberculosis* fbpB gene into *M. bovis* BCG (Horwitz *et al.*, 2000). This recombinant strain shows better protection against virulent *M. tuberculosis* infection than does the parent BCG strain in a guinea pig model. This vaccine strategy has not been used with the *M. tuberculosis* fbpA gene, but presumably this will be done, given the reported virulence phenotype of the fbpA mutant. Analyses of differential gene expression following exposure to isonicotinic acid hydrazide (INH) and the effects of antimicrobial agents have demonstrated recently (Garbe *et al.*, 1996).

Treatment and Vaccination

Treatment of asymptomatic or doubtful sub-clinical TB in high TB prevalence countries such as India can be justified only in the presence of a significant risk of progression, disease transmission or loss of function of an organ. The disease has no pathogenic signs or symptoms and, hence, most often, the treatments are given empirically. Currently, TB is treated with multiple antibiotics, given to patients for a minimum of 6 months, and in most cases treatment lasts from 1-2 years (Blumberg *et al.*, 2005). Since antibiotics only destroy actively replicating microorganisms, or at the very least microorganisms that are synthesizing proteins, the fact that *M. tuberculosis* may reside in the host in an inactive dormant or latent state is a major complicating factor that requires such prolonged treatments. Patient adherence to antibiotic regimens is notoriously poor, and in TB with such prolonged treatment, it is common for patients to have incomplete treatment. This ultimately results in drug-resistant *M. tuberculosis* strains circulating in the human population. The frequency of these events is startling and has led to the dramatic surge in multiple drug-resistant *M. tuberculosis* (MDR-TB), extremely drug-resistant TB (XDR-TB) and totally drug-resistant TB (TDR-TB) (Espinal 2003, Velayati *et al.*, 2009). In many cases MDR-TB and TDR-TB are impossible to treat successfully or occurs in places where the necessary treatment is either unavailable, or too costly (Espinal, 2003; Velayati *et al.*, 2009). Moreover, the drugs like kanamycin and amikacin can cause ototoxicity in the fetus. Ethionamide and prothionamide are potentially teratogenic and should be avoided in women of child-bearing age. A four- drug regimen consisting of isoniazid, ethambutol, rifampicin and pyrazinamide are used in the treatment of Genital TB.

The Bacille Calmette-Guèrin (BCG) vaccine was developed in the early 1900s by Albert Calmette and Camille Guèrin. BCG is made of a live, attenuated strain of *M. bovis*. Many countries use BCG vaccine as part of their TB control programmes, especially for infants. The protective efficacy of BCG for preventing serious forms of TB (*e.g.* meningitis) in children is greater than 80 per cent ; its protective efficacy for preventing pulmonary TB in adolescents and adults is variable, ranging from 0 to 80 per cent. (Fine, 1995) A recent meta-analysis suggested an overall protective effect of 51 per cent in preventing tuberculosis disease. However, protection against meningitis was 64 per cent and versus disseminated disease it was 78 per cent. There could be many reasons for this such as methodological differences among the clinical trials, genetic differences within and among host populations, endogenous reactivation of persistent infection, exogenous re-infection, and effects of environmental mycobacteria on the host immune response to BCG. Furthermore, there have been reports about the influence of helminth infections that divert Th1 immunity towards Th2, resulting in reduced protection (Elias *et al.*, 2005). Today, the BCG vaccine is not considered as a secured vaccine against pulmonary TB. Although the modified live BCG vaccines or recombinant BCG vaccine have been found to be attractive (Pym *et al.*, 2003), the major concern for the clinical use of this kind of vaccine is safety. Introduction of missing genes to the BCG vaccine might include the possibility of reactivation of virulence.

Subunit vaccines contain purified antigens rather than whole organisms. However, almost all of the single subunit proteins with adjuvants used for vaccination showed a certain level of protection that is even lower than the BCG vaccination (Parra *et al.*, 2004). However, a major challenge in developing a subunit vaccine is the requirement of a safe and effective adjuvant.

DNA vaccine is injected into muscle cells usually with a "gene gun" that uses compressed gas to blow the DNA. Some muscle cells express the inoculated DNA and are able to stimulate the immune system. Although DNA vaccines are probably a good alternative, they have been disappointing so far when tested in larger animals like guinea pigs and non-human primates (Baldwin *et al.*, 1998). With the knowledge from different types of vaccines and the context of current global BCG vaccination, it has increasingly been realized that a combination of BCG or rBCG, DNA vaccines, and subunit proteins therapy may provide greater levels of protection among patients without TB. However, major challenges in developing such combinations are still not sufficient to elicit protective immunity against TB (Andersen and Doherty, 2005).

Cost-Effective Analysis

Cost-effectiveness analysis is a method for evaluating the diagnostic outcomes and costs of different diagnostic methods and procedures relative to one another. It is a decision-making assistance tool. It refers to the consideration of decision alternatives in which the costs, time constraint and consequences are taken into account in a systematic way. It is designed for the economic analysis of the operational objectives at different levels. It identifies the economically most efficient way to fulfil an objective.

The number of diagnostics tests and (bio) markers available in medical rehearsals has been increasing rapidly over the past decades. Consequently, there is growing concern about the overutilization of diagnostic tests and markers, the potential negative health consequences due to over testing, and the steeply rising costs for diagnostic testing (Welch, 2009). To avoid these problems proper evaluation of the downstream consequences or benefits, in terms of improved decision making and patient outcomes, as well as on the cost-benefits of diagnostic testing, is required (Bossuyt *et al.*, 2006, 2012; Ferrante *et al.*, 2012). However, the evaluation of diagnostic tests and markers typically stops after quantifying the accuracy of the test or marker as compared to the prevailing reference standard (Van den Bruel *et al.*, 2007, Bossuyt *et al.*, 2012, Ferrante *et al.*, 2012). Till date, operational data are inadequate on the impact and cost-effectiveness of programs performing FGTB diagnosis in resource-limited settings. Before investing an additional infrastructure, it is important to assess whether other, more immediately accessible, FGTB diagnostic tests might be cost-effective. Therefore, it is important to estimate the cost-effectiveness of different diagnostic laboratory tests and time constraints associated with the different diagnostic methods in the detection of FGTB.

All these methods target the organism attempting to directly demonstrate its presence in tissue or reveal morphologically characteristic lesions caused by the bacilli. However, these methods have poor sensitivity and specificity for the diagnosis of FGTB throughout the sub-clinical stages. These indicate that there are no reliable confirmatory investigatory procedures to ascertain the cause of infertility. Therefore, early detection of the disease and development of inexpensive methods are of current importance. The role of a single method is doubtful in early detection of the disease because all these methods are more or less useful in the diagnosis of FGTB. Keeping these views in mind we have proposed to summarize the current status of conventional and molecular methods useful in diagnosis of FGTB, this gives scope to suggest the possible diagnostic method in early detection of FGTB without any uncertainty. This study aims to review the accuracy of basic diagnostic methods in ascertaining the clinical suitability and cost-effectiveness in detecting both the presence of disease as well as the causative agents among infertile women suspected of suffering from FGTB. It is a prerequisite not only for accurate diagnosis, but also for effective treatment, correlation of clinical effectiveness and design of better vaccines. In addition, this help in identifying of biomarkers with more sensitivity and specificity. They also determine patient management strategies thus avoiding unnecessary procedures.

Methods for Detection of FGTB among Infertile Patients

Female Genital Tuberculosis (FGTB) which is commonly implicated as a cause of infertility is a symptom-less, rare disease with non-specific, mild clinical manifestation and low index of clinical suspicion. *Mycobacterium tuberculosis* the most common cause of human tuberculosis (99 per cent) and *M. bovis*, are capable of producing both a progressive disease and an asymptomatic latent infection. It generates disturbing effects by causing irreversible damage to the fallopian tube, endometrium and other genital organs, consequential in infertility which is hard to treat both by medicinal and surgical methods. FGTB normally occurs in women less than 40 years of age (Chaudhary *et al.*, 1996) and may simulate advanced ovarian malignancy (Lantheaume *et al.*, 2003). The pathogenicity and mechanism of host response to FGTB is very controversial and still unclear. Actually, the bacilli reach the genital tract by three principal routes. The haematogenous spreading from an extra genital sources (Chavan *et al.*, 2004; Sebitloane *et al.*, 2005) such as pulmonary route (90 per cent), lymphatic spread, descending direct spread (Akhan and Pringot, 2002) and through sexual contact (Richards and Angus, 1998; Gatongi *et al.*, 2005). Primary infection of the genitalia may rarely occur from direct inoculation during sexual intercourse (Gatongi *et al.*, 2005) with an infected partner suffering from tuberculous lesions of the genitalia (Angus *et al.*, 2001, Alan *et al.*, 2006). Ascending spread of infection from the vagina, cervix and the vulva has been reported (Lamba *et al.*, 2002, Duggal *et al.*, 2009). The seeding of bacilli usually occurs immediately after puberty as the blood supply to the pelvic organs increases and, as a result, more bacilli can reach the sex organs and infect them (Crofton *et al.*, 1992). Once the immunity to MTB contains and overrides the growth of a small number of disseminated TB bacilli after primary infection, the infection may remain silent throughout life until lowered immunity or overwhelming re-infection precipitates the disease (Blanca and Restrepo, 2007, Arora *et al.*, 2003). Increased circulation and hormone dependence of female genital organs after sexual maturity may, in part, explain why the genital system is vulnerable to this infection after sexual maturity

(Chaudhary *et al.*, 1996). The risk of developing the disease can also observed among immuno-compromised individuals, including patients with old age, malnutrition or coinfection with HIV, severe psychiatric dysfunction, multiple sclerosis and other autoimmune disorders, women with diabetes, genetic mutations and other medical disorders like hypertension (Blanca and Restrepo, 2007; Lawn and Zumla, 2011). The signs, symptoms and altered immune responses of FGTB patients mimic those of immuno-suppressed individuals, hence diagnostic awareness may prevent unnecessary treatment and morbidity (Eastwood *et al.*, 2001).

Diagnosis is indefinable and a high index of suspicion is very essential in the routine diagnostic process (Simon *et al.*, 1977). There are no reliable confirmatory investigative procedures to ascertain the cause of infertility (Mani *et al.*, 2003, Jassawalla, 2006). There are no accepted guidelines for diagnosing EPTB in view of the low sensitivity of bacteriological tests and the poor specificity of most immunological and serological investigations (Tripathy and Tripathy 2002, Ramachandaran and Paramasivan, 2002). Constant attempts have been made to develop definitive diagnostic criteria due to limitations in the available diagnostic tests to make a conclusive diagnosis of genital TB. Moreover, inefficacy of laboratory diagnostic tests and inaccessibility to reproductive clinics has resulted in underreporting of GTB. It is estimated that at least 11 per cent of the patients lack symptoms and FGTB is often detected in diagnostic workup of women attending infertility clinics. Thangappah *et al.* (2011) revealed that 57 per cent of infertile women in whom the presence of TB was suspected on clinical grounds showed a positive endo-TB-polymerase chain reaction (PCR) test, whereas only 9.5 per cent tested positive for the test with no clinical ground for suspicion. Therefore, a high degree of suspicion assisted by intensive investigation is significant in the diagnosis of this disease.

Studies have shown high variability in human scoring of chest X-rays with wide ranges of sensitivity and specificity. Sensitivity of the chest X-ray ranges from 53.3 per cent to 72 per cent (Abebe *et al.*, 2013, Padmapriyadarsini *et al.*, 2013), while specificity ranges from 22 per cent to 72.9 per cent (Davis *et al.*, 2009, Huerga *et al.*, 2012). Erythrocyte sedimentation rate (ESR) is a nonspecific marker of inflammation and is elevated in a number of infectious and non-infectious conditions. Khanna *et al.* (2011) have found ESR to be 57.69 per cent sensitive and 63.51 per cent specific in the diagnosis of GTB. The Mantoux test is usually nonspecific, not an ideal reference standard because the test is confounded with BCG (Bacillus Calmette–Guérin) vaccination, non-tuberculous mycobacteria (NTM) that leads to false-positive results (Puri and Bansal, 2009). It was reported to be 61.5 per cent sensitive and 66.21 per cent specific in diagnosing tuberculosis-polymerase chain reaction (TB-PCR) positive cases (Khanna *et al.*, 2011). Raut *et al.* (2001) have found Mantoux test to be 55 per cent sensitive and 80 per cent specific in diagnosing genital tuberculosis laparoscopically. Khanna *et al.* (2011) found that hysterosalpingography (HSG) showed 76.90 per cent sensitivity and 52.70 per cent specificity. Sakar *et al.* (2008) showed the sensitivity and specificity of HSG to be 63 per cent and 89.3 per cent respectively, and the accuracy ratio 72 per cent.

Laparoscopy is an invasive technique used for obtaining tissue samples for various investigations. Sellors *et al.* (1991) found laparoscopy to be 50 per cent and 80 per cent sensitive and specific, respectively. Not all hospital operating rooms can afford to offer laparoscopy facilities because of high cost and non-availability of trained doctors. Laparoscopy cannot always be performed on everyone. Some patients with prior operations may have a dense scar tissue within the body that a safe operation cannot be done. The range of Z-N stain positivity reported in earlier studies varies between 0 per cent and 44 per cent. However, Mustafa *et al.* (2006) found that the specificity of Z-N staining was 100 per cent, and the sensitivity was 61 per cent. Smear sensitivity varies among different investigators from 22 per cent to 49.7 per cent. In diagnosing spinal tuberculosis, histopathogical examinations yielded 82 per cent sensitivity and 100 per cent specificity. (Rasit *et al.*, 2011) Careful histologic examination of serial sections of fallopian tubes during autopsy resulted in an increased diagnosis of tubal TB from 7.7 per cent to 20 per cent. The other source of material generally available for culture or biopsy of the female genital tract without resorting to diagnostic laparoscopy or laparotomy is the endometrium, menstrual discharge, pelvic aspirated fluid, urine and sputum. However, small inoculum and slow growth of mycobacteria reaching the endometrium from the tubes reduces the chance of obtaining positive samples from a single endometrial tissue biopsy or menstrual culture. Since, the fallopian tubes cannot be removed for the study, sampling from the ovaries and endometrium was suggested for the detection of FGTB (Punnonen *et al.*, 1983). Use of menstrual blood for bacteriologic or molecular diagnosis has been recommended (Abebe *et al.*, 2004) but was reported to show low sensitivity (Simon *et al.*, 1977). Studies on serial sections of tissues are needed because the lesions are frequently erratic and positive endometrial culture for TB was found only in 25 per cent of cases of tuberculous endometritis as the endometrium is often focal and due to cyclical shedding of the endometrium, granulomas do not have enough time to develop (Kapoor *et al.*, 2013). In such cases, the granulomatous endometrium may not show evidence of tuberculosis in all the cycles. A negative endometrial biopsy does not rule out the involvement of the pelvis since sampling errors are common and the disease may have involved other pelvic organs without association of endometritis. Part of the endometrium obtained should be examined bacteriologically, as this may be positive for tuberculosis when histologic examination is negative (Gatongi *et al.*, 2005, Puri and Bansal, 2009). Culture of bacteria on Löwenstein–Jensen's (L-J) egg based solid media showed a sensitivity of 6 per cent and a sensitivity of 100 per cent in detecting spinal tuberculosis (Shetty *et al.*, 2006, Rasit *et al.*, 2011). However, Kidenya *et al.* (2013) showed that micro broth culture was reliable in detecting *M. tuberculosis* in sputum with greater sensitivity (89 per cent vs. 77 per cent) and specificity (95.9 per cent vs. 93.4 per cent). The rate of mycobacterial species recovery from the L-J culture system ranges from 53.6 per cent to 95.9 per cent (Monterola *et al.*, 1998).

Conventional/phenotypic methods have slow and low detection rates and have limitations due to secondary nature of genital tuberculosis. Sampled sites may not represent the infected area and the infected site can be simply missed due to sparse number and paucibacillary nature of mycobacteria (Thangappah *et al.*, 2011). Tissue reactions in those having tuberculosis may at times be atypical and bacteriologically mute (Bhanu *et al.*, 2005). Thus, these methods have poor sensitivity and specificity for the diagnosis of FGTB throughout the sub-clinical stages. However, tests like interferon gamma release assays (IGRAs) may not differentiate latent from active infection. In endemic areas, where BCG vaccination is a nationwide prevention policy, a meta-analysis of the pooled sensitivity of IGRA for tuberculosis was 70 per cent to 78 per cent and the specificity was 99 per cent among patients who did not receive BCG vaccination and 96 per cent among BCG-vaccinated persons (Pai *et al.*, 2008). Song *et al.* (2009) reported that the sensitivity and specificity of the IGRA for EPTB were 69 per cent and 82 per cent, respectively.

Nucleic acid (NA) based detection of pathogens, initiated approximately 25 years ago, is still ongoing and continues to evolve (Wilson, 2011). After Watson and Crick (1953) elucidated the structure of DNA, it took another thirty years for the first molecular diagnostic tests to appear in the microbiology laboratory. In general, molecular diagnostic testing consists of three stages: i) making NA available for detection, ii) amplification (organism, signal, or NA), and iii) identification of amplification products. However, the means to perform these three common stages and the sequence in which they are performed are subject to great diversity. The methods can be divided roughly into 3 main groups: i) probe hybridization assays through fluorescent *in situ* hybridization (FISH) colony count ii) signal amplification assays through branched DNA (bDNA) hybrid capture, and iii) NA amplification assays through PCR, nucleic acid sequence-based amplification (NASBA), transcription mediated amplification (TMA), strand displacement amplification (SDA), Qβ replicase amplification (QβA), ligase chain reaction (LCR), rolling circle amplification (RCA) and many of their modified methods.

Development of diagnostic molecular microbiology really speeded up in the late 1980s, when Kary Mullis and coworkers described the *in vitro* synthesis of specific DNA by a polymerase-catalysed process, the polymerase chain reaction (PCR) (Mullis and Faloona, 1987; Saiki *et al.*, 1985). This PCR technology initiated a revolution in the diagnosis of infectious diseases. Indeed, spectacular results were obtained shortly after development of the PCR. In recent times, polymerase chain reaction (PCR) has been found to be the most sensitive technique for rapid diagnosis (Rivasi *et al.*, 2007, Singh *et al.*, 2007). PCR-based methods have been used for the rapid detection and differentiation of *M. tuberculosis* complex (MTC) and nontuberculous mycobacteria (NTM). The diagnosis and differentiation of NTMs is necessary to treat the patients accordingly (Sankar *et al.*, 2008). The sensitivity of approved PCR for pulmonary TB is 97 per cent and the specificity is 76 per cent (Cousins *et al.*, 1992). However, the efficacy of PCR for the diagnosis of EPTB, including genitourinary TB, is not conclusive. Sharma *et al.* (2013) recently reported the sensitivity and specificity of multi-targeted PCR for diagnosis of presumed tubercular uveitis at 77.7 per cent and 100 per cent, respectively. Other studies showed sensitivity and specificity for the PCR assay ranging from 70.4 per cent to 79.5 per cent with specificity greater than 98 per cent when compared to culture examination and conventional microscopy (Bergmann and Woods 1996, Devallois et al., 1996) and sensitivity generally increasing to 75-98 per cent for acid fast bacilli (AFB) positive specimens (Bergmann and Woods, 1996).

Apart from conventional techniques, molecular techniques like PCR have been developed for the detection of *M. tuberculosis* (Clarridge *et al.*, 1993, Kidane *et al.*, 2002, Bhanu *et al.*, 2005, Thangappah *et al.*, 2011) and for the detection of other *Mycobacterium* species (Fauville-Dufaux *et al.*, 1992, Kidane *et al.*, 2002, Ka¨ser *et al.*, 2009). Over the last 20 years, various gene targets have been used in PCR with varying results. However, conventional PCRs have the limitation of detecting only one target gene. *Mycobacterium tuberculosis* (MTB), the causative pathogen of TB has co-existed and co-evolved from very early human life on earth. MTB capably adapted for its survival against environmental, host immune system and other factors. These major evolutionary changes have been phenotypic as well as genotypic by diversifying into various lines of descent or lineages (Coleman *et al.*, 2001, Comas *et al.*, 2009). However, appropriate scientific evidence for such an adaptation is lacking mainly due to difficulty in separating the biological factors from the socio-economic and other confounding factors. Nevertheless, there is increasing evidence that the genetic differences amongst the MTB strains are relevant to the outcome of TB infection and disease management (Coleman *et al.*, 2001). This knowledge of strain diversity has special contemplation during TB epidemics or sporadic outbreaks where only a few homogenous strains or types are found to be responsible for such events (Chatterjee *et al.*, 2010). In order to determine the strain diversity of MTB, molecular genotyping tools have been used extensively in the last couple of decades. Among these, IS6110 restriction fragment length polymorphism (RFLP) was widely used but it has a major limitation that in several regions, *e.g.* South India, a high proportion of MTB strains will carry a very low copy number or are devoid of IS6110 (Das *et al.*, 1995, Siddiqi *et al.*, 2001). This typing method also has a relative lack of portability, which hampers comparison between two separate studies. (Braden *et al.*, 2002)

As with all new technologies, although exiting and promising results prevailed, also arose new problems for the clinical microbiology laboratory. Unfortunately, the major drawback of these methods was the lack of sensitivity when applied directly to clinical specimens including tissues, cells, stools, and cerebrospinal fluid (CSF) (Brooks *et al.*, 1988; Rotbart, 1991; Yang and Rothman, 2004). Quality assessment programs showed that during the early 1990s sensitivity and specificity problems were surprisingly common among laboratories performing routine molecular diagnostic testing. Between 43-100 per cent (13-23 per cent of all negative specimens) and 55-100 per cent (13-40 per cent of all positive specimens) of the participating laboratories reported false-positive and false-negative results, respectively (Damen *et al.*, 1996, Livak *et al.*, 1995, Noordhoek 1996). PCR using single target gene alone is not sufficient for the detection of all strains of *M. tuberculosis*, therefore use of multiple target genes was considered to be more appropriate (Sujatha *et al.*, 2001, Sharma *et al.*, 2013). Improvement in the sensitivity of PCR was reported using different set of target genes for the detection of extrapulmonary tuberculosis (Del Portillo *et al.*, 1996, Sujatha *et al.*, 2001). The increase in PCR sensitivity and decrease in false negative results were achieved using dual targets for the detection of *M tuberculosis* (Barani *et al.*, 2012).

Recently, we have developed a multi-gene/multi-primer PCR targeting mycobacterial genus and species-specific gene targets (Bhanothu *et al.*, 2014a) in the simultaneous detection and differentiation of *Mycobacterium* sp. directly from clinical samples. The use of a multi-gene PCR system based on the simultaneous amplification of the species-specific 19-kDa antigen gene, MTB complex specific TRC4 element and MPB64 antigen gene and genus specific 32-kDa protein/MPT59 α (alpha)–antigen gene in a single tube- single step reaction identified MTB and distinguished it from other nontuberculous mycobacteria. The 19-kDa antigen (lpqH/Rv3763) gene (Ashbridge *et al.*, 1989, Cole *et al.*, 1998), TRC4 element (located in ORF Rv0697) (Sujatha *et al.*, 1997; Cole *et al.*, 1998) and MPB64 protein gene (Harboe, 1986; Yamaguchi *et al.*, 1989; Li *et al.*, 1993) are markedly species specific and widespread in mycobacterial genome (Cole *et al.*, 1998) and routinely used in the diagnosis of FGTB by the multi-gene PCR method. We have demonstrated that multi-gene PCR showed a significant advantage over the conventional techniques where as a minimum detection limit of single solid bacilli (or 10^1 colony forming unit) per gram (or ml) of tissue sediments without the use of radioisotopes, without the use of costly and complex equipment and above all three target genes could be studied at a time (Kidane *et al.*, 2002). Advanced nucleic acid-based methods such as multi gene PCR can be utilized not only for bacteriological presence but also in the clinical findings of host in response to infectious agents.

This has great potential in the laboratory diagnosis of FGTB, particularly in latent and paucibacillary conditions as well as in active tuberculosis. The multi-gene PCR reveals its potential in the quick and precise diagnosis of tuberculosis of any organ. This method can detect the mycobacterial infection and can also differentiate between its different species in a single tube-single reaction and in a single gel electrophoresis run, so that the clinician can choose the appropriate chemotherapy for the patient and can decide whether anti tuberculosis therapy (ATT) is required or not. Multi-gene PCR method is more useful in terms of cost and equipment needed in resource-limited settings, where modern culture facilities and costly tests such as Gene Xpert are not available. The amount of reagents required per reaction is the same as conventional PCR, except for the requirement of four sets of primers. But the advantage outweighs the minimal cost and time. The method is not only a rapid and sensitive tool, but it also demands less skill as compared to laparoscopy, hysteroscopy, and histopathology, which are the standard methods used in developing countries at present. Othman *et al.* (2012) reported that the cost of X-ray film per patient was US$ 0.80. The cost of an AFB test preparation for each patient was US$ 2.2. The estimated overheads cost per patient was US$ 1.20 for extra-pulmonary TB cases. However, for laboratory tests/X-rays, the cost per patient was US$ 182.0 for extra-pulmonary TB (Othman *et al.*, 2012). The diagnostic cost (including the costs of testing all individuals with suspected TB) per TB case detected is US$ 28–49 for the base case and increases significantly to US$ 133–146 (Vassall *et al.*, 2011). A single sputum smear examination costs between US$ 1.13 and US$ 1.63. The unit costs of culture ranges from US$ 13.56 to US$ 18.95. The calculated cost of our study is unmatched with others and much lower than that reported in Malaysia (US$916.40), South Africa (US$ 890.50), Uganda (US$ 403.20), Pakistan US$ 310.00 (Khan *et al.*, 2002, Elamin *et al.*, 2008) and even in India US$ 171 (Rajeswari *et al.*, 1999). The lower cost of our study may be due to exclusion of the cost of the laboratory building, instrumentations, manpower, furniture, pipettes and dispensers, vehicles, transportations, overheads and stationery charges. Moreover the study had included only patients living in urban areas, where patients have access to all local and advanced facilities. So, the estimated costs may be more than the real costs for rural residents. Thus, the expenditure to patients might be higher than that expected. The fact that the diagnostic tests affect short-term outcomes, rather than long-term patient outcomes makes evaluation of these tests more complicated than prevention of disease. Perhaps most important, diagnostic methods do not generally directly affect long-term patient outcomes. Instead, the results of diagnostic tests can influence the care of patients; in that way, diagnostic tests may affect long-term outcomes. Because of this, the benefits associated with the use of a specific diagnostic method will depend on the performance characteristics (*e.g.*, sensitivity and specificity) of the test, as well as other factors, such as prevalence of disease, costs of other diagnostic tests and effectiveness of available treatments for the disease in question. Most of the studies are reliance on published data for parameter estimates, many of which are subject to substantial variability, as well as the lack of direct data on the full costs (including purchase of equipment, laboratory scale-up, and training of staff) of the investigation procedures and therefore cannot be generalized.

Conclusion

Compared to Z–N staining and culturing on L-J media, multi-gene PCR improved the detection rate of suspected FGTB. FGTB could be diagnosed if multi-gene PCR is considered in the evaluation of infertile patients in areas where tuberculosis is endemic. Site specific sampling, irrespective of sample type and amplification of the 19-kDa antigen gene in combination with TRC4 element as a successful multi-gene PCR for the diagnosis of FGTB and differentiation of mycobacterial infection among endo-ovarian tissue biopsies and PAFs taken from infertile women are suggested. Taking different sampling sites for laparoscopic examination as the primary technique for the diagnosis of FGTB among infertile women is advisable. However, endo-ovarian tissue biopsies should not be considered free of infections in infertile patients until it has been studied even at ultra-structural levels (Sharma *et al.*, 2010). Increasing the awareness and importance of incorporating multiple genes, targeting different characteristics of infectious agents in a single tube-single step reaction using multi-gene PCR method is needed. Enhanced detection of FGTB cases can be possible due to multiple sampling by laparoscopic technique, from multiple pathological sites.

References

Abebe M, Lakew M, Kidane D, Lakew Z *et al.*, Female genital tuberculosis in Ethiopia. *Int. J. Gynaecol. Obstet.* 84: 241-246. 2004.

Abou-Zeid C, Ratliff TL, Wiker HG. Characterization of fibronectin-binding antigens released by *M. tuberculosis* and *Mycobacterium bovis* BCG. *Infect. Immun.* 56: 3046-51. 1988.

Ahmed N, Mohanty AK, Mukhopadhyay U, Batish BK *et al.*, PCR-based rapid detection of *Mycobacterium tuberculosis* in blood from immunocompetent patients with pulmonary tuberculosis. *J. Clin. Microbiol.* 36: 3094-5. 1998.

Akhan O, Pringot J. Imaging of abdominal tuberculosis. *Eur. Radiol.* 12: 312-23. 2002.

Alan JW, Louis RK, Andrew CN, *et al.*, editors. *Campbell-Walsh Urology. 9th ed.* New York: Saunders, Elsevier. 2006.

Ali AA, Abdallah TM. Clinical presentation and epidemiology of female genital tuberculosis in Eastern Sudan. *Int. J. Gynaecol. Obstet.* 118: 236-238. 2012.

Andersen P, Doherty TM. The success and failure of BCG - implications for a novel tuberculosis vaccine. *Nat. Rev. Microbiol.* 3(8): 656-62. 2005.

Angus BJ, Yates M, Conlon C, Byren I. Cutaneous tuberculosis of the penis and sexual transmission of tuberculosis confirmed by molecular typing. *Clin. Infect. Disease.* 33: 132–4. 2001.

Arora VK, Gupta R, Arora R. Female genital tuberculosis - need for more research. *Ind. J. Tuberc.* 50(9): 36-38. 2003.

Ashbridge KR, Booth RJ, Watson JD, Lathigra RB. Nucleotide sequence of the 19 Kda antigen gene from *Mycobacterium tuberculosis. Nucleic Acids Res.* 17(3): 1249–1249. 1989.

Baldwin SL, D'Souza C, Roberts AD *et al.*, Evaluation of new vaccines in the mouse and guinea pig model of tuberculosis. *Infect. Immun.* 66: 2951-9. 1998.

Bates JH. Diagnosis of tuberculosis. *Chest.* 76 (Suppl 6): 757–763. 1979.

Belisle JT, Vissa VD, Sievert T, Takayama K, *et al.*, Role of the major antigen of *M. tuberculosis* in cell wall biogenesis. *Science.* 276: 1420-1422. 1997.

Bergmann JS, Woods GL. Clinical evaluation of the Roche AMPLICOR PCR *Mycobacterium tuberculosis* test for detection of *M. tuberculosis* in respiratory specimens. *J. Clin. Microbiol.* 34(5): 1083-1085. 1996.

Bhanothu V, Theophilus JP, Kalyan Reddy P, Rozati R. Occurrence of female genital tuberculosis among infertile women: a study from a tertiary maternal health care research centre in South India. *Eur. J. Clin. Microbiol. Infect. Dis.* 33 (11): 1937–1949. 2014b.

Bhanothu V, Theophilus JP, Rozati R. Use of endo-ovarian tissue biopsy and pelvic aspirated fluid for the diagnosis of female genital tuberculosis by conventional versus molecular methods. *PLoS One.* 9(5): e98005. 2014a. doi: 10.1371/journal.pone.0098005

Blanca I, Restrepo. Convergence of the tuberculosis and diabetes epidemics: renewal of old acquaintances. *Clin. Infect. Disease.* 45(4): 436–438. 2007.

Blumberg HM, Leonard MK, Jasmer Jr RM. Update on the treatment of tuberculosis and latent tuberculosis infection. *JAMA.* 293: 2776-84. 2005.

Borremans M, De Wit L, Volckaert G, Ooms J *et al.*, Cloning, sequence determination and expression of a 32-kilodalton-protein gene of *Mycobacterium tuberculosis. Infect. Immun.* 57: 3123-3130. 1989.

Bossuyt PM, Irwig L, Craig J, Glasziou P. Comparative accuracy: assessing new tests against existing diagnostic pathways. *BMJ.* 332: 1089-1092. 2006.

Bossuyt PM, Reitsma JB, Linnet K, Moons KG. Beyond diagnostic accuracy: the clinical utility of diagnostic tests. *Clin. Chem.* 58(12): 1636-1643. 2012.

Botha MH, van der Merwe FH. Female genital tuberculosis. *SA Fam Pract.* 50(5): 12- 16. 2008.

Braden CR, Crawford JT, Schable BA. Quality assessment of *Mycobacterium tuberculosis* genotyping in a large laboratory network. *Emerg. Infect. Dis.* 8(11): 1210e5. 2002.

Brightbill HD, Libraty DH, Krutzik SR, Yang RB, *et al.*, Host defense mechanisms triggered by microbial lipoproteins through toll-like receptors. *Science.* 285(5428): 732–736. 1999.

Brisson-Noel A, Aznar C, Chureau C *et al.*, Diagnosis of tuberculosis by DNA amplification in clinical practice evaluation. *Lancet.* 338: 364–366. 1991.

Brooks Jackson J, Balfour Jr HH. Practical diagnostic testing for human immunodeficiency virus. *Clin. Microbiol. Rev.* 1: 124-138. 1988.

Broune AW, Willium LM. *Genital tuberculosis: recent advances in obstetries/gynaecology. 2nd edition,* 10th Vol.: 1962. London. 1962.

Centres for Disease Control and Prevention (CDCP). Nucleic acid amplification tests for tuberculosis. *MMWR Morb. Mortal. Weekly Rep.* 45: 950–952. 1996.

Chakrabarti AK, Sen S, Banerjee A, Roy K. Female genital tuberculosis- a retrospective study. *Ind. J. Tub.* 45: 101-3. 1998.

Chakravorty S, Dudeja M, Hanif M, Tyagi JS. Novel multipurpose methodology for detection of mycobacteria in pulmonary and extrapulmonary specimens by smear microscopy, culture, and PCR. *J. Clin. Microbiol.* 43: 2697-702. 2005.

Chatterjee A, D'Souza D, Vira T, Bamne A, *et al.*, Strains of *Mycobacterium tuberculosis* from Western Maharashtra, India, exhibit a high degree of diversity and strain-specific associations with drug resistance, cavitary disease, and treatment failure. *J. Clin. Microbiol.* 48(10): 3593e9. 2010. http: //dx.doi.org/10.1128/ JCM.00430-10.

Chaudhary M, Gupta S, Khare S, Lal S. Diagnosis of tuberculosis in an era of HIV pandemic: a review of current status and future prospects. *Ind. J. Med. Microbiol.* 28(4): 281–289. 2010.

Chaudhary NN. Overview of tuberculosis of the female genital tract. *J. Ind. Med. Assoc.* 94: 345-61. 1996.

Chavan GB, Hira P, Zachira TT, Chawla A *et al.*, Female genital tuberculosis; hysterosalpingographic appearances. *Br. J. Radiol.* 77: 164-9. 2004.

Cheng VCC, Yam WC, Hung IFN, Woo PCY *et al.*, Clinical evaluation of the polymerase chain reaction for the rapid diagnosis of tuberculosis. *J. Clin. Pathol.* 57: 281–285. 2004.

Clarridge JE, RM Shawar, TM Shinik, BB Plikaytis. Large-scale use of polymerase chain reaction for detection of *Mycobacterium tuberculosis* in routine mycobacteriology laboratory. *J. Clin. Microbiol.* 31: 2049–2056. 1993.

Closs O, Harboe M, Axelsen-Christensen NH, Magnussen M. The antigens of *Mycobacterium bovis*, strain BCG, studied by cross-immuno-electrophoresis: a reference system. *Scand. J. Immunol.* 12: 249-263. 1980.

Cole ST, Brosch R, Parkhill J, Garnier T *et al.*, Deciphering the biology of *M. tuberculosis* from the complete genome sequence. *Nature.* 393: 537-544. 1998.

Coleman PG, Perry BD, Woolhouse ME. Endemic stability-a veterinary idea applied to human public health. *Lancet.* 357(9264): 1284e6. 2001.

Collee JG, Fraser AG, Marmion BP, Simmons A, (Eds.). *Mackie and McCartney Practical Medical Microbiology, 14th Edition,* Churchill Livingstone. 1996.

Comas I, Homolka S, Niemann S, Gagneux S. Genotyping of genetically monomorphic bacteria: DNA sequencing in *Mycobacterium tuberculosis* highlights the limitations of current methodologies. *PLoS One.* 4(11). 2009.

Cousins DV, Wilton SD, Francis BR, Gow BL. Use of polymerase chain reaction for rapid diagnosis of tuberculosis. *J. Clin. Microbiol.* 30: 255–258. 1992.

Crofton J, Horne N, Miller F. *Clinical tuberculosis.* 1st ed. London: Macmillan Education Ltd. pp. 502-10. 1992.

Dam P, Shirazee HH, Goswami SK, Ghosh S *et al.*, Role of latent genital tuberculosis in repeated IVF failure in the Indian clinical setting. *Gynecol. Obstet. Invest.* 61(4): 223-227. 2006.

Damen M, Cuypers HT, Zaaijer HL, Reesink HW *et al.*, International collaborative study on the second EUROHEP HCA-RNA reference panel. *J. Virol. Methods.* 58: 175-185. 1996.

Das S, Paramasivan CN, Lewis DB, Prabhakar R *et al.*, IS6110 restriction fragment length polymorphism typing of clinical isolates of *M. tuberculosis* from patients with pulmonary tuberculosis in Madras, South India. Tubercle. *Lung Dis.* 76: 550-554. 1995.

Davis JL, Worodria W, Kisembo H, Metcalfe JZ *et al.*, Clinical and radiographic factors do not accurately diagnose smear-negative tuberculosis in HIV-infected in-patients in Uganda: a cross-sectional study. *PLoS One.* 5(3): e9859. 2009.

Del Portillo P, Thomas MC, Martínez E, Maranón C *et al.*, Multi primer PCR system for differential identification of mycobacteria in clinical samples. *J. Clin. Microbiol.* 34: 324-328. 1996.

Devallois A, Legrand E, *et al.*, Evaluation of AMPLICOR MTB test as adjunct to smears and culture for direct detection of *Mycobacterium tuberculosis* in the French Caribbean. *J. Clin. Microbiol.* 34(5): 1065-1068. 1996.

Duggal S, Duggal N, Hans C, Mahajan RK. Female genital TB and HIV co-infection. *Ind. J. Med. Microbiol.* 27: 361-372. 2009.

Eastwood JB, Corbishley CM, Grange J. *M. tuberculosis* and the kidney. *J. Am. Soc. Nephrol.* 121: 307–314. 2001.

Eisenach KD, Cave MD, Bates JH, Crawford JT. Polymerase chain reaction amplification of a repetitive DNA sequence specific for *Mycobacterium tuberculosis*. *J. Infect. Dis.* 161: 977–981. 1990.

Eisenach KD, Sifford MD, Cave MD, Bates JH *et al.*, Detection of *Mycobacterium tuberculosis* in sputum samples using a polymerase chain reaction. *Am. Rev. Respir. Dis.* 144: 1160–1163. 1991.

Elamin EI, Ibrahim MI, Sulaiman SA, Muttalif AR. Cost of illness of tuberculosis in Penang, Malaysia. *Pharm. World Sci.* 30(3): 281–286. 2008.

Elias D, Akuffo H, Pawlowski A, Haile M *et al.*, *Schistosoma Mansoni* infection reduces the protective efficacy of BCG vaccination against virulent *Mycobacterium tuberculosis*. *Vaccine.* 23: 1326-34. 2005.

Espinal MA. The global situation of MDR-TB. *Tuberculosis (Edinb).* 83: 44-51. 2003.

Fauville-Dufaux M, Vanfleteren B, De Witt L, Vincke JP *et al.*, Rapid detection of tuberculous and non-tuberculous mycobacteria by polymerase chain reaction amplification of a 162 bp DNA fragment from antigen 85. *Eur. J. Clin. Microbiol. Infect. Dis.* 11: 797–803. 1992.

Ferrante Di Ruffano L, Hyde CJ, McCaffery KJ, Bossuyt PM *et al.*, Assessing the value of diagnostic tests: a framework for designing and evaluating trials. *BMJ.* 344: e686. 2012.

Fifis T, Costopoulos C, Radford AJ, Bacic A, *et al.*, Purification and characterization of major antigens from a *Mycobacterium bovis* culture filtrate. *Infect. Immun.* 59: 800-807. 1991.

Fine PE. Variation in protection by BCG: implications of and for heterologous immunity. *Lancet.* 346: 1339-45. 1995.

Garbe TR, Hibler NS, Deretic V. Isoniazid induces expression of the antigen 85 complex in *Mycobacterium tuberculosis*. *Antimicrob. Agents Chemother.* 40: 1754–1756. 1996.

Gatongi DK, Gitau G, Kay V, Ngwenya S, *et al.*, Female genital tuberculosis. *Obstet. Gynaecol.* 7: 75-9. 2005.

Gennaro ML. Immunologic diagnosis of tuberculosis. *J. Infect. Dis.* 30 (3): 243–246. 2000.

Ghosh SK, Mondal R. Quick diagnosis of female genital tuberculosis using multiplex fast polymerase chain reaction in Southern Assam, India. *Int. J. Gynaecol. Obstet.* 118: 72–73. 2012

Gupta N, Sharma JB, Mittal S, Singh N *et al.*, Genital tuberculosis in Indian infertility patients. *Int. J. Gynaecol. Obstet.* 97: 135–138. 2007.

Harboe M, Nagai S, Patarroyo ME, Torres ML *et al.*, Properties of proteins MPB64, MPB70, and MPB80 of *Mycobacterium bovis* BCG. *Infect. Immun.* 52(1): 293–302 1986.

Helen A Fletcher, Helen D Donoghue, Michael Taylor G, Adri GM van der Zander *et al.*, Molecular analysis of *Mycobacterium tuberculosis* DNA from a family of 18th century Hungarians. *Microbiology*. 149: 143–151. 2003.

Horwitz MA, Harth G, Dillon BJ, Maslesa-Galic S. Recombinant bacillus calmette-guerin (BCG) vaccines expressing the *Mycobacterium tuberculosis* 30-Kda major secretory protein induce greater protective immunity against tuberculosis than conventional BCG vaccines in a highly susceptible animal model. *Proc. Natl. Acad. Sci. USA*. 97: 13853– 13858. 2000.

Huerga H, Varaine F, Okwaro E, Bastard M *et al.*, Performance of the 2007 WHO algorithm to diagnose smear-negative pulmonary tuberculosis in a HIV prevalent setting. *PLoS One*. 7(12): e51336. 2012.

Jassawalla MJ. Genital tuberculosis - a diagnostic dilemma. *J. Obstet. Gynecol.* 56 (3): 203-204. 2006.

Jensen KA. Rinzuchtung und typenbestim mung von tuberkelbazillentammen zentralbl. bakteriol. parasitenkd. infektionskr. *Hyg. Abt. I. Orig.* 125: 222-239. 1932.

Ka¨ser M, Hauser J, Small P, Pluschke G. Large sequence polymorphisms unveil the phylogenetic relationship of environmental and pathogenic mycobacteria related to *Mycobacterium ulcerans*. *Appl. Environ. Microbiol.* 75(17): 5667. 2009. doi: 10.1128/aem.00446-09

Kadival GV, D' Souza CD, Kulkarni SP, Samuel AM. A highly specific polymerase chain reaction for detection of *M. tuberculosis*. *Indian J. Tuberc.* 43: 151-4. 1996.

Kapoor N, Pawar S, Sirakova TD, Deb C *et al.*, Human granuloma *In-vitro* model, for TB dormancy and resuscitation. *PLoS One*. 8: e53657. 2013.

Kent PT, GP Kubica. Public health mycobacteriology: a guide for the level III laboratory. USDHHS, Center Disease Control, Atlanta. 1985.

Khan MA, JD Walley, SN Witter, A Imran *et al.*, Costs and cost effectiveness of different DOT strategies for the treatment of tuberculosis in Pakistan cost. *Health Policy Planning*. 17: 178–186. 2002.

Khanna A, Agrawal A. Markers of genital tuberculosis in infertility. *Singapore Med. J.* 52(12): 864-7. 2011.

Kidane D, Olobo JO, Habte A, Negesse Y *et al.*, Identification of the causative organism of tuberculous lympadenitis in Ethiopia by PCR. *J. Clin. Microbiol.* 11(40): 4230-4234. 2002.

Kidenya BR, Kabangila R, Peck RN, Mshana SE *et al.*, Early and efficient detection of *Mycobacterium tuberculosis* in sputum by microscopic observation of broth cultures. *PLoS One*. 8(2): e57527. 2013.

Kitaura H, Ohara N, Matsuo K, Tasaka H *et al.*, Cloning, sequencing and expression of the gene for the alpha antigen from *M. intracellulare* and use of PCR for the rapid identification of *M. intracellulare*. *Biochem. Biophys. Res. Comun.* 169: 1466-1473. 1993.

Sharma K, Vishali Gupta, Reema Bansal, Aman Sharma *et al.*, Novel multi-targeted polymerase chain reaction for diagnosis of presumed tubercular uveitis. *J. Ophthal. Inflamm. Infect.* 3: 25. 2013.

Lamba H, Byrne M, Goldin R, Jenkins C. Tuberculosis of the cervix: case presentation and review of the literature. *Sex. Transm. Inf.* 78: 62–63. 2002.

Lantheaume S, Soler S, Issartel B, Isch JF *et al.*, Peritoneal tuberculosis simulating advanced ovarian carcinoma: a case report. *Gynecologie. Obstetrique. Fertilite.* 31(7-8): 624–626. 2003.

Lawn SD, Zumla AI. Tuberculosis. *Lancet.* 378(9785): 57-72. 2011.

Lee BY, Horwitz MA. Identification of macrophage and stress-induced proteins of *Mycobacterium tuberculosis*. *J. Clin. Invest.* 96: 245–249. 1995.

Leung CC Yam, Yew WC, Ho WW *et al.*, T-Spot. TB outperforms tuberculin skin test in predicting tuberculosis disease. *Am. J. Respir. Crit. Care Med.* 6: 834-40. 2010.

Li H, Ulstrup JC, Jonassen TØ, Melby K, *et al.*, Evidence for absence of the MPB64 gene in some substrains of *Mycobacterium bovis* BCG. *Infect. Immun.* 61: 1730-1734. 1993.

Livak KJ, Flood SJA, Marmaro J, Giusti W *et al.*, Oligonucleotides with fluorescent dyes at opposite ends provide a quenched probe system useful for detecting PCR product and nucleic acid hybridization. *PCR Methods Appl.* 4: 357-362. 1995.

Lowenstein E. Die zachtung der tuberkelba zillen aus dem stramenden blute. zentralbl. bakteriol. parasitenkd. infektionskr. *Hyg. Abt. I. Orig.* 120: 127. 1931.

Mani R, Nayak S, Kagal A, Deshpande S *et al.*, Tuberculous endometritis in infertility: a bacteriological and histopathological study. *Ind. J. Tuberc.* 50: 161. 2003.

Matsuo K, Yamaguchi R, Yamazaki A, Tasaka H *et al.*, Cloning and expression of the *Mycobacterium bovis* BCG gene for extracellular α-antigen. *J. Bacteriol.* 170: 3847-3854. 1988.

Mazurek GH, LoBue PA, Daley CL *et al.*, Comparison of a whole-blood interferon gamma assay with tuberculin skin testing for detecting latent *Mycobacterium tuberculosis* infection. *JAMA.* 286: 1740-7. 2001.

Medzhitov R, Preston-Hurlburt P, Janeway Jr CA. A human homologue of the drosophila toll protein signals activation of adaptive immunity. *Nature.* 388: 394–397. 1997.

Minden P, Houghten RA, Spear JR, Shinnick TM. A chemically synthesized peptide which elicits humoral and cellular immune responses to mycobacterial antigens. *Infect. Immun.* 53: 560-564. 1986.

Monterola JM, Gamboa F, Padilla E *et al.*, Comparison of a nonradiometric system with Bactec 12B and culture on egg-based media for recovery of mycobacteria from clinical specimens. *Eur. J. Clin. Microbiol. Infect. Dis.* 17: 773–777. 1998.

Morgagni JB. De sedibus et causis meorboram. *Epistola.* 38: 34. 1744.

Mullis KB, Faloona FA. Specific synthesis of DNA *In-vitro* via a polymerase-catalyzed reaction. *Methods Enzymol.* 155: 335-350. 1987.

Mustafa AS, Abal AT, Chugh TD. Detection of *Mycobacterium tuberculosis* complex and non-tuberculous mycobacteria by multiplex polymerase chain reactions. *East Mediterr. Health J.* 5(1): 61-70. 1999.

Mustafa AS, Ahmed A, Abal AT, Chugh TD. Establishment and evaluation of a multiplex polymerase chain reaction for detection of mycobacteria and specific identification of *Mycobacterium tuberculosis* complex. *Tuber. Lung Dis.* 76 (4): 336-43. 1995.

Mustafa T, Wiker HG, Mfinanga SG, Mørkve O *et al.*, Immunohistochemistry using a *Mycobacterium tuberculosis* complex specific antibody for improved diagnosis of tuberculous lymphadenitis. *Mod. Pathol.* 19: 1606-14. 2006.

Nagai S, Wiker HG, Harboe M, Kinomoto M. Isolation and partial characterization of major protein antigens in the culture fluid of *Mycobacterium tuberculosis. Infect. Immun.* 59: 372-382. 1991.

Nakamura RM, Velmonte MA, Kawajiri K, Ang CF *et al.*, MPB 64 mycobacterial antigen: a new skin test reagent through patch method for rapid diagnosis of active tuberculosis. *Int. J. Tuberc. Lung. Dis.* 2: 541–546. 1998.

Namavar Jahromi B, Parsanezhad ME, Ghane-Shirazi R. Female genital tuberculosis and infertility. *Int. J. Gynaecol. Obstet.* 75: 269-272. 2001.

National committee for clinical laboratory standards (CLSI/NCCLS). *Approved guideline protection of laboratory workers from occupationally acquired infections.* 2nd ed. NCCLS, Wayne, Pa. M29-A2. 2001.

Neonakis IK, Spandidos DA, Petinaki E. Female genital tuberculosis: a review. *Scand. J. Infect. Dis.* 43: 564-572. 2011.

Neyrolles O, Gould K, Gares MP, Brett S *et al.*, Lipoprotein access to MHC class I presentation during infection of murine macrophages with live mycobacteria. *J. Immunol.* 166: 447–457. 2001.

Noordhoek GT, van Emden JDA, Kolk AH. Reliability of nucleic acid amplification for detection of *Mycobacterium tuberculosis*: an international collaborative quality control study among 30 laboratories. *J. Clin. Microbiol.* 34: 2522-2525. 1996.

Noss EH, Pai RK, Sellati TJ, Radolf JD *et al.*, Toll-like receptor 2-dependent inhibition of macrophage class II MHC expression and antigen processing by 19-Kda lipoprotein of *Mycobacterium tuberculosis. J. Immunol.* 167: 910– 918. 2001.

Oettinger T, Andersen AB. Cloning and B-cell-epitope mapping of MPT64 from *Mycobacterium tuberculosis* H37Rv. *Infect. Immun.* 62: 2058–2064. 1994.

Ohmen JD, Barnes PF, Grisso CL, Bloom BR *et al.*, Evidence for a super antigen in human tuberculosis. *Immunity*. 1: 35. 1994.

Othman GQ, Ibrahim MIM, Raja'a YA. Costs associated with tuberculosis diagnosis and treatment in Yemen for patients and public health services. *East Mediterr. Health J.* 18 (4): 393-398. 2012.

Padmapriyadarsini C, Tripathy S, Sekar L, Bhavani PK *et al.*, Evaluation of a diagnostic algorithm for sputum smear-negative pulmonary tuberculosis in HIV-infected adults. *J. Acquir. Immune. Defic. Syndr.* 63(3): 331-8. 2013.

Pai M, Ramsay A, O'Brien R. Evidence-based tuberculosis diagnosis. *PLoS Med.* 5: e156. 2008.

Parikh FR, Naik N, Nadkarni SG, Soonawala SB *et al.*, Genital tuberculosis: a major pelvic factor causing infertility in Indian women. *Fertil. Steril.* 67: 497– 500. 1997.

Parra M, Pickett T, Delogu G, Dheenadhayalan V *et al.*, The mycobacterial heparin-binding hemagglutinin is a protective antigen in the mouse aerosol challenge model of tuberculosis. *Infect. Immun.* 72: 6799-805. 2004.

Punnonen R, Kiilholma P, Meurman L. Female genital tuberculosis and consequent infertility. *Int. J. Fertil.* 28(4): 235-8. 1983.

Puri S, Bansal B. Diagnostic value of polymerase chain reaction in female tuberculosis leading to infertility and conception rate after ATT. *J. Obstet. Gynecol. Ind.* 59(1): 67-70. 2009.

Pym AS, Brodin P, Majlessi L *et al.*, Recombinant BCG exporting ESAT-6 confers enhanced protection against tuberculosis. *Nat. Med.* 9: 533-9. 2003.

Rajeswari R, Balasubramanian R, Muniyandi M. Socioeconomic impact of tuberculosis on patient and family in India. *Int. J. Tuberc. Lun. Disease.* 3: 869–877. 1999.

Ramachandaran R, Paramasivan CN. What is new in the diagnosis of tuberculosis? *ICMR. Bulletin.* 32: 69–76. 2002.

Barani R, Gopalsamy Sarangan, Tessa Antony, Soundararajan Periyasamy, *et al.*, Improved detection of *Mycobacterium tuberculosis* using two independent PCR targets in a tertiary care centre in South India. *J. Infect. Dev. Ctries.* 6(1): 46-52. 2012.

Rasit AH, Ibrahim SF, Wong CC. The role of polymerase chain reaction (PCR) in diagnosis of spine tuberculosis after pre-operative anti-tuberculosis treatment. *Malays. Orthopaed. J.* 5(1): 8-12. 2011.

Raut VS, Mahashur AA, Sheth SS. The mantoux test in the diagnosis of genital tuberculosis in women. *Int. J. Gynaecol. Obstet.* 2: 165–9. 2001.

Reddi PP, Talwar GP, Khandekar PS. Molecular cloning and characterization of continually located repetitive and single copy sequences of *Mycobacterium tuberculosis*: development of PCR based diagnosis assay. *Int. J. Lepr.* 61: 227-35. 1993.

Richards MJ, Angus D. Possible sexual transmission of genitourinary tuberculosis. *Int. J. Tuberc. Lung Dis.* 2: 439. 1998.

Rivasi F, Curatola C, Garagnani L, Negri G. Detection of *Mycobacterium tuberculosis* DNA by polymerase chain reaction from paraffin samples of chronic granulomatous endometritis. *Histopathology*. 51: 574–578. 2007.

Romero Ramos R, Romero Gutierrez G, Abortes Monroy I, Medina Sanchez HG. [Risk factors associated to female infertility]. *Ginecol. Obstet. Mex.* 76(12): 717-21. 2008.

Rotbart HA. Nucleic acid detection systems for enteroviruses. *Clin. Microbiol. Rev.* 4: 156-168. 1991.

Ruiling Fu Chun Wang, Chunwei Shi, Mengji Lu, Zhengming Fang *et al.*, An improved whole-blood gamma interferon assay based the CFP21-MPT64 fusion protein. *Clin. Vaccine Immunol.* 16: 686–691. 2009.

Saiki RK, Scharf S, Faloona F, Mullis KB *et al.*, Enzymatic amplification of beta-globulin genomic sequences and restriction site analysis for diagnosis of sickle cell anemia. *Science*. 230: 1350-1354. 1985.

Sakar MN, Gul T, Atay AE, Celik Y. Comparison of hysterosalpingography and laparoscopy in the evaluation of infertile women. *Saudi. Med. J.* 29(9): 1315-8. 2008.

Sankar MM, Gopinath K, Singla R, Singh S. *In-vitro* antimycobacterial drug susceptibility testing of non-tubercular mycobacteria by tetrazolium microplate assay. *Ann. Clin. Microbiol. Antimicrob.* 11: 7–15. 2008.

Saracoglu OF, Mungan T, Tanzer F. Pelvic tuberculosis. *Int. J. Obstet. Gynaecol.* 37(2): 115–20. 1992.

Saraswat P, Swarankar ML, Bhandari A, Soni RR. Detection of active female genital tuberculosis by molecular method. *Int. J. Pharma. Bio. Sci.* 1: B328-B334. 2010.

Sebitloane MH. HIV and gynaecological infections, best practice and research. *Clin. Obstet. and Gynaecol.* 19(2): 231–241. 2005.

Sellors JW, Mahony J, Goldsmith C *et al.*, The accuracy of clinical findings and laparoscopy in pelvic inflammatory disease. *Amer. J. Obstetr. Gynecol.* 164 (11): 113–120. 1991.

Shafer RW, Edlin BR. Tuberculosis in patients infected with human immunodeficiency virus: perspective on the past decade. *Clin. Infect. Dis.* 22: 683. 1996.

Sharma JB, Mohanraj P, Roy KK, Jain SK. Increased complication rates associated with laparoscopic surgery among patients with genital tuberculosis. *Int. J. Gynecol. Obstet.* 109: 242–244. 2010.

Sharma JB, Roy KK, Pushparaj M, Kumar S. Hysteroscopic findings in women with primary and secondary infertility due to genital tuberculosis. *Int. J. Gynaecol. Obstet.* 104: 49-52. 2009.

Sharma K, Sharma A, Sharma SK, Sen RK *et al.*, Does multiplex polymerase chain reaction increase the diagnostic percentage in osteoarticular tuberculosis? a prospective evaluation of 80 cases. *Int. Orthop*. 36: 255–259. 2011.

Shetty J, Kumar P, Ramkumar V *et al.*, Management of female genital tuberculosis: re-appraised. *Obstet. Gynaec. Today*. 11: 506-9. 2006.

Siddiqi K, Lambert ML, Walley J. Clinical diagnosis of smear-negative pulmonary tuberculosis in low-income countries: the current evidence. *Lancet Infect. Dis.* 3(5): 288-96. 2003.

Siddiqi N, Shamim M, Amin A, Chauhan DS *et al.*, Typing of drug resistant isolates of *Mycobacterium tuberculosis* from India using the IS6110 element reveals substantive polymorphism. *Infect. Genet. Evol.* 1(2): 109e16. 2001.

Simon HB, Weinstein AJ, Pasternak MS, Swartz MN *et al.*, Genitourinary tuberculosis: clinical features in a general hospital population. *Am. J. Med.* 63(3): 410–420. 1977.

Singh KK, Nair MD, Radhakrishnan K, Tyagi JS. Utility of PCR assay in diagnosis of en-plaque tuberculoma of the brain. *J. Clin. Microbiol.* 37: 467-70. 1999.

Singh N, Sumana G, Mittal S. Genital tuberculosis: a leading cause for infertility in women seeking assisted conception in North India. *Arch. Gynecol. Obstet.* 278: 325-327. 2008.

Singh S, Gopinath K, Shahdad S, Kaur M *et al.*, Non-tuberculous mycobacterial infections in Indian AIDS patients detected by a novel set of ESAT-6 polymerase chain reaction primers. *Jpn. J. Infect. Dis.* 60: 14–18. 2007.

Soini H, Agha SA, El-fiky A, Viljanen MK. Comparison of AMPLICOR and 32 kilo dalton PCR for detection of *Mycobacterium tuberculosis* from sputum specimens. *J. Clin. Microbiol.* 34: 1829-30. 1996.

Song KH, Jeon JH, Park WB, Kim SH *et al.*, Usefulness of the whole-blood interferon-gamma release assay for diagnosis of extrapulmonary tuberculosis. *Diagn. Microbiol. Infect. Dis.* 63: 182–187. 2009.

Stackebrandt E, Frederiksen W, Garrity GM, Grimont PA *et al.*, Report of the ad hoc committee for the re-evaluation of the species definition in bacteriology. *Int. J. Syst. Evol. Microbiol.* 52: 1043–1047. 2002.

Stenger S, Modlin RL. Control of *M. tuberculosis* through mammalian toll-like receptors. *Curr. Opin. Immunol.* 14: 452. 2002.

Sudre P, Rieder H, Bassetti S, Hirschel BJ *et al.*, HIV infection, tuberculosis and tuberculin test in Switzerland. The swiss HIV cohort study. *Schweiz. Med. Wochenschr.* 126(47): 2007-12. 1996.

Sujatha N, Vijayalakshmi P, Narayannan PR, Venkatesan P *et al.*, Evaluation of PCR using TRC4 and IS6110 primers in detection of tuberculous meningitis. *J. Clin. Microbiol.* 39: 2006-2008. 2001.

Sujatha N, Sahadevan R, Narayanan PR. Isolation and characterization of an insertion element-like repetitive sequence specific for *M. tuberculosis* complex. *Curr. Sci.* 73: 259-266. 1997.

Surcel HM, Troye-Blomberg M, Paulie S, Andersson G *et al.*, Thl/fh2 profiles in tuberculosis, based on the proliferation and cytokine response of blood lymphocytes to mycobacterial antigens. *Immunology.* 81: 171-176. 1994.

TB CARE I. International standards for tuberculosis care (ISTC), 3rd edition. 2014 Available at URL: www.istcweb.org

Thangappah RBP, Paramasivan CN, Narayanan S. Evaluating PCR, culture and histopathology in the diagnosis of female genital tuberculosis. *Ind. J. Med. Res.* 134: 40–46. 2011.

Thoma-Uszynski S, Stenger S, Takeuchi O, Ochoa MT *et al.*, Induction of direct antimicrobial activity through mammalian toll-like receptors. *Science.* 291: 1544–1547. 2001.

Tinelli A, Malvasi A, Vergara D, Roberta Martignago *et al.*, Abdominopelvic tuberculosis in gynecology: laparoscopical and new laboratory findings. *Aus NZ. J. Obstet. Gynecol.* 48: 90–95. 2008.

Tripathy SN, Tripathy SN. Gynaecological tuberculosis -an update. *Indian J. Tuberc.* 45: 193-7. 1998.

Tripathy SN, Tripathy SN. Infertility and pregnancy outcome in female genital tuberculosis. *Int. J. Gynaecol. Obstet.* 76(2): 159-63. 2002.

Van den Bruel A, Cleemput I, Aertgeerts B, Ramaekers D *et al.*, The evaluation of diagnostic tests: evidence on technical and diagnostic accuracy, impact on patient outcome and cost-effectiveness is needed. *J. Clin. Epidemiol.* 60: 1116-1122. 2007.

van Soolingen D, DeHaas PEW, Hermans PWM, Groenen PMA *et al.*, Comparison of various repetitive DNA elements as genetic markers of strain differentiation of epidemiology of *Mycobacterium tuberculosis*. *J. Clin. Microbiol.* 31: 1887-95. 1993.

Varma TR. Genital tuberculosis and subsequent fertility. *Int. J. Gynecol. Obstet.* 35: 1–11. 1991.

Vassall A, van Kampen S, Sohn H, Michael JS *et al.*, Rapid diagnosis of tuberculosis with the Xpert MTB/RIF assay in high burden countries: a cost-effectiveness analysis. PLoS Med. 8(11): e1001120. 2011. doi: 10.1371/journal.pmed.1001120

Velayati AA, Masjedi MR, Farnia P, Tabarsi P *et al.*, Emergence of new forms of totally drug-resistant tuberculosis bacilli: super extensively drug-resistant tuberculosis or totally drug-resistant strains in Iran. *Chest.* 136: 420–5. 2009.

Vijaya Bhanu N, Singh UB, Chakraborty M, Suresh N *et al.*, Improved diagnostic value of PCR in the diagnosis of female genital tuberculosis leading to infertility. *J. Med. Microbiol.* 54: 927–931. 2005.

Walter JB, Israel MS. *General pathology* (7th Edi.) 5th lid. Churchill Livingstone, Edinburgn, p240. 1996.

Wang Z, Potter Belinda M, Gray Amanda M, Sacksteder Katherine A, Geisbrecht Brian V, *et al.*, The solution structure of antigen MPT64 from *M. tuberculosis* defines a new family of beta-grasp proteins. *J. Mol. Biol.* 366(2): 375–381. 2007.

Watson JD, Crick FH. Molecular structure of nucleic acids; a structure for deoxyribose nucleic acid. *Nature.* 171: 737-738. 1953.

Welch HG. Overdiagnosis and mammography screening. *BMJ*. 339: b1425. 2009.

Wiker HG, Sletten K, Nagai S, Harboe M. Evidence of three separate genes encoding the proteins of the mycobacterial antigen 85 complex. *Infect. Immun.* 58: 272-274. 1990.

Wilson ML. Recent advances in the laboratory detection of *Mycobacterium tuberculosis* complex and drug resistance. *Clin. Infect. Dis.* 52(11): 1350-1355. 2011.

World health organization (WHO; Country Office for India). Standards for TB care in India. (STCI). 2014. Available at URL: http: //www.tbcindia.nic.in

Yamaguchi R, Matsuo K, Yamazaki A, Abe C *et al.*, Cloning and characterization of the gene for immunogenic protein MPB64 of *Mycobacterium bovis* BCG. *Infect. Immun.* 57: 283-288. 1989.

Yang S, Rothman RE. PCR-based diagnostics for infectious diseases: uses, limitations, and future application in acute-care settings. *Lancet Infect. Dis.* 4: 337-348. 2004.

Young DB, Garbe TR. Lipoprotein antigens of *Mycobacterium tuberculosis*. *Res. Microbiol.* 142: 55–65. 1991.

Index

C

F

G

H

N

O

S

T

U

V

W

X

www.ingramcontent.com/pod-product-compliance
Ingram Content Group UK Ltd.
Pitfield, Milton Keynes, MK11 3LW, UK
UKHW022216051026
15624UKWH00001B/185